W9-CMK-204

THIS IS YOUR BRAIN ON FOOD

THIS IS YOUR BRAIN ON FOOD

An Indispensable Guide to the Surprising Foods That Fight Depression, Anxiety, PTSD, OCD, ADHD, and More

UMA NAIDOO, MD

Little, Brown Spark
New York Boston London

Little, Brown Spark
Hachette Book Group
1290 Avenue of the Americas, New York, NY 10104
littlebrownspark.com

First Edition: August 2020

Little, Brown Spark is an imprint of Little, Brown and Company, a division of Hachette Book Group, Inc. The Little, Brown Spark name and logo are trademarks of Hachette Book Group, Inc.

Printing 11

ISBN 978-0-316-53682-0
LCCN 2019957287

LSC-C

Printed in the United States of America

This book is dedicated to my beloved late father and Pinetown Granny,

to my mom (who gave me the most important piece of advice in my life),

and to my husband, without whom this book would never have materialized.

Contents

THIS IS YOUR BRAIN ON FOOD

Introduction

Nutrition and psychiatry may not seem like the most natural fit. When you picture Dr. Freud with his pipe and his leather couch, he's probably not scribbling a recipe for baked salmon on his prescription pad. Indeed, in my experience psychiatrists send their patients home with prescription drugs or referrals to other types of therapy, but no guidance on how food can help them with the challenges that brought them to the analyst's couch. And though many conscientious modern eaters think constantly about the food we're eating—how it will affect our hearts, the environment, and most of all our waistlines—we don't think about its influence on our brains.

While this relationship between nutrition and mental health may not feel intuitive at first glance, it's key to understanding twin epidemics in modern health care. Though medical knowledge and technology are better than they have ever been, both mental health disorders and bad health outcomes caused by poor dietary choices are disturbingly common. One in five American adults will have a diagnosable mental health condition in any given year, and 46 percent of Americans will meet the criteria for a diagnosable mental health condition sometime in their life. Thirty-seven percent of Americans are considered obese, with an additional 32.5 percent considered overweight, making a total of roughly 70 percent of the population above an optimal weight. An estimated 23.1 million Americans have a diabetes diagnosis, with another 7.2 million estimated to be undiagnosed. That's a total of 30.3 million people, almost 10 percent of the population.

Much like the intricate relationship between the gut and brain that forms the basis of this book, diet and mental health are inextricably linked, and the connection between them goes both ways: a dearth of good dietary choices leads to an increase in mental health issues, and mental health issues in turn lead to poor eating habits. Until we solve nutritional problems, no amount of medication and psychotherapy is going to be able to stem the tide of mental issues in our society.

While fixing the broken relationship between diet and mental health is certainly important on a societal level, it can also make a crucial difference on an individual level—and not just for those who suffer from diagnosed mental conditions. Whether or not you have ever visited a mental health professional for depression or anxiety, every one of us has felt sad and nervous. We all have experienced obsession and trauma, large or small. We all want to keep our attention and memories sharp. We all need to sleep and have a satisfying sex life.

In this book, I want to show you ways in which you can use diet to achieve well-being in every aspect of your mental health.

When people learn that I am a psychiatrist, a nutritionist, and a trained chef, they often assume that I have been cooking since I was young and that my medical interests came later. But I actually learned to cook relatively late in life. I grew up in a large South Asian family surrounded by grandmothers, aunts, a mother, and a mother-in-law who were all exceptional cooks. I didn't need to cook! My mom, a double-boarded physician and excellent cook and baker, did get me interested in baking, and it was through the exact measuring of ingredients that the roots of my love for science took hold. Otherwise, I was happy to let others handle things in the kitchen.

When I moved to Boston to train in psychiatry at Harvard, I felt ripped from the love and warmth of my extended family and the delicious food that signified home. I knew I had to learn how to cook in order to carve out a home in this new place. My husband, being the brilliant person he is, already knew how to cook, but I banished him from the kitchen (at least so he likes to joke—in reality he was an invaluable guide and brutally honest taste tester) and began to try out a few recipes that I'd been taught.

For inspiration, I channeled memories of Pinetown Granny, as we called my maternal grandma. While my mom attended medical school during the day, I hung out with her and watched her cook. At three years old I'd peer into the kitchen, not allowed to step anywhere near the hot stove and oven, and observe her closely. We'd start the day by picking fresh vegetables from the garden, then prepped fresh vegetables for lunch, set the table, told stories, and took an afternoon nap.

Since cable was an unaffordable luxury as we were getting on our feet in Boston, I also watched public television and met the magnificent Julia Child, dropping omelets and teaching me about French cuisine. She inspired great confidence in my cooking and kept me company during many lonely hours when my husband was completing his fellowship. Slowly and steadily, cooking became a part of me and a space in which I could decompress once I began residency.

Even after I began to work as a practicing psychiatrist, my passion for cooking stayed strong, and my husband suggested I spend some time at the Culinary Institute of America. I loved taking classes at the CIA but couldn't sustain the commute while actively working as a doctor in Boston. So I enrolled in an amazing local school, Cambridge School of Culinary Arts, and pledged to keep myself committed to both psychiatry and cooking.

I quickly learned that unlike the sexy medical dramas on TV, which are a far cry from the real-life medical world, professional-level cooking as it is depicted onscreen is really how it is—a lot of screaming and yelling from the head chef, although they're not usually as foul-mouthed as Gordon Ramsay. Though it is stressful, nothing beats the gratifying feeling when your meringue comes together perfectly, or when you appreciate the depth and flavor of a perfectly executed consommé, or when your pâte is the texture of buttercream before it sets.

All the while, I was still actively practicing at the hospital. Thinking back, I am not sure how I managed it. There were many times when I took my books to dinner to study for my written culinary exams. There were also long hours catching up with work, emails, prescriptions, and telephone calls after school. Somehow I got through. I see now that my passion for both worlds drove me, for I truly love psychiatry as much as I do cooking.

During this phase I also became more fascinated with the nutritional value of food. I began speaking actively to my patients about how much cream and sugar went into their 20-ounce Dunkin' Donuts coffee when they complained about weight gain they attributed to their antidepressants. To augment my knowledge of nutrition and confidence in bringing dietary advice to my clinical work, after I graduated culinary school, I also completed a program in nutritional science.

Armed with my knowledge of psychiatry, nutrition, and the culinary arts, I continued to integrate my clinical work with nutritional and lifestyle techniques, and I honed my own holistic and integrated approach to psychiatry. That method has become the blueprint for my work, culminating in the founding of the Nutritional and Lifestyle Psychiatry program at Massachusetts General Hospital, the first clinic of its kind in the United States.

Even after so much training and experience in my fields, my education in nutritional psychiatry wasn't complete until I witnessed its power firsthand. A few years ago, I was in a luxurious hotel room in

Beverly Hills, glancing at sun speckles dancing on the wall, remembering how good it felt to read a book and slide comfortably into an afternoon nap. My husband and I were enjoying a long-awaited and much-deserved long weekend to celebrate his birthday—an event that had gradually evolved into an annual opportunity to get away from our lives to relax and reset.

As I settled myself in to nap, I moved the book, brushing against an odd spot on my chest that I would not normally have reason to touch. I felt a bump. At first, I thought I was just tired, but as I examined myself I shot up in bed, stunned. It was definitely a lump. Cancer. I wanted to doubt the accuracy of my clinical skills, but I could not.

Back in Boston, I was diagnosed within seven days. That week was a whirlwind of tests and appointments that flew by at lightning speed. I felt blessed for having access to some of the best medical care in the world. Despite immense support from colleagues and friends, for the first time in my life I was facing something I had not anticipated. No one wakes up thinking it might be the day they get cancer. I felt completely helpless. I kept thinking about what I might have done wrong, but my strong Hindu roots helped me reframe my situation. As my grandmother and mother had taught me growing up: "This is part of the karma you must face; approach it and handle it with grace, have faith in God, and it will all be okay." While my family and I were all devastated and in tears, those words rang true.

Still, I struggled to work through my emotions; my professional training as a psychiatrist didn't make it any easier to master the roil of feelings that swirled through my brain. For the first time in my life as a doctor I could not control the outcome of this disease. It was out of my hands. I could do nothing but stretch out my forearm for blood tests and know that soon I would be doing the same for the massive IV bolus treatments of chemotherapy. I went from feeling desperate and panicked to feeling like my emotions were suspended.

There was no laughter or tears, no fear or joy. There was only a bone-chilling numbness.

As I got up the morning of my first treatment, I decided I should have a calming cup of turmeric tea. I kept replaying how life had instantly taken a 180-degree turn. I was nervous and afraid and trying to be brave. I knew intimately all the traumatic side effects I might face, even if my treatment was ultimately successful. Yet something about turning the switch on the electric tea kettle metaphorically set off that light bulb in my head: "I know how to cook, I know about my body, and I can help myself through how I eat."

That may seem like an elementary conclusion for a nutritional psychiatrist to reach, but it's quite different to be the patient rather than the clinician, especially since I had always been lucky enough to be healthy. But I resolved that I was going to take care of my mind and body through eating healthy food, no matter what the cancer threw at me.

What transpired over the next sixteen months was an intense cycle of chemotherapy, surgery, and radiation. Every chemotherapy appointment, the oncology fellow who worked with me would ask what I had brought to eat that day. I would pull out my lunch bag with a nutrient-dense smoothie made from probiotic-rich yogurt, berries, almond milk, kefir, and dark chocolate. Because of how I ate, I was never nauseous. My weight fluctuated as the side effects of different medications made my appetite increase and decrease, but I ate foods I loved even when medication changed their flavor.

Through all of this oncologic assault on my body, I felt surprisingly healthy, and I found ways to keep my energy up even as the constant round of treatments should have left me totally drained. It was admittedly a greater challenge to stay on top of my mental health, but once again, the food I ate was crucial to keeping an even keel and positive emotional outlook. I cut back on coffee and gave up wine; I ate fresh fruit that I washed, cleaned, and prepared at home. I made soothing high-protein, high-fiber Indian lentil soups (dal) loaded with folate-rich spinach (page 271). I made a healing and delicious hot chocolate from scratch once a week as a treat on Thursday nights, giving me something to look forward to after treatments. I was careful to make smart food choices that were not loaded with unhealthy calories. Fatigue prevented me from working out, so I chose to take brisk walks regularly; this also uplifted my mood, as exercise does raise endorphins. I ate to lower my anxiety around weekly Thursday chemo treatments and help lift my mood when the dark, wintry days of Boston closed in on me during chemotherapy.

It gave me strength to see how my mental health was bolstered by incorporating the same recommendations I was making to my patients. I truly needed to "walk the walk," as they say. I had to test myself to see if these strategies could quell my anxiety, soothe me to sleep, and lift my mood. I was not sure I would be a success story, but I felt I owed it to my patients and myself to give my own treatment plan a real fighting chance.

Cancer also made me embrace mindfulness and think more deeply about my own lifestyle. I grew up around regular meditation practice kept up by my parents and extended family; Ayurvedic principles were incorporated daily, and ballet, dance, and exercise were also routine. Yet cancer made me realize that after studying and working so intensely for many years, I'd allowed some of those healthy habits to slip. My mom reminded me to start meditating regularly; my husband and my best friend reminded me about my early years as a ballet dancer, which helped me to return to adult ballet classes and barre-style gym classes. The stress of my busy years had taken a toll on me on a cellular level, and so I now know on the deepest level how important lifestyle techniques are to helping us thrive and flourish. It is not one dimension or one thing; we are each a whole person, and holistic practice is key. While nutritional psychiatry is central to healing, the lifestyle aspects are vital too.

Until writing this, I hadn't spoken widely about my struggle with cancer. I have now completed treatment, my hair is back (thank goodness!), and I walk through each day hoping to reach remission while remembering that what I eat truly impacts how I feel.

All this experience—my background, my schooling, my clinical experience, my time in kitchens, my illness—has inspired me to write this book. I hope that in its pages I can not only introduce you to the exciting field of nutritional psychiatry, but also give you advice on how to eat to maximize the awesome power of your brain.

CHAPTER ONE

The Gut-Brain Romance

There aren't many things that keep me up at night. I like my sleep. But on occasion, I find myself tossing and turning because I think that in psychiatry, and in medicine as a whole, we have completely missed the forest for the trees.

Granted, we've come a long way from the cold showers and shackles of the seventeenth and eighteenth centuries. In those early barbaric years, "madness" was considered a sinful state, and the mentally ill were housed in prisons. As civilization progressed, mentally ill patients were moved to hospitals.[1] The problem is, as we became more and more focused on the troublesome thoughts and emotions of mental illnesses, we stopped noticing that the rest of the body was also involved.

This wasn't always the case. In 2018, historian Ian Miller pointed out that eighteenth- and nineteenth-century doctors were clued in to the fact that the body's systems are connected.[2] That's why they talked about the "nervous sympathy" among our different organs.

However, in the late nineteenth century, doctors changed this perspective. As medicine became more specialized, we lost track of the big picture, only looking at single organs to determine what was wrong and what needed fixing.

Of course, doctors did recognize that cancers might spread from one organ to the next, and that autoimmune conditions like systemic lupus erythematosus could affect multiple organs in the body. But they neglected to see that organs that were seemingly quite separate in the body might still profoundly influence one another. Metaphorically speaking, illness could come from a mile away!

Compounding the problem was that, rather than working collaboratively, physicians, anatomists, physiologists, surgeons, and psychologists competed with one another. As one British doctor wrote in 1956, "There is such a clamour of contestants for cure that the patient who really wants to know is deafened rather than enlightened."[3]

This attitude prevails in medicine even today. That's why so many people are oblivious to the fact that when mental health is affected, the root of the problem is not solely in the brain. Instead, it's a signal that one or more of the body's connections with the brain has gone awry.

We know that these connections are quite real. Depression can affect the heart. Pathologies of the adrenal gland can throw you into a panic. Infections darting through your bloodstream can make you seem like you have lost your mind. Maladies of the body frequently manifest as turbulence of the mind.

But while medical illness can cause psychiatric symptoms, we now know that the story goes even deeper. Subtle changes in distant parts of the body can change the brain too. The most profound of these distant relationships is between the brain and the gut. Centuries ago, Hippocrates, the father of modern medicine, recognized this connection, warning us that "bad digestion is the root of all evil" and that "death sits in the bowels." Now we are figuring out how right he was. Though we are still on the forefront of discovery, in recent years the gut-brain connection has provided one of the richest, most fertile research areas in medical science and the fascinating nexus of the field of nutritional psychiatry.

ONCE UPON A TIME . . .

Watching a developing embryo differentiate is like looking through a kaleidoscope.

Once upon a time, a sperm made its way to an egg. They were not ships passing in the night. They connected. And when the union was successful, you were conceived. Warmly ensconced in your mother's uterus, you, as this fertilized egg (called a zygote), started to change.

At first, the zygote's smooth outer surface developed ripples like a mulberry. As time went on, the magical egg, under the spell of biological instructions, started to change its configuration until your baby body took shape. Eventually, after nine long months, you were armed with a heart, gut, lungs, brain, limbs, and other nifty things, ready to announce yourself to life.

But before all that, before you emerged ready to take on the world, before your gut and brain became distinct entities, they were one. They came from the same fertilized egg that gave rise to all the organs in your body.

In fact, the central nervous system, made up of the brain and spinal cord, is formed by special cells known as neural crest cells. These cells migrate extensively throughout the developing embryo, forming the enteric nervous system in the gut. The enteric nervous system contains between 100 million and 500 million neurons, the largest collection of nerve cells in the body. That's why some people call the gut "the second brain." And it's why the gut and brain influence each other so profoundly. Separate though they may appear to be, their origins are the same.

LONG-DISTANCE RELATIONSHIP

I once had a patient who was confused as to why I talked about her gut while treating her mind. To her, it seemed irrelevant. "After all," she said, "it's not like they are actually next to each other."

While your gut and brain are housed in different parts of your body, they maintain more than just a historical connection. They remain physically connected too.

The vagus nerve, also known as the "wanderer nerve," originates in the brain stem and travels all the way to the gut, connecting the gut to the central nervous system. When it reaches the gut, it untangles itself to form little threads that wrap the entire gut in an unruly covering that looks like an intricately knitted sweater. Because the vagus nerve penetrates the gut wall, it plays an essential role in the digestion of food, but its key function is to ensure that nerve signals can travel back and forth between the gut and the brain, carrying vital information between them. Signals between the gut and brain travel in both directions, making the brain and gut lifelong partners. That is the basis of the gut-brain romance.

CHEMICAL ATTRACTION

So how does your body actually transmit messages between the gut and the brain via the vagus nerve? It's easy enough to imagine the gut and the brain "talking" to each other over some kind of biological cell phone, but that doesn't quite do justice to the elegance and complexity of your body's communication system.

The basis of all body communications is chemical. When you take a pill for a headache, you usually swallow it, right? It enters your mouth, then makes its way to your gut, where it is broken down. The chemicals from the pill travel from your gut to your brain through your bloodstream. And in your brain, they can decrease the inflammation and loosen your tense blood vessels too. When the chemicals you swallow successfully exert their effects on the brain, you feel relief from that pain.

In the same way as the chemicals in that pill, chemicals produced by the gut can also reach your brain. And chemicals produced by your brain can reach your gut. It's a two-way street.

In the brain, these chemicals originate from the primary parts of your nervous system (with an assist from your endocrine system): the central nervous system, which comprises the brain and spinal cord; the autonomic nervous system (ANS), which comprises the sympathetic and parasympathetic systems; and the hypothalamic-pituitary-adrenal axis (HPA-axis), which comprises the hypothalamus, pituitary gland, and adrenal gland.

The central nervous system produces chemicals such as dopamine, serotonin, and acetylcholine that are critical for regulating mood and processing thought and emotion. Serotonin, a key chemical deficient in the brains of depressed and anxious people, plays a major role in regulating the gut-brain axis. Serotonin is one of the most buzzed-about brain chemicals because of its role in mood and emotion, but did you know that more than 90 percent of serotonin receptors are found in the gut? In fact, some researchers believe that the brain-serotonin deficit is heavily influenced by the gut, an idea we'll dig deeper into later on.

The autonomic nervous system (ANS) is in charge of a broad range of essential functions, most of which are involuntary: your heart keeps beating, and you keep breathing and digesting food because of your ANS. When your pupils dilate to take in more light in a dark room, that's the ANS. Perhaps most crucially for our purposes, when your body is under duress, your ANS controls your fight-or-flight response, an instinctual reaction to threat that sends a cascade of hormonal and physiological responses through your body in dangerous or life-threatening situations. As we'll see later on, the gut has a profound effect on fight or flight, particularly through the regulation of the hormones adrenaline and noradrenaline (also known as epinephrine and norepinephrine).

The HPA-axis is another crucial part of the body's stress machine. It produces hormones that stimulate release of cortisol, the "stress hormone." Cortisol amps the body up to handle stress, providing a flood of extra energy to deal with difficult situations. Once the threat passes, the cortisol level returns to normal. The gut also plays an important role in cortisol release and is instrumental in making sure the body responds to stress effectively.

In a healthy body, all these brain chemicals ensure that the gut and brain work smoothly together. Of course, as in all delicate systems, things can go wrong. When chemical over- or underproduction disrupts this connection, the gut-brain balance is thrown into disarray. Levels of important chemicals go out of whack. Moods are upset. Concentration is disrupted. Immunity drops. The gut's protective barrier is compromised, and metabolites and chemicals that should be kept out of the brain reach the brain and wreak havoc.

Over and over again throughout this book, we are going to see how this chemical chaos gives rise to psychiatric symptoms, from depression and anxiety to loss of libido to devastating conditions like schizophrenia and bipolar disorder.

In order to correct those chemical imbalances and restore order to brain and body, you might assume that we would need a barrage of sophisticated, carefully engineered pharmaceuticals. And to a degree, you'd be right! Most drugs used to treat mental conditions do seek to alter these chemicals to return the brain to a healthy state—for example, you may have heard of selective serotonin reuptake inhibitors (most commonly referred to as SSRIs), which boost serotonin in order to fight depression. Modern mental health medications can be a godsend to patients who struggle with a variety of disorders, and I don't want to downplay their importance as a therapy in many circumstances.

But what sometimes gets lost in discussions about mental health is a simple truth: the food you eat can have just as profound an effect on your brain as the drugs you take. How can something as basic and natural as eating be as potent as a drug that cost millions of dollars to develop and test? The first part of the answer lies in bacteria.

WHY SMALL THINGS MATTER

Behind the scenes of the gut-brain romance is a huge collection of microorganisms that reside in the gut.[4] We call this panoply of different bacterial species the microbiome. The gut microbiome — in both humans and other animals — is another type of romance, with both parties relying on each other for survival. Our guts provide the bacteria with a place to live and thrive, and in return they perform crucial tasks for us that our bodies can't perform on their own.

The microbiome is made up of many different types of bacteria, with a much greater diversity of species in the gut than anywhere else in the body. Each individual gut can contain up to a thousand different species of bacteria, though most of them belong to two groups — *Firmicutes* and *Bacteroides* — which make up about 75 percent of the entire microbiome.

While we won't spend too much time discussing individual species in this book, suffice it to say that when it comes to bacteria, there are good guys and bad guys. The microorganisms that inhabit the gut are normally good guys, but it's inevitable that some bad ones get mixed in. This isn't necessarily a concern, as your body generally makes sure that the good and bad bacteria stay at the right balance. But if diet, stress, or other mental or physical problems cause changes in gut bacteria, that can cause a ripple effect that leads to many negative health effects.

The idea that the microbiome plays such an essential role in bodily function is relatively new in medicine (think about how often you've heard of bacteria as "germs that will make you sick" rather than as a helpful team of microorganisms that performs a vital service), particularly when it comes to bacteria's influence on the brain. But over the years, the science has been building that gut bacteria can affect mental function.

About thirty years ago, in one of the most compelling studies that first made us aware that changes in gut bacteria could influence mental function, researchers reported on a series of patients with a kind of delirium (called hepatic encephalopathy) due to liver failure. In hepatic encephalopathy, bacterial "bad guys" produce toxins, and the study showed that these patients stopped being delirious when antibiotics were administered by mouth. That was a clear sign that changing gut bacteria could also change mental function.

In the years since, we've accumulated a huge amount of knowledge about how the gut microbiome affects mental health, and we'll unpack that knowledge throughout this book. For instance, did you know that functional bowel disorders like irritable bowel syndrome and inflammatory bowel disease also come with mood changes due to bacterial populations being altered?[5] Or that some clinicians feel that adding a probiotic as part of a psychiatric medication treatment plan can also help to lower anxiety and depression? Or that if you transfer the gut bacteria of schizophrenic humans into the guts of lab mice, those mice also start to show symptoms of schizophrenia?

The primary reason gut bacteria have such a profound effect on mental health is that they are responsible for making many of the brain chemicals we discussed in the last section. If normal gut bacteria are not present, production of neurotransmitters such as dopamine, serotonin, glutamate, and gamma-aminobutyric acid (GABA)—all critically important for the regulation of mood, memory, and attention—is impacted. As we'll see, many psychiatric disorders are rooted in deficits and imbalances of these chemicals, and many psychiatric drugs are tasked with manipulating their levels. Therefore, if your gut bacteria are intimately involved with producing these vital chemicals, it stands to reason that when your gut bacteria are altered, you risk doing damage to this complex web of body and brain function. That's a lot of responsibility for a group of microscopic organisms!

Different collections of bacteria affect brain chemistry differently. For instance, changes in proportions and function of *Escherichia, Bacillus, Lactococcus, Lactobacillus,* and *Streptococcus* can result in changes in dopamine levels and may predispose one to Parkinson's disease and Alzheimer's disease.[6] Other combinations of abnormal gut bacteria may result in abnormally high concentrations of acetylcholine, histamine, endotoxin, and cytokines, which can damage brain tissue.

In addition to regulating neurotransmitter levels, there are various other ways in which microbiota influence the gut-brain connection. They are involved in the production of other important compounds like brain-derived neurotrophic factor, which supports the survival of existing neurons and promotes new neuron growth and connections. They influence the integrity of the gut wall and the gut's barrier function, which protect the brain and the rest of the body from substances that need to be confined to the gut. Bacteria can also have an effect on inflammation in the brain and body, particularly influencing oxidation, a harmful process that results in cellular damage.

A TWO-WAY STREET

As I mentioned earlier, the gut-brain connection works both ways. So if gut bacteria can influence the brain, it is also true that the brain can change gut bacteria.

All it takes is two hours' worth of psychological stress to completely change the bacteria in your gut.[7] In other words, a tense family Christmas dinner or unusually bad traffic can be enough to upset the balance of your microbiome. The theory is that the ANS and HPA-axis send signaling molecules to gut bacteria when you are stressed, changing bacterial behavior and composition. The results can be damaging. For example, one kind of bacterium changed by stress is *Lactobacillus*. Normally, it breaks down sugars into lactic acid, prevents harmful bacteria from lining the intestine, and protects your body against fungal infections. But when you are stressed, *Lactobacillus* fails on all these fronts due to how stress disrupts its functioning, leaving you exposed to harm.

The brain can also affect the physical movements of the gut (for example, how the gut contracts), and it controls the secretion of acid, bicarbonate, and mucus, all of which provide the gut's protective lining. In some instances, the brain affects how the gut handles fluid. When your brain is not functioning well—for example, when you have depression or anxiety—all these normal and protective effects on the gut are compromised. As a result, food is not properly absorbed, which in turn has a negative effect on the rest of the body since it's not getting the nutrients it needs.

WHEN THINGS GO SOUTH

So to recap, your brain needs the proper balance of gut bacteria to make the chemicals it needs to stay stable and healthy. The gut needs your brain to be stable and healthy so that it can maintain the proper balance of gut bacteria. If that cyclical relationship is disrupted, it means trouble for both the gut and the brain. An unhealthy gut microbiome leads to an unhealthy brain, and vice versa.

A quick illustration of these issues is provided by a survey Mireia Valles-Colomer and her colleagues conducted in April 2019 of more than a thousand people, in which they correlated microbiome features with well-being and depression.[8] They found that butyrate-producing bacteria were consistently associated with higher quality-of-life indicators. Many bacteria were also depleted in people with depression, even after correcting for the confounding effects of antidepressants. They also found that when the dopamine metabolite 3,4-dihydroxyphenylacetic acid, which helps gut bacterial growth, is high, mental health is improved. GABA production is disturbed in people with depression too.

That's just the tip of the iceberg. In each chapter of this book, we will go into specific gut-brain disturbances that map out the relationships between the microbiome and individual disorders. In the pages to come, we will see how depression, anxiety, post-traumatic stress disorder, attention deficit hyperactivity disorder, dementia, obsessive compulsive disorder, insomnia, decreased libido, schizophrenia, and bipolar disorder might all be associated with an altered microbiome. For each condition, I will walk you through where we stand with research today and give you an idea where there may be room for further study.

FOOD FOR THOUGHT

In addition to exploring how disruptions in gut bacteria can cause these kinds of mental issues, we're also going to keep our eyes peeled and our appetites sharp for foods that can help encourage a healthy gut and a healthy brain.

Food influences your brain directly and indirectly.[9] When food is broken down by the microbiota into fermented and digested materials, its components directly influence the same kinds of neurotransmitters we've been discussing, such as serotonin, dopamine, and GABA, which travel to the brain and change the way you think and feel. When food is broken down, its constituent parts can also pass through the gut wall into the bloodstream, and certain metabolites can act on the brain that way as well.

As we've already touched on, food's most profound effect on the brain is through its impact on your gut bacteria. Some foods promote the growth of helpful bacteria, while others inhibit this growth. Because of that effect, food is some of the most potent mental health medicine available, with dietary interventions sometimes achieving similar results to specifically engineered pharmaceuticals, at a fraction of the price and with few if any side effects.

On the other hand, food can also made you sad—certain food groups and eating patterns can have a negative effect on your gut microbiome and your mental health.

Throughout the book, we will examine foods that both help and hurt mental health. You will learn how to use healthy, whole foods to ensure that your brain is working at peak efficiency. In chapter 11, I will provide you with sample menus and recipes that will boost your mood, sharpen your thinking, and energize your whole life.

THE CHALLENGE IN PSYCHIATRY

The idea of using food as medicine for mental health is central to nutritional psychiatry, and in my opinion, it's crucial to finding meaningful, lasting solutions to mental health problems.

As I said at the beginning of the chapter, we've come a long way since the seriously mentally ill were confined to asylums or hospitals without much understanding of their suffering. But mental health is still in a crisis. More than 40 million Americans are dealing with a mental health concern—more than the populations of New York and Florida combined.[10] Mental disorders are among the most common and costly causes of disability.[11] Depression and anxiety are on the rise. Suicide is a staple on lists of top causes of death, no matter what age-group. We're in a mental health mess, no matter how many people are in denial about it.

It has been challenging to find treatments that help people manage their moods, cognition, and stress levels. Historically, we turned to evidence-based medications and talk therapies that worked for specific conditions. For example, for someone who was depressed, we might have tried a selective serotonin reuptake inhibitor like

Prozac. For someone who was panicky, we might have used cognitive behavioral therapy. Those kinds of treatments are still in wide use and can be effective. But for some people, the positive effects last only a short period of time, and they do not completely eliminate symptoms. Sometimes patients develop side effects from the medications and stop taking them. Other times they are afraid of becoming "dependent" on a medication and ask to be taken off it. Some patients who come to see me do not meet the criteria for a disorder such as depression or anxiety. They struggle with symptoms but not enough to warrant a medication intervention.

My own view of where we went wrong is this: psychiatric diagnoses have no statistical validity, and the conditions have no biomarkers of specific diseases.[12] "Diagnoses" are simply lists of symptoms. We assume that when a person presents with psychological symptoms, the problem rests solely in the brain. Given what we have reviewed so far, it is clear that other organs such as the gut play a role in how we think and feel. We need to examine the whole person and their lifestyle in order to better treat them.

The problem is bigger than psychiatry, extending to medicine as a whole. Despite the huge number of health issues that relate to diet, it may sound far-fetched, but many patients don't hear food advice from their doctors, let alone their psychiatrists. Medical schools and residency programs do not teach students how to talk to patients about dietary choices. Nutrition education for doctors is limited.

Thankfully, we are inching toward a moment in health care when medicine is no longer strictly about prescriptions and a single line of therapy. Thanks to the wealth of medical knowledge accessible to the general public, patients are more empowered and informed than ever. It feels as though all my colleagues are experiencing a similar movement in their specialties, with patients eager to explore a diverse range of ways to feel better. One of my success stories of nutritional treatment was a referral from an infectious disease colleague. Another time, an orthopedic colleague reached out to me to ask more about the data on turmeric as an anti-inflammatory, as his patient with severe knee pain wanted to delay surgery until he'd tried this nutritional intervention.

In psychiatry, we are finally beginning to talk about the power of food as medicine for mental health. The body of research on the microbiome and how food impacts mental health is growing. In 2015, Jerome Sarris and his colleagues established that "nutritional medicine" was becoming mainstream in psychiatry.[13]

The goal of nutritional psychiatry is to arm mental health professionals with the information they need so that they can offer patients powerful and practical advice about what to eat. With this book, my goal is to offer you, the reader, the same kind of information. That doesn't overshadow the importance of working with your doctor, since medication and the appropriate therapy remain a part of the journey to improved mental health. A better diet can help, but it's only one aspect of treatment. You cannot eat your way out of feeling depressed or anxious (and in fact, as we'll see, trying to do so can make things worse). Food is not going to relieve serious forms of depression or thoughts of suicide or homicide, and it is important to seek treatment in an emergency room or contact your doctor if you are experiencing thoughts about harming yourself or someone else.

As I found in my battle with cancer, it is also extremely important to look after your mental health with strategies of mindfulness, meditation, exercise, and proper sleep. The literature on these topics is vast, with methods both ancient and modern (and sometimes a combination of the two!). I won't go into detail about those topics in this book, but I encourage you to explore them on your own.

That being said, in addition to taking guidance from your doctor and encouraging mental wellness in other ways, you should support your treatment by paying attention to how and what you eat. The relationship linking food, mood, and anxiety is garnering more and more attention. In the chapters that follow, I will guide you through the exciting science of food and its connection to a variety of common mental health challenges.

HOW TO USE THIS BOOK

To better guide you through the science behind how food affects mental health, I'm going to explore ten different mental conditions over the course of this book. Of course, no one reader will need every chapter—you see a lot as a clinical psychiatrist, but thankfully, even I haven't seen a patient who is suffering from every condition we will discuss. It's important to me that readers be able to skip around to the chapters that apply to them most, so I've arranged each chapter to be as self-contained as possible. If you're reading straight through, you'll likely start to notice trends in the advice as we see how various foods and eating patterns affect different conditions in similar ways. Since all the conditions we will talk about are rooted in the gut-brain connection, there is naturally overlap in the foods that worsen and improve them, so be aware that you will see the same recommendations come up multiple times. In each chapter, I will present the studies that support eating or avoiding foods for the given condition.

As you read the book, I encourage you to do so with an open mind. Nutritional psychiatry is just one part of a complex puzzle, and the amount of evidence differs for different foods. Most of the evidence showing that microbiome changes affect the brain comes from animal studies. But several human studies have now also demonstrated the key connection between microbiota and mental health, and I'll include as many human studies as possible in our discussions.

It's also important to note that in many of the studies we cover in the book, researchers supplied the nutrients they studied through dietary supplements. Supplements can help fill in nutritional gaps, but I believe you should always try to get your nutrients from your daily diet first. If you do want to incorporate supplements into your routine, always consult your doctor to ensure you're getting the dosages correct and there are no interactions with medications you are taking. For example, many people don't realize that the innocent grapefruit and related food products like grapefruit juice interact with many medications due to a chemical compound that blocks certain liver enzymes.

Conventionally, good evidence in medicine means that there have been at least two double-blind clinical trials showing that a treatment has efficacy over a placebo control. A double-blind, placebo-controlled study means that the clinical trial participants may receive the real medication or an inactive substance that looks exactly like the medication (called a placebo). Neither the participant nor the researcher will know which medication (real or placebo) they are receiving. That's the only way to make certain that the real drug is effective.

The problem with double-blind trials is that they give you data on a group of individuals, not the individuals themselves. The group's characteristics may not reflect each unique brain. The only way to truly know what works for you is to experiment on your own. While you should never experiment with medication or even dietary supplements without consulting a doctor, as long as you are sticking to healthy, whole foods, I encourage you to try eating different things to see what diet makes you feel best. This book is intended to be a rigorous but realistic guide on how to choose foods based on your current mental health challenges. In each chapter, I will provide guidelines on each food's or diet's efficacy and safety and give you an idea of the current research and data that support my suggestions.

Of course, this information will likely change as time goes on, as medical knowledge shifts with the release of new studies and research. It doesn't make things easier that nutritional epidemiology has a tendency toward problematic data interpretation. For example, as I write this book, a recent series published in the *Annals of Internal Medicine* is dominating headlines with the claim that there are no health benefits for reducing red meat consumption. I cannot realistically support the conclusions reached by these articles, and I will just reiterate that in making the carefully balanced guidelines presented in this book, I have steered clear of sensationalized nutrient research and outcomes.

Finally, I want to emphasize that psychiatry is a complicated and individualized field. I am by no means suggesting that every patient who suffers from the conditions we are about to explore will find total relief solely through diet. It's important to work with a mental health professional to develop the right mix of psychotherapy and antidepressant medication when necessary. But no matter what, the food you eat will be an important part of the puzzle.

THE WAY TO A PERSON'S BRAIN

There's a proverb that states that the way to a man's heart is through his stomach. We might have stumbled upon a great truth with slight modification: for both men and women, the food that enters our stomachs can warm our hearts and change our brains.

May this book help bring you greater clarity, calmness, energy, and happiness. Let the exploration begin!

CHAPTER TWO

Depression: Probiotics, Omega-3s, and the Mediterranean Eating Pattern

Let's face it, Doc, there's nothing a great meal can't fix, right?" Ted said to me during his first visit to my office. Ted was thirty-nine, a highly successful entrepreneur who found himself feeling depressed—unhappy with his weight and stressed out by his job and countless responsibilities at home—and using food to help him cope and feel happier. While he was able to function in his day-to-day life, his mood was low, and food seemed to ease the pain he felt. Every night, after working long hours, he'd eat dinner, promptly followed by a bowl of ice cream. Then he'd sit down, watch the news, and mindlessly munch on chocolate or whatever else he could raid from his kids' snack cupboard. All the while enjoying a glass of wine, or two, or three.

When he discussed his symptoms during his annual physical, his primary care doctor suggested he start taking Prozac. While he was open to the idea of an antidepressant, he first wanted to explore other options such as nutritional strategies to help him feel better. That was when he reached out to me for an appointment.

I think Ted was surprised to hear me commiserate with him

about how tempting it can be to chase away bad feelings by eating unhealthy food. Even though I'm a doctor, I'm also a human being who knows the allure of "eating your feelings." But I also understand that even if it makes you feel better in the moment, staving off bad moods with junk food means you'll eventually pay the price both physically and mentally. The physical toll of Ted's depression-induced eating was clear—he had gained 30 pounds, despite trying to eat healthily at his main meals—but the mental toll was even more profound. While Ted thought that his eating habits were combatting his depression, they were actually deepening it.

Ted was right about one thing: food can be powerful medicine. If you make the right dietary choices, a great meal *can* "fix" almost anything, including how you feel about yourself and your life. In this chapter we are going to dive into all the ways that food can harm and heal your moods and learn how to eat in order to live your happiest life.

DEPRESSION AND YOUR GUT

When stress is skyrocketing and your mood is plunging, it's only natural to turn to comfort food. How many of you, like Ted, have found yourselves in a funk, sinking into a couch in front of the TV, with a chocolate bar, tub of ice cream, or bag of potato chips in hand? It's not surprising that in 2018, a cross-sectional research study of depressed college students found that 30.3 percent ate fried foods, 49 percent drank sweetened drinks, and 51.8 percent ate sugary food two to seven times per week.[1] Women were found to be even more susceptible to eating unhealthy food when depressed.

Of course, not everyone who is depressed binges on junk food, because depression can have a variety of effects on appetite.[2] For some, depression dulls their appetite. For others, it makes them ravenous. Many depressed people will skip meals and make poor food choices, which makes sense given that depression is associated with waning levels of mood-regulating neurotransmitters such as serotonin. This can make self-care, like fixing healthy meals, a real challenge. All you can think is, *I want to feel better,* and convenient junk foods like candy bars and potato chips in the moment seem to do the trick.

But here's the thing: they really don't. As you'll come to learn later in this chapter, high sugar intake can contribute to and worsen depression, as well as increase the odds that depression will recur in your life. Luckily, there are foods that can boost and improve mood. How? In part, thanks to the fascinating and complex relationship between the gut and the brain. When discussing depression and the gut with my patients, I often use the phrase "blue bowel," a lighthearted name for the very serious relationship between depression and your gut.

As we discussed in chapter 1, food changes the types of bacteria present in your gut microbiome. Your gut bacteria may become less diverse as a result of your diet, which may cause the bad bacteria to outgrow the good bacteria, triggering a cascade of negative health effects. Food can also influence the chemical messages these bacteria send from your gut up to your brain along the vagus nerve—signals that can make you feel either depressed and drained or uplifted and energized.

Animal research first led scientists to theorize that people who are depressed have different populations of gut bacteria than those who are not depressed. For instance, in mice, when the brain's main center for smell is surgically removed, the mice exhibit depression-like behavior. These changes were accompanied by alterations in gut bacteria. In other words, inducing depression in mice changes their gut activity and bacteria.

Studies in humans appear to confirm this hypothesis. In 2019, psychiatrist Stephanie Cheung and her colleagues summarized findings from six studies[3] that looked at gut health in patients with depression. They reported that patients with major depressive disorder had at least fifty types of bacterial species in their gut microbiome that were different from those of control subjects without major depressive disorder. Recent research suggests that bacterial species associated with higher quality-of-life indicators are depleted in depressed subjects, while bacteria that cause inflammation are often found in higher numbers in people suffering from depression. This tells us that inflammation and depression are closely linked.

Fighting Depression with Probiotics and Prebiotics

If you're suffering from gut-induced depression, how do you reset your gut microbiome to steer you back to a healthy mental state? The key is to increase probiotics and prebiotics in your diet. Probiotics are live bacteria that convey health benefits when eaten. Probiotic-rich foods contain beneficial bacteria that help your body and brain. An animal study in 2017 from the University of Virginia School of Medicine indicated that *Lactobacillus*, a single gut bacterium commonly found in live cultures in yogurt, can reverse depression in rats. This bacterium is often an ingredient in human probiotic supplement formulations. More recently, similar findings have been established in humans as well.

Prebiotics are essentially food for helpful bacteria, certain types of fiber that we cannot digest but the good bacteria in our guts can. For probiotics to be effective, it is helpful for them to have prebiotic foods available in the gut to digest. Probiotics break down prebiotics to form short-chain fatty acids that help reduce gut inflammation, block the growth of cancerous cells, and help the growth of healthy cells.

In 2010, Michael Messaoudi and his colleagues studied fifty-five healthy men and women who were randomly assigned to receive either a daily probiotic formula or a placebo for thirty days.[4] Before and after treatment, the research subjects filled out questionnaires about their mood. They also provided urine samples so that their levels of cortisol, the body's main stress hormone, could be checked.

Compared to the placebo group, those in the probiotic group reported less depression, and urinary levels of cortisol were lower, indicating that their brains were less depressed *and* less stressed.

Why was this the case? Certain species of gut bacteria have the ability to boost levels of brain chemicals such as gamma-aminobutyric acid, which may speed relief from depression and other mental health conditions.[5]

Probiotics are available in supplements, but it's preferable to increase your levels of friendly bacteria through dietary sources. Yogurt with active cultures is one of the best sources of probiotics; just avoid fruited yogurts high in added sugars. Other probiotic-rich foods include tempeh, miso, and natto (fermented soybean products); sauerkraut; kefir (soured yogurt); kimchi (Korean pickle); kombucha (a fermented tea drink); buttermilk; and select cheeses such as cheddar, mozzarella, and Gouda. Examples of prebiotic-rich foods include beans and other legumes, oats, bananas, berries, garlic, onions, dandelion greens, asparagus, Jerusalem artichokes, and leeks.

For an example of the power of probiotics, consider my patient Rosa. Rosa read about my work in nutritional psychiatry in a feature on probiotics in the *Wall Street Journal* and asked her pulmonologist to refer her to me. She had severe asthma and had been in and out of inpatient units suffering from serious bacterial, viral, and fungal chest infections. Her doctors could not get ahead of the infections. She was treated with multiple antibiotics and other medications that she believed had disrupted her microbiome.

While Rosa was by no means terminally ill, she arrived in a frail, emotionally depleted state, feeling as though life was not worth living. She had lost her appetite, had lost weight, and had struggled with eating hospital food when she was in treatment. Given that her microbiome was likely quite disrupted by the medications she had been taking for several lung infections, I spoke to her about using both probiotic- and prebiotic-rich foods in her daily diet and bulking up on fresh fruit and vegetables.

She switched her breakfast chocolate croissant out for a plain Greek yogurt topped with berries, cinnamon, and a drop of honey. She followed my recipe for making a creamy salad dressing using kefir and added this to a healthy green salad with beans, dandelion greens, and radish for lunch. She added onions and garlic to all her vegetable side dishes and leeks to her soups. She began drinking kombucha and used my recipe for miso-glazed sweet potatoes (page 279) as a side to her baked salmon dinner (page 248). In fact, she liked the taste of miso paste so much that she began to use it on her daily vegetable side dish (her favorite was grilled asparagus), thereby incorporating another probiotic food source.

Although it took time to heal her microbiome, she began to feel brighter, less fatigued, and less "foggy" two to three weeks after we adjusted her diet. I am delighted to report she is now thriving, is eating healthier, has not been readmitted to the hospital for infections this year, and, most important, is no longer depressed and is feeling like herself again.

FOODS THAT DULL YOUR MOOD

There are many other ways that the food you eat can affect your mood. As evidenced by a 2019 study by Heather M. Francis and her colleagues, there is strong evidence that poor diet is connected to depression.[6] Whether you want to say goodbye to depression symptoms you're currently experiencing or prevent the blues from creeping up on you, be sure to leave the following foods on the grocery store shelf.

Sugar

While scientific literature backs the long-held notion that feeling down in the dumps can lead you to overindulge in sugary treats, it also suggests the opposite to be true: the more sugar you eat, the more likely you are to be depressed. In 2002, Arthur Westover and

Lauren Marangell found a profound correlation between people who ate sugar and those with depression.[7] Statistically speaking, a perfect correlation is 1. Researchers almost never hit this mark, because there are always exceptions. But in their study, these researchers reported the correlation between eating sugar and having depression at 0.95—that's pretty close to 1. And this was true across six countries!

In 2019, a meta-analysis of ten previously published observational studies including 37,131 people with depression concluded that consuming sugar-sweetened beverages put people at a higher risk for depression. If they drank just over a 12-ounce can of soda a day (about 45 grams of sugar) they increased their risk by 5 percent. But if they drank two and a half cans of soda a day (about 98 grams of sugar), their risk jumped to 25 percent.[8] In other words, more sugar consumed also meant a greater risk of depression. Pay attention to the sugar content of what you drink.

Why might sugar cause depression? The brain relies on glucose, a type of sugar, from the food we eat in order to survive and to function. Over a twenty-four-hour period, the brain needs only 62 grams of glucose to do its job, an incredible display of energy efficiency considering the brain has at least 100 billion cells. You can easily meet this need through healthy, whole foods. Consuming unhealthy processed foods like baked goods and soda, which are loaded with refined and added sugars, often in the form of high-fructose corn syrup, floods the brain with too much glucose. This "sugar flood" can lead to inflammation in the brain and may ultimately result in depression.

Research also shows that higher blood-glucose levels are linked to lower levels of brain-derived neurotrophic factor (BDNF) in rats. BDNF is a protein found in the brain, gut, and other tissues that is critical to helping the brain grow and develop, as well as helping the brain adapt to stress.[9] So you won't be surprised to hear that studies have found low levels of BDNF in women with depression.[10]

BDNF may also improve the effect of antidepressant drugs, another indicator that it plays an important role in preventing depression.[11]

High-Glycemic-Load Carbohydrates

Even if high-carbohydrate foods—for example, bread, pasta, and anything else made from refined flour—don't taste sweet, your body still processes them in much the same way it does sugar. That means they can also raise your risk for depression. Don't panic, I'm not going to suggest eliminating carbs from your diet completely! But the quality of the carbs you eat matters.

In 2018, researchers sought to evaluate which particular carbohydrates, if any, had an association with depression.[12] They administered a questionnaire called the carbohydrate-quality index to 15,546 participants. "Better-quality" carbohydrates were defined as whole grains, foods high in fiber, and those ranked low on the glycemic index (GI). The GI is a measure of how quickly foods convert to glucose when broken down during digestion; the faster a food turns into glucose in the body, the higher its GI ranking.

Of the participants in this study, 769 people were found to be depressed. The researchers discovered that people who had the highest score on the carbohydrate-quality index, meaning they were eating better-quality carbs, were also 30 percent less likely to develop depression than those who were eating high-GI carbs. In other words, a high-GI diet appears to be a risk factor for depression.[13] High-GI carbs include potatoes, white bread, and white rice. Honey, orange juice, and whole-meal breads are medium-GI foods. Low-GI foods include green vegetables, most fruits, raw carrots, kidney beans, chickpeas, and lentils.

In order to minimize your chance for depression, you'll want to structure your diet to avoid high-GI foods while leaning more heavily on medium- and especially low-GI foods, with an emphasis on good sources of whole grains and fiber such as brown rice, quinoa, steel-cut oatmeal, chia seeds, and blueberries. However, a word of caution: you don't want to overindulge in medium- or low-GI foods either. A large quantity of any carbs, no matter what their GI, places what is called a high glycemic load on your body. Very simply, the glycemic load of a certain food is a number that estimates how much the food will raise your blood-glucose level after you eat it. Studies show that a high glycemic load can increase your chances of depression as well.

The take-home message? While you don't need to cut out carbs completely to improve or avoid depression symptoms, it's essential to make sure you're choosing the right carbs and eating them in reasonable quantities. To help out, I've included a chart in Appendix A of common foods with low-, medium-, and high-glycemic loads.

Artificial Sweeteners, Especially Aspartame

Saccharin (Sweet'N Low), aspartame (NutraSweet), sucralose (Splenda), and stevia (Truvia) are just a few of the most popular artificial sweeteners in use by food manufacturers today. Other lesser-known compounds are erythritol, lactitol, maltitol, sorbitol, and xylitol. These sugar replacements are increasingly common in foods that purport to be "healthy" by helping you cut down on calories.

That's alarming, because science implicates many artificial sweeteners in depression: one study showed that people who consume artificial sweeteners, mostly via diet drinks, are more depressed than those who don't consume such beverages.[14] Even worse, several studies have demonstrated that artificial sweeteners can be toxic to the brain, altering brain concentrations of mood-regulating neurotransmitters.[15]

Aspartame, the primary sweetener in many popular diet drinks, including Diet Coke, has been proven to be particularly damaging. In 2017, a review of the studies on aspartame found that it increases substances in the brain that inhibit the synthesis and release of the "happy" neurotransmitters dopamine, noradrenaline, and serotonin.[16]

In addition, aspartame causes oxidation, which increases harmful free radicals in the brain. We'll talk about the damaging effects of oxidation many times throughout the book. Oxidation is a chemical process that releases certain particles known as reactive oxygen species, including free radicals, which are unstable molecules prone to causing havoc in cells.[17] At low to moderate concentrations, reactive oxygen species are important to your brain cells because they help to maintain internal chemical balance. However, at higher concentrations, an imbalance between antioxidants (which fight free radicals) and the free radicals themselves triggers a condition called oxidative stress, which can cause cell loss or even brain damage and can render the brain more prone to depression.

Not all sweeteners are guaranteed to be harmful. However, there is mounting evidence that other sweeteners beyond aspartame, such as sucralose, could also be causing or worsening depression. A 2018 study showed that sucralose significantly alters gut bacteria in mice, increasing a type of bacteria that other studies show is increased in people who are depressed.[18] Sucralose also increases myeloperoxidase activity. Myeloperoxidase is a marker of inflammation, and one study found that twins with a history of depression had levels of myeloperoxidase 32 percent higher than those without depression.[19]

If you suffer from depression, I recommend avoiding all artificial sweeteners. Since you're also avoiding sugar, it may take time to wean yourself off of a sweet tooth, but the benefits will be well worth the effort.

Fried Foods

Tempura, empanadas, samosas, fish and chips, chicken-fried steak. Is your mouth watering? I get it. I often spend time on Cape Cod, where, every summer, the delectable aroma of fried pickles and French fries fills my nostrils and proves simply irresistible. I couldn't imagine never eating fried food again, even though I know all the associated health risks. Flavor matters to my quality of life! Still, when it comes to depression, it pays to reduce the amount of fried foods you eat.

A study in Japan looked at 715 Japanese factory workers and measured their levels of depression and resilience. It also documented their level of fried-food consumption. Sure enough, the research team found that people who consumed more fried foods were more likely to develop depression in their lifetime.[20]

Much like the findings associated with sugar consumption, this finding might seem counterintuitive. I mean, when was the last time eating French fries depressed you? Never, right? At least not while you're eating them. I'm betting a few hours after the last time you indulged in a fried-food feast you felt bad—like you had too much and overdid it. While we usually think these bad feelings are simply due to the guilt of overeating, they might be feeding into more serious feelings of depression over time.

If you're eating fried foods daily, switch to weekly. If it's a weekly habit, try enjoying them just once a month. If you don't eat fried foods, you're already on your way to happier times!

Bad Fats

Fried foods are likely such mood killers because they're usually fried in unhealthy fats. In recent years, the conversation around fat in the diet has changed from all fats being unhealthy to a clearer distinction between "bad fats" (for instance, margarine, shortening, and hydrogenated oils) known to cause cardiovascular disease and other woes, and "good fats" (for instance, avocados, almonds, and olive oil) that can help prevent disease and benefit well-being.

In 2011, Almudena Sánchez-Villegas and her colleagues reported on earlier research in which they had set out to determine if there was an association between fats and depression.[21] They enrolled 12,059 Spanish university graduates who were free of depression at the start of the study and had each answer a 136-item food-frequency questionnaire to estimate their consumption of specific culinary fats (olive oil, seed oils, butter, and margarine) in order to determine their intake of different categories of fats—saturated fatty acids, polyunsaturated fatty acids (PUFAs), trans-unsaturated fatty acids (trans fats), and monounsaturated fatty acids (MUFAs). During follow-up visits, participants were asked to note any new onset of depression.

After about six years, 657 new cases of depression were identified. The researchers found that the more trans fats in a participant's diet, the more likely they were to become depressed. On the other hand, the more MUFAs and PUFAs a participant consumed, the less depressed they were. In terms of individual culinary fats, the researchers concluded that olive oil—which consists largely of MUFA—significantly lowered depression risk.

To prevent or lower your chances of depression, shun all trans fats. Although the Food and Drug Administration banned trans fats in 2018, food manufacturers are permitted a transition period to comply with this regulation, so trans fats can still be found in certain foods including microwave popcorn, frozen pizza, refrigerated biscuit dough, fast food, vegetable shortening, and some margarines.

MUFAS should make up the majority of the fats in your diet. In addition to olive oil, MUFAs are found in nuts (almonds, walnuts) and nut butters (almond and cashew butter) as well as avocados.

While PUFAs are better than trans fats, not all sources of PUFAs are the best choices for depression. For example, corn, sunflower, and safflower oil in moderation in your diet may be okay, but in excess they can cause an imbalance in omega-3 and omega-6 fatty acids, which may impact emotional regulation and lead to depression (more on this shortly).[22]

Added Nitrates

Used as a preservative and to enhance color in deli slices and cured meats like bacon, salami, and sausage, nitrates may be connected with depression.[23] One recent study even suggests that nitrates can alter gut bacteria in such a way as to tip the scales toward bipolar disorder.[24] If you simply can't live without salami and sausages, seek out those containing buckwheat flour, which is used as a filler. Buckwheat flour contains important antioxidants that will counter some of the negative health effects of these meats.[25]

GOOD FOOD FOR GOOD MOODS

Now that you know the common dietary culprits for depression—the foods that can cause all those unpleasant symptoms, from guilt to sleep and appetite problems, difficulty concentrating, low energy, and a loss of interest in many things in life—it's time to look at the flip side. Here's what to eat in order to prevent the blues or kick them to the curb once and for all.

Foods Rich in Omega-3 Fatty Acids

We already discussed good fats for depression earlier in the chapter, but I want to give special attention to the importance of omega-3 fatty acids. Omega-3s are crucial to mental health, and we will discuss their benefits over the course of the book.

Omega-3s are important for normal body metabolism—they are a vital part of cell membranes and provide the starting point for making the hormones that regulate blood clotting, contraction and relaxation of artery walls, and inflammation. But since we cannot produce them on our own, we must get our omega-3s from our diet. This is why we call them *essential* fats.

The three main omega-3 fatty acids are alpha-linolenic acid, eicosapentaenoic acid (EPA), and docosahexaenoic acid (DHA). All three are important to the body, performing a number of tasks, especially in cell membranes. EPA and DHA are the two omega-3s that play the most critical role in mood disorders, so it's particularly important to ensure that you get enough of them.

While there is some argument about the importance of omega-3s in the fight against depression, most studies suggest they are instrumental, including a 2016 meta-analysis of thirteen randomized controlled trials of 1,233 patients with major depressive disorder. It found a beneficial overall effect of omega-3s in patients with major depressive disorder, especially in participants taking higher amounts of EPA and in those taking antidepressants.[26]

Omega-3s promote brain health by lowering inflammatory markers and protecting neurons from excessive inflammation. The key is to maintain a healthy balance between omega-3s and omega-6s, which are found in different foods. In a typical Western diet, omega-6s are quite common, while omega-3s are much rarer, leading to an omega-6 to omega-3 ratio of somewhere around 15 to 1. The ideal ratio is more like 4 to 1.[27] That means most Americans need to cut down on omega-6s while eating more omega-3s.

Indeed, studies have shown that people who consume foods high in omega-6 fatty acids have more than four times the risk of depression compared to those who consume foods high in omega-3s. This means that eating foods high in omega-6s like full-fat cheese, high-fat cuts of red meat, corn oil, and palm oil may increase your chances of depression. On the contrary, eating foods high in omega-3s like fatty fish, walnuts, vegetable oils, and dark, leafy vegetables may protect you against depression.

The very best source of omega-3s, especially EPA and DHA, is fish. In particular, cold-water fatty fish, such as salmon, mackerel, tuna, herring, and sardines, contain high amounts of omega-3s. Fish with a lower fat content, such as bass, tilapia, cod, and shellfish, aren't quite as rich in omega-3s but still have significant amounts. Farmed fish usually have higher levels of EPA and DHA than wild-caught fish, but it depends on the food they are fed. That's because fish themselves do not actually make the omega-3s. Instead, they are found in microalgae. When the fish consume phytoplankton, which consumes microalgae, they accumulate omega-3s in their tissues.

Omega-3s can also be found in other foods, though nothing is as good a source as fatty fish. Grass-fed beef contains more omega-3s than commercial beef. Alpha-linolenic acid is available from plant sources like edamame, walnuts, and chia seeds, and there are an increasing number of omega-3-fortified foods on the market, especially eggs, milk, and yogurt.

You can also improve your ratio of omega-6 to omega-3 by using certain oils in your cooking. For instance, rather than using plain vegetable oil, which is extremely heavy in omega-6, use canola oil. While canola oil is far from a perfect source of omega-3s, its ratio of omega-6 to omega-3 is roughly 2 to 1, making it a natural choice for a healthier alternative to similar oils.

Foods Rich in Helpful Vitamins

Many vitamins play key roles in preventing and easing depression. The most important are folate (B_9) and B_{12}. Their functions in the body are inextricably linked: a deficiency in vitamin B_{12} results in a folate deficiency, which can ultimately contribute to a loss of brain cells, chiefly those located in the hippocampus. Termed "hippocampal atrophy," this loss of brain cells is associated with depression. The hippocampus is a critical brain structure that plays an important role in learning and memory, so depressed patients may lose their ability to learn new ways to cope with their stress.

In patients with folate deficiency, depression is the most common symptom.[28] In fact, studies have demonstrated that the higher one's folate level, the lower one's level of depression.[29] In addition to its role in the hippocampus, folate may also affect serotonin synthesis, and in depression, serotonin is often low.[30]

Hence, both vitamin B_{12} and folate should be optimized to prevent or treat depression. Enjoy ample amounts of legumes, citrus fruits, bananas, avocados, leafy green and cruciferous vegetables, asparagus, nuts and seeds, and fish and shellfish.

Vitamins B_1 (thiamine) and B_6 (pyridoxine) are also key for preventing and easing depression, as they help the brain produce and synthesize the neurotransmitters involved in mood regulation. These vitamins are abundant in the foods mentioned in the previous paragraph, as well as in soybeans and whole grains.

Vitamin A facilitates proper brain function such as the growth and adaptation of neurons.[31] As with vitamin B_{12}, a deficiency of vitamin A may result in shrinkage of certain brain areas, disturbing how the brain responds to stress.[32] In 2016 a study found that vitamin A can significantly improve fatigue and depression in multiple sclerosis patients.[33] However, too much retinoic acid (a metabolite of vitamin A) has also been associated with depression and suicide.[34] The amount of vitamin A you would have to consume to suffer these ill effects is far beyond what you will eat in a healthy, varied diet, so feel free to eat vitamin A–rich foods such as sweet potatoes, carrots, spinach, and black-eyed peas.

Vitamin C is important for proper brain functioning, as it's responsible for the regulation of neurotransmitter synthesis.[35] Several observational studies have suggested a relationship between low levels of vitamin C and depression.[36] Get your vitamin C from citrus fruits, cantaloupe, strawberries, and cruciferous vegetables including broccoli, cauliflower, and Brussels sprouts.

We will talk about vitamins many times throughout the book, so if you need a refresher on what vitamins perform which brain functions, and what foods contain those vitamins, you can refer to Appendix B.

Foods Rich in Iron and Other Helpful Minerals

In the brain, iron helps make up the covering that protects neurons and helps control the synthesis of chemicals and chemical pathways involved in mood.[37] In fact, a large concentration of iron is found in the basal ganglia, a collection of brain cells that have been implicated in depression.[38] In clinical studies, low iron levels and depression have been linked.[39] Good food sources of iron include shellfish, lean red meats and organ meats (in moderation), legumes, pumpkin seeds, broccoli, and dark chocolate (though any sweet should be eaten in moderation).

Magnesium is also important for proper brain function. The first report of magnesium treatment for agitated depression was published in 1921, and it showed success in a whopping 220 out of 250 cases.[40] Since then, countless studies have suggested that depression is related to magnesium deficiency. Several case studies, in which patients were treated with 125–300 mg of magnesium, have demonstrated rapid recovery from major depression, often in less than a week. How can you get enough magnesium in your diet? Eat more avocados, nuts and seeds, legumes, whole grains, and some omega-3-rich fish (such as salmon and mackerel).

When it comes to potassium, the picture is not as clear, but some studies have shown that higher potassium intake can improve mood.[41] Sweet potatoes, bananas, mushrooms, oranges, peas, and cucumbers are all high in potassium.

Most evidence strongly supports a positive association between zinc deficiency and the risk of depression, with zinc supplements reducing depressive symptoms.[42] A meta-analysis of seventeen studies found that blood zinc concentrations were lower in depressed subjects than in control subjects.[43] Zinc probably helps because it reduces brain inflammation.[44] Find high concentrations of zinc in seafood (especially cooked oysters), lean beef, and poultry, with lower amounts found in beans, nuts, and whole grains.

Finally, several studies have also suggested that a diet high in selenium significantly improves mood scores.[45] Brazil nuts are packed with this nutrient.

Again, if you need a quick reference for what foods contain these minerals, see Appendix B.

Seasonings, Spices, and Herbs

What should you use to season that piece of nutrient-rich grilled fish or veggie sauté? The following spices and seasonings can help combat depression. Use them with the antidepressant foods shared previously for double the mood-boosting effect.

In general, one important benefit of spices is their antioxidant properties—in other words, they help the brain fight off harmful free radicals and therefore prevent oxidative stress, which can damage tissues. There is a measure of spices' antioxidant capacities called ORAC (oxygen radical absorbance capacity). I've included an ORAC chart in Appendix C showing which spices have the most antioxidant benefits. Make sure to prioritize those in your cooking as much as possible.

Saffron: In 2013, a meta-analysis of five previously published randomized controlled trials looked at the effects of saffron supplementation on symptoms of depression among participants with major depressive disorder.[46] In all these trials, researchers found that saffron supplementation significantly reduced depression symptoms compared to the placebo controls. A study in 2017 demonstrated that 15 mg of saffron was as effective as 20 mg of Prozac in decreasing depressive symptoms! Apparently saffron's secret power was known to Christopher Catton, a nineteenth-century English herbalist who once said, "Saffron has power to quicken the spirits, and the virtue thereof pierces by and by to the heart, provoking laughter and merriment."[47] While its precise mechanism of action is not known, in animals saffron increases levels of the good-mood neurotransmitters glutamate and dopamine.[48]

Per pound, saffron is more expensive than gold, and its flavor can overpower others, so you'll want to use a sprinkle and not a handful! After blooming a few threads (see San Franciscan Seafood Stew, page 289), add it to vegetable and rice dishes, such as saffron risotto or biryani. You can also find a supplement or extract, though as always with supplements, consult your doctor before taking it.

Turmeric: A meta-analysis in 2017 evaluated six clinical trials that tested the active ingredient in turmeric, called curcumin, for depression.[49] They concluded that curcumin was significantly more effective than placebo in reducing depressive symptoms. How is it capable of such profound effects? Simply put, it adjusts brain chemistry and protects brain cells against toxic damage that leads to depression.

The effective dose is 500–1,000 mg a day. While you will read that 1 teaspoon of turmeric contains about 200 mg of curcumin, that's not exactly accurate. Because turmeric contains approximately 2 percent curcumin by weight, 1 tablespoon (or 3 teaspoons) which weighs 6.8 grams, really contains about 0.136 grams of curcumin, or 136 mg. For any dish, more than 1 teaspoon of turmeric may be overwhelming, so making a few dishes with a teaspoon or two of turmeric a day is a potential solution: add a touch of turmeric to your soups and stews, or even add it to your smoothie. Make a hot tea with it or add a pinch to your salad dressing. Note that piperine, a constituent found in black pepper, increases the absorption and bioavailability of curcumin by 2,000 percent.[50] So when you use turmeric, always add some freshly ground pepper too.

Oregano: Carvacrol, an active ingredient in oregano, was found to have antidepressant activity in mice.[51] Other researchers have also connected carvacrol with neuroprotective and antidepressant effects in animals, although to date, there are no such studies in humans. That said, I believe it's likely to help protect brain tissue. Commonly used in many cuisines, it's a staple ingredient in my favorite Greek dressing, used to marinate olives and feta cheese, and delicious on oven-roasted vegetables.

I'll discuss lavender, passionflower, and chamomile in detail while discussing anxiety in chapter 3, but know that these herbs can all be helpful for depression too.[52] They're easiest enjoyed as teas.

I know that it may feel a bit overwhelming imagining yourself standing in a busy grocery aisle trying to remember exactly which foods are highest in which nutrients.

An even easier way to keep straight what you should and should not eat when fighting depression is to follow a broad diet that naturally steers you toward food that is healthy for your brain and away from food that can hinder your mood. Luckily, such a diet already exists!

THE MEDITERRANEAN EATING PATTERN

While the Mediterranean diet wasn't formulated expressly with mental health in mind, it incorporates all the depression-busting foods just mentioned, and in healthy ratios to help you achieve the nutrient balance needed for optimal brain functioning and mood regulation. And, of course, it's healthy for your body in many other ways.

As first described in 1957 by physiologists Ancel Keys and Francisco Grande Covián, and then refined by scientific studies that evaluated the impact of this way of eating on health outcomes, some daily foods in the original Mediterranean diet should include:

- 3–9 servings of vegetables
- ½–2 servings of fruit
- 1–13 servings of cereals (bread and other grains, preferably whole grains)
- Up to 8 servings of olive oil[53]

While those serving sizes look like broad ranges (particularly for cereals — 13 servings of carbs per day is not advisable in modern nutrition), the amounts translate to roughly 2,200 calories a day, broken down as 37 percent total fat (of which 18 percent is monounsaturated and 9 percent is saturated) and 33 grams of fiber.

Rather than adhering to the strict proportions of the traditional Mediterranean diet, I prefer to have my patients follow the

Mediterranean eating pattern (MEP), which confers the same protective effects on depression risk.[54] I sometimes describe this way of eating as a "Mediterranean lifestyle," because my patients often feel the word *diet* can sound negative. Diet is associated with restriction, while, truly, this dietary approach is all about the delicious foods you can *add* to your life to enhance your meals and feel better in the process. Plus, when you don't feel you're giving up food, you can avoid what inevitably occurs on restrictive diets: the pendulum swinging back, where you end up overeating the shunned foods anyway. The MEP is a plant-based diet that's abundant in locally grown seasonal fruits and vegetables and other foods that are minimally processed (e.g., beans, nuts, whole grains). Sweets are limited, and only high-quality fats are acceptable, with olive oil being the primary source of fat. The MEP includes low to moderate dairy intake, and protein is mainly seafood, with red meat and eggs consumed in smaller quantities and with low frequency. Wine is consumed in low to moderate amounts with meals, and herbs and spices are used instead of salt to add flavor to foods. In fact, there is plenty of flexibility with flavors. I always try to adapt the Mediterranean lifestyle to a patient's culture and tastes, so, for example, I might suggest South Asian recipes for chickpeas or adding Mexican oregano and fajita spices to hummus, depending on what the patient loves to eat.

It's worth noting that there is some controversy about whether the actual diet of the Mediterranean region can be adapted to other parts of the world, as the food preparation and sources of food differ.[55] But I believe it can, since the composition of the diet is much more important than preparation or flavors. After all, the antidepressant mechanism of the Mediterranean diet is in large part due to its emphasis on consumption of fruits and vegetables—produce contains high levels of antioxidants that reduce oxidative stress and may, in turn, reduce neuron damage—and olive oil, which is rich in antioxidants and other brain-healthy compounds.[56] Nutrient-dense fruits and veggies and high-quality olive oils are now more readily available in supermarkets and online. And of course, fish, nuts, and whole grains can be found at many grocery stores or farmers' markets as well.

The MEP in Action

For an example of the power of the MEP, consider my client Josephine, a fifty-one-year-old married woman dealing with weight issues and poor diabetes control—and depression as a result. When she arrived at our first meeting, she appeared exhausted even though it was only nine a.m.! Her eyes were sad and tired. She told me that she felt frazzled, like she was always making poor food choices. Despite her best efforts, she hadn't lost any weight, and she couldn't get her blood sugar under control. When I asked about her biggest stressor, she responded pointedly: trying to eat right. Her perceived lack of control over her diet saddened her to the point that she was considering taking an antidepressant.

I asked her to write out a food log for a few days, through which I discovered dietary red flags: she typically ate breakfast (Cheerios and low-fat milk), but she still felt "blue" and hungry when she arrived at work. She'd have a slice of toast with peanut butter later and remain on the edge of hunger most of the day, never feeling satiated or energized. Most important, she went to work unprepared, without any lunch or snacks, and instead relied on vending machines and options from her work cafeteria.

Over the course of several sessions, we discussed the Mediterranean eating pattern. I taught her how to build a healthy salad for lunch, jam-packed with nutrient-rich greens and fresh chopped veggies (broccoli, green beans, and red peppers), and topped with oven-baked salmon, chickpeas, almonds, or an avocado for healthy proteins and fats. In addition, she added chia seeds for fiber and more protein and made a simple homemade vinaigrette (fresh lemon juice, olive oil, salt, and pepper). I recall her look of delight as she said, "I didn't understand how filling that would be. Now I feel energized and full after my lunch, and I'm not running for peanut butter and crackers in the afternoon."

For breakfast, she started making overnight whole-grain oats with almond milk, cinnamon, and berries; she would portion out five breakfasts in mason jars, seal them, and leave them in her fridge. Every morning she would grab her oatmeal and eat it on the train. It saved her time, she felt healthier for making better food choices, and she felt her mood slowly lifting from those prior morning blues and low energy.

By her third visit, she had lost 5 pounds, the blood test number that her diabetologist tracked had lowered for the first time in years, and she was enjoying her meals and not feeling deprived. She noticed that by eating tasty but healthy options throughout the day, she did not crave chocolate or ice cream at night. In fact, she ate a small piece of extra-dark chocolate with a few strawberries at night and felt good. Overall she described feeling revitalized. Her husband and colleagues noticed a difference. She even had enough energy to start exercising again and to use mindfulness in ways she had learned in a meditation course. She could do all these things because her blue and somber mood had lifted, and she told me she felt as though the weight of her depression had been lifted off her shoulders.

What the Studies Say

A wealth of research confirms the Mediterranean eating pattern's ability to protect against diabetes, prevent heart disease, and confer longevity. And the literature backs up my clinical findings that it can help stave off depression and soothe depressive symptoms as well.

Perhaps one of the best-known studies is the SMILES (Supporting the Modification of Lifestyle in Lowered Emotional States) study. Dr. Felice Jacka, a colleague of mine and the director of the Food and Mood Centre at Deakin University in Australia, led a team that conducted a twelve-week trial to explore whether deliberate dietary intervention is effective as an add-on treatment in moderate to severe depression. The diet they used? You guessed it: a Mediterranean eating pattern, which they termed the Modi*Med*-Diet. Specifically, their approach focused on "increasing diet quality by supporting the consumption of the following 12 key food groups" with these recommended servings:

Whole grains	5–8 per day
Vegetables	6 per day
Fruit	3 per day
Legumes	3–4 per week
Low-fat and unsweetened dairy foods	2–3 per day
Raw and unsalted nuts	1 per day
Fish	at least 2 per week
Lean red meats	3–4 per week
Chicken	2–3 per week
Eggs	up to 6 per week
Olive oil	3 tablespoons per day
"Extras" foods	Wine (red preferred): up to 2 glasses per day, with meals No more than 3 per week: sweets, refined cereals, fried food, fast food, processed meats, and sugary drinks

At the end of twelve weeks, the researchers found that close to a third of the people in the dietary intervention group exhibited an improvement in their symptoms of depression, whereas only 8 percent of the people in the control group improved. The diet worked!

More recently, in 2019, a related study followed up on 15,980 adults who did not have depression at the start of the study or in the first two years of the study.[57] Researchers measured participants' food consumption at baseline and then documented, over a period of time, whether they followed the Mediterranean diet or another diet for comparison. Roughly ten years after the study began, 666 people had developed depression. Those who most closely followed the Mediterranean diet were significantly less likely to become depressed.

Note that most studies of this diet are observational, meaning researchers can only draw inferences. A trial by Almudena Sánchez-Villegas and her colleagues showed more definitively that the Mediterranean diet benefits depression.[58]

Other Dietary Strategies to Beat the Blues

Studies show that other "traditional" eating patterns are also effective dietary strategies for preventing depression, for example, the Norwegian diet, also known as the Nordic diet.[59] Like the MEP, the Nordic diet prioritizes plant foods over meats and animal products, foods from the sea and lakes, and foods from the wild countryside. The biggest difference between this diet and the Mediterranean diet is that it emphasizes canola oil rather than olive oil. In 2013, a review of twenty-five previously published studies examined how diet impacts depression. Researchers found that both the Norwegian and Mediterranean diets were associated with less depression, though the evidence was limited.[60]

Limited evidence also exists for the traditional Japanese diet and reduced risk of depression. This diet includes foods similar to those in both the Norwegian and Mediterranean diets, with the addition of pickled and fermented items, which, as we mentioned earlier, are rich probiotic foods.

A GREAT MEAL CAN FIX EVERYTHING

After our appointment, my patient Ted committed himself to following a personalized meal plan based on the MEP. For lunch at work, he bought a healthy salad with extra leafy greens topped with oven-baked salmon or roasted turkey breast. He replaced his afternoon vending-machine snack with snacks like almond butter on freshly sliced apples, walnuts with dark chocolate chips, hummus with celery and grape tomatoes, or a clementine with some grapes. He felt better, as he went to work with his own lunch bag and knew he would not be stressed about feeling hungry and making poor choices. He even learned to make these same healthy choices when traveling, steering clear of pizza and hot dogs at airports.

When he got home at night, he enjoyed his dinner of oven-baked salmon with kale pesto (page 248) and a nutrient-dense flavorful green salad, and because he had made filling food choices during the day, he no longer craved ice cream and cookies following dinner. Even though he was not sure he was losing weight, he noticed his pants fit more comfortably. His coworkers told him he appeared trimmer and asked him if he had joined the gym.

More important, he gradually felt the positive effects on his mood. He described feeling brighter and more energized, and he successfully managed to treat his mood symptoms without taking Prozac. Three years later, he is living at his goal weight and no longer feels depressed.

Ted is the perfect example of how you can put the principles of nutritional psychiatry to work, creating nutrition and lifestyle plans that offer a natural approach to staving off and easing depression.

Of course, depression is only one facet of mental health. It often comes hand in hand with its partner, anxiety. In the next chapter, we'll explore ways in which anxiety can also be overcome with a diet of healthy, delicious food.

DEPRESSION CHEAT SHEET

The Mediterranean eating pattern is a great guideline to give you a complete diet that will fight depression and keep your brain healthy.

Foods to Embrace:

- Probiotics: Yogurt with active cultures, tempeh, miso, natto, sauerkraut, kefir, kimchi, kombucha, buttermilk, and certain cheeses.
- Prebiotics: Beans, oats, bananas, berries, garlic, onions, dandelion greens, asparagus, Jerusalem artichokes, and leeks.
- Low-GI carbohydrates: Brown rice, quinoa, steel-cut oatmeal, and chia seeds.
- Medium-GI foods, in moderation: Honey, orange juice, and whole-grain bread.
- Healthy fats: Monounsaturated fats like olive oil, nuts, nut butters, and avocados.
- Omega-3 fatty acids: Fish, especially fatty fish like salmon, mackerel, tuna, herring, and sardines.
- Vitamins B_9, B_{12}, B_1, B_6, A, and C.
- Minerals and micronutrients: Iron, magnesium, potassium, zinc, and selenium.
- Spices: Saffron and turmeric.
- Herbs: Oregano, lavender, passionflower, and chamomile.

Foods to Avoid:

- Sugar: Baked goods, candy, soda, or anything sweetened with sugar or high-fructose corn syrup.
- High-GI carbs: White bread, white rice, potatoes, pasta, and anything else made from refined flour.

- Artificial sweeteners: Aspartame is particularly harmful, but also saccharin, sucralose, and stevia in moderation and with caution.
- Fried foods: French fries, fried chicken, fried seafood, or anything else deep-fried in oil.
- Bad fats: Trans fats such as margarine, shortening, and hydrogenated oils are to be avoided totally; omega-6 fats such as vegetable, corn, sunflower, and safflower oil should only be consumed in moderation.
- Nitrates: An additive used in bacon, salami, sausage, and other cured meats.

CHAPTER THREE

Anxiety: Fermented Foods, Dietary Fiber, and the Tryptophan Myth

It was a beautiful day in Boston, one of those perfect crisp fall days that make me a little euphoric. The leaves were a reddish golden hue, and apples and pumpkins decorated the city. As the sunlight streamed in through the window, Marisol, a thirty-nine-year-old mother of two sons named Josue and Fernando, walked into my office. Despite the beautiful weather, she burst into tears shortly after sitting down. Her anxiety had become overwhelming.

"I just can't take this anymore," she said. "Every day I get up with a knot in my stomach. Will Josue be hit by a bus on the way to school? Will Fernando be held back another year? Will there be a school shooting? I mean, it never stops. Even when they are at home, I am literally chewing my nails off. And to top it all, my belly aches and I'm constipated. It doesn't help that Thanksgiving is around the corner. I've got to get my act together because twenty people are coming over for dinner."

She went on to tell me that she couldn't sleep at night with her heart pounding in her chest. I knew immediately that Marisol was describing symptoms of generalized anxiety disorder, a condition that causes normal, everyday worries to feel overwhelming.

Marisol's story is not uncommon. Anxiety can take many different forms: generalized anxiety disorder, panic disorder, agoraphobia, social anxiety disorder, or a host of specific phobias. Though these conditions have different triggers and develop in different ways, they all lock the brain into unhealthy patterns that can lead to panic attacks, paralyzing fear, and an inability to lead a happy and satisfied life.

Anxiety disorders are the most common type of psychiatric disorder in the United States, with up to a third of the population suffering from one during their lifetime.[1] Even that might be an underestimation, since anxiety often goes undiagnosed and untreated. There is a tendency to accept anxiety as an inevitable part of living in a stressful modern world, and to a degree, it's true that it's impossible to totally escape worry. But that doesn't mean you have to let anxiety impinge on your living your best, most fulfilled life.

While there are several approaches to treating anxiety, only 50–60 percent of people respond to medication and psychotherapy, and only a quarter of patients have complete resolution of their symptoms. A crucial part of battling anxiety is making sure your diet is full of foods that are calming and free of foods that put you on edge.

Marisol had already completed several trials of medications that treat anxiety, without much success. We still had a few more medications to try, but that was not going to be enough. We needed to address her diet as well.

THE ANXIOUS GUT

Even if you don't suffer from an anxiety disorder, you probably intuitively understand that there is a connection between anxious feelings and your gut. Think about how your stomach feels when you are nervous. Maybe you've found yourself running to the bathroom before a big test in school. Maybe you've felt nauseated or had dry heaves when you're on edge about a presentation at work. The connection is even built into our language, as we talk about "butterflies in your stomach" for mild nervousness or "a pit in your stomach" for feelings of dread. Those figures of speech aren't mere coincidence. Whether we realize it or not, they're inspired by the complex bidirectional relationship between the gut and the brain.

In 2018, Gilliard Lach and his colleagues shed light on the physiological connection between anxiety disorders and bowel issues.[2] Their work centered around gut peptides, short chains of amino acids that are used by your body as signaling molecules, carrying information between the gut and the brain. In the gut, specialized cells called enteroendocrine cells produce more than twenty signaling molecules, including peptides.[3] The specific types of signaling molecules that are created are determined by your gut bacteria. By manipulating the gut bacteria of mice, and then monitoring the corresponding change in various kinds of peptides present in the guts and brains of the mice, Lach and his team were able to track how changes in the gut microbiome influenced symptoms of anxiety, proving that there is a profound connection between the two. Though the researchers weren't able to make any conclusions about how this knowledge could be applied to microbiome-based therapeutic strategies to combat anxiety in humans, that's certainly a possibility down the road.

One part of the brain that is especially affected by changes in the gut microbiome is the amygdala, a structure found deep in the brain that is a key part of the circuit that goes awry when you are anxious.[4] In fact, the connection between the microbiome and amygdala development is so strong that some researchers think we should be targeting the microbiome to stabilize amygdala activation and reduce anxiety.

Research has shown that germ-free mice (meaning they lack all microorganisms and therefore have no gut microbiome) have larger amygdalae than mice with normal microbiomes.[5] The amygdala is also hyperactive, working overtime in an unhealthy way.[6] When it comes to amygdalae, bigger and more active is most definitely not better; in humans, a hyperactive amygdala makes it difficult to control your emotions, as if your brain has an alarm that is constantly going off.[7] If the lack of gut bacteria can so profoundly influence the amygdala's form and function, that's a strong sign that the microbiome plays an important role in brain health.

In 2004, Nobuyuki Sudo and his colleagues found that germ-free mice also have an exaggerated hypothalamic-pituitary-adrenal axis (HPA-axis) response to stress.[8] Incredibly, the introduction of just one specific bacterial species into the mice's microbiome reversed this. It amazes me that changing just one bacterial species—one among a multitude in the gut—can improve how an organism responds to stress!

If you're doubtful that the brains of mice have much overlap with your stressful human life, rest assured that recent human studies have found similar results. In 2018, a study compared the microbiota in people with generalized anxiety disorder to those of healthy controls.[9] They found that the patients with generalized anxiety disorder had very different bacteria, which were both sparser and less diverse than those in their healthy counterparts. Specifically, bacteria that produce short-chain fatty acids—like the peptides we just discussed, which are a sign of a healthy gut—were scarce, and there was an overgrowth of "bad" bacteria. That's another clear example of how gut health affects brain health.

An interesting aspect of that study was that simply treating the anxiety disorder through nondietary methods did not cause a corresponding change in the patients' gut bacteria. In other words, while the gut has immense influence on the brain's behavior, the opposite may not be true—treating mental symptoms with antianxiety medication or psychotherapy doesn't mean that the imbalances in your gut will automatically fall in line. In order to address the root of the problem, you have to target the actual bacteria too.

Finally, irregularities in your microbiome can weaken your gut wall, which usually serves as a barrier preventing bacterial metabolites and molecules from entering the bloodstream.[10] Since a weakened gut wall allows bacteria to leak through the gut lining and into the blood circulation (and even into the brain), this is called leaky gut syndrome. While there are certainly compounds that need to travel into and out of our gut, in general we want to keep the bacteria of our microbiome confined there. When bacteria are allowed to escape, they can cause damage all over the body, including in the brain. For instance, we have evidence that a component of the bacterial cell wall called lipopolysaccharide causes anxiety-like behaviors in mice.[11]

Bowel Disorders

Given this constant interaction between your gut and your brain, it's no surprise that there is a strong correlation between anxiety and bowel disorders. Up to 60 percent of patients with anxiety have irritable bowel syndrome (IBS).[12] IBS is a chronic disorder that causes abdominal pain and changes in bowel habits, without any obvious physical cause. Marisol's constipation, for example, was a sign of IBS, but the condition can also manifest as gas, bloating, diarrhea, or all of the above. To make matters worse, the more severe the anxiety, the more severe the IBS.[13] That means when you have a stressor like hosting Thanksgiving dinner, your symptoms are likely to flare up.

IBS patients have brain changes too.[14] Studies have shown that in IBS sufferers, regions of the brain that usually help us attend to our daily tasks, feel emotions, and manage pain do not function as well as they do in most individuals. These brain abnormalities are similar to what we see in patients who have an anxiety disorder, like panic disorder or generalized anxiety disorder. This correlation implies that IBS and these anxiety disorders affect the gut and the brain in similar ways.

Anxiety also occurs more commonly in people with inflammatory bowel disease (IBD), which includes bowel disorders where there is underlying structural damage to the gut, such as ulcerative colitis and Crohn's disease. Up to 40 percent of people suffering from these disorders also have troublesome anxiety.

FOODS THAT INCREASE ANXIETY

Now that we have an understanding of the relationship between the gut and the brain that causes jittery bowel, let's take a look at some ways you can improve your diet to alleviate symptoms of anxiety. First, we're going to focus on foods to keep out of your diet.

The Western Diet

Though it may sound like it's describing whatever cowboys cook over their campfires, the Western diet actually refers to the standard American diet. Though plenty of Americans are as health-conscious as anyone else in the world, the Western diet is what you'd typically find in a fast-food meal—the major components are bad fats (saturated fats, trans fats, and unhealthy PUFAs like the vegetable oil commonly used for deep-frying) and high-GI carbs, which means lots of fried food, sweetened drinks (especially those sweetened with high-fructose corn syrup), and lots of red meat. While there's no question that this diet is bad for your physical health, we'll see its negative influence on mental health throughout this book. Anxiety is no exception.

Many animal studies indicate that high-fat and high-carbohydrate diets promote anxiety. For instance, in 2016, neuroscientist Sophie Dutheil and her colleagues demonstrated that rats on a high-fat diet were more prone to diabetes and anxiety.[15] In 2017, a research group confirmed that diets rich in saturated fats and fructose increase anxiety-like behaviors in rats.[16] And in mice, a lower-calorie diet has been shown to decrease anxiety while improving brain blood flow.[17]

There have been similar findings in humans, with several studies demonstrating that high-carb diets lead to obesity and anxiety.[18] While the exact brain chemistry associating high-fat and high-carb diets with anxiety is quite complex, it's likely that unhealthy diets cause brain serotonin to be reduced in some brain regions, thereby increasing the possibility of anxiety.[19] I don't want to oversimplify, as other genetic and chemical factors certainly play a role in anxiety.[20] Still, it's clear that serotonin levels do play an important role. Perhaps the most valuable takeaway here is that high-fat and high-carb diets can change your brain chemistry, potentially leading to anxiety.

Another reason it's a good idea to avoid the Western diet is that it's a prime culprit in weight gain and eventually obesity. Obesity is associated with being more anxious, with one study finding that obese people have a 25 percent increased chance of suffering from mood and anxiety disorders.[21] The chronic stress of anxiety can also increase visceral fat (fat that is stored in the abdominal cavity and around our organs), type 2 diabetes, and other metabolic complications.[22]

Obesity also leads to bacterial changes in your gut that lead to increased anxiety. In animal studies, obesity itself is not necessarily linked to anxiety—for example, obese mice were not found to be particularly anxious. However, when you give normal-weight mice microbiota from people on a high-fat diet, they become anxious even though they are not obese.[23] That's a strong indicator that the bacterial changes in your gut that come with obesity are responsible for the increased anxiety. Once again, we see how important our daily diet is in terms of taking care of our gut microbiome and hence the gut-brain balance.

While it's certainly a good idea to cut down on fats and

carbohydrates to lose weight if you're suffering from anxiety, it's also important that you don't go too far in the other direction. I've had patients come to see me who are eating very little—800 calories or fewer a day—and report spikes in anxiety. Those who have panic disorder or generalized anxiety disorder can also precipitate severe anxiety when they allow their blood sugar to plunge because they forget to eat.

As for how to structure your diet in order to maintain a healthy weight, I encourage you to follow the same principles we discussed with the Mediterranean eating pattern in chapter 2. When I talk about high-fat and high-carb diets, I don't mean that you have to cut out *all* fats or *all* carbs. As we've already covered, it's important to make sure that you are getting plenty of high-quality monounsaturated fatty acids and polyunsaturated fatty acids (especially omega-3s, which we will examine again shortly); low-GI carbohydrates are fine too. Most important is to use portion control to keep your calorie intake reasonable, and to strictly limit the amount of bad fats (such as trans fats and saturated fats), and high-GI carbs (such as refined flour and sugar).

For an example of how the Western diet can cause anxiety, consider my client Helen. Helen was pregnant, and though she had always been a calm person, during her pregnancy, she started to suffer from panic attacks. All of a sudden, her heart would start racing and she would get short of breath, break out into a sweat, and become so dizzy she'd have to sit down. Understandably, these panic attacks terrified her, even once she'd calmed herself down.

When I inquired about Helen's diet, I learned that prior to her pregnancy she ate cereals for breakfast, salad for lunch, and some kind of fish, chicken, or meat along with a side of vegetables for dinner. On occasion, she would indulge in a burger, pasta, or dessert. Overall, it sounded like an average, relatively healthy diet. But during her pregnancy, she became obsessed with gochujang, a Korean savory-sweet sauce, and kalbi, a kind of grilled fatty beef short ribs.

Now, if you've ever tasted gochujang, you'll understand how one could become obsessed with it. It's like a supercharged Korean ketchup—spicy, sweet, and savory. There's pretty much nothing that you couldn't slather it on. But sadly, that doesn't mean it's good for you. While there are a variety of recipes, the one Helen ate included rice powder, wheat flour, corn syrup, and a heap of sugar, all ingredients that should be avoided in large quantities. When you consider that she often ate this with kalbi, which consists of 71 percent fat, her diet quality was severely compromised.

Helen's poor diet choices were the root cause of her panic attacks, but they were also putting the mental health of her baby at risk. Animal studies teach us that when a mother's diet is high in fat, it can change the child's physiology as well. For instance, in 2012, Daria Peleg-Raibstein and her colleagues reported that rats demonstrated increased anxiety when their mothers were on high-fat diets.[24] In humans, epidemiological studies have shown a link between obesity in the mother and anxiety and other mental woes in the children. The mechanism is thought to be due to inflammation caused by the mother being overweight during pregnancy, which then affects the developing brain of the fetus.

For Helen, who was rapidly gaining weight in excess of what was normal for her pregnancy, major dietary changes were needed. Once we weaned her off gochujang and kalbi and back to a diet focused on vegetables and healthy fats, her panic attacks abated, and her baby was born healthy.

Caffeine

Caffeine can feel like a lifeline in a busy world, but it's important to realize that excess caffeine in your diet can precipitate or worsen anxiety. Caffeine overstimulates regions of the brain that process threat. In 2011 an experimental psychology research study gave fourteen healthy male volunteers either 250 mg of caffeine or placebo capsules.[25] They then examined brain blood flow in different regions as subjects looked at threatening or neutral faces. They found that caffeine activated the midbrain periaqueductal gray matter, a brain region that is typically activated when a predator is closing in on you.[26] To make things worse, caffeine also shuts down a brain region that typically helps you regulate your anxiety.

If you are feeling anxious, you don't need to quit caffeine entirely, but consider cutting down. Just make sure you wean yourself slowly—some of my patients who have suddenly stopped drinking coffee end up in my office with significant panic attacks and anxiety brought on by caffeine withdrawal.

How much caffeine can you drink before it becomes problematic? Most studies show that less than 100 mg of caffeine has little or no effect on anxiety.[27] For between 100 mg and 400 mg/day, the results are mixed; nine studies showed no effect on anxiety, whereas twelve studies have shown significant increases in anxiety. Above 400 mg/day, the majority of studies show a significant increase in anxiety.

Do your best to stay well under that 400 mg/day mark. To put this in context, one Starbucks venti (20 ounces) puts you over the daily limit (475 mg) by itself, so you'll need to stick to smaller sizes. On the other hand, one Nespresso capsule makes 1 ounce of coffee that packs only 50–80 mg of caffeine, so that is a good choice if you like to drink coffee throughout the day without overdosing on caffeine.[28] If you want to cut down on caffeine but still crave the taste of coffee, you can always switch to decaf, though even decaf coffee does contain small amounts of caffeine.

Alcohol

I often encounter people in my practice who live stressful lives. The "work hard, play hard" mind-set often leads to heavy drinking on the weekends as a way to relieve stress. While drinking might make them relax in the moment, they pay for their fun the next morning, when they wake up guilty, jittery, and jumping out of their skin, all symptoms of mild to moderate alcohol withdrawal. Plus, people who are anxious sleep more poorly if they drink alcohol regularly.[29] Add the fact that alcohol—and binge drinking—is one of the leading preventable causes of death in the United States, and it's fair to say that the "relaxation" alcohol provides comes with a significant price.[30]

For sufferers of social anxiety disorder, the cycle can be even more vicious. Those who get anxious in social situations tend to self-medicate with "liquid courage." They may feel like booze helps them socialize, but it can lead to deeper problems—social anxiety more than quadruples the risk of developing an alcohol use disorder.[31]

In general, men who consume more than 14 drinks per week or more than 4 drinks in a single day at least once a month are considered to be heavy drinkers, as are women who drink more than 7 drinks per week or 3 drinks per day.[32] But different people (and their brains) respond differently to alcohol abuse. When I work with anxious patients who drink, I always ask them to consider the contexts in which they might be using alcohol in an unhealthy way—for instance, using drinking as a means of coping with something they are trying to avoid—and to consider moderating the amount they drink. Of course, for patients who show signs of alcoholism, it's important to recognize the heightened anxiety that can come from withdrawing from alcohol. Developing a plan to safely manage the symptoms of alcohol withdrawal is essential and should be done with the help of a psychiatrist or doctor.

Gluten

Rex, age forty-five, was an electrician with a jolly outlook on life. But in the weeks before he first came to see me, he had begun to have panic attacks, especially when he was out in public. Out of the blue, he would get heart palpitations and shortness of breath, and he'd feel like he was going to faint. After I ruled out medical causes of anxiety—like an excess of thyroid hormone and a primary heart condition—I started him on antianxiety medications. Unfortunately, the medication only mildly improved his symptoms.

On one occasion, Rex came to see me directly after the Fourth of July, and I asked him how he had enjoyed the day. He told me that even though he was surrounded by family and friends, he still had flare-ups of his anxiety. When I asked him what he had eaten, he listed sausages, baked beans, and hot dogs with ketchup. His drink of choice was vodka. Upon hearing this, I realized that every one of those foods has gluten in it. I referred him to a gastroenterologist, and within a few weeks, he was diagnosed with celiac disease. He was surprised at the diagnosis since he hadn't had any of the more common bowel symptoms. But celiac disease can be "silent," causing damage with no obvious signs. Once he stopped eating gluten-containing foods, he started feeling better, and within five months, his anxiety had disappeared.

While going gluten-free was absolutely the right choice for Rex, the overall science on anxiety in celiac patients is a little conflicted. In 2011 Donald Smith led a meta-analysis that examined whether people with celiac disease have a higher rate of anxiety than those without it.[33] Researchers found that anxiety is neither more common nor more severe in adults with celiac disease than in healthy adults. However, another study demonstrated that after being on a gluten-free diet for one year, patients with celiac disease were less anxious.[34] And yet another study demonstrated that being on a gluten-free diet is less helpful in reducing anxiety for women with celiac disease than it is for men.[35]

Not everyone with gluten sensitivity has celiac disease, and even among celiac sufferers, the effect on the brain is complex.[36] However, if you're suffering from anxiety, I do recommend getting tested for celiac disease, or even testing yourself by going on a gluten-free diet temporarily to see if it reduces your symptoms. For my patients who have gone gluten-free on a trial basis, the difference in anxiety was obvious quite early, which led them to get more testing.

Artificial Sweeteners

As we saw in chapter 2, when you use artificial sweeteners that have no nutritional value, they can increase "bad" gut bacteria and therefore negatively affect mood and anxiety. Sweeteners like aspartame have been more directly linked with anxiety in research studies and should be avoided, or at the very least used in moderation.[37]

FOODS THAT RELIEVE ANXIETY

Just as there are foods that amplify anxiety, there are also foods that help tamp it down, so make sure to add these to your diet.

Dietary Fiber

In 2018, Andrew Taylor and Hannah Holscher found that diets rich in dietary fiber may reduce the risk of depression, anxiety, and stress.[38] Dietary fiber is a broad category of food ingredients that are nondigestible by our natural gut enzymes. However, though our guts themselves can't break down fiber, different types of gut bacteria can. When dietary fiber can be broken down by bacteria, we call this being "fermentable." Fermentable dietary fiber promotes the growth of "good" gut bacteria. For example, when dietary fiber is broken down into certain smaller sugar molecules, the "good" bacteria *Bifidobacterium* and *Lactobacillus* increase, which has a positive effect on mood by activating brain pathways and nerve signaling that can alleviate anxiety.[39]

Fiber can also assist with anxiety by keeping your weight down through a number of mechanisms. Since fiber-rich foods take longer to chew, you tend to eat them more slowly, which means your body has more time to recognize it's full. Fiber can also fill up your stomach without contributing a lot of calories, which helps you feel more satiated with less food. It also takes a longer time to pass through the stomach and small intestine, which makes you feel full for longer.[40]

Dietary fiber also decreases inflammation throughout the body, including the brain. There is considerable evidence that brain (and body) inflammation is elevated in patients with anxiety.[41] In 2016 Vasiliki Michopoulos and her colleagues found that people with anxiety disorders have elevated levels of certain markers that denote inflammation.[42] Inflammation in the brain has been shown to affect areas that are linked to anxiety (for example, the amygdala), and dietary fiber can help by calming down the brain's and body's inflammatory responses.[43]

You'll find rich dietary fiber in the "five Bs": beans, brown rice, berries, bran, and baked potato with the skin on. If you have bran and fruit for breakfast and brown rice and beans for lunch, then you'll have this covered. The "B" you'll want to eat sparingly is the baked potato—potatoes are high in carbs, and we tend to dress them with high-fat condiments. As we covered earlier, neither a high-carb nor a high-fat diet is good for anxiety.

Other high-fiber foods include pears, apples, bananas, broccoli, Brussels sprouts, carrots, artichokes, almonds, walnuts, amaranth, oats, buckwheat, and pearl barley.

Omega-3s

We talked about the power of omega-3s to combat depression in chapter 2, and they're important in the fight against anxiety as well.

In 2011, Janice Kiecolt-Glaser and her colleagues tested the effects of omega-3s on sixty-nine medical students, measuring their anxiety levels during lower-stress periods and again just before an exam.[44] They found that subjects who were given high levels of omega-3s had 20 percent less anxiety than a control group. What's more, the high-omega-3 group had 14 percent less inflammation in their bodies (as measured by an inflammation marker called interleukin-6).

In 2018, a study found that, specifically, the more omega-3 fatty acid eicosapentaenoic acid people consumed, the less anxiety they had. The study also found that a higher ratio of omega-6s to omega-3s led to increased levels of anxiety. Also in 2018, researchers conducted a meta-analysis of nineteen clinical trials, including 2,240 participants from eleven countries, which showed that omega-3s were associated with a reduction in anxiety symptoms.[45]

In general, the reduction in anxiety caused by omega-3s is thought to occur via anti-inflammatory and neurochemical mechanisms that affect the brain.[46] One potential mechanism for the beneficial effects of omega-3s may occur via the brain's dopamine pathway. When the brain is inflamed, IL-1, an inflammatory marker, can increase dopamine levels in the nucleus accumbens, a collection of brain cells implicated in human anxiety. Studies have shown that omega-3s can suppress this effect in both animals and humans.[47]

I first saw the dramatic effects of omega-3s in a patient named Amber, a twenty-three-year-old woman who suffered from social anxiety, avoiding staff meetings, presentations, and social events. Medications were only partially helpful. For her, simply adding more fish and seafoods rich in omega-3s and switching from vegetable to canola oil to lessen the omega-6 load and balance out the ratio (as we discussed in chapter 2) made all the difference in the world. Within three months of making these changes, her anxiety symptoms improved significantly.

Aged, Fermented, and Cultured Foods

Fermented foods, like plain yogurt with active cultures and kimchi, are a great source of live bacteria that can enhance healthy gut function and decrease anxiety.[48] In the brain, fermented foods may confer several advantages. Fermented foods have improved human cognitive function in several studies.[49] A recent review of forty-five studies indicated that fermented foods might protect the brain in animals, improving memory and slowing cognitive decline.[50] While the mechanism is not yet clear, three potential effects are highly likely: chemical by-products of intestinal bacteria and bioactive peptides may protect the nervous system; the changing gut bacteria might suppress the stress response through the HPA-axis; and neurotransmitters and "brain tissue builders" such as brain-derived neurotrophic factor, gamma-aminobutyric acid, and serotonin may be increased.

In 2015, Matthew Hilimire and his colleagues questioned 710 people about their fermented-food consumption, social anxiety, and neurotic traits.[51] You've probably heard the term "neurotic" used in a number of different ways colloquially, but in medical literature, studies show that neurotic people typically are angrier, more anxious, self-conscious, irritable, emotionally unstable, and depressed than the average person.[52] Neuroticism is regarded as a fundamental trait that people often inherit from their parents. Hilimire's study found that eating fermented food frequently correlated with having fewer symptoms of social anxiety in neurotic patients. Taken together with previous studies, the results suggest that fermented foods that contain probiotics may have a protective effect against social anxiety symptoms for those at higher genetic risk.

Probiotic-rich yogurt can be a powerful part of your diet, but it's important to note that yogurt that undergoes heat treatment does not have the same benefits. One such example is yogurt-covered raisins—these aren't going to help your anxiety, as the heat-treated yogurt has no beneficial bacteria left. Also, you should ensure that the yogurt you consume does not have added sugar. Cereal bars that say "made with real yogurt" may contain only small amounts of yogurt powder and will not help your anxiety.

Going back to Helen, my gochujang- and kalbi-addicted patient, one thing I did tell her was to continue eating kimchi—a delicious kind of fermented Korean cabbage. Kimchi is prepared by fermenting baechu cabbage with lactic acid bacteria. Like kefir and sauerkraut, kimchi is one of those fermented foods associated with less social anxiety.

Other sources of fermented foods include kombucha, miso, tempeh, and apple-cider vinegar. You can also ferment vegetables like carrots, cauliflower, green beans, radishes, and broccoli. You can find recipes for okra pickles and miso-glazed sweet potatoes in chapter 11.

Tryptophan

Even if you think you couldn't name an amino acid to save your life, I'm going to bet you've heard of tryptophan (TRP). Every year as we're digging into Thanksgiving dinner, someone is bound to bring up the idea that the TRP in the turkey is going to lull everyone into a post-meal nap.

To medical researchers, however, tryptophan is more than just a well-worn holiday talking point. Since TRP is a precursor of serotonin, scientists have theorized that a high-tryptophan diet could help raise the low serotonin levels in anxious brains. In animal studies, TRP reaches brain regions that can increase or decrease anxiety.[53] In humans, taking a supplement of purified TRP will increase brain serotonin.[54]

In 2014, Glenda Lindseth and her colleagues conducted a study to test how a high-TRP diet over four days could change the anxiety levels in study participants.[55] Twenty-five healthy individuals were given two diets, with a two-week period in between. The first contained 5 mg/kg of tryptophan (the current US recommended daily allowance) for four days. The second diet contained double that dose for four days. Sure enough, the study found that participants consuming higher levels of tryptophan had significantly less depression, irritability, and anxiety.

Before you dedicate yourself to eating a Thanksgiving meal every day of the year to cure your anxiety, there's a wrinkle: although purified TRP increases brain serotonin, foods containing TRP do not.[56] This is because tryptophan is actually the least abundant amino acid in protein, and it's carried into the brain by a transport system that prioritizes other amino acids. So, after the ingestion of a meal containing protein, tryptophan gets crowded out, keeping it from crossing over into the brain.

If this is the case, how do we explain the findings in the Lindseth study? There is a body of evidence that suggests that eating carbohydrates along with protein can increase the tryptophan available to the brain.[57] When you eat carbohydrates (like the mashed potatoes at Thanksgiving), the body produces insulin. This insulin diverts other amino acids to your muscles but leaves tryptophan untouched. As a result, tryptophan can cruise through into the brain.

Though that sounds logical, some experts question this rationale. So if you're trying to increase tryptophan, you should probably take it in supplement form. One study showed that, after just fifteen days, purified TRP made participants (particularly men) more agreeable and helped them feel better.[58]

While the tryptophan benefits of Thanksgiving dinner may be up for debate, there are other sources of tryptophan that may surprise you. For instance, try chickpeas. Some people refer to chickpeas as the ancestors of Prozac. To ensure tryptophan absorption, chickpeas can be made into hummus and combined with whole wheat pita bread, which provides the carbs. For breakfast or a snack, you could also try my recipe for avocado hummus (page 250) on healthy whole-grain toast.

Vitamin D

Studies have demonstrated that adults with depression and anxiety have lower blood levels of vitamin D. In 2019, Siavash Fazelian and his colleagues tested fifty-one women with diabetes and vitamin D deficiency to see whether taking a vitamin D pill every two weeks would change their anxiety levels.[59] After sixteen weeks, compared to people who took placebo, people who took the vitamin D were significantly less anxious. In another study, when vitamin D was administered as part of a micronutrient intervention to more than eight thousand people who were depressed and anxious, keeping vitamin D levels high was protective against anxiety.

Vitamin D is increasingly recognized as a necessary substance called a neurosteroid, which crosses the blood-brain barrier and enters brain cells.[60] While it's in the brain, it decreases inflammation and toxic destruction of cells and controls the release of nerve growth factor, which is essential for the survival of hippocampal and cortical neurons. The hippocampus plays a crucial role in providing feedback to the HPA-axis when there is stress, and it is also intricately connected to the amygdala.[61] The cortex, too, is involved in how we respond to anxiety and stress. Given that abnormalities in all these brain regions may lead to anxiety, vitamin D has an important role in protecting their tissues.

About 80 percent of our vitamin D comes from exposing our skin to direct sunlight; it's important to remember that sunlight streaming through our windows does not have the same effect, since glass absorbs all ultraviolet B radiation. With indoor lifestyles being so prevalent today, our skin is often left in the dark. As a result, vitamin D deficiency is occurring in epidemic proportions worldwide.[62]

Aside from sun exposure, fortified milk and other products such as egg yolk, salmon, sun-dried mushrooms, and cod liver oil are all rich sources of vitamin D. That means that if you have a strict vegan diet, or suffer from milk allergies, you may be more predisposed to vitamin D deficiency, and you need to be extra-conscientious about getting enough of it in your diet or through sun exposure.

Other Vitamins

Vitamin D isn't the only important vitamin for brain health. In fact, cells would not be able to live or breathe without a broad range of vitamins. These vitamins are an intrinsic part of many chemical reactions necessary for sustaining an energetic life and a good mood. They are essential for the formation and synthesis of neurotransmitters and the metabolism of brain lipids, and they protect the brain from toxins, boost immunity, and regulate many chemicals that make us more or less anxious.[63]

Adam, a thirty-five-year-old patient of mine, was struggling with severe anxiety and binge eating. While he maintained a normal diet during the week, on the weekends, when he would come home intoxicated, he would aggressively binge eat popcorn, cookies, and ice cream. Over time, he developed chronic fatigue, insomnia, nightmares, depression, worsening anxiety, and recurrent headaches accompanied by frequent nausea, vomiting, diarrhea, and abdominal pain. After a full medical workup, we could not find the cause of his symptoms, but his anxious nature together with the binge eating and history of alcohol abuse made me wonder if he might be deficient in thiamine, another name for vitamin B_1. I suggested that he take thiamine more regularly, along with additional therapy. Within six months, despite the occasional alcohol binge, his symptoms improved drastically.

Up to 250 mg of thiamine has been shown to be effective for anxiety.[64] In animal studies, thiamine appears to reduce stress-like responses because it protects the hippocampus.[65]

Other B vitamins have specific antianxiety properties too. In older women and women suffering from premenstrual stress, vitamin B_6 may provide significant relief.[66] And many other studies have demonstrated that vitamin B complex can reduce anxiety, possibly by reducing oxidative stress in the brain.[67]

The positive effects of vitamins on anxiety extend beyond the vitamin B group as well. In 2012, researchers measured the levels of the antioxidant vitamins A, C, and E in the blood of patients with generalized anxiety disorder.[68] They found that levels of all three were low, and after six weeks of supplementation, anxiety symptoms improved. In other studies, multivitamins have been shown to reduce stress and anxiety after twenty-eight days, and in one study, to reduce stress in three hundred people after thirty days of supplementation.[69] A 2013 meta-analysis confirmed the stress-relieving effects of multivitamins.[70]

Given what we know, adding a multivitamin to your daily routine will likely help fight anxiety.

Magnesium

In humans, magnesium deficiency is associated with high anxiety levels. When people are anxious while taking a test, they excrete more magnesium than usual in their urine. And when magnesium levels are low, this can worsen anxiety.[71]

In 2017, Neil Bernard Boyle and his colleagues reviewed the effects of magnesium supplementation on anxiety.[72] They found that magnesium supplementation can help especially if you are vulnerable to anxiety, likely because of the way that magnesium can ease stress responses, changing levels of harmful stress chemicals in the brain.[73]

Dietary intake of magnesium is poor in Western populations. For example, 68 percent of Americans and 72 percent of middle-aged French adults consume inadequate amounts of magnesium in their diets. Foods rich in magnesium include almonds, spinach, cashews, and peanuts. Cooked black beans, edamame, peanut butter, and avocado also have relatively high amounts of magnesium.

Most studies show a difference in levels of anxiety after an intake of magnesium over six to twelve weeks.[74] As an added bonus, magnesium helps muscle cells relax after contracting. When magnesium levels are low, your muscles may contract too much and cause your body to experience muscle cramps, spasms, or tightness.

Nutritional and Herbal Supplements

Certain nutritional and herbal supplements can help you manage anxiety. In 2010, Shaheen Lakhan and Karen F. Vieira explained that there is strong evidence that herbal supplements containing extracts of herbs such as passionflower or kava and combinations of amino acids like L-lysine or L-arginine reduce anxiety.[75] Passionflower increases the neurotransmitter gamma-aminobutyric acid, which in turn decreases anxiety. One of the advantages of passionflower over traditional anxiety medications is that it causes less sedation—a frequent side effect of pharmaceutical treatments.

Passionflower has been shown to specifically reduce anxiety after surgery too.

Forty-five drops of passionflower liquid extract taken daily or a specific tablet formulation of 90 mg/day has been shown to be effective. However, those of you on blood thinner medications (Coumadin or Plavix) or on the type of antidepressants called monoamine oxidase inhibitors (commonly referred to as MAOIs, for example, Nardil or Parnate) should avoid passionflower.

Other foods and nutrients that decrease anxiety include selenium (found in Brazil nuts), potassium-rich foods (e.g., pumpkin seeds), flavonoids (e.g., dark chocolate), and theanine (e.g., green tea).[76] Foods that contain high amounts of lysine such as lean beef and lamb, tempeh, seitan, lentils, black beans, and quinoa can also be helpful. On the other hand, avoid wheat bran since it contains phytic acid, which blocks zinc absorption and causes anxiety.

When it comes to spices that reduce anxiety, the standout is turmeric. The active ingredient in turmeric, curcumin, decreases anxiety and changes the corresponding brain chemistry, protecting the hippocampus. Curcumin's positive effect on anxiety has been confirmed by animal studies and three trials in humans.[77]

Chamomile is an herb that comes from the daisy-like flowers of the Asteraceae plant family. It has been consumed for centuries as a natural remedy for several health conditions, and it has been shown in several studies to help lower anxiety.[78] Though it can be taken in capsule form, I recommend getting chamomile the traditional way, in tea. One to 3 cups a day is generally safe unless you are taking blood thinner medications or are about to have surgery. Pregnant women should consult their doctors before consuming chamomile tea.

Oral lavender oil preparation has also been shown in several studies to lower anxiety.[79] Lavender oil is available as a supplement, but you can also drink lavender tea or even use lavender in aromatherapy. For supplements I suggest consulting with your doctor first.

Lastly, hydration is not something to be ignored when you're anxious. Although we need more evidence to convincingly follow this recommendation, I have had patients who experience worsening of anxiety or even full-blown panic attacks when they are dehydrated and do not realize it. So it's worth staying hydrated for general good health as well as to keep anxiety in check.

CALMING AN ANXIOUS GUT

My patient Marisol worked diligently with me to reshape her diet, focusing on eating foods that could help target her anxiety, while excluding those that worsened it. As an added bonus, the recipes that we developed together were full of nutritious foods, so they were good for her whole family. By lowering her anxiety and improving her sleep, she had the energy to be able to plan her days and weeks with both food and family activities. She loved her children fiercely, and being free of her pervasive worries about them opened up space that allowed her to genuinely enjoy their company rather than being consumed by anxiety. After six months she was eating better, sleeping better, and living a calmer life, no longer waking up with a knot in her stomach.

Even if your anxiety doesn't approach the level of Marisol's, I am confident that following the guidelines we've established in this chapter will help you calm your mind and free yourself from the anxieties of daily life.

ANXIETY CHEAT SHEET

Foods to Embrace:

- High-fiber foods: Beans, brown rice, berries, bran, pears, apples, bananas, broccoli, Brussels sprouts, carrots, artichokes, almonds, walnuts, amaranth, oats, buckwheat, and pearl barley.

- Aged, fermented, and cultured foods: Yogurt, kombucha, miso, tempeh, apple-cider vinegar, and pickled vegetables.
- Tryptophan: Turkey, other meats, and chickpeas, especially when combined with carbohydrates.
- Vitamins D, B_1, B_6, A, C, and E.
- Minerals: Magnesium, potassium, and selenium.
- Spices: Turmeric.
- Herbs: Lavender, passionflower, and chamomile.

Foods to Avoid:

- The components of the Western diet: Foods high in bad fats (red meat, fried foods) and high-GI carbs (white bread, white rice, potatoes, pasta, and anything else made from refined flour).
- Caffeine: Keep caffeine consumption under 400 mg/day.
- Alcohol: For men, stay under 14 drinks per week and no more than 2 drinks in any single day; for women, stay under 7 drinks per week and no more than 1 drink in any single day. By cutting back slowly, you will help lower anxiety.
- Gluten: If you have celiac disease or non-celiac gluten sensitivity, avoid all wheat products, such as bread, pizza, pasta, and many alcoholic drinks.
- Artificial sweeteners: Aspartame is particularly harmful, but also saccharin. Use sucralose and stevia in moderation and with caution.

CHAPTER FOUR

PTSD: Glutamates, Blueberries, and "Old Friends" Bacteria

My patient Letitia worked as a lawyer, protecting the rights of young women who had been domestically abused. Even on the best days, her job was stressful, both from the high-pressure environment of the legal profession and from the emotional weight of helping clients at such a difficult, vulnerable time. But one terrifying day, a gunshot nearly put an end to her journey. She was visiting a client at her house but never made it inside; the client's husband opened the door and was enraged at the sight of her. He pulled out a gun and shot her in the leg.

Thankfully, she was able to make a full physical recovery from the wound, but she still carried the emotional scars from that horrible day. Her work suffered because she could no longer bring herself to visit her clients at their homes. Even when she entered her own office, she lived in fear that a client's partner was lurking, waiting to attack her. Rationally, she knew that this was unlikely, but she was at the mercy of her fear. Despite an initial response to medication, and weekly psychotherapy sessions, Letitia still had residual symptoms, and the memory of that day continued to intrude on her life.

Letitia's story is typical for people who suffer from post-traumatic stress disorder (PTSD). While there is no surefire way to cure PTSD quickly, there are many ways in which a good diet can help improve its symptoms, especially when combined with psychotherapy and medication. Of course, there are also ways in which a bad diet can exacerbate PTSD and make recovery even harder. In this chapter, we'll explore how trauma affects the body and brain and how PTSD sufferers can eat to manage their symptoms and keep themselves firmly on the path to recovery.

TRAUMA AND YOUR GUT

Most of us suffer some kind of trauma in our lives. The death of a loved one, a natural disaster, a sexual assault, or a difficult breakup may all take their toll on our lives. Whether the damage stems from a single event or unfolds over time, traumatized individuals are at risk for PTSD.[1] Thankfully, most people who experience a traumatic event do not go on to develop PTSD.[2] But those who do often have to wrestle with this condition for a long time; although symptoms may subside eventually, in many cases that can take well over a decade.[3] Furthermore, PTSD symptoms do not always materialize immediately. Sometimes, they are suddenly triggered even years after the traumatic event.

PTSD can cause a variety of symptoms, as we saw with Letitia. Some people might experience recurrent memories of the event, for example, or disturbed dreams. Some may even disassociate entirely, flashing back to a time of trauma in a way that feels like reality. They may have an exaggerated startle response, which means they overreact to startling noises with great shock and fear. These symptoms have been shown to be connected with excessive amygdala activation and a lack of activity in the frontal cortex and hippocampus—all parts of the brain that play a crucial role in fear response, trauma processing, and memory. Essentially, the fear and memory circuits of your brain talk to each other in harmful ways, trapping the brain in a cycle of reexperiencing traumatic events.[4]

Traumatic situations naturally trigger the brain's fight-or-flight system via the hypothalamic-pituitary-adrenal axis (HPA-axis), as your instincts help your body determine how best to deal with the stress. Since PTSD causes traumatic moments to resurface again and again, that creates constant disruption in the HPA-axis. As we've learned, the HPA-axis is one of the pathways through which the gut and brain are connected, which means the gut isn't spared from trauma.[5] In fact, of all the psychiatric syndromes we will discuss in this book, PTSD has one of the strongest brain-body relationships, with repeated cycles of trauma adding to the wear and tear on delicate tissues.[6] Physical problems stemming from PTSD range from stomach ulcers to gall bladder diseases and bowel disruption. For example, in 2018, a meta-analysis of eight studies found that people with PTSD have more irritable bowel syndrome than those without it.[7] While these physical symptoms were once dismissed as imagined due to emotions gone awry, research shows a real connection here, which has been very validating for my patients.

Just as we've seen with other psychiatric conditions, a major factor in reversing trauma's effects has to do with making sure that gut bacteria are flourishing and healthy. When you feed a traumatized mouse one of two specific types of normal gut bacteria, *Lactobacillus rhamnosus* or *Bifidobacterium longum*, the mouse becomes calmer.[8] This modification of gut bacteria also changes its brain chemistry. In particular, brain-derived neurotrophic factor and N-methyl-D-aspartate receptor expression improves, allowing these receptors, which govern brain growth and adaptability, to start functioning normally again.

Think of your gut bacteria like a cushion against the harmful effects of trauma. If they are flourishing healthily, they can help your body react appropriately. Without them, stress that is transmitted to the rest of your body is uncontrolled.

PTSD and "Old Friends" Bacteria

In 2018, Sian Hemmings and her colleagues found that the types of gut bacteria in people exposed to trauma were similar whether they developed PTSD or not.[9] However, one subtle difference was that people with PTSD had fewer Actinobacteria, Lentisphaerae, and Verrucomicrobia, three bacteria that have long been considered "old friends" of ours.

The "old friends" hypothesis posits that in past societies, humans lived in a way that promoted certain beneficial bacteria that protected us from inflammatory diseases like allergies and asthma.[10] As our society has urbanized, those friendly bacteria have dwindled significantly due to our loss of interaction with soil, animals, and outdoor environments, leading to a growing epidemic of a wide variety of inflammatory diseases (this basic idea is known as the "hygiene hypothesis").[11] Perhaps the most troubling subset of those diseases is mental health disorders, ranging from developmental disorders such as autism and schizophrenia to stress-related disorders like anxiety and PTSD.

In the absence of "old friends" bacteria, inflammation can get out of control, compromising our brains and leaving us more vulnerable to PTSD. Furthermore, PTSD itself may cause greater brain inflammation, which only deepens the cycle of destruction.[12] For instance, even six months after a motor-vehicle accident, children and adolescents who developed PTSD had elevated levels of interleukin-6 and cortisol, both of which are indicators of the body's excessive inflammatory response. In other words, when you feel emotional pain, your brain has to rally. But too much rallying causes inflammation, which can hurt your brain even more.

Even though they're not as plentiful as they once were, the three "old friends" bacteria are an important part of controlling your brain's rallying processes. In their absence, your brain has to deal with recovering from emotional pain on its own, and it all becomes too much.

In addition to limiting inflammation in the brain, these "old friends" bacteria act as gatekeepers in the gut wall.[13] But when stress knocks them out, the gut-brain barrier is no longer as effective, and a host of chemical changes result (as we saw with "leaky gut" in chapter 3). Depression, anxiety, and PTSD are three possible consequences, depending on an individual's vulnerability.

Much of that vulnerability is determined by what you do and do not eat. In the rest of the chapter, we will explore foods that worsen PTSD and your reaction to trauma, and those that help fortify your gut and brain against their effects.

FOODS THAT DEEPEN TRAUMA

For an example of how not to eat if you have PTSD, let's go back to my patient Letitia. The first time she came to see me, I had a strong hunch that she wasn't eating well for her condition. When I took a dietary history, I noticed that she was a newly diagnosed diabetic. Much like many other working mothers with busy lives, she had little time to cook for herself. She often ate out, and her top choice was Chick-fil-A. At least three times a week, dinner was a quick Chick-fil-A Deluxe Sandwich, a large order of fries, and a 20-ounce diet soda.

Although the Chick-fil-A Deluxe Sandwich is 500 calories, 41 percent of that is fat, and 34 percent is carbohydrate. Only a quarter is protein. The large fries add another 460 calories, of which more than 90 percent are fat and carbs. Add that up, and you're talking about roughly 1,000 calories in one meal—about double what is recommended, especially if you're diabetic.

Letitia knew that her dinner choices were not the healthiest, but she had trouble weaning herself off a routine that was convenient and felt satisfying in the moment. Whether she was conscious of it or not, I suspected that her PTSD was also contributing to her poor diet. When you don't have trauma to deal with, you have enough brain capacity to take the time to make healthy choices. But a brain that is under fire from fear and painful memories has an entirely different agenda. All it wants is a little break. Fast foods and soda can act as a form of self-soothing, providing comfort in an almost automatic reaction that is difficult to stop.

Since there was no way Letitia was going to cut out Chick-fil-A entirely, I recommended that she switch to the Grilled Chicken Sandwich, which has 300 calories, only 17 percent of which are fat. I also suggested that she consume fewer than five fries, just for the taste, and then wean herself off entirely. Although the 20-ounce diet soda sounded harmless, it had more than 100 mg of caffeine in it. As we learned in chapter 3, caffeine can worsen anxiety, so I suggested that she either downsize to the 12-ounce or try sparkling water instead. Again, I had her wean herself off the soda slowly so that she did not precipitate caffeine withdrawal, which might make her anxiety worse.

Letitia followed this plan, fully embracing the idea that she needed to change her dietary habits. She began to buy rotisserie chicken seasoned only with salt and pepper, which she adapted into various meals for her family. For example, she might serve half a rotisserie chicken with a side of steamed broccoli or sliced chicken breast atop a healthy and tasty green salad with almonds, adding segments of clementine, which her children loved. If she had any chicken left over she took it for lunch in a lettuce wrap. Using a store-bought but healthily prepared chicken was a transition to eventually cooking more at home, eliminating unhealthy fats and eating good carbs such as those in raw or steamed veggies.

Just months later, Letitia noticed a significant reduction in anxiety symptoms. After several months she felt calmer, no longer waking up at night with sweats and fear. As a result, she felt rested in the morning. Between her new diet and a steady flow of talk therapy with her regular therapist, over about six months she was able to get back to her important work at full efficiency, no longer paralyzed by the trauma she experienced.

High-Fat Diets

You'll probably recognize Letitia's Chick-fil-A habit as having two major aspects of the Western diet we discussed in chapter 3—high fat and high-glycemic-index (high-GI) carbohydrates. The Western diet is particularly destructive to PTSD patients, so let's first consider the effects of the abundance of fat (as always, when I talk about high-fat diets, I mean diets high in unhealthy fats like saturated fat, trans fats, and fats used in fried food, rather than healthy fats such as omega-3s or those found in olive oil).

When animals consume a typical Western high-fat diet, it makes them more susceptible to PTSD. In 2016, Priya Kalyan-Masih and her colleagues demonstrated this by first modeling "trauma" in mice by exposing them to the odor of cats.[14] They fed one group of mice a Western high-fat diet while the control group was fed a lower-fat diet. One week later, the mice that consumed the high-fat diet were much more anxious than the control group. And the hippocampus was significantly smaller in the high-fat group. Since research has shown that the hippocampus is already shrunken in brains suffering from PTSD, this study shows that high-fat diets further complicate symptoms.[15] In its shrunken state, the hippocampus is less effective at managing stress hormones and the brain's response to fear. Similar associations between high-fat diets and PTSD have been demonstrated in other animal studies.[16]

In human studies, it is clear that PTSD affects metabolism in a way that promotes overeating and obesity.[17] For instance, a whopping 84 percent of US male Vietnam War veterans are overweight or obese, a much higher rate than in the general population.[18] I have seen this firsthand in my work with veterans and their families. In 2017, I had the privilege of consulting with a hospital program that works directly with veterans. I developed a culinary program for them that included live cooking classes based on easy and healthy recipes to encourage home cooking. (Some of the recipes I wrote, tested, and taught for those classes, like Baked Salmon with Walnut Kale Pesto, Chocolate-Dipped Strawberries, and Oven-Roasted Miso-Glazed Sweet Potatoes, are shared in chapter 11.)

John Violanti is a researcher who specializes in police stress (and was a New York State trooper for twenty-three years himself). In 2006, he and his colleagues did a study looking at the incidence of metabolic syndrome in police officers.[19] Metabolic syndrome is a cluster of conditions that occur together, increasing your risk of heart disease, stroke, and type 2 diabetes. These conditions include increased blood pressure, high blood sugar, excess body fat around the waist, abnormal cholesterol or triglyceride levels, and obesity. The results of the study showed that officers with severe PTSD had almost three times the rate of metabolic syndrome as those with milder forms of PTSD. In a similar study in 2007, Victor Vieweg and his colleagues found that male military veterans with PTSD had a higher body mass index (BMI) than those without PTSD, often reaching the obesity range.[20]

In 2016, Erika Wolf and her colleagues examined this PTSD–metabolic syndrome connection to determine how it affected the brain.[21] Wolf's team evaluated the brain structure of 346 US military veterans who had been deployed to Iraq or Afghanistan. Specifically, they examined whether the thickness of the brain's outer layer, the cortex, correlated with PTSD symptoms and/or metabolic syndrome. When they examined the data, they found that people with metabolic syndrome had thinner cortices and that PTSD conferred an additional risk for this.

So if you have PTSD, you are at risk for metabolic syndrome and premature brain aging. A high-fat diet might ease your symptoms in the short term, but it will only worsen your health problems. In my work with war veterans, I have felt a sense of surrender from these patients, as if the trauma of war had weakened their will to live. Not only were they tortured by their flashbacks and anxiety, but some let their bodies go as well. Others were struggling with the side effects of psychiatric medications—such as weight gain. On the one hand, I didn't like recommending that they cut down on the foods that comforted them. Why take away the one source of comfort they had? On the other hand, eating a high-fat diet amounts to self-sabotage, damaging your brain in multiple ways.

The best way for PTSD sufferers to improve their diet is to think about comfort foods as a taste addiction that they simply have to beat in order to feel less anxious and preserve their brains. When I work with PTSD patients, I tell them to think of the fat in their diets as brain sludge, gumming up all the delicate folds and crevices of their precious gray matter. This image is usually vivid enough to help them cut down on fats.

Sugar and High-GI Carbs

Sugar and high-GI carbs are also destructive to the traumatized brain. In 2010, Bettina Nowotny and her colleagues examined the effect of acute psychological stress on glucose metabolism in fifteen overweight Bosnian war refugees with PTSD.[22] They found that acute stress increased cortisol and blood glucose after a meal. This was consistent with another study that demonstrated that women with PTSD had twice the risk of type 2 diabetes compared to women without PTSD.[23] And twin studies have confirmed that PTSD could be a marker of vulnerability to type 2 diabetes.[24] In fact, the association between PTSD and obesity is so common, researchers are beginning to think that PTSD is a metabolic disorder like diabetes. That's likely why it's not uncommon to see patients like Letitia who have both diabetes and PTSD.

Given this propensity for diabetes in PTSD patients, it stands to reason that drinking soda and other high-sugar beverages is problematic. Unfortunately, in 2011, Jacqueline Hirth and her colleagues found that among a sample of 3,181 women, those with PTSD were more likely to consume more than 1 serving of soda per day.[25]

High blood sugar affects the ability of the hippocampus to react to stress.[26] As a result, when people are dealing with trauma, eating sugary foods may compromise the brain's ability to deal with that stress. But as we learned in chapter 2, sweet foods aren't the only ones that can spike blood sugar. High-GI carbohydrates, like potatoes, white bread, and white rice, can have a similar effect. Foods with a low glycemic index (low GI) can help prevent sudden spikes in blood sugar. It's important to know which foods increase blood glucose more than others. For example, a banana increases blood glucose more than an apple, which has the same amount of carbohydrates. And a boiled sweet potato increases blood glucose more than a boiled carrot.

But while knowing the glycemic index of individual foods is a good first step, food is combined in meals and, when combined, can affect glucose levels differently. For instance, in 2019, Jiyoung Kim and her colleagues found that although rice is a high-GI food, when it is eaten as part of a mixed meal with egg, sesame oil, and bean sprouts, the different components of the meal result in the rice having a lower GI index than it would in an unmixed meal with the same amount of carbohydrate. This is especially important for cultures that rely on carbohydrates like rice as a staple.

I saw this concept in action in Kushal, a patient of mine who was a Sri Lankan doctor suffering from PTSD. In 2004, a deadly tsunami swept through the southern coast of Sri Lanka as a result of the Indian Ocean earthquake, killing close to thirty thousand people. After that disaster, Kushal moved to Boston and came to see me for a number of symptoms. The slightest rumble of any kind would send him spiraling into a panic. He insisted on staying as far away from the ocean as he could, which disrupted his life with his family.

As a doctor, Kushal was familiar with PTSD, but he had had limited success with medications and psychotherapy. When he came to see me, I took a full dietary history, and I could see how distraught he was from trying to follow a Mediterranean-style diet. I asked him why he was staying away from traditional Sri Lankan food, and he said he was trying to avoid rice because of the connection between PTSD and diabetes. Sri Lankan food can be intense and spicy, and he couldn't enjoy it without rice. I admired how committed he was to changing his diet, but it clearly wasn't working for him.

When I talked to him about how mixed meals can alter the GI of individual foods, he started to cheer up. I explained that you can reduce the GI of foods like rice by adding foods rich in dietary fiber, or by adding vinegar or bean or dairy products.[27] In fact, one study found that you can reduce the GI of white rice by 20–40 percent in this way.[28]

Relieved, he went home and prepared his favorite Sri Lankan rice dish. He also began to use brown rice. On some days he made my recipe for cauliflower rice (page 268), which added more vegetables to his diet. You can't imagine his delight when he next visited me. He had gone back to eating his traditional food a few times a week, and he was astounded by how it relieved his anxiety and PTSD over time. In addition after three years of follow-up appointments, he had no sign of diabetes or other metabolic syndrome, and his weight has remained stable.

While it's hard to know the GI for every meal combination, I hope you see why it's not sufficient to simply tally up the GI of individual foods. Of course, even in a mixed meal, you still have to watch your carbohydrate intake and make healthy choices. But Kushal's story is an important reminder that food genuinely is an important source of comfort, especially in people who have suffered from trauma. As long as you make an effort to understand how it affects your body and brain, consider your individual sensitivities, and eat unhealthy foods only in moderation, finding ways to integrate your favorite foods into your diet will ultimately have a positive effect.

Glutamates

Glutamate has been used to enhance the flavor of food for more than twelve hundred years.[29] It imparts a unique taste known as umami. Though umami is not as instantly recognizable as sweetness, sourness, bitterness, or saltiness, it is the fifth basic taste that our tongues have the capacity to perceive. Though glutamates naturally occur in many foods, the most common way to impart an umami flavor in a dish is to cook with the additive monosodium glutamate (MSG).

There has been considerable controversy over the years about whether MSG is toxic or not. However, that matter is considered close to settled in modern nutrition circles: extensive scientific studies have demonstrated that MSG is safe at ordinary levels, and some studies show that it may even promote digestion and metabolism of food in the gut.[30] Ten grams of MSG for an average adult does not increase glutamate levels. As a result, many experts believe that the MSG dangers are all hype.[31]

However, in sensitive individuals, MSG may cause problems including brain toxicity. PTSD patients are particularly likely to be vulnerable to excess glutamates, leading to increased brain inflammation and the destruction of brain cells.[32] Glutamate is an excitatory neurotransmitter, which means that it generates an electrical impulse in nerve cells. If you have too many of these impulses, the connection between nerve cells can be disrupted. This disruption is especially prominent in the hippocampus and medial prefrontal cortex, regions that help modulate the stress response.

In 2019, Elizabeth Brandley and her colleagues reported on how a low-glutamate diet may impact PTSD.[33] They studied Gulf War veterans with PTSD and gave half of them a low-glutamate diet while the other half ate normally. Preliminary analyses indicated that the low-glutamate diet was effective in reducing anxiety and symptoms of PTSD.

Foods that contain MSG and other glutamates include fish sauce, oyster sauce, tomato sauce, miso, Parmesan cheese, savory snacks, chips, ready-to-eat meals, mushrooms, and spinach. Glutamic acid, a precursor of glutamate that has similar effects, is also found in seaweed, cheeses, soy sauce, fermented beans, tomatoes, and high-protein foods like meats and seafood. (Be aware that many high-glutamate foods also contain the amino acid tyramine, which can interfere with MAOI antidepressants. See chapter 9 for more details.)

You shouldn't assume that all these foods will definitely worsen symptoms, but sufferers of PTSD would be wise to eliminate some of them to see if there is any improvement. Even if you're not suffering from the effects of trauma, while it's not necessary to cut out glutamates entirely, follow the Goldilocks principle: not too much, not too little, but just enough.

SOOTHING FOODS

Thankfully, dietary treatments for trauma aren't all about food that should be left out of your diet. Let's consider foods that might help traumatized brains get back to normal function.

Blueberries

In 2016, Philip Ebenezer and his colleagues examined the anti-inflammatory effects of blueberries in rats with inflammation and free-radical damage in the prefrontal cortex and hippocampus due to PTSD.[34] One group of rats was given a blueberry-enriched diet, while the control group ate a regular, blueberry-free diet. The study found that a blueberry-enriched diet increased serotonin levels in the brain and reduced free radicals and inflammation.

A closer look at the findings in a series of studies done by the same group revealed that the anti-inflammatory effects of blueberries may be even more dramatic than we think, with important implications for human mental health. The PTSD-induced rats in the study showed very low expression of the gene *SKA2*. That same gene also has low expression in humans who commit suicide. While we can't question rats about suicidal feelings, it seems likely that the similarity isn't coincidental. Remarkably, when the investigators had the rats eat a blueberry-rich diet each day, *SKA2* levels increased in the blood and brain compared to the rats on a normal diet.

In other words, blueberries may impact the downregulation of genes. We need more studies in humans to be sure, but it can't hurt to add more blueberries to your diet. They are delicious and healthy in many ways. I'd suggest adding ½ cup to 1 cup per day. Frozen blueberries are just as good as fresh as long as they don't have added sugars, juice, or preservatives.

Omega-3 Fatty Acids

We've already seen a few ways in which omega-3s can be good for mental health, and PTSD is no exception. Multiple studies have shown the efficacy of omega-3s in fighting PTSD: in 2019, Laiali Alquraan and her colleagues found that omega-3s protected the brains, particularly the hippocampus, of rats with PTSD.[35] In a randomized controlled trial of fish oil in rescue workers after the Great East Japan Earthquake, omega-3s also decreased PTSD symptoms.[36] In 2013, Yutaka Matsuoka and his colleagues examined three hundred people who had suffered from PTSD after a motor vehicle accident to see if blood levels of omega-3s correlated with PTSD symptoms.[37] Once again it was found that the higher the levels of omega-3s, the lower the levels of PTSD.

I saw the power of omega-3s to fight PTSD in my patient Leslie. When I first met Leslie, I didn't know she was suffering from PTSD, only that her anxiety was at an all-time high. She worked as a sous-chef in a busy hotel kitchen. If you've ever worked in a kitchen like this, you know how noisy they can be. Pots and pans sizzle, and there is a cacophony of communication among staff. Dishes are plonked on the tables, and glasses come crashing down. Working in that environment was becoming untenable for Leslie; the noise was unbearable, and sudden noises made her jump out of her skin.

As we talked, I realized that there was more going on than just job stress. She broke into tears as she recounted being sexually abused by her father between the ages of eight and thirteen. Although she was able to escape him when she went to college, she had never confronted him or told anyone except her therapist about her trauma. She began to soothe her anxiety by eating more and making poor food choices, which led to weight gain. Several times a week, she had flashbacks and nightmares, making it difficult to sleep at night. This, in turn, made it almost impossible to go to work the next day. While medications and therapy had been helpful, she was still struggling.

Leslie's story was heartbreaking, but sadly childhood sexual abuse is more common than most people realize.[38] Worldwide, 8–31 percent of girls and 3–17 percent of boys are sexually abused, and victims often end up suffering from PTSD.

When I took a dietary history from Leslie, she described herself as a "meat and potatoes gal." She rarely ate fish because she had a strong aversion to its smell. This posed a real challenge because I knew that she needed omega-3s, and as we've already learned, fish are the richest source of them.

I recommended plant oils such as flaxseed, canola, and soybean oils. I told her that a key type of omega-3 called alpha-linolenic acid could be obtained from plants like edamame, walnuts, chia seeds, and radish seeds, though you won't find other omega-3s such as eicosapentaenoic acid or docosahexaenoic acid in these sources. I encouraged her to switch to grass-fed beef, which has higher levels of omega-3s (though no beef is a great source of them). I also pointed her toward foods that are fortified with omega-3s, like egg, milks, and yogurt.

When looking to bolster your omega-3s, general rules of thumb to remember are:

- Eat fish, especially farmed, fatty fish from reliable sources.
- If you eat beef, use grass-fed beef.
- If you're vegetarian, use organic canola oil and seek out foods fortified with omega-3s.

Vitamin E

In chapter 2, I introduced you to the damage that free radicals can inflict on your brain, causing oxidative stress. Free radicals may arise from normal physiological processes, stress, or inflammation, but they may also arise when you are exposed to X-rays, ozone, cigarette smoke, air pollutants, or industrial chemicals. Just think about that for a second. Every time you expose yourself to stress, it can damage the cells in your body the same way that powerful environmental pollutants can. Chronic PTSD means your brain is constantly stressed and therefore flooded with free radicals.[39]

Vitamin E is part of the body's defense system against free radicals. In 2019, Camila Pasquini de Souza and her colleagues found that vitamin E turned down the anxiety levels in mice with PTSD significantly, likely by mopping up free radicals.[40] We've also seen encouraging results in human trials. Many studies of patients who have brain trauma show that vitamin E can help to prevent further brain damage.[41] That feels like a strong reason to recommend vitamin E to those struggling with PTSD.

Just 1 tablespoon of wheat germ oil a day will give you your total vitamin E requirement. Other sources of vitamin E include sunflower seeds, dry-roasted almonds, hazelnuts, peanut butter, spinach, broccoli, and raw tomatoes.

Spices and Natural Supplements

Ginkgo biloba is a natural product that comes from a tree of the same name. One of its important effects is preventing cell damage by free radicals.[42] Because of that, it can protect the brain in much the same way as vitamin E.

A study by Jamal Shams and his colleagues reported on findings from a twelve-week trial that compared ginkgo biloba to placebo in people who met the criteria for PTSD after experiencing a magnitude 6.3 earthquake in Bam City, Iran.[43] They found that 200 mg of ginkgo biloba was more effective than placebo for reducing anxiety, depression, and symptoms of PTSD. Since there is no way to get the active chemical of ginkgo biloba in regular food, you'll have to take it as a supplement, with your doctor's approval. It's available at pharmacies and health food stores.

It may also be helpful to incorporate our old friend turmeric into your diet to get the benefits of its active ingredient, curcumin. When rats consume curcumin, they form fewer fear-based memories and activate fewer of those memories.[44] While no curcumin studies have been done in humans with PTSD yet, given all the benefits we've already explored, it's worth a try.

Don't forget a pinch of black pepper in dishes with turmeric, since as discussed earlier pepper activates it.

OVERCOMING TRAUMA ONE MEAL AT A TIME

It is always fulfilling to help patients in my clinic improve their diets to strengthen their mental health, but that's particularly true with patients like Letitia, Kushal, and Leslie, who have overcome such devastating personal trauma. It is truly an inspiration to see their resilience in the face of hardship, and it's an honor to play a role in their journey to heal their brains and souls. I hope that this chapter helps you understand the crucial role that food plays in that journey, and that you can apply these same principles to recovering from traumas you may have suffered.

The human brain is remarkable in its ability to recover from painful experiences, but don't forget to give it the tools it needs to build itself back up—a healthy diet and a helping hand from the trusty gut.

PTSD CHEAT SHEET

Foods to Embrace:

- Blueberries: ½–1 cup per day.
- Omega-3 fatty acids: Fish, especially fatty fish like salmon, mackerel, tuna, herring, and sardines.
- Vitamin E.
- Spices: Turmeric.
- Supplements: Ginkgo biloba.

Foods to Avoid:

- The components of the Western diet: Foods high in bad fats (red meat, fried foods) and high-GI carbs (white bread, white rice, potatoes, pasta, and anything else made from refined flour).
- Sugar: Baked goods, candy, soda, or anything sweetened with sugar or high-fructose corn syrup.
- MSG, other glutamates, and glutamic acid: Fish sauce, oyster sauce, tomato sauce, miso, Parmesan cheese, savory snacks, chips, ready-to-eat meals, mushrooms, spinach, seaweed, cheeses, soy sauce, fermented beans, tomatoes, and high-protein foods like meats and seafood. You have seen in earlier chapters that some of these foods also have positive impacts. It is all about working out a personalized nutrition plan.

CHAPTER FIVE

ADHD: Gluten, Milk Caseins, and Polyphenols

Sanjay was a thirty-year-old computer programmer who was referred to me because of debilitating worry and panic attacks. He was constantly getting into trouble at work. He had missed several deadlines, and when he was asked about his performance, he was too terrified to say that he was struggling mentally. As a result, he often skipped work entirely, but of course his absenteeism just made the situation worse. His team leaders chalked his issues up to laziness and questioned his ability to perform his duties. He was at risk of losing his job.

Medications helped his anxiety somewhat, but he still found himself procrastinating whenever he had a task to complete. As I talked to him about his problems with work and life, I began to suspect that Sanjay was suffering from attention deficit hyperactivity disorder (ADHD). In fact, as we delved into his history, it seemed likely that he had been suffering from symptoms of the condition since high school, but his teachers and peers had written off his struggles as stubbornness, insubordination, or, worse, lack of intelligence.

Starting him on a stimulant medication (Ritalin) and making

several changes to his diet eventually saved his job and maybe even his life. He stopped drinking alcohol impulsively, he felt less depressed and anxious, and the world started to feel manageable again. He began eating whole foods instead of junk food, processed fast foods, and soda. He could focus on tasks at work and became a valuable member of the team. Most of all, he was relieved that people no longer thought of him as "dumb."

Stories like Sanjay's are not uncommon. We live in an age where our attention is constantly under attack. Notifications dinging on our phones, the endless chatter of social media, and the barrage of information at work and in our personal lives make it difficult to stay focused. Having email on your phone also means that your work world has access to you 24/7. All of this can make for a frustrating day, even for people with perfectly healthy brains. When you have to deal with these daily distractions while suffering from ADHD, you can feel overwhelmed and isolated.

The core features of ADHD include difficulty paying attention, hyperactivity, and impulsivity, but patients present in a variety of ways.[1] For some, learning is a particular challenge, whereas for others, unstable mood, anxiety, and oppositional behavior are the primary symptoms.[2] ADHD is an increasingly common condition—one in twenty-five people have the diagnosis. Usually it begins in childhood (though it can begin later too), but it often persists for years—65 percent of people with childhood-onset ADHD have symptoms that last into adulthood.[3] As we have seen with Sanjay, ADHD can compromise your ability to function at work, at home, and in your social life.[4]

Although ADHD may be addressed through medication or psychotherapy, it is often highly resistant to treatment.[5] For this reason, dietary interventions can be helpful alongside other treatments. In this chapter, we will examine ADHD, take a look at the gut-brain interactions, and consider foods that may help or hurt.

One thing that distinguishes ADHD from the other conditions

we are studying is that it is quite often diagnosed in children. While I see plenty of adult ADHD patients like Sanjay, ADHD can certainly take hold early on and cause many challenges for children who suffer from it. The same is true for two closely related conditions: sensory processing disorder and autism spectrum disorder. Part of the reason I'm able to share this book with you is my clinical experience with adult patients. Though some of the studies cited in this chapter were performed on children, since I am not a child psychiatrist, I won't delve into childhood ADHD or these other conditions specifically in this book. Still, the benefits of eating a whole, healthy diet apply to both children and adults.

ADHD AND YOUR GUT

When you have ADHD, the connections between different brain regions are disrupted, specifically between the prefrontal cortex, the "thinking" brain, and the striatum, the part of the brain that deals with reward behaviors. Additionally, your brain chemistry is affected, particularly your levels of dopamine, the brain's "reward" chemical, and noradrenaline, a fight-or-flight hormone.[6]

Although medications used to improve ADHD symptoms generally increase the levels of dopamine and noradrenaline, we are learning that treating ADHD isn't as simple as boosting the levels of these chemicals, as other brain chemicals such as gamma-aminobutyric acid and serotonin are also involved. While a full explanation of how brain chemistry impacts ADHD is beyond the scope of this book, it's clear that attention is regulated by a delicate balance of factors.

So, if ADHD is caused by chemical imbalances in your brain, what role does your gut play? Larger molecules such as dopamine and noradrenaline cannot cross the blood-brain barrier, which means that they are confined solely to your brain. But they are made of precursor molecules—building blocks—that can. And where are these precursor molecules made? You guessed it: the gut.

Gut bacteria play an important role in ADHD, synthesizing many of these chemical precursors.[7] Different bacterial species in the gut produce different chemicals, which means that if gut bacteria change, the brain's chemical stability can be upset.[8] And as we've seen with other conditions, a reduction in the diversity of gut bacteria can be particularly problematic.[9]

In 2017, Esther Aarts and her colleagues examined the differences in the microbiome between patients with ADHD and healthy individuals.[10] Compared to controls, people with ADHD had more bacteria that made phenylalanine, a building block necessary for dopamine and noradrenaline synthesis.

The investigators then looked at how the brains of each group responded to reward. Decreased anticipation of brain reward is a hallmark of ADHD—in other words, studies show that people with ADHD aren't motivated as strongly by incentives to behave in a certain way.[11] Sure enough, the researchers found that the ADHD subjects showed less brain activation in response to being rewarded. Furthermore, the less their brains responded to the reward, the more phenylalanine-producing bacteria were present in their guts. The researchers concluded that ADHD subjects had to make more bacteria that produce phenylalanine to compensate for how their brains responded.

That's a highly simplified view of how chemical and bacterial mechanisms interact, but it gives you an idea of the important scientific research being done with respect to ADHD. In fact, even in this major study, the investigators recognized that the only sure conclusion they could draw was simply that gut "disturbances" correlate with brain "disturbances."

In addition to the serious neurological symptoms, ADHD can come with physical symptoms as well. In 2018, another research study found an increase in two gastrointestinal symptoms—constipation and flatulence—in children with ADHD when compared to control subjects.[12] Yet again, this study correlated the gastrointestinal dysfunction in ADHD with changes in the microbiome.

Fighting ADHD takes a combination of proper medications and a proper diet. Let's talk about some foods that harm and hinder patients who are striving to restore their focus.

FOODS THAT WORSEN ADHD

I recently evaluated a twenty-year-old college senior, Suzy. Suzy was a bright and hardworking student. However, even though she was conscientious and generally cheery, her grades began to fall during her senior year, and she started to feel depressed. She also constantly had an upset stomach, which she had just accepted as a way of life. She'd had an ADHD diagnosis since she was younger, but while Ritalin had helped her focus on her work in the past, the effect seemed to be dwindling as she built up a tolerance.

Suzy assumed that the cause of her troubles was that her dorm had become too distracting, but she also admitted that there had been no significant changes in her living environment since her more successful semesters. I noted that her diet seemed to have shifted toward more comfort food. She told me that her standard breakfast was instant oatmeal with milk. Lunch frequently included bread and pasta. She snacked on cubes of cheese throughout the day, and she had pizza for dinner at least three times a week.

It doesn't take a nutritionist to see that she was eating a lot of dairy and gluten, and it's no coincidence that both of these dietary components can exacerbate the symptoms of ADHD.

Gluten

Just as we saw in chapter 3 on anxiety, there is also a well-established link between ADHD and gluten intolerance or celiac disease. In 2006, Helmut Niederhofer and Klaus Pittschieler assessed a sample of people across a broad age range to test the association between ADHD and celiac disease.[13] The participants' ADHD symptoms were measured before they started a gluten-free diet and six months after. The study found that people who had celiac disease were more likely to have ADHD, and a gluten-free diet improved their symptoms after the initial six-month period.

Suzy's celiac test came back negative, but you don't have to have celiac disease to be sensitive to gluten. This condition is called non-celiac gluten sensitivity.[14] While the association between non-celiac gluten sensitivity and ADHD is by no means conclusive, various studies point to a connection between the two. In some instances, as we saw in chapter 3 with my "silent celiac" patient Rex, gluten sensitivity may cause neurologic and psychiatric symptoms without any corresponding digestive symptoms.[15] People typically associate gluten sensitivity with digestive issues, so in the absence of upset stomach or bowel symptoms, gluten isn't on the radar as a factor that can worsen ADHD.

The exact reason that gluten sensitivity and brain dysfunction are connected is not fully understood. In 2005, Päivi A. Pynnönen and her colleagues assessed adolescents with celiac disease and behavioral problems.[16] They found that adolescent celiac disease patients had significantly lower tryptophan concentrations in their blood.

Three months after patients started a gluten-free diet, the researchers found a significant decrease in patients' psychiatric symptoms compared to their baseline condition, coinciding with significantly decreased celiac disease activity and prolactin levels and with a significant increase in L-tyrosine, L-tryptophan, and other amino acids known to be precursors of brain chemicals such as serotonin. The authors concluded that it was possible that behavioral problems, such as those that occur with ADHD, may in part be due to certain important precursor amino acids not being available until people stopped eating gluten. In certain individuals, gluten-free diets can help the body increase levels of the precursors to make serotonin, which is one neurotransmitter involved in ADHD.

I encouraged Suzy to go on a gluten-free diet, and she quickly saw benefits. Most of the gluten Suzy was eating came from bread, pizza, and pasta, but it can also be found in a huge range of processed foods and alcohol. Thanks to an increase in awareness of gluten-free diets, there is a wealth of options for eating gluten-free, and it wasn't difficult for Suzy to cut out gluten without cutting out her favorite foods. After kicking her gluten habit, Suzy was able to get her senior year back on track and graduate as expected.

Dairy

Suzy's diet was also high in dairy. Eating a lot of dairy means you eat a lot of casein, which may worsen ADHD.[17] Casein is the main protein found in dairy products such as milk, cheese, yogurt, and ice cream, but it can be a factor even in foods that are thought of as dairy substitutes, like nondairy creamer and margarine.

Not all casein is the same. The main form is called beta-casein, of which there are two major types, A1 and A2. Most regular milk contains both types, but research suggests that A1 proteins may be harmful to the gut in ways that A2 proteins are not.

In 2016, a team led by Sun Jianqin studied forty-five participants who consumed milk containing both A1 and A2 milk proteins, and then milk containing only A2 protein.[18] The researchers found that when subjects drank milk containing A1 protein, they had more gastrointestinal inflammation, their thinking was slower, and they made more errors on an information-processing test. It was as if the A1 protein muddied their thinking, something that ADHD patients can ill afford. The study even suggested that lactose intolerance may be caused by sensitivity to A1 caseins rather than lactose itself.

Although more research is under way about whether A1 milk causes any adverse effects except occasional digestive problems, it's clear that sufferers of ADHD should be cautious about the kind of casein they consume.[19]

Luckily there is milk available that only has A2 proteins. Milk from breeds of cows that originated in Northern Europe is generally high in A1 protein. These breeds include Holstein, Friesian,

Ayrshire, and British shorthorn. Milk that is high in A2 protein is mainly found in breeds that originated in the Channel Islands and southern France. These include Guernsey, Jersey, Charolais, and Limousin cows.[20] Of course, it's not often practical to choose what kind of cows your milk comes from! However, there are now A2-only milks available in many grocery stores and online.

While it's great to have A2 protein milk available, since much of the dairy we consume is in the form of cheese, yogurt, butter, and prepared foods, cutting out A1 caseins still requires significant dietary changes. It's worth noting that sheep's and goats' milk is generally A2 milk, which makes cheese and yogurt choices a bit easier. You can also try nut milks and milk nut yogurts as a way to avoid casein.

Sugar

You've probably heard that sugar makes people (especially children) "hyper." That's created a common perception that sugar causes or triggers ADHD. It's true that sugar can have an effect on ADHD through several pathways. For instance, because it can increase adrenaline, a hormone that increases heartbeat and blood sugar levels, sugar may cause more hyperactivity.[21] And because it reduces dopamine sensitivity in the brain, sugar can amplify impulsive reward-seeking behavior that is common in ADHD.[22] Still, while many parents and teachers swear by limiting kids' sugar intake to improve their behavior, recent research indicates that the idea that sugar causes ADHD is a misperception.

In 2019, Bianca Del-Ponte and her colleagues investigated whether high sugar intake was associated with ADHD in a study of children between the ages of six and eleven years old.[23] Through interviews and diet monitoring, the researchers were able to calculate the actual sucrose consumption of all the children in the study. Trained interviewers collected data on whether children met the criteria for ADHD or not.

Although they found that high sucrose consumption was more

common in six-year-old boys with ADHD compared to those without ADHD, this effect was not seen in children of other ages in either gender. Changing sucrose consumption between six and eleven years of age also did not affect the incidence of ADHD in boys or girls. Overall, the researchers concluded that sugar consumption does not lead to ADHD. If there is any correlation, children with ADHD may simply consume more sugar.

Although there are other studies that have demonstrated that sugar consumption (especially sugar-sweetened beverages)[24] is associated with ADHD, a large majority of recent studies back up the idea that sugar does not cause ADHD.

Still, while the evidence of sugar's role in hyperactivity may not be as damning as popular perception would indicate, sugar is never good for mental or physical health, so I always recommend that ADHD patients of all ages limit how much they eat.

Food Colorings, Additives, and the Few Foods Diet

The earliest research on the effect of food on ADHD can be traced back forty years, when pediatric allergist Benjamin Feingold hypothesized that both artificial food additives (colorings and flavors) and foods rich in salicylates might make children more inattentive and restless.

Salicylates are chemicals found naturally in some fruits, vegetables, coffee, tea, nuts, spices, and honey. They are synthesized for use in medications like aspirin, Pepto-Bismol, and other products.

In 1976 Feingold formulated a diet that eliminated food additives and salicylates, which would come to be known as the Feingold diet.[25] Some people refer to it as the Kaiser Permanente diet. It was popular in its early days, though the effects were poorly understood. The studies by Dr. Feingold were followed by other studies investigating the effects of eliminating artificial food coloring and eventually led to a diet eliminating many foods and additives, called the few foods diet. This diet is essentially an elimination diet, a category of diets pioneered in 1926 by food allergy specialist Albert Rowe and still in use today.[26] In this approach, you remove one potentially offending food at a time and carefully record any changes in symptoms, before adding foods back in one at a time.

In 1983, a meta-analysis found that the effect of the Feingold diet on ADHD was actually quite weak, casting doubt on the efficacy of elimination diets in improving ADHD in general.[27] However, in 2004, another meta-analysis of only the higher-quality studies demonstrated that eliminating food colorings seemed to make a difference in parents' observations of children with ADHD, but not in teachers' or other caretakers' observations.[28]

Just as in our discussion of sugar, this gives us another example of how parents' conceptions of triggers for ADHD don't always agree with studies. While it is possible that parents may make erroneous associations and have strong biases, I don't believe that we can just throw out parents' findings.

A 2012 meta-analysis by Joel Nigg and his colleagues and a 2017 meta-analysis by Lidy Pelsser demonstrated that a restriction diet that eliminated food-coloring additives benefited some children with ADHD, determining that between 10 and 30 percent of people with ADHD would likely respond.[29]

While none of these elimination diets are ironclad ways to eradicate ADHD, they are still worth considering if symptoms don't respond to less drastic dietary measures.

FOODS FOR FOCUS

Preliminary research indicates that certain foods may improve the symptoms of ADHD. Before diving into specific nutrients, it's worth noting that research has shown that overall diet intervention has been effective at staving off ADHD—in other words, it's important to eat healthily over a broad spectrum of food.[30] For example, several studies have shown that ADHD responds well to the Mediterranean eating pattern, which we discussed in chapter 2. In 2017, Alejandra Ríos-Hernández and her colleagues studied 120 children and adolescents and found that those who did not stick to the Mediterranean diet were more likely to have ADHD.[31] Other studies have confirmed that low adherence to the Mediterranean diet is associated with ADHD.[32]

Beyond the Mediterranean diet, there are several specific foods and nutrients that can help fight ADHD.

Breakfast

Breakfast is an important meal for all of my patients, so that they are adequately fueled to jump-start their brains (and bodies) every morning. But for ADHD patients, stimulants can take a toll on appetite, so being hungry in the morning may not be a given.[33] My patients often find that creating a routine around breakfast can be helpful.

In 2017, David O. Kennedy and his colleagues explored what morning nutrients could be helpful for ADHD sufferers.[34] They compared the cognition of ninety-five people after they ate a noncommercial nutrient-enriched breakfast bar made for this study (containing alpha-linolenic acid, L-tyrosine, L-theanine, vitamins, minerals, and 21.5 mg of caffeine) versus a control bar for fifty-six days. Then they examined how cognitive function differed before eating the bars and at 40 and 160 minutes after eating the bars. They found that in all tests, people who ate the nutrient-enriched bars were more alert and attentive, and they could process information more rapidly.

It's unclear which specific nutrients in the test bars helped, and of course, you won't be able to find breakfast bars that are exactly the same as those used in the study, since they were specially formulated. And since commercially available breakfast bars tend to be packed with sugar and refined carbs, a better way to start the day when you can't eat whole foods is to make a smoothie. The

Chocolate Protein Smoothie on page 261 is designed to give you nutrients similar to those in the bars used in the study to give your morning the right boost to fight ADHD.

Caffeine

One notable factor in the breakfast bar study discussed in the previous section was the caffeine. In animals, caffeine has been shown to have beneficial effects on attention and memory, and a 2011 study demonstrated that tea might be an effective treatment for adult ADHD.[35] Presumably, the caffeine in tea increases people's motivation, alertness, vigilance, efficiency, concentration, and cognitive performance. On the other hand, caffeine may cause overexcitability too, so it's important not to overdo it.[36]

As we discussed in the anxiety chapter (chapter 3), the amount of caffeine that you consume matters. Again, our guideline is no more than 400 mg of caffeine per day for adults. I do not recommend giving children caffeine, even if it could be beneficial—it's just too hard to determine a safe dose for their smaller bodies.

Polyphenols

In 2018, Annelies Verlaet and her colleagues found that natural antioxidants like dietary polyphenols could be useful in combating ADHD, helping to alleviate oxidative stress on the brain.[37]

Studies have shown that people with ADHD are at a greater risk of oxidative stress in brain tissue.[38] This can lead to damaged brain cells and altered neurotransmitter levels (like dopamine) and electrical-signal transmission, which can make ADHD worse. Since ADHD sufferers appear to lack some of the natural ability to fight off oxidative stress, it is particularly important for them to get as many antioxidants as possible through food in order to alleviate their symptoms and prevent brain cell damage.

One crucial type of antioxidant is polyphenols. Polyphenols are chemical weight lifters for the body's immune response. They act as low-dose toxins that train the body to mount an immune response in a process called hormesis. Polyphenols can also exert other biological effects that are helpful to the brain; for example, they influence the survival and regeneration of neurons.

The richest sources of polyphenols are berries, cherries, eggplant, onions, kale, coffee, and green tea.

Dietary Micronutrients

Some animal and human studies have indicated that when there is a deficiency of zinc, hyperactivity may occur.[39] Indeed, zinc deficiencies are associated with ADHD in children, in part because its absence reduces the activity of reward pathways that rely on dopamine.[40]

Other studies have shown that children with ADHD have lower levels of iron and magnesium than controls, both of which are involved in dopamine synthesis.[41]

In 2017, Jin Young Kim and her colleagues studied 318 healthy children to see if their diets impacted their cognition. They used the Symbol Digit Modalities Test (SDMT), a test of speed of information processing, to see which dietary elements were beneficial.[42] They found that the consumption of vitamin C, potassium, vitamin B_1, and nuts all increased performance on the SDMT. In addition, the more mushrooms people ate, the better they were able to reason, while noodles and fast food decreased SDMT scores.

A FOCUS ON FOOD

It's clear that being able to focus is incredibly important to success, whether you're a kindergartner developing the skills to read and reason and socialize, a college student like Suzy studying for exams and writing papers, or an adult like Sanjay who is struggling to succeed at a fast-paced, high-pressure job. While ADHD drugs like Ritalin and Adderall can be godsends for those who really need them, they don't come without risks. They can be habit-forming and easily abused.[43]

If you struggle with mild ADHD symptoms, I encourage you to alter your diet in the ways we've talked about to see if your mind becomes clearer through strengthening the natural pathways between your brain and your gut. And even if medication is right for you, know that these dietary principles will work alongside your other treatments to clear and calm your mind.

ADHD CHEAT SHEET

As with depression, the Mediterranean eating pattern is a great overall diet to follow for improving ADHD symptoms.

Foods to Embrace:

- Breakfast: It's important for ADHD sufferers to get the day started right, so try starting with a smoothie like the one on page 261.
- Caffeine: While caffeine can be beneficial to ADHD, keep consumption under 400 mg/day.
- Polyphenols: Berries, cherries, eggplant, onions, kale, coffee, and green tea.
- Vitamins C and B_1.
- Minerals: Zinc, iron, potassium, and magnesium.

Foods to Avoid:

- Gluten: If you have celiac disease or non-celiac gluten sensitivity, avoid all wheat products, such as bread, pizza, pasta, and many alcoholic drinks.

- Dairy, specifically A1 milk caseins: Drink and cook with products made from A2 milk, nut milk, or goat's or sheep's milk.
- Sugar: While sugar is unfairly vilified as a cause of ADHD, it's still best to limit intake; avoid baked goods, candy, soda, or anything sweetened with sugar or high-fructose corn syrup.
- Food colorings and additives: Colorings and additives can be eliminated by following diets such as the Feingold diet or the few foods diet if ADHD symptoms don't respond to less radical diet changes.

CHAPTER SIX

Dementia and Brain Fog: Microgreens, Rosemary, and the MIND Diet

More than twenty years ago, I met Brian, a wildly brilliant sixty-year-old professor who came to see me about his anxiety. It was both exciting and a little daunting for a young psychiatrist to treat a mind that had been deemed a possible Nobel laureate in medicine, but we developed a good rapport over the course of our weekly meetings, and I came to look forward to each appointment.

It was in March, as he was struggling with anxiety about preparing his taxes, when I first noticed that he seemed to be fading away. The effect was subtle; it wasn't as if he just came in one day without the ability to remember. But slowly, week after week, I saw an ever-so-slightly vacant look on his face, a tremor so subtle that I couldn't tell if it came from having too much coffee, and slips of the tongue so minor that I would have ignored them had I not noticed the other signs. At first, I wrote the symptoms off as stress, but eventually, this triad of vacancy, tremor, and oddities in speech raised my suspicion that something was amiss.

I referred him for a thorough neurological examination, which included detailed tests of his memory and attention. The results showed that he was in the early stages of Parkinson's disease. Parkinson's is known for causing physical tremors, but it is often accompanied by dementia as well, and given the decline I'd seen in him, I feared the worst. The news was devastating for him, for me, and for the world.

Parkinson's has no cure, which meant we had only symptomatic treatments in our arsenal. I desperately searched the nutritional literature for possible diet and lifestyle alterations we might try. At that time, the field of nutritional psychiatry was in its infancy—in fact, the term "nutritional psychiatry" didn't even exist yet—and there was not much to turn to. We were stuck.

Brian succumbed to complications of Parkinson's disease some ten years later, and, sadly, for eight of those ten years, his memory was almost totally gone. After the initial slow fade, he lost both his long-term memory and the ability to form new short-term memories.

Had I known then what I know now, I would have been much more aggressive with nutritional recommendations. We don't have a nutritional cure for dementia today, but there are now many studies that indicate different ways in which food may play a significant role in preventing or slowing cognitive decline. In this chapter, I will explain how our food choices can help us preserve our memories, and how they can clear our minds from the brain fog that sometimes disrupts the clarity of our daily lives.

Dementia comes in many forms. For example, vascular dementias occur due to blockages in blood vessels that stop blood from feeding brain tissue. Frontotemporal dementias are a general group of regional brain abnormalities that cause memory loss. Others, like Alzheimer's disease, are less well understood. Even though we see distinct abnormalities in Alzheimer's brains—most notably buildups of protein among nerve cells called amyloid plaques that disrupt nerve-cell function—we still do not fully understand the mechanics of the disease or the best ways to treat it.

While these conditions all stem from different parts of the brain and different causes, food can have a profound effect on all of them. As with all the other conditions we've discussed so far, understanding why starts with understanding the gut-brain connection.

YOUR GUT AND MEMORY

As we saw with anxiety, it's not difficult to feel the connection between your gut and your memory. If you see an old partner who cheated on you, you might instantly become nauseous. If you drive down a street where you ate a delicious meal, you may start to salivate and your stomach might grumble. Given that your gut "remembers," it should come as no surprise that it works hand in hand with your brain's memory systems. The key to that connection lies in the chemicals that make your brain and body function, many of which are regulated by your gut.

For example, the stress hormone cortisol can disrupt your ability to recall long-term memories, and as we've covered before, your gut bacteria affect blood cortisol levels by regulating the hypothalamic-pituitary-adrenal axis.[1] That means that the wrong balance of gut bacteria can lead to a spike in cortisol, which in turn can put a damper on your ability to recall memories.

Memory is also affected by levels of other neurochemicals, such as noradrenaline, serotonin, and dopamine.[2] For instance, we now know that noradrenaline enhances memory, especially when emotions are running high.[3] And studies have identified a close association between a serotonin-dopamine imbalance and changes in brain tissue that lead to learning and memory impairment. Once again, all these neurochemicals are dependent upon gut bacteria to produce the necessary precursors to keep them at healthy levels.

The vagus nerve can enhance memory when stimulated because it connects to brain structures like the amygdala and hippocampus, which are central to memory formation.[4] Since gut bacteria can change vagus nerve activation, that's another way in which they affect your memory.[5]

The most telling sign that there is a strong connection between the gut and memory is that the composition of gut bacteria changes in patients afflicted with several memory-related diseases. For instance, in Parkinson's disease patients like Brian, there is a significant decrease—77.6 percent—of the specific gut bacterium Prevotellaceae compared to controls.[6] And the microbiomes of Alzheimer's patients have decreased Firmicutes, increased Bacteroidetes, and decreased *Bifidobacterium*.

Sometimes the relationship can run the other way, with changes in gut bacteria altering the course of these diseases. Rosacea is known primarily as a skin condition in which people blush or flush more easily, but rosacea patients also have a slightly increased risk of developing dementia, particularly Alzheimer's disease.[7] Changing gut bacteria can make a huge difference for rosacea patients. In 2009, Andrea Parodi and colleagues demonstrated that when you eradicate small-intestine bacterial overgrowth common in rosacea, the skin condition goes away.[8] This microbiome-based treatment can last up to nine months, and with the rosacea in remission, the risk of dementia is likely reduced.

Researchers also believe that gut bacteria trigger metabolic processes and brain inflammation that impact memory,[9] and they may also compromise blood flow in the brain. In addition, changes in gut bacteria may increase amyloid deposits, thereby contributing to Alzheimer's disease.[10] Modification of the gut microbiome by diet or by using probiotics may offer new preventive and possible therapeutic options for Alzheimer's.

All this evidence points to the idea that we may be able to reduce the possibility of dementia by avoiding foods that compromise our gut bacteria and eating foods that enhance them.

FOODS THAT WEAKEN MEMORY

In order to understand which foods are helpful or detrimental to memory, it's important to note that there are many different memory systems in the brain. For example, procedural memory systems help us to learn tasks such as playing the piano, typing, or playing golf. Relational memory includes remembering facts and events such as a new acquaintance's name or facts about the world. Working memory is short-term memory that we need to remember phone numbers or directions for how to get somewhere we've never been.

With all that in mind, let's look at how different foods and diets can harm or help these different kinds of memory.

The Western Diet

Once more we see the destructive effects of the Western diet.[11] High-fat and high-glycemic-index (high-GI) foods can alter brain pathways necessary for learning and memory, with neurons in the hippocampus and prefrontal cortex especially affected.[12]

The hippocampus is the part of the brain most involved in forming relational memories. Fascinatingly, hippocampal size actually changes when you practice remembering. For example, the hippocampus is bigger in London taxi drivers, who have to memorize extensive and complicated routes through the streets of London.[13] However, when diets high in fats and sugar damage the hippocampus, it tends to shrink, which impedes memory. Furthermore, the hippocampus is responsible for regulating how much food we eat. Damage to this region makes portion control more difficult, which in turn can lead to overeating, creating a cycle that can be hard to break.[14]

High-fat and high-GI diets can affect the hippocampus in a variety of ways. First, the Western diet can hamper the expression of critical growth factors like brain-derived neurotrophic factor and other hormones that promote healthy function in the hippocampus.[15]

Second, poor diets can affect insulin signaling and insulin sensitivity in the body's tissues. It's unclear exactly what insulin's role is in the hippocampus, but studies have indicated that it likely impacts memory. One recent study showed that high saturated fat intake in male rats interfered with insulin signaling in the hippocampus, which led to interference with hippocampal function and corresponding relational memory abilities.[16]

Third, a diet high in saturated fat and refined sugar in male rats showed increased oxidative stress, which damages brain cells and reduces the efficacy of cell-to-cell communication in the hippocampus.[17]

Looking beyond the hippocampus and relational memory, a study from 2019 showed that obesity caused by a poor diet can lead to changes in cognitive control and the function of the prefrontal cortex and its impact on working memory as well.[18]

In addition to these direct effects on the brain, the Western diet compromises the blood-brain barrier, which is tasked with keeping toxic substances out of the brain.[19]

Dietary components such as saturated fat may also exacerbate inflammation in the brain, which has been linked to cognitive decline in aging and risk of developing Alzheimer's disease.[20] Inflammation disrupts many of the chemical pathways instrumental in memory formation, such as those that rely on dopamine and glutamate.[21] The nerves themselves become sluggish and information travels far more slowly.

There is also some indication that high-fat diets have different effects at different ages. Chloé Boitard and her colleagues demonstrated that while juvenile exposure to a high-fat diet decreases memory and brain growth in mice, the same effects were not observed in adult mice.[22] Human studies, however, indicate that high fat consumption is detrimental to memory in adults as well.[23] It's worth noting that the developing brain in children and adolescents is particularly sensitive, which means we should be extra-vigilant about the foods they are eating.

Thankfully, it appears that the damage done by a high-fat diet can be undone. In 2016, Boitard and her team found that in adolescent rats, these brain changes are reversible by switching from the high-fat, high-sugar diet to a more standard and well-balanced diet. And in 2019, Paul Loprinzi and his colleagues found that in seventeen studies, sustained exercise in rodents reduced high-fat-diet memory impairment.[24] So, cutting back on bad fat, bad carbs, and sugar; eating a healthy, whole-foods diet; and exercising regularly are likely to help reverse the damage and enhance your brain's ability to remember.

Gluten

Several types of dementia are associated with celiac disease and non-celiac gluten sensitivity.[25] When patients have celiac disease, they often report sudden, intermittent memory difficulties as well as problems recalling words.[26] Some patients may develop a more severe form of dementia, with symptoms such as confusion and an inability to calculate simple math.

Though some studies show that avoiding gluten will heal the gut lining and restore memory, there is also evidence that once dementia sets in, the damage is done even if you avoid gluten thereafter.[27] So, if you are planning to cut out gluten, do it sooner rather than later. You can also remove it from your diet and see how you feel and if your thinking is clearer and sharper. In my work, the clinical feedback I get from my patients is an important factor that helps guide their personalized nutritional strategies.

PROTECTING MEMORY THROUGH DIET

The idea that certain foods can enhance your memory goes back centuries. Think of Ophelia in *Hamlet* saying, "There's rosemary, that's for remembrance." Let's explore how modern science has shown that eating—and, in fact, eating a little less—can aid in memory and fight dementia.

Calorie Restriction

In a certain sense, all foods can contribute to memory loss. That's not because of any specific nutrients, but because eating more calories overall seems to have a negative effect on memory. In 2009, Veronica Witte and her colleagues demonstrated that restricting calories by 35 percent improved memory in healthy elderly patients after three months.[28] While the exact mechanisms underlying the memory benefits of calorie restriction are unknown, in this study, memory improvements correlated with decreases in insulin and the inflammatory marker C-reactive protein. In other studies, low insulin and high inflammation have been correlated with better cognition.

The benefits of calorie restriction may extend to people who have Alzheimer's disease. In mouse models, eating fewer calories resulted in less brain amyloid, and other studies have shown that individual brain cells are protected too.[29]

It's not just the elderly who can benefit. In 2019, Emilie Leclerc and her colleagues conducted a clinical trial in which they compared working memory in healthy middle-aged adults who restricted their calorie intake by 25 percent over two years with others who ate whatever they wanted.[30] After twelve months and up to two years later, there was a significant improvement in working memory in calorie-restricted individuals compared to people in the other group. At the end of the study, the improvement in memory was shown to correlate most strongly with lower protein intake compared to other macronutrients. In other words, eating too much protein was correlated with memory loss.

If you plan to cut down significantly on your calories, it is important that you work with your doctor to explore healthy ways to do so. A few studies have demonstrated that dieting to lose weight can actually worsen memory, possibly because dieters obsessively focus on their food and weight, which takes up brain space necessary for memory.[31] But if you work with your doctor to formulate a responsible plan to reduce your total calorie intake by about 25 percent, your memory may improve.

Soy

Soy products are often mentioned as being good for memory and cognition, but the reality isn't quite that simple. First of all, it's important to define what soy products we're talking about. There is a huge range of soy products, and they each have different effects on the brain. Although all "soy" products come from soybeans, soy sauce, tofu, fermented tofu, miso, tempeh, and soy isolates are all different foods with different tastes and different nutritional profiles.

Isoflavones are a type of phytoestrogen, a plant-derived compound that mimics the activity of the human hormone estrogen (more on estrogen in chapter 10).[32] Soybeans and soy products are the richest source of isoflavones in the human diet, but they are also found in beans, chickpeas, split peas, peanuts, walnuts, and sunflower seeds. A 2015 meta-analysis of ten placebo-controlled randomized clinical trials involving 1,024 participants found that soy isoflavones favorably affected cognitive function and visual memory in postmenopausal women.[33]

Not all studies of isoflavones have been in agreement about their benefits. One theory for conflicting results is that people metabolize soy differently.[34] In regard to isoflavone metabolism, only about 25 percent of non-Asians and 50 percent of Asians host the intestinal bacteria that can metabolize isoflavones at all, meaning that any positive or negative effects are lost on much of the population.[35]

Fresh soybeans, generally known as edamame when eaten whole, contain thiamine and may help cognition in people with Alzheimer's disease. Soybeans have other micronutrients that can improve memory, for instance, phosphatidylserine, a lipid that is abundant in the brain. When soy-derived phosphatidylserine is consumed it improves cognitive function relative to placebo.

While the effects of various soy products are population- and individual-specific, there is enough evidence to recommend eating them in moderation. Certainly, fresh edamame is a healthy snack and offers you brain-boosting thiamine. Of course, you should consult with your doctor if you have any concerns.

Alcohol

In 2018, Karina Fischer and her colleagues examined a broad range of single foods, exploring whether there are universally applicable patterns of foods that are protective against Alzheimer's disease and memory decline.[36] They looked at the effect on memory of red wine, white wine, coffee, green tea, olive oil, fresh fish, fruits and vegetables, red meat, and sausages. They found that only red wine had an impact—at least in men. For women, drinking red or white wine increased their risk of memory decline.

However, in 2019, Jürgen Rehm and his colleagues reviewed twenty-eight studies on the connection between alcohol use and dementia performed between 2000 and 2017.[37] Overall, Rehm found that light to moderate alcohol use in middle to late adulthood was associated with a decreased risk of cognitive impairment and dementia. However, heavy alcohol use increased the risk of all types of cognitive impairment and dementia.

Archana Singh-Manoux and his colleagues followed 9,087 people over twenty-three years to see how alcohol related to the incidence of dementia. In 2018 in the *British Medical Journal*,[38] they reported that people who had abstained from alcohol completely or who consumed more than 14 drinks per week had a higher risk of dementia compared to those who drank alcohol in moderation.

Though international recommendations for alcohol use vary widely, according to the Centers for Disease Control, light alcohol use refers to fewer than 3 drinks per week. Moderate alcohol use refers to more than 3 but fewer than 14 drinks per week for men and fewer than 7 drinks per week for women. Heavy alcohol use refers to more than 14 drinks per week for men and more than 7 drinks per week for women. However, given the findings of the studies mentioned here, for maximum memory protection I recommend staying between light drinking and moderate drinking guidelines. For my patients, that means roughly 3 drinks per week for women and 5 drinks per week for men.

Of course, alcohol can have many negative health effects as well, so drinking according to either the CDC's recommendations or the guidelines I suggest only makes sense after talking to your primary care physician about other risk factors.

Coffee

In 2017, Boukje van Gelder and her colleagues reported on 676 elderly men they had studied over ten years to see if coffee protected them from cognitive decline.[39] They found that men who drank coffee had less cognitive decline than those who didn't. The greatest effect was seen in those who drank 3 cups of coffee a day, with those who drank more or less seeing less dramatic effects.

In 2009, Marjo Eskelinen and her colleagues reported on a group of people they had followed over twenty-one years to see if coffee helped cognition.[40] They found that coffee drinkers at midlife had a lower risk of dementia and Alzheimer's disease later in life compared with those who drank no coffee or up to 2 cups per day. The lowest risk of dementia was found in people who drank 3–5 cups of coffee per day.

There are a number of ways in which coffee might protect the brain.[41] Caffeine, which increases serotonin and acetylcholine, may stimulate the brain and help stabilize the blood-brain barrier. The polyphenols in coffee may prevent tissue damage by free radicals as well as brain blood vessel blockage. Trigonelline, a substance found in high concentration in coffee beans, may also activate antioxidants, thereby protecting brain blood vessels.

However, not every substance in coffee is helpful. Unfiltered coffee contains natural oils called diterpenes, which increase LDL cholesterol levels, potentially resulting in thickening and hardening of the walls of the arteries in the brain (though they do have some helpful anti-inflammatory properties).[42] Acrylamide, a chemical formed when coffee beans are roasted, can inhibit neurotransmission, destroy dopamine neurons, and increase oxidative stress. The amount of acrylamide in coffee can vary; dark-roasted, fresh coffee beans generally have the lowest amount.

The wide range of chemicals in coffee is probably why current researchers do not believe that the protective effect of coffee against dementia is conclusive enough to make a formal recommendation.[43] However, know that there are more good effects than bad of moderate coffee consumption (about 2–4 cups per day) and that it could have benefits later in life. Remember to keep your overall caffeine consumption under 400 mg/day.

Olive Oil

Many animal and laboratory studies have found that extra-virgin olive oil (EVOO) protects cognition. Olive oil is a source of at least thirty phenolic compounds, such as oleuropein, oleocanthal, hydroxytyrosol, and tyrosol, all of which act as strong antioxidants and brain protectors.

EVOO also enhances the extraction of polyphenols and carotenoids from vegetables. In 2019, José Fernando Rinaldi de Alvarenga and his colleagues examined the effects of EVOO using the *sofrito* technique.[44] The technique's name may sound exotic, but pretty much every culture has its version of it—while ingredients vary among cultures, it's simply sautéeing vegetables (often onion and garlic, and sometimes bell peppers, tomatoes, or chilies) in EVOO. *Sofrito* is used as a starter for many different dishes because of the savory depth of flavor it adds. The researchers found that when you use this technique with EVOO, brain-protective polyphenols such as naringenin, ferulic acid, and quercetin migrate from the other ingredients into the EVOO.

While not every study agrees on olive oil's cognitive benefits, given that it is a great source of healthy fats, I recommend using it, especially in a *sofrito* preparation as part of the MIND diet, which we will discuss at the end of the chapter.

Spices

Marina, age sixty, visited my office during a struggle with memory loss. After doing a battery of neuropsychological and brain-imaging tests, we found that her memory and brain were objectively healthy. However, on detailed psychological inquiry, I learned she was suffering from long-standing depression, which she had previously attributed to merely feeling "blah" as she aged.

People who suffer from depression can appear to be suffering from dementia, a condition we call pseudodementia.[45] Unlike "real" dementia, when you treat the depression, the memory problems go away. While Marina did recover, the shock of feeling like she was losing her memory prompted her to ask about preventive factors for dementia. Naturally, I was happy to talk to her about nutrition.

Marina already followed a diet similar to the Mediterranean diet, and she had no interest in following the MIND diet we will discuss shortly. My suggestion was to use spices that have been shown to improve memory function.

Turmeric, pepper, cinnamon, saffron, rosemary, ginger, and many other spices have been shown to enhance memory. While most of these need more research to definitively establish their benefits, many controlled studies and plentiful anecdotal evidence indicate that they are worth trying. After all, they have little downside, and they can amp up the flavors in your cooking without adding calories. For Marina, introducing new spices into her diet was a welcome change, and after just six months she reported that she felt sharper and that her mind felt refreshed. Try the following spices to improve your memory.

Turmeric: Once again, turmeric and its active ingredient, curcumin, are front and center. Curcumin has antioxidant, anti-inflammatory, and neurotrophic activities. In fact, one recent review of thirty-two animal and laboratory studies showed that it can reverse some brain damage caused by Alzheimer's.[46] A 2019 review of curcumin studies also showed improvement in attention, overall cognition, and memory.[47]

The effective dose of curcumin is not clear, partly because when you consume curcumin, very little of it is absorbed into the blood. However, as we've seen, black pepper may help curcumin absorption (and in fact, black pepper may improve cognition on its own; see the following text).[48] Curcumin is also made more available to your body through cooking. This all adds up to interesting recipes for dishes like Spicy Shrimp—sautéed with turmeric and black pepper—which you can find on page 276.

Turmeric is also used in Indian curries, which may confer some of their own protective effects. A 2006 study on the relationship between curry consumption and cognitive function in the elderly found that elderly participants who "often" (once a month or more) or even "occasionally" (once or more in six months) consumed curry had superior cognitive function compared to those who "rarely" (less than once in six months) consumed curry.[49] Scientists have also reported the incidence of Alzheimer's disease for people aged seventy to seventy-nine to be four times lower in India than in the United States.[50]

It's very difficult to eat too much curcumin, so feel free to use up to 4 teaspoons daily. In addition to cooking with turmeric, you can add a teaspoon or two to a soup or a smoothie. Golden Milk made with turmeric (page 280) is also a delicious and soothing treat.

Black pepper and cinnamon: When winter arrives and you have to be outside in the cold for a long time, studies show that low temperatures can impair your cognition. But black pepper and cinnamon are two spices that can reverse this decline in thinking ability.[51]

Besides suppressing inflammatory pathways, these spices may act as antioxidants; increase the availability of acetylcholine, which improves memory; and help clear amyloid deposits, which as we've seen is an important factor in Alzheimer's disease.

Saffron: In 2010 Shahin Akhondzadeh and his colleagues tested whether saffron could impact cognition.[52] They administered either 15 mg capsules of saffron or a placebo twice daily to people with mild to moderate Alzheimer's disease. After sixteen weeks, saffron produced a significantly better outcome on cognitive function than placebo.

Rosemary: One of my favorite things to do is to pluck fresh rosemary and then run my index finger and thumb down the woody stem so that the leaves drop off. The aroma is intoxicating. It's a boost to the senses, and I feel sharper and calmer all at once.

It turns out that this is not just about my personal love for the scent. One study indicated that the aroma of rosemary changes brain waves so that people become less anxious, more alert, and better able to compute math problems.[53]

In 2012, Mark Moss and Lorraine Oliver examined the effect of rosemary on cognitive function.[54] They asked twenty people to sit in cubicles that were infused with the scent of a rosemary essential oil and gave them a number of tests of thinking ability, including arithmetic and pattern recognition. Higher levels of the scent correlated with better attention and executive function (the ability to retain information, be flexible with it, and organize it). In an earlier study, Moss had found that rosemary improved working memory too.[55]

Rosemary, like coffee, contains diterpenes. While we already discussed some downsides to diterpenes, they are anti-inflammatory and can protect cells from oxidative death. Rosemary can also boost acetylcholine, which is instrumental in memory.

While we need more studies to have full confirmation, at this point you can assume that rosemary will help boost memory, attention, and well-being. Try using rosemary with roasted vegetables, oven-baked potatoes, or a roast chicken dinner, or even add it to spice up some nuts. (Add a little olive oil to help the rosemary stick to these foods.)

Ginger: Ginger has also been shown to enhance working memory in middle-aged healthy women.[56] In animals, it has increased the levels of adrenaline, noradrenaline, dopamine, and serotonin contents in the cerebral cortex and hippocampus, so it is possible that it works through these brain chemicals to enhance memory in key parts of the brain.

In rats with Alzheimer's-type disease, gingerroot has also been shown to improve memory. This effect is currently being investigated in humans.[57]

Sage: Due to its rich array of pharmacological constituents, sage can influence cognition. Sage decreases inflammation in the brain, reduces amyloid deposits, decreases oxidative cell damage, increases acetylcholine, and helps neuronal growth.[58]

Studies have demonstrated that sage can enhance memory, attention, word recall, and speed of memory in healthy adults.[59] Sage can also make people feel more alert, content, and calm and can improve cognition.[60]

The benefits of sage can be attained by cooking with fresh or dried sage, or by essential oils using aromatherapy.

THE MIND DIET

If all this information about what foods to embrace or avoid to improve memory feels overwhelming, you'll be happy to know that researchers have pinpointed a diet that combines all these principles to offer maximum cognitive protection. The MIND diet (MIND stands for **M**editerranean-DASH **I**ntervention for **N**eurodegenerative

Delay)[61] has been shown to be effective at reversing and protecting against cognitive decline and Alzheimer's disease.

As the name hints, the MIND diet is a combination of two diets, the Mediterranean diet and the DASH diet. We're already familiar with the Mediterranean diet from our discussion in chapter 2, but the important features here are that it is low in saturated fats and high in healthy oils, with red meat eaten infrequently.

DASH stands for **D**ietary **A**pproaches to **S**top **H**ypertension. It typically includes 5 daily servings of vegetables, 5 servings of fruit, about 7 servings of carbohydrates, 2 servings of low-fat dairy products, 2 or fewer servings of lean meat products, and nuts and seeds two to three times per week.[62]

Earlier studies of these individual diets had demonstrated that each may protect patients from cognitive decline on their own. However, in 2015, Martha Clare Morris and her colleagues developed the MIND diet as a powerful combination of the two for long-term brain health.[63] Based on previous research, they put together a list of diet components that were either positive or negative for cognition. They named ten brain-healthy food groups: green leafy vegetables, other vegetables (like peppers, carrots, and broccoli), nuts, berries, beans, whole grains, seafood, poultry, olive oil, and wine. They also named five unhealthy food groups: red meats, butter and margarine, cheese, pastries and sweets, and fried or fast food.

Each of these components was assigned a MIND diet score, which allowed researchers to quantify how well participants were following the diet. For example, a participant would get 0 points for eating fewer than 2 servings of leafy greens per week, .5 point for eating between 2 and 6 servings per week, and 1 point for eating more than 6 servings per week. For the unhealthy foods, the scoring scale was reversed: a participant eating 7 or more meals of red meat per week would get 0 points, while 4–6 meals of red meat per week would yield .5 point, and fewer than 4 meals of red meat per week would get the full point.

Study participants were tested for five different dimensions of "cognitive impairment": episodic memory (long-term recall of personal facts), working memory (short-term recall of information that is still being acted upon), semantic memory (memory of facts and knowledge about the world), visuospatial ability (the ability to see and understand the size and space of our surroundings), and perceptual speed (how fast things are seen).

Morris's team tracked participants' MIND scores and cognitive scores over a number of years (the average participant was tracked for 4.7 years) and then correlated the cognitive scores with the MIND diet scores over time. The results were clear: the higher the MIND diet scores, the slower the rate of cognitive decline. Participants who were in the highest third of the MIND score category were seven and a half years younger in cognitive age than those in the lowest third. These associations held up for the total cognitive score as well as each of the five cognitive domains, though the associations were strongest for episodic memory, semantic memory, and perceptual speed. The MIND diet was also associated with a reduced incidence of Alzheimer's disease.

Since Morris's initial study, there have been a bevy of studies that support her findings and show how the MIND diet affects individual diseases. In 2019, Diane Hosking and her colleagues in Australia also found that the MIND diet was more likely to prevent progression to Alzheimer's disease over twelve years.[64] And in 2018, Puja Agarwal and her colleagues found that the MIND diet was associated with a reduced incidence and delayed progression of Parkinsonism in old age.[65]

In short, experts now believe that the MIND diet offers the best evidence for protection of memory, so it's well worth integrating as many aspects of it as possible into your daily eating habits. You don't necessarily need to work yourself up to a full MIND diet score every week as long as you focus on the ten "good" foods.

MIND Diet "Good" Foods and Their Optimal MIND Score Serving Sizes[66]	
Green leafy vegetables (kale, collards, greens, spinach, lettuce/tossed salad)	6 or more servings per week
Other vegetables (green/red peppers, squash, carrots, broccoli, celery, potatoes, peas or lima beans, tomatoes, tomato sauce, string beans, beets, corn, zucchini/summer squash/eggplant)	1 or more servings per day
Berries (strawberries, blueberries, raspberries, blackberries)	2 or more servings per week
Nuts	5 or more servings per week
Olive oil	Use olive oil as your primary oil
Whole grains	3 or more servings per day
Fish (not fried, particularly high-omega-3 fish such as salmon)	1 or more meals per week
Beans (beans, lentils, soybeans)	More than 3 meals per week
Poultry (chicken or turkey)	2 or more meals per week
Wine	1 glass per day (it's important to note that 1 glass of wine per day resulted in a higher MIND score than any more or less)

I want to highlight the importance of green leafy vegetables, which contain folate, vitamin E, carotenoids, and flavonoids, nutrients that protect against dementia and cognitive decline. When I tell my patients that leafy greens make a difference, they often turn up their noses at the idea. But "leafy greens" do not just include half-dead lettuce. When you go to the supermarket or farmers' market, experiment with different types of leafy greens.

For instance, microgreens are vegetable greens that are harvested very young, soon after they've sprouted. They are a delicious alternative to standard leafy greens, and they are extremely nutrient dense, containing up to forty times the nutrients of their mature counterparts. They are packed with vitamins C, E, and K. Microgreens can be grown from many vegetables, even ones for which you don't necessarily think of eating the leaves. For example, popular microgreens include arugula, chives, cilantro, red cabbage, kale, and basil, but also broccoli, radish, and sunflower. Another great thing about microgreens is that you can grow them in your own home. All you need is an inch of potting soil in a shallow tray, microgreen seeds (which you can buy at your local nursery or online), and clean water in a spray bottle to mist the seeds. Seven to fourteen days after they've germinated, they will be ready to harvest and eat. You can use them in a salad, on avocado toast, or over tacos as a garnish.

BRAIN FOG

While dementia is the most serious, life-altering form of memory loss, it's not the only condition that can cause gaps in your cognition. "Brain fog" occurs when you cannot think clearly, when you cannot concentrate or multitask, or when you lose short-term and long-term memory. Sometimes brain fog is associated with more serious dementia; for example, people with early Alzheimer's disease often have brain fog. It also commonly occurs in autism-spectrum disorders, chronic fatigue syndrome, and fibromyalgia. However, in my experience, brain fog can happen to anyone, even without an underlying condition.

While we do not know for certain what causes brain fog, researchers believe that it is due to excessive brain inflammation. Much like other conditions we've seen, brain fog is most efficiently alleviated by the kind of basic, whole-foods-oriented diet we've talked about throughout the book. I recommend following a diet similar to the Mediterranean eating pattern or the MIND diet we just discussed.

Beyond those basics of diet, here are some tips on how to eat in order to fight that inflammation and restore sharp thinking and decision-making.

Luteolin: In 2015, Theoharis Theoharides and his colleagues showed that luteolin, a type of flavonoid, has numerous neuroprotective properties that decrease brain fog.[67] As an antioxidant and anti-inflammatory agent, this substance prevents toxic destruction of nerve cells in the brain.

Foods that contain luteolin include juniper berries, fresh peppermint, sage, thyme, hot and sweet peppers, radicchio, celery seeds, parsley, and artichokes. Oregano is also one of the best sources of luteolin, but you should buy dried Mexican oregano. While fresh oregano contains roughly 1 mg/100 g of luteolin, dried Mexican oregano contains 1,028 mg/100 g.

Probiotics are not always helpful: Since probiotics are all the rage—and we've discussed them as beneficial to promoting good gut bacteria several times in this book—you might understandably think they are always good for you, with no exceptions. However, in 2018, Satish Rao and his colleagues found that regular use of probiotics was associated with slower digestion, which led to brain fog.[68] If you're taking a probiotic and finding your thoughts sluggish, consider switching supplements (since every gut is unique and the effects of different supplements vary from person to person) or, better yet, getting your probiotics from dietary sources like yogurt with active cultures.

Gluten: In 2018, Lucy Harper and her colleague Justine Bold showed that gluten can cause brain fog.[69] After consuming gluten, some people find themselves thinking less clearly and wanting to sleep all day. If you are suffering from brain fog, cut out gluten to see if you improve. It may turn out that you have celiac disease or non-celiac gluten sensitivity.

Phosphatidylserine (PS): PS is required for healthy nerve cell membranes and coverings, and its protective effects can prevent brain fog. In 2010, Akito Kato-Kataoka explained that six months of soybean-derived PS improved memory function in elderly Japanese adults.[70]

PS is available in supplement form, but it's also present in soybeans. PS isn't very common otherwise, but you can try including white beans, eggs, and dairy products in your diet.

Citicoline: While it may be tough to figure out on your own what the cause of your brain fog may be, studies show that if your brain fog is due to acetylcholine and dopamine depletion, you can consider eating citicoline in foods such as beef liver and egg yolks.[71]

MEMORIES AND YOUR GUT

Memories are a cornerstone of human identity. They are an intrinsic part of the way we learn, document our histories, and benchmark our progress as we course through this life. Without our memories, we would be unable to do our jobs successfully, brush our teeth, drive home, or recognize people whom we have known throughout our lives. That's why we cherish our memories, and it is why we mourn the loss of them when dementia or brain fog sets in.

I wish that I had known what I know now when I treated Brian all those years ago, so that we could have put him on a robust eating plan full of foods that could have extended his memory for at least a few more years. No matter how old you are, it's never too late or too early to start eating in a way that gives you the best possible chance of staving off dementia as you age and making sure that you feel fresh, sharp, and capable every day.

MEMORY CHEAT SHEET

The MIND diet is the most comprehensive eating plan for ensuring a healthy memory. Eat green leafy vegetables, colorful vegetables, berries, nuts, olive oil, whole grains, fish, beans, poultry; drink red wine.

Foods and Strategies to Embrace:

- Calorie restriction: Work with your doctor to make a plan to reduce your total calorie intake by about 25 percent.
- Alcohol: Don't abstain totally or drink too much; 3–5 drinks per week is ideal for women, and 5–7 drinks is ideal for men.
- Coffee: Coffee is beneficial, but keep total caffeine consumption under 400 mg/day.
- Olive oil: Olive oil is protective, especially when used in a *sofrito* preparation.
- Herbs and spices: Turmeric, black pepper, cinnamon, saffron, rosemary, ginger, sage.
- For brain fog: Luteolin-rich foods (juniper berries, fresh peppermint, sage, thyme, hot and sweet peppers, radicchio, celery seeds, parsley, artichokes, and dried Mexican oregano); phosphatidylserine (PS)-containing foods (white beans, eggs, and dairy); citicoline-rich foods (beef liver, egg yolks).

Foods to Avoid:

- The components of the Western diet: Foods high in bad fats (red meat, fried foods) and high-GI carbs (white bread, white rice, potatoes, pasta, and anything else made from refined flour).
- Gluten: If you have celiac disease or non-celiac gluten sensitivity, avoid all wheat products, such as bread, pizza, pasta, and many alcoholic drinks.

CHAPTER SEVEN

Obsessive-Compulsive Disorder: NAC, Glycine, and the Dangers of Orthorexia Nervosa

We all know that nagging feeling when we leave our homes and wonder if we left the stove on or if we actually locked the door. But imagine what it feels like when you cannot escape those thoughts. No worry ever leaves your mind, and no matter how hard you try, nothing is ever complete. That's what it's like to have obsessive-compulsive disorder (OCD), and it is absolute torture.

When Adam entered my office, he appeared to be a confident young man. But once he let his guard down, all the compulsions and repetitive checking behaviors came pouring out. His rituals, including checking the handbrake on his car, rescrewing the cap onto his toothpaste, and making sure the trash can lid in his kitchen was shut, consumed hours of his day. Sometimes he was late for work because he was afraid to start his car.

We worked on small ways to improve his symptoms. He followed my advice and used a ride-share service to work, which encouraged him to leave home without finishing his rituals, as he didn't want to make the driver wait. We found a trash bin online that had an automatic lid that shut every time you used it. This calmed him down to a degree, but when he drove to our appointments, he still went back to his car and would stay there for hours, obsessing over whether he ought to release the handbrake or not. What if he did and the car rolled backward? What if he hit the gas harder than he should and hit someone by mistake? The thoughts would spin around in his mind relentlessly like a hamster on a wheel.

For many years, OCD was considered an anxiety disorder.[1] Only recently has it been put in a class of its own, along with other disorders on what is called the OCD spectrum. In my opinion, the differences between OCD and anxiety are debatable, because many patients with OCD also suffer from terrible anxiety—technically speaking, up to 30 percent of people with OCD also experience generalized anxiety disorder during their lifetime.[2]

OCD is closely related to several other mental health disorders. Tic disorders such as Tourette's syndrome are also considered to be on the OCD spectrum, as are body dysmorphic disorders, trichotillomania (hair pulling), excoriation disorder (skin picking), pathological gambling, kleptomania, sexual compulsivity, and other conditions. People with OCD also share personality traits with people with eating disorders such as anorexia nervosa or binge-eating disorders, and there is often overlap in patients.

When I was treating Adam, about fifteen years ago, the only available treatments were a few medications and cognitive behavioral therapy. Now there are controlled trials and many case histories that can help guide nutritional interventions as well. In this chapter I will explain the nutritional interventions for OCD and related conditions and how those who are trapped by these symptoms can find relief.

THE OCD GUT

As we've seen with related conditions like anxiety, the gut-brain connection is a factor in OCD. Changing gut bacteria can change the course of the disease, and gut bacteria change when OCD symptoms emerge.

For example, Pranish Kantak and his colleagues at the University of North Dakota induced OCD-like behaviors in mice and then tested whether probiotics altered their symptoms. In the first experiment, mice were pretreated with either a probiotic or saline for two or four weeks. After OCD-like behaviors were induced, the researchers observed that they were significantly less extreme in the probiotic-treated mice than in the controls, which received only saline.[3]

In the second experiment, an additional group of mice was included in the analysis. These mice had been pretreated with fluoxetine, commonly known as Prozac, for four weeks. Selective serotonin reuptake inhibitor (SSRI) antidepressants are used as first-line treatment for OCD. Sure enough, the drug worked to lessen OCD symptoms, but the probiotic group had results very similar to those of the fluoxetine group. In other words, probiotics fought OCD just as well as the primary pharmaceutical treatment.

To demonstrate the gut-brain connection working in the opposite way, in 2018 Tony Jung and his colleagues at McMaster University administered a drug to induce OCD-like symptoms in rats and then monitored the rats' gut bacteria.[4] Their investigation determined that the rats' gut bacteria did indeed change as OCD set in. The researchers concluded that the change in gut bacteria was precipitated by the time taken and energy used in compulsive behaviors (for instance, think about how much time and energy my patient Adam was expending).

The results of those animal studies have been substantiated by human studies. For example, in a general survey about the psychological effects of probiotics in healthy humans, it was demonstrated that participants who used probiotics for thirty days reported that obsessive-compulsive symptoms were reduced.

In 2015 psychologist Jasmine Turna and her colleagues explained that OCD symptoms may be a result of the bidirectional relationship between the gut and brain.[5] Altered gut bacteria impact the hypothalamic-pituitary-adrenal axis (HPA-axis), starting a cascade of hormonal and immune responses that result in OCD.

There is considerable evidence that the HPA-axis is not working as it should in OCD. For instance, take the behavior of the stress hormone cortisol in OCD patients. In healthy individuals, cortisol levels have a low baseline. When these individuals experience stress, cortisol levels spike as the body releases the hormone to respond to crisis. In OCD patients, however, the baseline cortisol level is elevated, but when there is a crisis, there is no corresponding cortisol spike.[6] In fact, cortisol levels often go *down* when OCD patients are put under stress, the exact opposite of what we expect. It's as if the HPA-axis is overwhelmed due to the constant stress of OCD, and the brain cannot fight external stressors the way it would in a healthy person.

As for what causes the changes in gut bacteria that might precipitate OCD, in 2014, cognitive psychologist Jon Rees explained that stress and antibiotics can both alter the gut microbiome.[7] A wide variety of stresses might trigger changes in the gut microbiome and therefore OCD, and studies indicate that they do not need to be major, life-changing events.[8] Health-related worry, school stress, or loss of a loved one can all trigger OCD even when they are not traumatic. Even pregnancy can alter gut microbiota and lead to OCD-type symptoms.

In children, a variant of OCD called PANDAS—which stands for pediatric autoimmune neuropsychiatric disorders associated with streptococcus—has long been thought to be associated with streptococcal infections and immune dysfunction. However, now experts wonder if it's not the strep itself that leads to PANDAS, but rather the antibiotic used to treat the strep. The antibiotics that fight strep can disrupt the gut microbiome, triggering OCD symptoms.

All in all, these findings indicate that OCD symptoms arise

when gut bacteria change, and vice versa. As we know by now, the way to ensure that you have healthy gut bacteria is to make sure you're getting the proper nutrients in your diet and avoiding foods that might upset the balance of your microbiome.

FOODS THAT CAN WORSEN COMPULSION

Since OCD is so intertwined with anxiety, I always recommend that patients stick to the basic tenets of eating for anxiety. Beyond avoiding foods that we discussed in chapter 3, here are a few dietary factors to steer away from when suffering from OCD.

Glutamate

As we saw in chapter 4 when discussing PTSD, glutamate is a substance that is common in many natural foods and used as an additive in prepared dishes to add umami flavor. Dietary glutamates are generally regarded as healthy in normal amounts for most individuals, but sufferers of OCD should be very careful about their glutamate intake. That's because glutamate plays an important role in your brain as a neurotransmitter that is deeply intertwined with OCD symptoms.

In 2018, Kathleen Holton and Elizabeth Cotter presented a case of a fifty-year-old man who had suffered from daily OCD symptoms for thirty-nine years, with no improvement from any pharmacological treatment.[9] In addition to OCD, the man also had fibromyalgia (a chronic pain condition) and irritable bowel syndrome, which ended up being the source of a breakthrough discovery about how diet affects OCD.

This man was enrolled in a randomized double-blind placebo-controlled clinical trial to test the effects of a low-glutamate diet on fibromyalgia and irritable bowel syndrome. After one month on the diet, not only were his fibromyalgia and irritable bowel syndrome symptoms reduced, but he also had significant improvement in his OCD. Holton and Cotter concluded that glutamate must be involved in the chemical abnormalities underlying OCD.

In 2017, Přemysl Vlček and his colleagues presented extensive evidence showing a key role of glutamate pathway abnormalities within the brain circuits involved in OCD.[10] Glutamate is the major excitatory neurotransmitter in the central nervous system; that means that its role is encouraging neurons to spring into action.[11] Though the exact role glutamate abnormalities play remains unclear, OCD is at least partially caused by a malfunction of the system that tells your cells to act, and excess dietary glutamate can worsen the damage.

Excess glutamate is not the only piece of the puzzle, however. In 2019, Yan Li and his colleagues explained that OCD was most likely caused by increases in both excitatory glutamate and one of its counterparts, the inhibitory neurotransmitter gamma-aminobutyric acid (GABA).[12] As you might expect, inhibitory neurotransmitters do the opposite of excitatory ones, discouraging neurons from action.

The effect of having surpluses of both glutamate and GABA is that the brain is getting stop and go signals at the same time. OCD brains are in constant chaos due to the mixed messages being sent to their neurons. No wonder they get stuck! The full story behind GABA-glutamate abnormalities is much more complex than this simplified explanation, but the key point is that OCD patients can see relief by cutting down on glutamates in their diet.

There are two types of dietary glutamate. Bound glutamate is usually eaten as part of a protein, and thus it can be digested and absorbed well. Free glutamate is not bound to other amino acids, which means that it can cause spikes of glutamate in the blood. You want to avoid these spikes.

Free forms of glutamate are found in cured meat, Roquefort and Parmesan cheese, fish sauce, soy sauce, ripe tomatoes, broccoli, grape juice, caviar, salami, miso, and bone broths. As we discussed in chapter 4, glutamate is also found in monosodium glutamate (MSG), an ingredient in many kinds of packaged, processed, and prepared foods. For instance, it is used in Chick-fil-A nuggets, as well as in stocks, instant meals, and soy and yeast extracts. Patients suffering from OCD or OCD-like symptoms should try to cut down on these foods as much as possible to see if an improvement is made. (I have already guided you to be aware that many high-glutamate foods also contain the amino acid tyramine, which can interfere with MAOI antidepressants. See chapter 9 for more details.)

Gluten

In 2018, gastroenterologist Luis Rodrigo and his colleagues conducted a study to see if reducing gluten intake could reduce OCD symptoms in children with both OCD and Tourette's syndrome.[13] Indeed, after one year on a gluten-free diet, patients found that their obsessions interfered less with their lives and that they experienced less distress.

The precise reasons for this improvement in OCD symptoms after removal of gluten are not known. In prior chapters I have explained how the celiac brain is prone to autoimmune brain cell destruction as well as glutamate-GABA imbalances.[14] This likely contributes to OCD symptoms.

While there isn't airtight evidence that a gluten-free diet can help people with OCD, this study and other case reports suggest that it's worth going on a gluten-free diet to see if symptoms improve.

FOODS AND SUPPLEMENTS TO FIGHT COMPULSION

Vicky was a fifty-year-old chief human resources officer for a Fortune 500 company. At work, she was meticulous about being on time and on task. But at home, she was frustrated and struggling with the fact that her last child was about to leave for college.

She was cheerful and upbeat when we chatted about most topics, but she became anxious when speaking about her marriage. She eventually admitted that she was unsure whether to stay married or not. On the one hand, she had no major issues or fights with her husband. On the other hand, she felt that he was too set in his ways. She was ready to travel the world, and he did not want to make changes in his life.

In order to try to cope with her anxiety and desire to do something, she read *The Life-Changing Magic of Tidying Up* by Marie Kondo. At first she loved it; Kondo's philosophy of decluttering gave her an outlet for her stress. Before long, she had not only cleared out her closets and basement but also started to arrange all her shoes and clothing by color.

Her husband found her constant tidying annoying, and when she moved on to his clothes, he lost it. Even her children locked their doors when they came home for fear that she would come in and start rearranging things in their rooms. Gradually, her tidying habits started infringing on other parts of her life. She would be late for work because she was tidying, and when she got to the office it was all she could think about.

I recognized that she was developing OCD. Although OCD usually starts earlier in life, it can begin later too, with a small proportion of cases beginning in people over fifty.[15] Vicky was resolute that she did not want to try medication, but through our therapy sessions together, she started to see how her obsessional behaviors were replacing her anxiety about wanting to leave her marriage.

Given her reluctance to take medication, I decided to try some dietary interventions with her. In particular, I wanted to try two different treatments that have been shown to reduce OCD symptoms without accompanying SSRIs—N-acetylcysteine (NAC) and myoinositol (MI).

Through a combination of diet, supplements, and therapy, after three months, Vicky was able to think more clearly. She had fewer obsessive thoughts and they were less intrusive, allowing her to function better. Her compulsive tidying was reduced considerably, and though it was a difficult decision, after a year, she decided that a trial separation from her husband was in order. Eighteen months after that, they got an amicable divorce.

I have continued to see Vicky, and whenever she goes off her diet, she starts to obsess again — sometimes about whether she did the right thing with her marriage, and sometimes she goes back to cleaning. However, when she restarts her nutritional interventions, these symptoms go away.

Let's explore NAC and MI, along with other dietary interventions that have been shown to help patients struggling with OCD.

N-Acetylcysteine

N-acetylcysteine is a dietary supplement used to treat a number of non–mental health illnesses, but it has also been shown to be a helpful treatment for OCD. NAC inhibits the release of glutamate between nerve cells in many brain regions, including the cortex, amygdala, hippocampus, and striatum, all of which are affected in OCD.[16] In addition, NAC reduces oxidative stress and inflammation in the brains of people with OCD.[17]

A 2017 study demonstrated that NAC amplified the effects of the antidepressant citalopram in improving resistance to compulsions and enhancing control of them in children and adolescents with OCD.[18] Another case report of a fifty-eight-year-old woman who controlled her OCD with the antidepressant fluvoxamine found that a supplementary course of NAC resulted in a significant improvement in OCD, with improvements beginning just one week into NAC treatment.[19]

NAC has also been shown to be effective in treating trichotillomania, an OCD-spectrum disorder in which individuals repetitively pull out their own hair. In 2009, Jon Grant conducted a double-blind randomized placebo-controlled trial to assess the efficacy of 1200–1400 mg/day of NAC in participants with trichotillomania over a twelve-week period.[20] Patients in the NAC treatment group were found to have a significantly greater reduction in hair-pulling symptoms compared to placebo.

There are case histories showing that NAC is helpful for compulsive nail-biting and skin-picking behavior too. More controlled studies are needed, but overall, the results of trials so far favor the use of NAC over placebo.[21] NAC is also considered safe, with no major side effects.

NAC isn't found in any natural foods, so it must be taken as a supplement. However, once in the body, it converts to the amino acid cysteine. Though all the research on NAC's effects on OCD is based on supplements, patients in my clinic have also achieved promising results by eating foods rich in cysteine. Meat, grains, and eggs all contain cysteine, as do ricotta cheese, cottage cheese, yogurt, broccoli, red pepper, and onion.

Myoinositol

Myoinositol is a variant of glucose that is made naturally in the body but can also be consumed through foods. There's a ton of MI in the brain, particularly in brain cell membranes, where it helps control which substances enter and exit the cells.[22] MI is a precursor of phosphoinositide, a type of lipid that facilitates cellular responses in many neurochemical pathways, including the serotonin and dopamine pathways implicated in OCD.[23]

Some researchers believe that MI has a mechanism of action on the brain similar to that of SSRIs.[24] Sure enough, a number of studies and trials have demonstrated that MI is helpful in OCD too. For example, in 1996, psychiatrist Mendel Fux and his colleagues studied thirteen patients with OCD, noting that 18 g/day of MI for six weeks resulted in a significant reduction in OCD symptoms compared to placebo.[25]

Despite the efficacy of MI on its own, it has not proven to be helpful as an add-on to standard treatments for OCD, such as SSRIs. Also, mild gastrointestinal side effects such as diarrhea, flatulence, and nausea have been noted. Still, those downsides are minor compared to the benefits it can provide.[26]

MI is plentiful in fruits, beans, grains, and nuts. Fresh vegetables contain much more MI than frozen or canned versions. For breakfast, grapefruit and bran flakes are rich sources of MI, and coffee has a trace. Just remember to check with your doctor before adding grapefruit to your diet, because of possible drug interactions. For lunch and dinner, steer toward navy beans or green beans. Brussels sprouts and lima beans are also high in MI, and carrots and corn have lower levels. Peanut butter (with no added sugar) is rich in MI, as is whole wheat bread. In general, whole-grain breads are higher in MI than refined breads. Cantaloupe and citrus fruits have an extraordinarily high amount of MI, so snack on them whenever you can.

Glycine

Glycine is another amino acid that impacts glutamate function in the brain, and studies indicate that it may be helpful in OCD due to its interaction with a type of glutamate receptor found in the brain known as an N-methyl-D-aspartate (NMDA) receptor.[27] While glycine is also an inhibitory neurotransmitter, it does not butt heads with glutamate the same way GABA does, and it helps calm the conflict in OCD patients' brains.

In 2009, William Greenberg and his colleagues administered 60 mg/day of glycine or placebo to patients with OCD, then monitored their symptoms at four, eight, and twelve weeks after starting the trial.[28] In the test subjects who received glycine, there was a strong trend toward reduction of OCD symptoms.

Again in 2009, William Louis Cleveland and his colleagues reported on another case that highlights the importance of glycine.[29] The patient in the case study was diagnosed with OCD and body dysmorphic disorder at age seventeen, and his symptoms were severe enough that he had to stop school. At age nineteen, he was housebound and had no social contact except with his parents. Several lines of treatment—SSRI antidepressants, antipsychotic drugs, and intravenous therapy—proved fruitless.

At age twenty-two, his symptoms worsened after he received antibiotic treatment for *H. pylori,* a bacteria that causes stomach ulcers. His clinicians concluded that his NMDA receptors were not working properly. The doctors started him on glycine, to stimulate NMDA. Over five years, treatment with glycine led to a robust reduction of his OCD and body dysmorphic disorder symptoms, with partial relapses occurring whenever the treatment was stopped. Thanks to his new glycine treatment, the patient was able to resume school and social life.

Although this is just a single trial, the results are quite dramatic, and along with the results of the controlled trial, it is solid evidence that glycine can be highly effective in treating OCD.

You don't have to rely on supplements to get glycine. It's present in meat, fish, dairy products, and legumes. Turkey is a richer source of glycine than beef, which is in turn a richer source than pork or chicken. The best sources of glycine are collagen and gelatin. Since bone broth contains both glycine and glutamate, it may feel contradictory to eat it. I have my clinical patients test out adding or excluding bone broth to see how their OCD symptoms respond. If bone broth has a negative effect on an individual patient, we simply stay with plant-based options like spinach, kale, cauliflower, cabbage, pumpkin, and fruits like bananas and kiwi, all of which also contain glycine.

Milk Thistle

Milk thistle (*Silybum marianum*), a member of the same family of flowers that includes sunflowers and daisies, has been used as a medicinal plant for centuries. According to ancient folklore, its signature violet flowers and white-veined leaves came from the Virgin Mary's milk.

The component of milk thistle that helps people with OCD is the flavonoid silymarin, which is a natural antioxidant. One of the main actions of silymarin is to inhibit monoamine oxidase (MAO), an enzyme that (among other functions) removes serotonin from the brain.[30] Inhibiting MAO increases serotonin, and as a result, OCD symptoms ease. (We've mentioned MAOI antidepressant medications already, which work in roughly the same way.)

When Mehdi Sayyah and his colleagues compared the effects of milk thistle extract (600 mg/day) with fluoxetine (30 mg/day) in patients with OCD, they found that the two treatments were similarly effective, and the side effects were similar as well.[31] While more studies are needed to convincingly recommend milk thistle as a treatment for OCD, since the potential for negative side effects is low, it's worth a try.

Supplements are the only way to incorporate milk thistle into your routine. As always, consult with your doctor before starting to take them.

Vitamin B_{12}

Vitamin B_{12} (cobalamin) is essential for the production of many brain chemicals, including serotonin. One study demonstrated that 20 percent of patients with OCD have low vitamin B_{12}, and this finding has been corroborated by other studies.[32] Though it's unclear whether low vitamin B_{12} is a cause or consequence of OCD, we know that it plays a role.

In 2012, Vivek Sharma and Devdutta Biswas reported on a case of a middle-aged man presenting with OCD who had low levels of B_{12} and a family history of vitamin B_{12} deficiency.[33] His OCD symptoms resolved when his levels were raised by taking methylcobalamin, a form of B_{12}. That's a good sign that it's worth trying to replace vitamin B_{12} in OCD patients.

Vitamin B_{12} is mostly found in meat, fish, and chicken, so most omnivores don't have too much trouble getting enough. If you're a vegetarian, B_{12} can also be found in dairy products. If you're a vegan, you can look for vitamin-fortified cereals and other foods.

But there are also out-of-the-box options like the fermented soybean product tempeh, which has high levels of vitamin B_{12}. Another rich vegetarian source of B_{12} is nori, a type of edible seaweed.

I once had a thirty-five-year-old vegetarian patient named Ashwariya. She had come to see me because of a collection of behaviors that were interfering with her life. For instance, she found herself trimming the fringe on her bedspreads, staying up all night to ensure that they were absolutely "perfect." She was obsessed with flaws in her skin, even when there were none. When she came to my office, she would sit down and then rearrange herself in the chair, sometimes making an embarrassed admission that she felt she was getting too fat to be able to comfortably seat herself, even though I could see she was of normal weight and that the chair was more than large enough for her to sit however she wanted.

After taking a detailed history, I recognized that she had OCD and body dysmorphic disorder. After doing some basic labs, I saw that her vitamin B_{12} was low, so I suggested that we try to improve this. Three months later, her distressing behaviors were still present and her B_{12} levels were still low despite taking supplements. When I asked her what form of B_{12} she was taking, she told me *Chlorella* tablets, which allegedly have significant amounts of vitamin B_{12}. However, she did not know that you have to check the nutrition label to see which version of *Chlorella* you are getting. Commercial preparations contain varying amounts of vitamin B_{12}, and hers did not contain much at all.[34]

She switched to *Spirulina*, a supplement made from blue-green algae. However, studies have shown that many dietary supplements like *Spirulina* contain pseudovitamin B_{12}—variants of B_{12} that are inactive in humans.[35]

Once more, her symptoms did not improve, so eventually, she started eating the dried seaweed product nori, which is rich in B_{12}, in vegetarian sushi. While nori does contain glutamates, Ashwariya didn't suffer ill effects from it. (If she had, I would have suggested wakame, a brown seaweed often enjoyed in miso soup, which has high B_{12} levels with a negligible amount of glutamate.) Within three months, her symptoms started to improve. While replacing vitamin B_{12} is not an ironclad way to treat OCD symptoms in every instance, in some cases it can be a lifesaver.

Turmeric

In 2010, Drs. Jithendra Chimakurthy and T. E. Gopala Krishna Murthy explored the value of curcumin in OCD.[36] As we've seen in previous discussions, curcumin has long been known to impact serotonin, dopamine, and noradrenaline metabolism, so the researchers felt it was likely to have an impact on the underlying neurochemical changes in OCD.

To study this, the team induced OCD-like behavior in rats before treating them with either curcumin or paroxetine (an SSRI). Rats treated with 5 mg/kg and 10 mg/kg of curcumin increased their blood dopamine levels, but only the 10 mg/kg preparation of curcumin increased serotonin levels. Paroxetine-treated animals showed an increase in serotonin but no changes in dopamine. Both curcumin and paroxetine decreased compulsive behaviors.

While human studies of turmeric's effects on OCD are still being researched, turmeric is generally so good for mental health that I recommend it as part of your regular diet.

SPECIAL CONSIDERATIONS

Orthorexia Nervosa

One big challenge of working with patients with OCD is being careful not to worsen their symptoms by giving them new fodder for their obsessions. With minds that are constantly churning through different stresses and compulsions, you never want to be piling on to the problem. In particular, you have to ensure that you don't precipitate orthorexia nervosa.

In 1997, physician Steven Bratman and his colleague David Knight coined the term orthorexia nervosa to describe individuals with an obsession for proper nutrition. This condition results from diets that are too restrictive, an obsessional focus on food preparation, and ritualized patterns of eating. In other words, people suffering from orthorexia nervosa are "health food junkies" to the extreme.

I admit that it may seem ironic for someone who is writing a whole book about eating well to caution against the pitfalls of being *too* focused on nutrition. But while it is a virtue to be conscious of what you're eating and do your best to ensure you're consuming food that is both nutritious and sustainable, there's no doubt this can cross over into obsession and feed other OCD tendencies.

I had a patient named Josue who traveled from far away for a consult with me after hearing of my work and my clinic. He expected to be given blood tests almost as soon as he entered the door, practically demanding an intricate medical solution to his problems. Yet on my initial interview, it was clear that his major issue was overly strict food choices, which left him nutritionally deficient. I began to address this by gently suggesting we talk about some healthy building-block recipes, but he scoffed and said my recommendations seemed "very pedestrian."

While I would love to tell you that I've gotten through to every single patient I've ever had, I don't think Josue followed my advice. He was not willing to accept the fact that the key to his mental health might be loosening his grip on a strictly regimented diet and focusing on eating a wide variety of healthy foods. Unfortunately, he never returned and I suspect his orthorexia prevented him from reaching his goals of a healthier weight and improved mood.

Of course there is a gray area here, and it's worth acknowledging that discussions surrounding foods change with time. I remember being at a restaurant in New York some years ago, not sure whether to be shocked or amused that several colleagues were asking the befuddled waiter questions about the cows' diet and whether pesticides were used on the vegetables. Nowadays, a preference for grass-fed beef and organic foods is commonplace, but back then, these preferences hadn't yet reached the mainstream.

I never want to discourage my patients from making healthy choices, but when their restrictive diets start to intrude upon their lives I begin to worry. Orthorexic individuals are often preoccupied with weight control, so I see that as a warning sign.[37]

In order to avoid symptoms of orthorexia nervosa, follow these rules of thumb when making changes in your diet:

- Start with changing one food at a time.
- If you fail to maintain that change, try another.
- Start with the least restrictive change so that your mood does not plummet.
- Plan ahead so your choices are automatic and you don't feel like you have to obsess over every meal.
- Measure your weight weekly rather than daily.
- Try limiting your social media exposure while changing your diet. In particular, studies have shown that Instagram use worsens orthorexia.[38]

These rules can be helpful for those with OCD tendencies and are good tips even for healthy individuals who are making diet changes.

Muscle Dysmorphia

Muscle dysmorphia is a variant of OCD in which people are obsessed with their musculature and often compulsively exercise.[39] This can result in radical diets and the use of dietary supplements in order to find the perfect muscle mass and to reduce body fat mass.

Jason, for instance, was a thirty-year-old who came to see me because he felt directionless and wanted to jump-start his motivation. Within a short period of time, I realized that his relationship with his father was at the core of his conflicts. On the one hand, he worked for his father and loved the ease of that. On the other hand, his father was hard on him, and as he grew older, this left him feeling frustrated, as if he would never rise to the level of his father's success.

Unable to talk to his father about any of this, he worked out his frustration in the gym. Despite having less than 9 percent body fat and obvious muscular definition, he told me that he had to get leaner and stronger because he had decided to enter a bodybuilding competition. I told him I thought he was in good enough shape, and he looked at me like I was clueless.

In the following weeks, he kicked his workout up a few notches, radically changed his diet, and came in looking so lean that it was mildly disturbing. Even at 5 percent body fat, he could not stop. He increased his protein intake far beyond even the high levels recommended for resistance and endurance athletes.[40] He also added a number of supplements — branched chain amino acids, glutamine, and the growth-hormone-stimulating amino acids (lysine, ornithine, and arginine). Worst of all, he started anabolic steroids.

It wasn't hard for me to see that Jason had pushed himself too far, but I had difficulty making him understand. At my urging, we ran a battery of tests and discovered that he was on the verge of renal failure. Luckily, it was early enough that the test acted as a wake-up call. I recommended going back to square one, a healthy diet of fresh fruit, vegetables, lean protein (chicken breast, turkey, and salmon were his favorites), and sources of healthy fats like olive oil and avocados. With time and patience he gradually came to see the difference and feel better both emotionally and physically. While I continued to work with him on the nutritional aspects of his condition, he also started to see a therapist who was able to talk to him about his childhood and growing up around his powerful and successful father. Eventually he connected his extreme diet and exercise choices with his complicated feelings toward his father. Over a year, he began to show significant improvement in recovering a healthy lifestyle.

To address muscle dysmorphia, avoid radical dietary changes and always consult a doctor or nutritionist when changing protein consumption or taking a supplement. In particular, avoid supplements that you read about online and from unvetted sources. Give careful consideration to what you are adding to your diet. Finally, always be wary of underlying psychological causes that are driving an unhealthy approach to otherwise healthy pursuits.

FIGHTING OBSESSION THROUGH DIET

Through the stories of my patients, I hope I've impressed upon you that OCD can be a subtle condition that presents in a host of different ways. While there are certainly patients like Adam, who have classic compulsions and radical checking behaviors, that's not the only form OCD can take. Sometimes, as we saw with Vicky, OCD can arise out of an interest that initially appears to be healthy, or it can be an accumulation of small habits and concerns about your body as it was with Ashwariya. Or maybe, as in Jason's case, it can even be the result of too much focus on a healthy lifestyle.

With such a varied, insidious disease, it is paramount that you see a doctor if you feel you are suffering from OCD-like symptoms. While treatments need to be individualized for each patient, it is always a good idea to implement some of the nutritional strategies we've discussed in this chapter.

OCD CHEAT SHEET

Since OCD is so closely related to anxiety, the dietary recommendations in chapter 3 also apply here.

Foods and Supplements to Embrace:

- N-acetylcysteine: While NAC itself must be taken as a supplement, cysteine-rich foods can also be effective. Try meat, grains, eggs, ricotta cheese, cottage cheese, yogurt, broccoli, red pepper, and onion.
- Myoinositol: Fresh vegetables, especially navy or green beans, Brussels sprouts, and lima beans; peanut butter; whole wheat bread; cantaloupe; and citrus fruits.
- Glycine: Meat, fish, dairy products, legumes, spinach, kale, cauliflower, cabbage, pumpkin, bananas, kiwi.
- Milk thistle (*Silybum marianum*): Available as a supplement.
- Vitamin B_{12}.
- Spices: Turmeric with a pinch of black pepper.

Foods to Avoid:

- MSG, other glutamates, and glutamic acid: Fish sauce, oyster sauce, tomato sauce, miso, Parmesan cheese, savory snacks, chips, ready-to-eat meals, mushrooms, spinach, seaweed, cheeses, soy sauce, fermented beans, tomatoes, and high-protein foods like meats and seafood.
- Gluten: If you have celiac disease or non-celiac gluten sensitivity, avoid all wheat products, such as bread, pizza, pasta, and many alcoholic drinks.

CHAPTER EIGHT

Insomnia and Fatigue: Capsaicin, Chamomile, and Anti-Inflammatory Diets

Dumisani was a forty-year-old cop who came to me for help with depression—at least that's what she thought she needed help with. She and her husband had adopted a newborn baby from Kenya, and since her husband's job required him to work during the day, she took the night shifts on the force, regularly working until past dawn.

When it was time for her to get to sleep at the end of a long shift, she couldn't. The exhaustion that felt overwhelming when she was at work was nowhere to be found when she closed her drapes and got into bed. The stress of her shift kept her wound up. Her baby was overjoyed to see her and wanted to play. She just couldn't convince her body that it was time to sleep. As a result, she only managed to snooze a little here and there while her baby napped during the day. Of course, when she went back to work the next night she felt even worse, dragging herself through shifts buoyed by a constant stream of coffee before repeating the cycle again.

This pattern eventually got to her. Depression set in, and despite eating healthily, she gained 15 pounds. I could immediately tell that an antidepressant was not going to be the solution to her problems.

We decided that prior to trying medications, she should try a few lifestyle changes. We talked about how working the late shift was disrupting her gut bacteria, the importance of regular sleep patterns, and ways she could change her diet to better manage her energy.

She changed her schedule so that she didn't have to work the graveyard shift every night. Her husband also made changes to his schedule and was able to take the baby to work on certain days. She was diligent about following the eating plan we had developed, which helped her feel energized and sleepy at the right times.

It may seem like a lot of juggling, but the sum of these changes was that Dumisani and her husband were able to attend to their family much more successfully. She was still working some nights, so her sleep schedule wasn't totally ideal, but even with this imperfect solution, within three months she had a dramatic change in her mood.

Close to a third of the world's population has trouble sleeping.[1] Whether you have trouble going to sleep or trouble staying asleep, it can affect every organ system in your body.[2] Your brain, heart, lungs, kidneys, and general metabolism may all be off-kilter.

When all the soothing music and sedatives in the world will not help you sleep, what can you do? And when you're awake, how can you live your life with optimum energy? That's what we will discuss in this chapter, highlighting foods that help and hurt when insomnia and fatigue disrupt your life.

SLEEP AND YOUR GUT

Maintaining the delicate balance of bacteria in your gut is crucial for healthy sleep. The gut-brain connections we see with sleep should feel familiar by now: by interacting with the immune system, your hormones, and the vagus nerve directly, gut bacteria communicate with your brain to determine sleep patterns.[3] And once again, the interaction goes both ways, with the brain able to have an effect on gut bacteria as well.

You've probably heard about the circadian rhythm, a twenty-four-hour internal body clock that regulates when we sleep and when we're awake. When this sleep/wake cycle is disrupted, it leads to metabolic damage. In 2014, Sarah Davies, a research associate at Imperial College London, demonstrated that when twelve young, healthy men were sleep deprived, levels of twenty-seven metabolites—including some of our favorites, like serotonin and tryptophan—changed.[4] When you sleep normally, these metabolites rise and fall in specific rhythms throughout the day. However, when you do not get enough sleep, this rhythm is disturbed and chemical peaks and troughs become erratic. This has led to another emerging field of medicine called chrononutrition, in which researchers study how your body's internal clock affects your digestion and metabolism.[5]

What does this have to do with your gut? Well, it's not just humans who have a natural sleep cycle; all living things do, including the bacteria in your microbiome. Intestinal bacteria fall into a pattern of "sleeping" and "waking" as their physiological processes fluctuate throughout the day.[6] In fact, the circadian rhythms of your gut bacteria can affect the human circadian rhythm by changing the genes that help you go to sleep or stay awake.[7]

Gut bacterial internal clocks and human internal clocks are usually synchronized.[8] However, when your body's internal clock is thrown off—for instance, when you have too many late nights or you are traveling across time zones and suffering from jet lag—the composition and behavior of your gut bacteria can change.[9] The resulting misalignment of circadian rhythms can affect how you metabolize food, ultimately contributing to obesity.

There are many animal studies that demonstrate this close connection between gut bacteria and sleep patterns. For example, one study showed that breaking up sleep patterns changes gut bacteria in mice.[10] As a result, the colon linings of the mice were damaged, "leaking" out substances that increased inflammation in their bodies, causing altered insulin sensitivity and increased eating. Researchers found that when they transplanted feces from these sleep-deprived mice into germ-free mice, the germ-free mice started experiencing the same problems with inflammation and metabolism.[11] Probiotics reversed these changes.

In humans, we see the dangers of sleep disruption most clearly with shift workers like Dumisani, who work during normal sleeping hours. You may think that shift work is uncommon, but two in five workers in the United States are shift workers who don't work nine-to-five jobs (coincidentally, that's approximately the same rate as the obesity rate in the United States).[12] Overnight workers rarely get enough sleep, and as a result, their gut bacterial equilibrium is thrown off. Even when shift workers have diets identical to those of non-shift workers, they are not able to metabolize food normally, resulting in a tendency to be more overweight or obese.[13]

Eating for Sleep

The best recipe for sleep often lines up with a healthy diet. For example, in 2014, Ryoko Katagiri and her colleagues reported that women who ate more noodles and sweets and less vegetables and fish had worse sleep than those with healthier diets.[14] Poor sleep quality was also more common in people who consumed energy drinks and sugar-sweetened beverages, and those who skipped breakfast and ate irregularly.

Despite this negative effect of sugar, it has been shown that a high-glycemic-index carbohydrate meal will get you to sleep faster, though it will ultimately lead to sleep that is less satisfying.[15] Another study showed that high-sugar diets, as well as high-saturated-fat and low-fiber diets, will give you lighter, less restorative sleep.[16] In particular, high-fat and high-carbohydrate diets decrease slow-wave sleep, which is restorative, and REM sleep, which helps to consolidate memory.[17]

Other sleep studies can be harder to parse. A Japanese study found that low protein intake (less than 16 percent of energy from protein) was associated with poorer sleep quality and difficulty going to sleep, whereas higher protein intake (more than 19 percent) was associated with difficulty maintaining sleep. Rather than encouraging you to try to thread the needle to hit the perfect 16–19 percent energy from protein, it's safe to say that eating a moderate amount of protein is ideal. As the mantra throughout this book has been, eat even the good foods in moderation, and be conscious of the balance of how and what you eat.

Broadly speaking, I recommend you follow a healthy, whole-foods diet like the Mediterranean eating pattern, and make sure to include or exclude certain foods based on how they affect your sleep. One credible finding is that if your diet has a smaller variety of foods in it, you will likely have worse sleep, so try to mix in as many foods as possible.[18] Whether it helps sleep or not, that's good advice in general; it makes eating novel and fun and diversifies your opportunity to get a wide array of nutrients.

FOODS THAT DISRUPT SLEEP

Certain foods will disrupt your sleep and make it far more difficult for you to feel refreshed. Let's consider foods you should limit when you're focused on getting a good night's sleep.

Caffeine

It's not rocket science to know that caffeine will keep you up at night—after all, feeling awake and alert is why we drink it in the first place. Drinking caffeine is a double-edged sword. On the one hand, it does make you more alert. On the other, if it prevents you from sleeping well, you will be less alert the following day. Researchers refer to this as the "sleep sandwich" effect, where sleep is sandwiched between two days of caffeine consumption, getting slowly squeezed down to fewer hours. Unfortunately, the number of people who fall prey to this effect is increasing. Close to 33 percent of Americans sleep fewer than six hours per night.[19]

Caffeine acts on adenosine receptors in the brain, which are associated with sleep, arousal, and cognition.[20] Many studies have shown that caffeine can disrupt sleep considerably. In 2013, Christopher Drake and his colleagues gave 400 mg of caffeine (roughly 4 cups of brewed coffee) to three groups of people either just as they were going to sleep or three or six hours prior.[21] All caffeine groups experienced a disruption in their sleep compared to placebo.

However, as we've seen previously, there are net benefits of caffeine, so simply eliminating it isn't necessarily the best strategy. Extensive research indicates that having 3–4 cups of coffee daily may help you to live longer, and it may protect you from heart disease, cancer, and neurologic, metabolic, and liver conditions too.[22] So the optimal solution is to use caffeine wisely and learn to recognize when it is working against you.

I suggest following these guidelines: drink 3–4 small to medium cups of coffee or caffeinated tea a day, but stop all caffeine consumption by three p.m. to be safe. If you're extra-sensitive to caffeine, avoid decaffeinated beverages late in the day too—Starbucks' decaffeinated coffee may actually have up to 13.9 mg of caffeine per 16-ounce serving.

Alcohol

Aidan was an eighteen-year-old college student who came to see me because he was depressed. His grades were dropping, and whenever a test approached, his anxiety shot through the roof. When I took a history, he told me he drank heavily on weekends when he knew he could sleep in the next day but stayed sober on weeknights when he had to get up early the following morning. This pattern of alcohol use isn't unusual among college students or other social drinkers, and it sounds logical; feeling tired after drinking should be mitigated by getting extra sleep on the weekends, right? Well, it's not quite that simple.

I recommended a sleep study on one of Aidan's sober days, and even though he was not drinking, his sleep was very poor. In particular, his REM sleep was disrupted, which was probably hurting his ability to remember information during exams and contributing to his pre-test anxiety.

Since he was reluctant to take medication, I recommended that he try giving up drinking for a month. Though this was difficult for him, he managed it, and the results were remarkable. His anxiety dropped and his grades improved significantly. He did go back to drinking alcohol after his month off but he did so far less frequently, and he now understood the damage that it could do to his sleep.

Alcohol is a sedative, so in theory it will put you to sleep faster.[23] However, soon after you go to sleep, it disrupts the normal sleep cycle. If we looked at Aidan's brainwaves on a night when he'd had a few too many, in the first half of the night we'd see an increase in slow-wave sleep.[24] Slow-wave sleep is very deep, and under a normal sleep schedule it takes some time for your body to get there. Though alcohol gets you into deep sleep much faster, in the second half of the night, your sleep is of poor quality, leaving you feeling drained in the morning.[25]

Alcohol also suppresses REM sleep, which in turn leads to issues with mental performance—as we saw with Aidan's slipping grades. A lack of REM sleep can make it more difficult to cope with threatening situations too.[26] When you drink alcohol, it changes your gut bacteria in a way that increases inflammation in the gut and the brain and reduces the protective calming effects from the vagus nerve.[27] Also during both intoxication and withdrawal, the amygdala becomes activated, worsening anxiety.

People who abuse alcohol have sleep disturbances that occur even when they aren't drinking. That's why, like Aidan, weekend binge drinkers often report not feeling rested during the week when they're not drinking.

So if you're tempted to use alcohol as a sleep aid—even something as seemingly innocent as a glass or two of wine before bed to "wind down"—be cognizant that drinking may end up hurting more than it helps. Even if you don't think of yourself as a heavy drinker, if you're having trouble sleeping, try abstaining totally for a month or so and seeing if your sleep improves.

FOODS THAT HELP YOU SLEEP

Melanie was a thirty-six-year-old food blogger. She spent her days testing recipes, making videos, posting pictures on social media, and responding to online queries. From the time she started her morning exercise routine to the time she slipped under the covers, there wasn't a wasted minute. When she eventually turned her light off, however, she couldn't get to sleep. Sometimes it took her two to three hours before she could fall asleep, and she often struggled to stay asleep all night. Since she went to bed at eleven p.m. and woke up at six a.m. daily, she would regularly struggle through her days on four hours of sleep.

When she came to see me, she was really frustrated. She had tried turning the television off early, putting away her phone well before bed, avoiding caffeine, and counting sheep, but none of these things had worked. So we started talking about her diet.

First, we identified foods that were especially lacking. She had very little oily fish in her diet, so I suggested she add in salmon, fresh tuna, and sardines. I also suggested that she add blueberries to her morning cereal and make a calming chamomile and tart cherry juice drink before bedtime.

With these changes, Melanie was able to fall asleep much more easily, and she stayed asleep all night long. Let's take a closer look at the foods that can help you sleep better.

Omega-3s

You can add improved sleep to the long list of benefits of omega-3 polyunsaturated fatty acids. A number of studies in animals demonstrate that omega-3s decrease inflammation and normalize sleep and that they protect the brain from memory impairment in sleep-deprived mice.[28]

There are also an increasing number of studies that demonstrate the beneficial effects of omega-3s on human sleep. For instance, in 2018 Leila Jahangard and her colleagues conducted a study on fifty depressed patients.[29] Compared to those on a placebo, the participants who received omega-3s improved their depression, anxiety, and emotional control, and over time they improved their sleep as well.

Omega-3s exert a direct or indirect effect on a host of factors that are necessary for good sleep.[30] For example, some fatty acids are precursors of prostaglandins, sleep-promoting substances in the brain. Other fatty acids contribute to the development of melatonin, necessary for sleep.[31] Omega-3s increase sleep efficiency and REM sleep too.[32]

Melatonin

Melatonin is a hormone produced naturally in the brain that regulates the body's circadian rhythms. Several research studies have shown that melatonin can help people fall asleep and can be very useful for jet lag, when our internal time clocks get disrupted. Melatonin can also help those suffering from seasonal depression by regulating their sleep cycles.

Melatonin is available as a supplement, but it also occurs naturally in certain foods. Food sources include eggs, fish, milk, rice and other grains (barley and rolled oats), fruits (grapes, pomegranates), nuts (especially pistachios and walnuts), seeds (sunflower seeds, mustard seeds, and flaxseeds), and a variety of vegetables (asparagus, tomatoes, broccoli, and cucumber).

Tryptophan

As we discussed in chapter 3, the popular myth that the tryptophan in Thanksgiving turkey makes you sleepy isn't always true, since it's difficult for dietary tryptophan to reach the brain. But there's no doubt that when tryptophan does make it into your brain, it puts you right to sleep.[33] Tryptophan increases blood and brain serotonin and melatonin, both of which help you get to sleep more easily.[34]

Tryptophan can be used in sleep therapy; it is usually dosed as an "interval therapy," in which people take the drug for a few weeks, hold off for a few weeks, and then restart. Again, I want to emphasize that supplements like tryptophan should only be taken under the supervision of a doctor. In fact, although in the United States tryptophan is regulated as a dietary supplement, in Canada, it is regulated as a medication.

If you would rather not take a supplement and would like to get as much tryptophan as possible from food, remember our corollary to the Thanksgiving myth: while much dietary tryptophan isn't absorbed into the brain, it can help to combine good sources of tryptophan with carbohydrates, like turkey and mashed potatoes. That same nutritional sensibility applies to cereal with milk (make sure to choose a healthy, low-sugar, whole-grain cereal), peanut butter on whole-grain toast, or cheese and whole wheat crackers. All these snack combinations can help you go to sleep.

Tryptophan is also found in pumpkin and squash seeds, roasted soybeans, cooked lamb shoulder, and cooked tuna. Not all of these make for perfect bedtime snacks, but it can't hurt to increase some of these foods in your diet, along with carbs, at dinner if you're struggling to sleep.

L-Ornithine

As we've discussed before, there are nine essential amino acids that cannot be made by the body and therefore must come from food sources. Like tryptophan, L-ornithine is an essential amino acid that has the potential to improve sleep quality when you're fatigued.[35] It is produced in the body from foods containing L-arginine.

The simplest way to get L-arginine is to eat complete protein sources, which means they contain all nine essential amino acids, which the body cannot produce on its own. These include meat, poultry, fish, eggs, soybeans, and quinoa.

Chamomile

We discussed chamomile in chapter 3 when talking about herbs that could help lessen the effects of anxiety, but its most enduring use is as a sleep aid. I'm sure you have heard about chamomile tea helping you sleep, and with good reason: chamomile is one of the most ancient herbs in existence, and science has backed up its positive effects.

In 2017, Mohsen Adib-Hajbaghery and his colleague conducted a sleep study in people more than sixty years of age who received either 200 mg of chamomile extract capsules or a placebo daily for twenty-eight consecutive days.[36] The study found that consuming the chamomile improved sleep quality significantly. And in 2019, a meta-analysis of all studies on chamomile tea and sleep demonstrated that it was very effective for improving sleep quality.[37]

The sedative effect of chamomile is attributed mainly to one of its constituents, a flavonoid called apigenin, which binds to the same receptors in the brain as Valium and Xanax.[38]

The most common way to get chamomile is to simply drink chamomile tea (though technically speaking, it's an "infusion" since there is no actual tea in the drink). Different kinds of teas have different amounts of chamomile, but it can be difficult to tell how much chamomile is in a given cup. Still, I would recommend 1–3 cups (8 ounces per cup) per day. I suggest to my patients that they have their last cup in the early evening so that it mellows them down in preparation for bed but leaves enough time for them to use the bathroom if needed.

Before you start drinking chamomile tea, clear it with your doctor, since chamomile can interact with sedatives, blood thinners, and painkillers. Also, if you are allergic to ragweed, daisies, marigolds, or chrysanthemums, you should avoid drinking chamomile, as you may be allergic to it as well.

Other Micronutrients

In addition to chamomile, there are many other naturally occurring compounds that can improve sleep, including gamma-aminobutyric acid (GABA), calcium, potassium, melatonin, pyridoxine, and hexadecenoic acid. You can get supplements of many of these dietary additives, but there are foods that contain these and other helpful substances too.

Barley grass powder is rich in antioxidants, electrolytes such as potassium, and GABA, all of which protect the brain and help you go to sleep.[39]

Maca is a plant relative of radish that smells like butterscotch. Found in places like Peru and China, it contains calcium, potassium, and fatty acids that also help with sleep.[40]

The *Panax ginseng* flower and leaf stimulate GABA receptors in the brain that promote sleep.[41] *Panax ginseng* is known as Asian, Chinese, or red ginseng, not to be confused with its American counterpart (which can have the opposite effect, as we will discuss shortly).

Lingzhi is an oriental fungus, which also stimulates GABA receptors and promotes sleep.[42]

Lettuce contains a substance known as lactucin, which is thought to contribute to its sedative properties.[43]

Cherries are a rich source of polyphenols and vitamin C.[44] As a result, they decrease inflammation and promote sleep. Tart cherry juice is a preparation that has been shown to reduce insomnia.[45] In 2018, Jack Losso and his colleagues administered either cherry juice or placebo to eleven subjects for two weeks and found that cherry juice increased sleep time and sleep efficiency.[46] While this is a small study, it provided the first human evidence for cherry juice as a sleep aid. Cherry juice is thought to increase tryptophan availability and reduce inflammation.

FOODS THAT FIGHT FATIGUE

If you're not sleeping well, it's only logical that the most noticeable consequence is going to be fatigue. You're not going to be able to tackle life's highs and lows with energy. But lack of sleep is far from the only reason that you might feel fatigued; there are lots of reasons why your body and brain may not be operating at peak efficiency.

If you are persistently fatigued, it is important to see a doctor, as fatigue can be rooted in many serious medical conditions such as heart and thyroid disease. When these have been ruled out, nutrition is a good place to start thinking about how to raise your energy levels.

Anti-inflammatory Foods

One reason for fatigue is chronic low-grade inflammation, which can be caused by several factors, including obesity, depression, and chronic pain.

When inflammation is present in the body, less energy is available to the brain. That's because low-grade inflammation flips off a metabolic switch in the chemical pathway that produces energy. The result is not only lower energy but an increase in toxic free radicals that damage brain tissue and reduce insulin sensitivity.

Because of this cycle, foods that increase inflammation can decrease your energy availability. To reduce inflammation, it is important to eat an anti-inflammatory diet.[47] We've covered plenty of anti-inflammatory foods thus far in the book, but the central tenets of an anti-inflammatory diet are as follows:

- Your brain is made up of 60 percent fat. In order to perform at its best, it requires a constant supply of omega-3 fatty acids—at least 2–3 g combined of eicosapentaenoic acid and docosahexaenoic acid per day.

- Reducing omega-6 fatty acids is key to maintaining the correct balance of omega-3s to omega-6s. Eating an excess of omega-6s can trigger the body to produce chemicals that spike inflammation. These fatty acids are found in oils such as corn, safflower, sunflower, grapeseed, soy, peanut, and vegetable. That means you should cut down on mayonnaise, many salad dressings, and most processed and fast foods.
- A diet rich in colorful, nonstarchy vegetables adds polyphenols, which fight inflammation through a number of processes. Other sources of polyphenols include: cloves, star anise, cocoa powder (natural, non-alkalized), Mexican oregano, dark chocolate, chestnuts, and flaxseed meal.[48] Black and green tea, blackberries, muscadine grape seeds, apple-cider vinegar, cinnamon, and superfruits such as the maqui berry may also help to decrease inflammation.[49]
- When you are on an anti-inflammatory diet, you must stabilize insulin by eating whole, plant-based foods rich in healthy fat (avocados, dark chocolate, olives, chia seeds, coconut, almonds, pecans, and walnuts) and natural chemicals.[50] Eat vegetables such as cauliflower, green beans, and broccoli.

If you follow these tenets, your body will be less inflamed and you will feel more energized and rejuvenated.[51]

Magnesium and Zinc

More than two decades ago, researchers realized that patients with chronic fatigue syndrome had low magnesium levels in their red blood cells. When their magnesium was replaced, they felt more energized.[52]

Magnesium decreases inflammation and relaxes the nervous system. For example, when you exercise, lactate accumulates in your blood, which leads to tired and achy limbs. However, magnesium can prevent this lactate accumulation, which in turn helps relieve fatigue.[53]

Food sources of magnesium include dry roasted almonds, boiled spinach, dry roasted cashews, soy milk, cooked black beans, and edamame.

Low zinc levels are also a hallmark of chronic fatigue syndrome, and increasing zinc can improve and prevent fatigue.[54] Zinc deficiency is very common, with about half of the world's population prone to zinc deficiencies due to dietary patterns. To get more zinc, incorporate lamb, pumpkin seeds, hemp seeds, grass-fed beef, and chickpeas into your diet.

Vitamins

Vitamins play an essential role in protecting the brain and energizing you. While you can certainly take a multivitamin to help bolster your levels of many vitamins, I encourage you to get as much as you can through natural sources. That means a balance of meat, fish, eggs, fruits, and vegetables. When I see patients with vitamin deficiencies, I usually see a glaring gap in their diets. Either they eat no meat or they eat few fruits and vegetables. If you feel this might be the case for you, examine your weekly diet to see where the gaps are. Then reflect on how you might increase the diversity of nutrients. For instance, over the years I have encountered many patients whose energy levels quickly improved after adding citrus fruits back into their diets.

Here are how specific vitamins work to provide you with the energy you need (for common food sources of these vitamins, see Appendix B):

Thiamine: Decreased thiamine levels (vitamin B_1) can result in altered mitochondrial activity. Since the mitochondria are the energy factory of your body's cells, that means reduced energy production.

Neurons have high energy requirements, which means they are especially vulnerable to a thiamine deficit.

B_6: Vitamin B_6, also called pyridoxine, is low in patients with chronic fatigue syndrome.[55] In the brains of animals, vitamin B_6 deficiency correlates with less glucose being utilized to produce energy.[56] A lack of vitamin B_6 also leads to a disruption of the connections among brain cells, decreasing efficient processing of information. Fatigue is a natural consequence.

Vitamin B_6 deficiency is more common in pregnant or lactating women, and it may also result from chronic alcoholism.

Folate: Vitamin B_9 is also known as folate. Like deficiency in other B vitamins, folate deficiency is associated with chronic fatigue syndrome.[57] Folate is also involved in cell development throughout the body. Without it, development is slowed down, and you are likely to feel fatigued from increased energy demands.[58]

The fatigue from folate deficiency may occur due to anemia. For instance, a forty-four-year-old man presented to a primary care internal medicine clinic with a one-month history of shortness of breath, fatigue, and numbness and tingling in his fingers.[59] After extensive investigations, his physicians found that he had a type of anemia called macrocytic anemia, which is commonly caused by folate deficiency. Anemia prevents you from having sufficient oxygen in your tissues, which leads to fatigue.

While there are other causes of fatigue besides anemia, I have seen many patients who simply have a lack of folate-rich foods in their diet.

B_{12}: Vitamin B_{12} (also known as cobalamin) deficiency has been associated with fatigue in certain instances, such as after a stroke.[60] We covered dietary sources of B_{12} in chapter 7, but in certain cases, for example, if patients suffer from gastritis, anemia, or Crohn's disease, those sources may not be sufficient. Although there is some controversy as to whether oral vitamin B_{12} is sufficient to increase

levels, many studies have shown that it is.[61] However, some people may need an injection to bring levels up. Your doctor will be able to help you monitor your B_{12} levels and determine your needs.

Vitamin C: Vitamin C is a crucial antioxidant in the brain,[62] and fatigue is a common symptom if you are low in vitamin C.

Vitamin D: When you do not have high enough levels of vitamin D, brain injury and inflammation ensue.[63] Vitamin D helps nerve growth and assists in the production of brain tissue. You can make your own vitamin D, but you need to expose your skin to the sun, and not through windows. Of course, excessive sun exposure poses its own risks, including skin cancer. Low SPF sunscreen appears not to affect vitamin D production, but higher SPF sunscreens may hamper it.[64] My dermatological colleagues would have some choice words for me if I told you not to wear sunscreen, so that's why nutritional sources are so important.

Vitamin E: Vitamin E (also known as alpha-tocopherol) can become deficient when there is malabsorption of fat, so deficiency is common in people who have digestive disorders or those who cannot absorb fat properly due to conditions such as cystic fibrosis or celiac disease.[65] It, too, is important for the developing nervous system, ensuring that the body's energy needs are met.

Capsaicin

Capsaicin is the compound in chili peppers that makes them spicy. In addition to adding a delicious burn to food, it has been shown to reduce fatigue in mice.[66] In humans, consuming 2.5 mg of capsaicin per meal (7.68 mg/day) has been shown to restore the energy balance in the body.[67]

Capsaicin affects energy because it impacts glucose metabolism in the body.[68] When capsaicin enters the gut, it triggers a vagal response to the brain, thereby regulating appetite by helping hormones from the brain's appetite regulation center more effectively detect when enough is enough.[69] There is increasing evidence attesting to its anti-obesity potential, which probably also helps fatigue.

The amount of capsaicin varies widely among different types of peppers, and it's proportional to how spicy the chili tastes. For example, the relatively mild jalapeño has only 0.165–0.33 mg of capsaicin. A serrano chili contains 0.396–1.518 mg of capsaicin. Spicier chilies like Thai bird's eye chilies and habaneros can be an efficient way to get capsaicin (if you can handle them!).

Rather than trying to add up capsaicin levels, I recommend that you try to incorporate more spicy food into your diet. Use extra cayenne pepper in your cooking, and if you order in Thai, Indian, or other spicy foods, order them one level spicier than you normally would.

Bear in mind that it's not just generic "spiciness" that matters, but the capsaicin itself. In other words, spicy foods that derive their burn from non-capsaicin compounds, like mustard, horseradish, black pepper, and ginger, do not affect energy balance in the same way.[70]

Other Spices

Black cumin: In one study in rats, *Nigella sativa* seed, commonly known as black cumin, helped fatigue after exhaustive swimming. It is known to be neuroprotective due to its antioxidant properties.[71] It also increases acetylcholine in the brain, which helps your muscles contract.

Though this is a very promising spice, we need more data, especially from human studies, before we can be sure it has a marked positive effect. Still, it can't hurt to integrate it into your food. You may see it sold as nigella seeds, onion seeds, or kalonji (the Hindi name). It can be used in Indian naan bread, Bengali potato stir-fry, and preserved lemons.

Turmeric: Our old friend curcumin, the active ingredient in turmeric, has been found to increase muscle glycogen content in mice.[72]

Glycogen is an important energy source. In humans, it may help in the management of exercise-induced inflammation and muscle soreness, thus enhancing recovery and performance in active people. Just 100 mg of curcumin can improve fatigue.

American Ginseng

Ginseng is often marketed as a supplement that increases energy levels and alleviates fatigue. There are some indications that this could be the case, since ginseng affects brain activity, specifically by increasing brain levels of dopamine, noradrenaline, and serotonin. It may also increase energy produced in the brain.

There are no food sources of ginseng, but it is sometimes added to drinks and foods, and it is available as a supplement.

FOOD IS ENERGY

I hope this chapter has proved to you that food is energy in more than one way. Of course, the calories you get through food provide the fuel that makes your biological systems go, but food can also be a key component in helping your body rest, allowing you to thrive with a clear mind and healthy attitude.

If you have trouble sleeping (or are fatigued while you're awake), I encourage you to try out the dietary strategies we've discussed. But it's also important to practice good overall sleep habits—sometimes called sleep hygiene. Make sure you're allowing yourself enough time for sleep, and keep a steady sleep routine. Ensure that your sleep environment is dark and peaceful, and avoid checking your phone, working on your computer, or watching TV at bedtime, since these can stimulate your brain and keep you awake. Avoid taking long naps during the day, which can disrupt nighttime sleep.

I know it can feel hard to prioritize sleep with all the demands of work, child care, and entertainment. But I promise you that getting a good night's sleep is fundamental to good overall health.

INSOMNIA AND FATIGUE CHEAT SHEET

Foods to Embrace:

- Omega-3 fatty acids: Fish, especially fatty fish like salmon, mackerel, tuna, herring, and sardines.
- Melatonin: Eggs, fish, milk, rice, barley and rolled oats, grapes, pomegranates, walnuts, sunflower seeds, mustard seeds, flaxseeds, asparagus, broccoli, and cucumber.
- Tryptophan: Turkey, other meats, and chickpeas, especially when combined with carbohydrates.
- L-ornithine: Meat, poultry, fish, eggs, soybeans, and quinoa.
- Chamomile tea.
- Foods containing helpful micronutrients: Lettuce, tart cherry juice, barley grass powder, maca, *Panax ginseng,* lingzhi, asparagus powder.

For Fatigue:

- Anti-inflammatory foods: Omega-3s, colorful vegetables for polyphenols.
- Minerals: Magnesium and zinc.
- Vitamins B_1, B_6, B_9, B_{12}, C, D, and E.
- Capsaicin-rich foods: Chili peppers including cayenne, serranos, and jalapeños.
- Spices: Black cumin and turmeric.

Foods to Avoid:

- Caffeine: You don't have to completely eliminate caffeine, but stick to the guideline of no more than 400 mg/day, and don't drink caffeine after three p.m.
- Alcohol: Though alcohol can put you to sleep, it also disrupts sleep.

CHAPTER NINE

Bipolar Disorder and Schizophrenia: L-Theanine, Healthy Fats, and the Ketogenic Diet

When it comes to serious psychiatric disorders, none are more recognizable than bipolar disorder (BD) and schizophrenia (SCZ). The two conditions have become so pervasive in the culture that they've been transformed into slangy adjectives in the modern lexicon. If something is "bipolar," it changes swiftly and violently — maybe the weather on a day that swings from chilly to warm or vice versa. If something is "schizophrenic," it has a split personality — perhaps an unpredictable boss who one moment is glowing with pride and the next fuming with anger.

Both of these popular usages are misrepresentations to a degree. While patients suffering from bipolar disorder do experience dramatic changes in mood, the up and down phases don't swing on a moment-to-moment basis, with manic episodes that generally last at least a week and depressive phases often lasting two weeks or more.

Despite the longtime association, SCZ does not have anything to do with "split personality," which is more likely a symptom of dissociative identity disorder. In medical literature, SCZ's symptoms are split into positive and negative. Positive symptoms include psychotic behavior not seen in the healthy population, like delusions and hallucinations. Negative symptoms are those that affect normal behaviors, like garbled speech or simply looking withdrawn and depressed.

Bipolar disorder and schizophrenia have parallels, and in fact some psychiatrists don't draw a clear distinction between the two conditions. Diagnosis in psychiatry can be controversial, and the criteria listed in the *Diagnostic and Statistical Manual of Mental Disorders* are not robustly based on research—relying instead on lists of symptoms. The categories aren't always satisfying to clinicians.[1] So while technically BD is classified as a mood disorder and SCZ is classified as a psychotic disorder, BD sometimes presents with psychotic symptoms such as hallucinations, which makes it difficult to tell them apart. On the other hand, someone with schizophrenia may also have a mood component, seeming irritable or angry, which may be interpreted as bipolar disorder.

In fact, some researchers don't believe that SCZ exists, while others see BD and SCZ as existing on a spectrum from mood swings to mood swings with psychosis to mostly psychosis.[2] In deference to the traditional idea that they are separate conditions, I will address them one by one in this chapter, but as you'll see, they benefit from many of the same dietary inclusions and exclusions.

BIPOLAR DISORDER

Nancy was a longtime patient of mine; I diagnosed her with bipolar disorder when she was twenty-one years old. She had been stable on 1200 mg of lithium and clonazepam for about a decade. Then she started a new job, and all hell broke loose.

She became stressed and stayed up at night with her mind racing. At work, she could not concentrate because her mind flitted from one subject to the next. She found herself putting together elaborate to-do lists that were an attempt to manage her time but ended up becoming a jumbled mountain of tasks that felt insurmountable. When she got home, instead of relaxing, she kept the lists going.

With an increase in distractibility, racing thoughts, and too much goal-directed activity, I recognized that she was hypomanic—hypomania is a less severe form of mania, but troublesome nonetheless. She had been stable on her medication for so long that I was hesitant to start changing it. So, before I made any adjustments, I checked on her dietary history. To my surprise, I found a number of things off-kilter. As she was stressed and always in a rush, she had switched from her regular protein shake for breakfast to bagels and muffins. She was drinking more coffee than usual so that she could concentrate at work. And at night, she was having a few glasses of wine, hoping they would help her go to sleep.

You're probably sensing familiar patterns in her eating habits that were harming her already delicate state of mind. To understand fully, let's consider the connection between the gut and brain in bipolar disorder.

THE BIPOLAR GUT

One of the key symptoms of BD is mood lability, a fancy way of saying that moods are prone to dramatic changes. For a week or so, people with bipolar disorder may be so hyperalert that they stay up all night, talk really fast, and struggle to focus on any one thing—they experience mania. After about a week they may plunge into depression, become withdrawn and worried, and have no interest in day-to-day activities.

The seriousness of BD goes beyond dramatic mood swings. People who have BD die prematurely from a variety of secondary medical causes. For instance, obesity occurs in 40 percent of adolescent youth with BD—twice the rate of the general population—which is exacerbated by the fact that many BD medications have weight gain as a side effect. BD patients also have more cardiovascular disease, diabetes, and autoimmune disease than the general population. That's why some researchers think of bipolar disorder not solely as a mental condition, but as a multisystem inflammatory disease.[3]

As we already know, the ongoing, low-grade inflammation in your body is often related to disruptions to your gut. When this widespread inflammation throughout the body occurs, the marker C-reactive protein increases. When BD patients are in either depressed or manic states, we also see an increase in C-reactive protein, an indicator that gut inflammation may also be associated with mood swings.

The links between BD and gut inflammation will likely sound familiar. For instance, patients with irritable bowel syndrome have more than twice the rate of BD compared to the general population.[4] There is also a rare condition called antibiomania, which is mania caused by antibiotics.[5] Indeed, the rising number of manic cases is thought to be in part due to an increase in prescriptions of new antibiotics that upset the balance of the gut microbiome.

We also see symptoms of leaky gut associated with BD. In BD patients, we can see gut chemicals in the blood by tracking a part of the gut-bacteria cell membrane called lipopolysaccharide. In healthy individuals lipopolysaccharide stays confined to the gut, but in BD patients, it leaks out, stimulating inflammation and promoting pro-inflammatory cytokines, which lead to greater depression and mood symptoms.[6]

The hypothalamic-pituitary-adrenal pathway is also affected in BD. When you are stressed, as is often the case in BD, a hormone called corticotrophin releasing factor is stimulated, presumably so that cortisol can be released from the adrenal gland to help the body cope with the stress. However, too much corticotrophin releasing factor can make the gut more "leaky" and sensitive.[7]

BD patients often have different types of gut bacteria, similar to the differences found in inflammatory bowel disease.[8] This leads to reduced levels of several familiar neurotransmitters produced by gut microbiota, including gamma-aminobutyric acid (GABA), noradrenaline, serotonin, dopamine, and acetylcholine. As we've seen so many times before, proper levels of these neurotransmitters are necessary for brain health.[9]

Given this evidence of the strong connection between BD and the gut microbiome, we know enough to start implementing dietary solutions. Let's talk foods that can impair and foods that can improve the bipolar brain.

FOODS AND EATING PATTERNS THAT WORSEN BIPOLAR DISORDER

Fluctuations between manic episodes and deep depression make it extra tricky to treat bipolar disorder with nutritional interventions. What may be good for mania may not be good for depression and vice versa, so it's important to tailor dietary treatments around the emotional seesaw. The foods that have an effect on bipolar depression mirror those that we discussed in chapter 2 on depression, so refresh your memory if you need to. Here, I will focus on studies that specifically address mania and bipolar disorder.

It's worth noting that several of the foods covered here may interact negatively with lithium.[10] Lithium has been used as the primary treatment for BD for decades, and it is so widely prescribed that it makes sense to consider the impact of different foods on its efficacy as well.

The Western Diet

Once again, we see the damaging effect of the Western diet.[11] Eating bad fats, refined carbohydrates, sugar, and meat with very few vegetables is destructive to the bipolar brain. In particular, as we saw with depression, BD patients consume more carbohydrate and high-energy foods.[12] Some researchers believe that eating sugar and comfort food is a form of self-medication for BD patients, but there is no doubt that an unhealthy diet ends up being physiological self-sabotage.

Switching to a diet like the Mediterranean eating pattern is helpful for BD.[13] However, it is difficult for BD patients to stick to healthier foods. Giving up a high-fat, high-sugar diet may be particularly challenging for sufferers of BD, because close to 10 percent of bipolar patients have binge-eating disorder, a condition that leads to out-of-control eating.[14] In 2017, Matias Melo showed that people with bipolar disorder also have night-eating syndrome, meaning they eat less during the day and binge at night, sometimes even waking up from a deep sleep to do so. That isn't a recipe for making healthy choices.[15]

With enough work and support it's possible for BD patients to change their eating habits. One study demonstrated that patients with BD could reduce their body mass index, and another demonstrated that having support from a nurse and lifestyle coach made a difference. Given the difficulty of implementing nutritional interventions with BD, it is important to have social support while doing so.[16]

While the Mediterranean eating pattern is a good alternative to the Western diet, there's another diet that has shown even more promise for treating BD. Preliminary data and case histories indicate that the ketogenic diet—which is high fat and low carbohydrate—has mood-stabilizing effects.[17] In 2019, Iain Campbell and Harry Campbell investigated how a ketogenic diet affected mood stabilization among individuals with bipolar disorder.[18] They analyzed text comments of 274 people in online forums about the mood effects of three types of diets: ketogenic, omega-3-enriched, and vegetarian. People reported stable moods far more often on the ketogenic diet than on any other diet.

There are many reasons for the keto diet's positive effects on BD, including its effects on glutamate/GABA transmission, in reducing oxidative stress, and in lowering overall inflammation.[19] Perhaps most important, the keto diet makes the mitochondria, your cells' energy makers, work better. Mitochondrial dysfunction has been associated with bipolar disorder.[20]

The ketogenic diet is high fat, moderate protein, and very low carbohydrates. I won't go into detail on how to implement a keto diet; it's currently in vogue for weight loss, so there is a wealth of information about how to make the switch. I recommend checking out *Keto Diet* by Dr. Josh Axe for a full rundown.

Beware that the keto diet has both short- and long-term side effects. After starting the keto diet, you may experience nausea, vomiting, headache, fatigue, dizziness, insomnia, difficulty in exercise tolerance, and constipation. This group of symptoms is sometimes referred to as keto flu and may last a few days to a few weeks. Ensuring adequate fluid and electrolyte intake can help counter some of these symptoms. Long-term adverse effects include fatty liver, low protein in the blood, kidney stones, and vitamin and mineral deficiencies. If you want to try the keto diet, it is important to consult your doctor.

Caffeine

Randy, a twenty-year-old literature major, was considering transitioning his gender (he preferred to use male pronouns when I treated him). This was a challenging time for him, and his stress was a factor in precipitating a manic episode during which he stayed up all night for most of three weeks, jumped over a highway median, and had delusions that he was Jesus come to save the world. He was eventually hospitalized, and I saw him six months after hospitalization.

By the time I started treating him, he was stable enough on medications to begin to process his gender dysphoria. But two months into treatment, he started to rev up again, acting over-energized and developing a tremor in his hands—something that concerned me because hand tremors can be caused by toxicity from high lithium levels. Part of me wondered if we should slow down the deep processing of an issue that had tortured him his entire life, but as we talked one day, he confessed that he had been drinking energy drinks. It wasn't just 1 or 2 a day. He had been consuming about 8–10 cans a day.

Energy drinks are not uncommon among college students.[21] Red Bull, Amp, Monster, Rockstar, Rip It, Full Throttle, and the ostentatiously named Cocaine are all designed to give them energy highs to fuel both studying and partying. Each energy drink contains about 80–141 mg of caffeine per 8-ounce serving (and one can usually contains much more than 1 serving). That level of caffeine consumption is too much for anyone, but for someone with BD, it's a risk for mania. Several case histories have demonstrated the connection between energy drinks and mania in BD patients.[22]

Fortunately, Randy did not have a toxic level of lithium; his tremors were due to his system being jazzed up on all that caffeine. I asked Randy if he was willing to taper off his caffeine consumption under my direct guidance—something that has to be done carefully because caffeine withdrawal can lead to a spike in lithium levels as well. He agreed and, slowly, over the next eight weeks, reduced his caffeine use from 8–10 energy drinks a day to 1 cup of coffee in the morning. His manic symptoms disappeared, and, even without the caffeine, he was able to focus better on his work because he stopped having the hand tremor, which had made it difficult to take notes and engage in his studies.

It's not hard to understand why caffeine might be bad for BD patients in manic states. In low doses, it elevates mood, most likely due to the interaction between dopamine and adenosine receptors in the brain, but in large doses it can lead to dangerous mood elevation.[23] Caffeine also disrupts sleep patterns, another factor that makes mania more likely.[24]

Unfortunately there have been no controlled trials on the

negative effects of caffeine in BD patients. As in Randy's case, though, using common sense and doing a trial discontinuation may pay off in the long run. For most BD patients, our standard routine of no more than 400 mg/day of caffeine is fine. When cutting down, remember that patients must wean themselves off caffeine gradually. Rapidly stopping can throw an already vulnerable brain into a tailspin and pose a danger for patients taking lithium.

Changes in Sodium Levels

Maurice was a forty-five-year-old Jamaican American man who came to see me about his BD. Within a few short weeks, we got his mania under control, and lithium seemed to be working wonders. His lithium blood level was at 1, which was a perfectly respectable number, since the ideal range is between 0.6 and 1.2.

Unbeknownst to me, after I'd been seeing him for about six months, Maurice was also diagnosed with hypertension. His primary care physician asked him to follow a low-salt diet. From the perspective of treating the hypertension, this made sense. However, a low-sodium diet may enhance lithium reabsorption in the kidneys, causing lithium blood levels to shoot up. This eventually worsens kidney function, which is especially problematic in a person who is prone to high blood pressure.

Maurice developed a tremor and diarrhea. I suspected lithium toxicity. Testing showed that his blood level was 1.5. Balancing lithium's effects in a hypertensive patient can be tricky, so we switched medications and tapered the lithium off slowly. His tremor went away, and he could reengage in his low-salt diet without negative consequences.

Maurice's case was not unusual; bipolar patients often have hypertension. In fact, there are some preliminary data that indicate that mania and hypertension have a lot of overlap.[25] There are even some case histories indicating that antihypertensive drugs such as verapamil and beta-blockers may help people with mania. Both disorders are associated with a greater incidence of stroke, thyroid disease, and diabetes.

Still, if you are taking lithium, it's important to keep sodium levels consistent. And if you're seeing multiple medical professionals about multiple conditions, make sure to keep everyone informed of each treatment you undergo.

Gluten

Recent studies have found elevated gluten-related antibodies in patients with bipolar disorder and have indicated that manic episodes may be associated with increased serum levels of antibodies against gliadin, a class of proteins present in wheat.[26] In other words, patients with BD are more likely to have celiac disease or non-celiac gluten sensitivity.

One study demonstrated that ASCA, a marker that is associated with both inflammatory bowel disease and celiac disease, was elevated in bipolar disorder.[27] Patients who were ASCA-positive were three to four times more likely to have bipolar disorder. In other words, there is evidence that the immune system in bipolar disorder is off-kilter, and when the bowel lining is compromised, foods including gluten and dairy caseins may instigate immune responses.

Since the case histories and basic science indicate that going gluten-free may be helpful, I often ask my patients to consider a week of gluten-free eating to observe if their mood stability improves.

Alcohol

In 2006, Benjamin Goldstein and his colleagues conducted a study in which they examined the relationship between alcohol use and BD in 148 patients.[28] None of the study participants were heavy drinkers; men consumed fewer than 4 drinks per week, and women consumed fewer than 1.5 drinks per week. Despite this low level of alcohol use, men with BD who drank closer to 4 drinks per week had more manic episodes and visited the emergency room more often over the course of their lives than those who drank less. Consuming spirits put them especially at risk. For women, the more alcohol they drank, the greater the likelihood of depression and hypomania.

Other studies have indicated that heavy alcohol consumption placed BD patients at risk for depression and that alcohol use put patients at greater risk of not adhering to their medication regimens.[29] Drinking too much alcohol may make for a slow recovery from bipolar depression, and it increases the chances of a manic episode.[30]

Together, these studies are strong evidence that patients suffering from BD should abstain from alcohol or, at the very least, severely restrict its use.

Grapefruit Juice, Tyramine, and Other Foods That May Interfere with Medication

As we've touched on earlier in the book, though grapefruit juice may seem like a tart, harmless way to start the day, it can inhibit the enzyme system that metabolizes certain drugs in the liver, thereby increasing the blood levels of medication.[31] This includes certain antidepressants, antianxiety medications, mood stabilizers, stimulants, and antipsychotics. All these types of drugs are commonly used in the treatment of BD.

For BD patients who are on MAOI antidepressants, it is important to avoid foods that contain the amino acid tyramine, which may inhibit the drug's function and cause a serious spike in blood pressure that requires emergency treatment.

Foods rich in tyramine include aged cheese, aged or cured meats, fava beans, Marmite (concentrated yeast extract), sauerkraut, soy sauce, and tap beer. A doctor can help you track many other relevant foods.

MOOD-STABILIZING FOODS AND SUPPLEMENTS

Omega-3s

We've seen many ways in which omega-3 fatty acids enhance mental health by protecting the brain, and there are some encouraging signs for bipolar disorder. In 2003, psychiatrists Simona Noaghiul and Joseph R. Hibbeln found that people who ate more seafood—a major source of omega-3s—had a lower prevalence of BD.[32] In 2011, David Mischoulon and colleagues conducted a meta-analysis of six clinical trials in which patients randomly received omega-3 supplementation or placebo.[33] They demonstrated a significant positive effect on depressive symptoms, though there was no improvement in manic symptoms. This should come as no surprise, given what we learned in chapter 2 about the power of omega-3s to fight depression. Even if they are only aimed at depressive symptoms, I recommend that BD patients eat a steady diet of omega-3s, given their broad-ranging benefits.

N-Acetylcysteine

In 2018, Jair Soares and his colleagues reported that when BD patients were given a combination of aspirin and the supplement N-acetylcysteine (NAC), their depressive symptoms resolved after sixteen weeks, an improvement over placebo.[34] This confirmed findings from earlier studies showing that NAC on its own was effective for bipolar depression. However, a more recent study could only partially confirm this effect, suggesting that NAC augmentation may not work for every patient.[35]

As we saw in our discussion of OCD in chapter 7, NAC is a derivative of the amino acid cysteine. It has antioxidant properties and protects brain tissue from damage by free radicals by decreasing inflammation. NAC is not found in food sources, but in the body, it converts into cysteine. Cysteine itself is found in onions, garlic, egg yolks, oats, Brussels sprouts, broccoli, red peppers, wheat germ, yeast, and dairy products like ricotta cheese, cottage cheese, and yogurt.

Folate and Folic Acid

In 2017, my Massachusetts General Hospital colleague Andrew Nierenberg and his co-investigators conducted a trial of L-methylfolate, a form of folate (vitamin B_9), in patients with bipolar depression.[36] The majority of patients had more than 50 percent improvement in depressive symptoms.

Another study demonstrated that in BD patients being treated with lithium, 200 mcg of folic acid protects them from relapsing.[37] However, a subsequent trial found that although folic acid supplementation may decrease the time to onset of symptoms, it doesn't prevent mood disorder any better than placebo.[38] That said, when folic acid is added to sodium valproate, a medication used to treat mania, it confers additional improvement.[39]

Some good food sources of folate include asparagus, leafy greens, bananas, legumes (cooked lentils and kidney beans), citrus fruit (oranges, lemons, limes, though remember to avoid grapefruit), beets, eggs, avocados, wheat germ, almonds, and flaxseeds.

Magnesium

In 1999, Angela Heiden and her colleagues administered intravenous magnesium sulfate to patients with severe, therapy-resistant manic agitation for seven to twenty-three days.[40] During the infusion, the subjects needed much less of their standard BD medications to feel stable. More than half of the patients showed marked clinical improvement, with no prohibitive side effects.

Two years prior to this, an oral magnesium preparation was found to have results equivalent to lithium in at least 50 percent of patients.[41]

Both of these studies are consistent with others that demonstrate that unmedicated BD patients have low levels of magnesium. It's also worth noting that lithium increases magnesium levels in the blood, which is possibly part of why it's an effective treatment for BD.

Though the evidence for magnesium's efficacy in treating BD isn't airtight, it's worth considering dietary supplementation with nuts, spinach, black beans, edamame, peanut butter, and avocado.

Zinc

In 2016, Marcin Siwek and his colleagues found that people with BD have decreased zinc during the depressive phase of their illness.[42] Another study indicated that for women with BD, lower zinc concentrations correlated with more severe depression.[43] When they were manic, hypomanic, or in remission, zinc levels were normal.

This squares with our discussion of zinc as a way to fight depression in chapter 2. I highly recommend that BD patients make sure to eat enough zinc, especially during depressive phases. Dietary sources of zinc include seafood (especially cooked oysters), lean beef, poultry, and egg yolks, with lower amounts in beans, nuts, and whole grains.

SCHIZOPHRENIA

Alice, a twenty-eight-year-old patient of mine, suffered from schizophrenia. When I first started treating her, she told me she believed that the Hells Angels were after her. At a Bruce Springsteen concert, she was convinced that men in leather jackets and sunglasses were in the crowd taking photographs of her. They also (allegedly) pursued her at Grateful Dead and Rolling Stones concerts. When I asked her why they might do this, she looked over both shoulders and said, "I've been sworn to secrecy. I'm sorry. I can't tell you."

It sounds outlandish, but at the time, her story was not that unusual. I had seen many patients, both male and female, who believed that they were in trouble with the Hells Angels, a particular version of a symptom called a paranoid delusion. When I started her on an antipsychotic called clozapine, she recovered. Although the symptoms never completely went away, they no longer held her back. She stopped hearing voices in her head, and she was able to function properly with less fear. Within a short period of time, she completed her GED and started working as an administrative assistant.

She stayed healthy for ten years. Then she started dating someone. Within a short period of time, I noticed the psychotic symptoms returning. I was shocked and wondered if her new relationship was troubling her. But when I took a dietary history, I noticed one big change. She and her boyfriend ate out a few times a week. She told me that they would often eat the bread at restaurants, whereas previously she ate very few wheat products. She was also drinking more, up to a few glasses of wine every night.

Hearing warning bells again? Before we dive into the specific ways Alice's new eating patterns were harming her, let's consider the gut-brain connection in schizophrenia.

THE GUT IN SCHIZOPHRENIA

Whether medicated or unmedicated, people with schizophrenia have less diversity of gut bacteria, and they even have some unique bacteria that aren't found in healthy guts.

One study demonstrated that when human feces from SCZ patients are transplanted into mice, the mice showed signs of SCZ compared to controls.[44] The mice also displayed behaviors similar to behaviors of other mice who had SCZ-like symptoms induced in another way. This animal study is powerful evidence that changes in gut bacteria can change brain chemistry.

As we saw with BD, SCZ patients have more gut problems than the general population. They have more inflammation, food intolerances, and defects of the gut wall leading to leaky gut. One postmortem study of gastrointestinal inflammation associated with

SCZ in eighty-two individuals found that 50 percent had gastritis, 88 percent had enteritis, and 92 percent had colitis, all signs of serious gut inflammation. And 20 percent of patients with irritable bowel syndrome have schizophrenia too.[45]

Due to the differences in gut function and gut bacteria, SCZ patients may have poor immunity. This means, for instance, that people with schizophrenia are more prone to bacterial infections, which leads to a greater rate of antibiotic prescriptions, potentially killing off normal gut bacteria.[46]

It's not just gut bacteria that are different in SCZ. There are also differences in the bacteria of the mouth and throat—something we don't see in the other conditions we've discussed.[47] If you think of the digestive system as one long, convoluted road from the mouth to the anus, you could say that the entire digestive highway is affected.

So, once again, diet matters in schizophrenia. Let's start with foods to avoid.

FOODS THAT WORSEN SCHIZOPHRENIA

The Western Diet

In 2015, Koji Tsuruga and his colleagues compared 237 patients diagnosed with either SCZ or schizoaffective disorder (similar to SCZ, but with additional symptoms of depression or BD) with healthy controls to see if their eating patterns put them at risk for their mental illnesses.[48] To explore whether diet correlated with illness, they divided groups into two dietary patterns. One group followed a vegetable dietary pattern and the other followed a cereal dietary pattern. People who followed the vegetable dietary pattern ate a lot of green leafy vegetables, seaweed, potatoes, and soybean products such as tofu and natto. By contrast, people who followed the cereal dietary pattern consumed a lot of rice, breads, and confectioneries.

When the researchers looked at the results, an interesting

pattern emerged. The cereal dietary pattern was associated with schizophrenia, and within this group, schizophrenia correlated to a higher ratio of unhealthy fats to total calories.

Another study shows that patients with schizophrenia tend to consume meals that contain substantially more unhealthy oils and fats. While there are many potential reasons for this, one leading idea is that SCZ patients have insufficient energy supply in the brain, and as a result fats are broken down at an increased rate.[49]

Any of this sound familiar? A combination of high levels of bad fats along with high-glycemic-index carbs and sugar is the calling card of our old friend the Western diet. Once again, we see how unhealthy it is for the brain. SCZ patients would be well served by switching to a diet heavy in vegetables and good fats, like the Mediterranean eating pattern that we have discussed.

Gluten

The idea that SCZ might be connected to gluten goes back to 1966, when physician and endocrinologist Francis Dohan reported a correlation between wheat consumption and SCZ during World War II.[50] Modern research has continued to explore the connection.

The presence of celiac disease in SCZ patients is almost double the rate of the general population. About one-third of patients with SCZ have antigliadin antibodies—about triple the rate of the general population—which can lead to both celiac disease and non-celiac gluten sensitivity.[51]

In 2018, Anastasia Levinta and her colleagues reviewed studies to determine whether being on a gluten-free diet was helpful to SCZ patients.[52] Six of nine studies demonstrated improved functioning and decreased symptom severity.

In 2019, Deanna Kelly and her colleagues conducted a study of sixteen patients with SCZ or schizoaffective disorder, all of whom had elevated antigliadin antibodies but did not have celiac disease.[53] Over five weeks, they received standardized gluten-free meals and a shake each day containing either 10 grams of gluten flour or 10 grams of rice flour.

Compared with participants who ate gluten, gluten-free participants demonstrated overall clinical improvement, better attention, fewer gastrointestinal side effects, and improvement in negative symptoms such as social withdrawal and apathy. There were no improvements in positive symptoms such as hallucinations, and cognitive symptoms were not better, but the overall effects were impressive.

Clearly, all patients with SCZ should at least try a gluten-free diet. We've already discussed eliminating gluten in chapters 3 and 5, so I won't go into detail here, but obvious foods to avoid include regular bread products, pasta, pizza, and cereals. Gluten may also show up unexpectedly in foods such as soy sauce, canned soups, licorice, imitation crabmeat, meat broths, beer, and products made with malt vinegar, malt flavoring, and malt extract.

Sugar

Eating refined sugar is a risk factor for SCZ. It has been shown to lead to poor outcomes in SCZ patients over a two-year timeframe, and SCZ patients have a greater prevalence of diabetes than the general population.[54]

Of ten studies that assessed refined sugar, breakfast cereals, and sweetened drinks, all found that the more patients ate these somewhat toxic substances, the greater the likelihood of psychosis.[55] These studies were mostly observational, so they aren't definitive, but still, SCZ patients should be encouraged to cut down their sugar intake as much as possible.

Alcohol

Drinking alcohol complicates the clinical picture of SCZ. More than 6 percent of schizophrenic patients have a history of hazardous alcohol consumption. Alcohol use usually starts after the earliest symptoms of the disease, so it is not thought to be a cause of SCZ per se, but alcohol abuse may be a result of the negative symptoms patients experience.[56]

One study looked at how alcohol abuse affected SCZ patients who were being treated with regular injections of an antipsychotic medication called fluphenazine.[57] It found that people who drank more than 20 drinks per week had more relapses of SCZ symptoms than those who drank occasionally or not at all. They also had more frequent positive symptoms like hallucinations and delusions. Other studies have confirmed that alcohol use can increase suspiciousness, and SCZ patients typically report more hallucinations and paranoia after drinking alcohol.[58]

Alcohol worsens symptoms of schizophrenia because it amplifies the negative effects of abnormalities that already exist in schizophrenic brains. For instance, people with SCZ have reduced white matter volume and changes in hippocampal anatomy that can be worsened by alcohol.[59] My advice to SCZ patients is to drink little to no alcohol. I find if I insist on complete abstinence they feel unfairly restricted, so I compromise by recommending no more than 1 drink per week, perhaps with Saturday dinner.

REALITY-RESETTING FOODS

Omega-3s

In 2009, Paul Amminger and his colleagues studied eighty-one people at "ultra-high risk" of a psychotic disorder.[60] These subjects were not being treated with antipsychotics. Over twelve weeks, participants were given a supplement of omega-3 polyunsaturated fatty acids or a placebo, followed by a phase of monitoring. By the end of the study, which lasted twelve months, two of forty-one individuals (4.9 percent) in the omega-3 group and eleven of forty (27.5 percent) in the placebo group developed a psychotic disorder. Omega-3 polyunsaturated fatty acids also significantly reduced positive and negative symptoms compared with placebo. This was a powerful demonstration of the protective effects of omega-3 in psychoses like SCZ.

This dramatic result hasn't been replicated in every study, but a recent review has agreed that omega-3s can be beneficial to those with schizophrenia.[61] I certainly encourage my schizophrenic patients to increase omega-3 consumption in their diets.

N-Acetylcysteine

SCZ patients have abnormal brain metabolism that leads to oxidative stress.[62] The release of free radicals damages brain tissue and sabotages the brain's normal defense systems, causing brain physiology to go awry. Antioxidants are particularly important for SCZ patients to help fight the negative effects of oxidative stress.

Glutathione is an important antioxidant that is low in patients with SCZ. Giving a dose of straight glutathione isn't helpful, since it is poorly absorbed and does not reach the brain easily. However, N-acetylcysteine (NAC) has been shown to successfully raise plasma glutathione levels and thus protect the brain.[63]

In a case study of a twenty-four-year-old woman with chronic and worsening paranoid-type schizophrenia that did not respond to antipsychotic treatment, NAC supplementation spurred improvement in seven days.[64] Improvements were seen in schizophrenia-specific symptoms as well as in spontaneity, social skills, and family relations.

These findings were supported by another study in which forty-two SCZ patients with acute symptoms who were being treated with an antipsychotic received either NAC or a placebo for eight weeks.[65] The researchers saw significant improvements in negative symptoms in the NAC treatment group compared to controls, though there was not significant improvement in all symptoms or frequency of symptoms.

In another study, 140 SCZ patients randomly received either placebo or NAC supplementation in addition to antipsychotic medication over twenty-four weeks.[66] People who received NAC supplementation improved on all symptoms.

Taken together, these studies give reasonable evidence that NAC supplementation could help treat schizophrenia. As we've discussed, NAC itself is not available from dietary sources, but I encourage SCZ patients to eat foods containing the amino acid cysteine, which are described in the section on bipolar disorder earlier in this chapter.

Alpha-lipoic Acid

Alpha-lipoic acid is a common ingredient in multivitamin formulas and antiaging supplements.[67] It plays a key role in chemical reactions of the cell's energy source, the mitochondrion. Like NAC, it is an antioxidant and protects the brain from excessive inflammation.

A 2017 research study in SCZ patients found that alpha-lipoic acid may reduce overall symptoms of SCZ and improve cognition as well.[68] It was also helpful in counteracting weight gain and movement abnormalities caused by antipsychotic medication.[69]

Alpha-lipoic acid is commonly found in vegetables (spinach, broccoli, tomato) and meats, especially organ meats like heart, kidney, and liver. While organ meats may not sound appealing, certain dishes like steak and kidney pie, liver and onions, and various types of pâté are delicious.

Vitamins

Vitamin C: In one study, forty patients with SCZ showed lower levels of a marker associated with SCZ after receiving a course of vitamin C.[70] SCZ symptoms also improved significantly in the experimental group compared to those receiving a placebo. Other studies have confirmed that vitamin C may be helpful in SCZ patients.[71]

B vitamins: B vitamins play an essential role in cellular

metabolism. Low blood levels of B vitamins are a relatively consistent finding in patients with schizophrenia. Folate has been of particular interest, since folate deficiency may interfere with DNA synthesis and repair and overall cellular function in the brain.[72]

In one study of Dutch SCZ patients, investigators noted that there were lower levels of serum vitamin B_{12} in SCZ patients compared to healthy controls.[73] There were no differences in folate and vitamin B_6 levels between the groups, although an earlier trial found differences in folate levels that correlated with an increased risk of SCZ.[74]

A former Massachusetts General Hospital colleague, Donald Goff, and his research group also reported low folate levels in ninety-one SCZ outpatients.[75] They found that higher folate levels correlated with a decrease in negative symptom severity among nonsmoking patients.

Several studies have demonstrated that B vitamin supplementation may be effective in SCZ. In one study, seventeen SCZ patients with low folate levels[76] received daily methylfolate supplementation (15 mg/day) in addition to their pharmacologic treatment for six months. They showed improvements in their symptoms and social abilities, allowing them to reintegrate back into society.

In one of the largest randomized controlled trials examining vitamin supplementation, Massachusetts General Hospital psychiatrist Josh Roffman and his colleagues randomly assigned 140 patients with schizophrenia on antipsychotic medication to a sixteen-week treatment of either a combination of folic acid (2 mg/day) and vitamin B_{12} (400 mcg/day) or placebo. The folate-plus-B_{12} group showed significant improvement in negative symptom severity, but treatment response was strongly influenced by each individual patient's genetics, which determined how well they absorbed folate.[77]

In 2017, Roffman and his colleagues found that folic acid supplementation does in fact improve symptoms in patients with SCZ.[78] While genetic variants played a role, improvement in negative symptoms occurred regardless of genes.

As discussed previously, vegetables and fortified whole-grain, low-sugar cereals are high in folate, and meat and dairy products are high in vitamin B_{12}. Green leafy vegetables, dark green vegetables such as broccoli and Brussels sprouts, beans, and other legumes all contain folate.

L-Theanine

L-theanine is a unique amino acid present almost exclusively in the tea plant, from which most varieties of tea are produced. It enhances alpha brain waves ("relaxation" waves), decreases excitatory chemicals in the brain, and boosts calming brain chemicals such as GABA.

One rigorous study found that L-theanine augmentation of antipsychotic therapy relieved several symptoms in SCZ and schizoaffective disorder patients. Another study found that L-theanine relieves positive symptoms and insomnia in SCZ patients.[79] While more studies are needed for these results to be conclusive, these provide good reason to drink tea.

Regular varieties such as green, black, and oolong tea contain theanine, but they also contain caffeine, so too much of these teas will rev you up. With SCZ patients, it's always best to look for a decaffeinated alternative. Herbal teas aren't made from traditional tea leaves, so they do not contain theanine. Fortunately decaf green, black, and oolong teas do.

Melatonin

Melatonin, the "sleep hormone," which we discussed in chapter 8, has been shown to be effective for insomnia in patients with SCZ. It may also augment the effects of antipsychotics through its anti-inflammatory and antioxidant effects.[80]

Eggs and fish are good sources of melatonin, as are nuts. Asparagus, tomatoes, olives, grapes, barley, oats, walnuts, and flaxseeds are also good sources.

SERIOUS MENTAL ILLNESS REQUIRES SERIOUS MEDICINE

Pharmaceuticals like lithium and antipsychotics are powerful weapons in fighting BD and SCZ. But equally powerful are the changes to diet that can work alongside medications to help people suffering from these debilitating illnesses.

My bipolar patient Nancy switched back from the Western diet to a ketogenic diet, cutting out carbs. She slowly cut her coffee down to 1 cup in the morning. And we added the protein shake for breakfast, this time with additional peanut butter.

For lunch, she avoided gluten, eating a salad with plenty of onions for cysteine, and avocados, lettuce, spinach, and red kidney beans for folate. For dinner, she increased the oily fish in her diet. For instance, she really liked baked salmon, so she had this regularly with different seasonings. Her favorite was olive oil, black pepper, oregano, and thyme, and she topped this with an onion sauté. She stopped drinking wine on weekdays. In about six weeks, her symptoms resolved, and she returned to baseline.

My schizophrenic patient Alice cut out bread and alcohol. Within seven weeks, her symptoms resolved, and she was able to function again. Her fiancé, spooked at first by her social withdrawal and hallucinations, was relieved to see that she was back to her normal self. She was able to discuss her problems with him, and since he observed what a difference alcohol and bread made, he was totally on board to help her cut both out of her diet. Now, a few years later, she is about to get married.

Both Nancy and Alice are inspiring examples of how maintaining mental health isn't always straightforward. It can require dedication to keep up with the latest recommendations. Both were stable on medication when something new in their life threw a wrench into their routines, sending them into a spiral of problems they thought they'd resolved. But with patience and determination and the right support, they were able to change their diets to help fill in the gaps that their medication didn't cover.

BIPOLAR DISORDER CHEAT SHEET

The keto diet has been shown to be a good whole-diet approach for patients with bipolar disorder.

Foods to Embrace:

- Omega-3 fatty acids: Fish, especially fatty fish like salmon, mackerel, tuna, herring, and sardines.
- N-acetylcysteine: While NAC itself must be taken as a supplement, cysteine-rich foods can also be effective. Try meat, grains, eggs, ricotta cheese, cottage cheese, yogurt, broccoli, red pepper, and onion.
- Vitamin B_9 (folate).
- Minerals: Magnesium, zinc.

Foods to Avoid:

- The components of the Western diet: Foods high in bad fats (red meat, fried foods) and high-glycemic-index carbs (white bread, white rice, potatoes, pasta, and anything else made from refined flour).
- Caffeine: Keep caffeine consumption under 400 mg/day.
- Sodium: For patients treated with lithium, it's important to keep sodium levels constant.
- Gluten: If you have celiac disease or non-celiac gluten sensitivity, avoid all wheat products, such as bread, pizza, pasta, and many alcoholic drinks.

- Alcohol: BD patients should totally abstain from or heavily restrict alcohol use.
- Complications with medicine: Grapefruit juice and foods containing tyramine (aged cheese, aged or cured meats, fava beans, Marmite, sauerkraut, soy sauce, and tap beer) can interfere with some medications prescribed for BD.

SCHIZOPHRENIA CHEAT SHEET

Foods to Embrace:

- Omega-3 fatty acids: Fish, especially fatty fish like salmon, mackerel, tuna, herring, and sardines.
- N-acetylcysteine (NAC): While NAC itself must be taken as a supplement, cysteine-rich foods can also be effective. Try meat, grains, eggs, ricotta cheese, cottage cheese, yogurt, broccoli, red pepper, and onion.
- Alpha-lipoic acid: Spinach, broccoli, tomato, and meats, especially organ meats like heart, kidney, and liver.
- L-theanine: Green, black, and oolong tea.
- Melatonin: Eggs, fish, milk, rice, barley and rolled oats, grapes, pomegranates, walnuts, sunflower seeds, mustard seeds, flax-seeds, asparagus, broccoli, and cucumber.
- Vitamins B_9, B_{12}, and C.

Foods to Avoid:

- The components of the Western diet: Foods high in bad fats (red meat, fried foods) and high-glycemic-index carbs (white bread, white rice, potatoes, pasta, and anything else made from refined flour).

- Gluten: If you have celiac disease or non-celiac gluten sensitivity, avoid all wheat products, such as bread, pizza, pasta, and many alcoholic drinks.
- Sugar: Baked goods, candy, soda, or anything sweetened with sugar or high-fructose corn syrup.
- Alcohol: SCZ patients should try to abstain from or heavily restrict alcohol use.

CHAPTER TEN

Libido: Oxytocin, Fenugreek, and the Science of Aphrodisiacs

Living in the modern world, it's difficult to avoid products designed to enhance your libido. Every day we're inundated with pharmaceutical ads for erectile dysfunction drugs showing vibrant middle-aged couples on their way to romantic weekends. Racks of drugstore and gas station "supplements" making dubious (and possibly dangerous) claims of the sexual supremacy they will deliver. Magazines full of tips to get in the mood and please your partner. It's safe to say that the genuine, factual advice on the subject is watered down with snake oil and attention-grabbing sensationalism, but there's no doubt that people are seeking ways to enrich their sex lives and improve their libidos.

What is a libido anyway? While the word is generally equated with sexual desire, in psychological theory, it has broader implications. Sigmund Freud, founder of psychoanalysis, described it as "the motive force of the sexual instincts," a fundamental drive for humans to seek pleasure. The psychiatrist and psychoanalyst Carl Jung, however, believed that libido could be separated from sexual instincts and was more akin to a vital life force that the philosopher Henri Bergson called élan vital.[1] And the psychoanalyst Ronald Fairbairn described libido as "primarily object seeking," downplaying the pleasure-centric Freud viewpoint in favor of thinking of libido as a way of relating and connecting with other people.[2]

Though there is no universally agreed definition, in all these interpretations of libido, the common thread is that it is an essential human drive.[3] In fact, libido has many similarities to another human drive: hunger.

Like hunger, libido is an instinctual state. They can both affect the way you behave, making you prioritize them above all else. There's not much thinking involved in either one, but we are programmed so that satiating hunger and satiating sexual desire are both rewarding, activating overlapping brain circuitry focused on pleasure.

Hunger and libido also involve similar chemicals, with dopamine playing a major role in both, and sex hormones like estrogen, testosterone, and progesterone influencing food intake and appetite.[4] The two even have an evolutionary similarity, since the ability to overeat and store the extra energy as glycogen and lipids conferred a reproductive advantage by allowing animals time to look for mates without worrying about constantly seeking food.[5]

Given all these connections, it's no surprise that food can influence your sex drive. In this chapter, we will look at how certain foods affect your libido, and how eating the right foods can help you optimize your sexual function.

Of course, it's important to remember that all psychological challenges come in a specific context. For some people, depression, stress, or anxiety may reduce libido. For others, the culprit could be the antidepressants used to treat those conditions—many psychiatric medications, from SSRI antidepressants to antipsychotics, decrease libido. As tempting as it is to believe you can fix sexual problems by eating certain foods, in my experience it's not that simple. So as you read through these tips, know that they are just one component of the solution. They are not quick fixes, but life and libido enhancers.

AROUSAL AND YOUR GUT

There are two main sex hormones—estrogen and testosterone. You probably know them as the "female" and "male" sex hormones, and indeed, estrogen is produced primarily by the ovaries and testosterone by the testes. Still, men and women have both estrogen and testosterone, and both are important to the sexual function of each gender. For example, while testosterone certainly plays a major role in male libido, estradiol (the main form of estrogen) has been shown to have a profound influence on libido, erections, and sperm creation.[6] And though there is some disagreement about the role testosterone plays in the female libido, it's clear that the connection is there.[7] Beyond sexual function, estrogen and testosterone are involved in the health of your bones, brain, and blood vessels.

Gut bacteria are yet again intimately involved in modulating libido because of their role in producing these two sex hormones. In 2014, veterinarian Theofilos Poutahidis and colleagues investigated whether gut bacteria can influence sex hormones in mice.[8] They gave mice a probiotic containing the gut bacterium *Lactobacillus reuteri* (*L. reuteri*), which has anti-inflammatory properties. Mice consuming *L. reuteri* in their drinking water produced more sperm and had more testosterone-producing cells in their testes compared to controls that were not exposed to this bacterium. This was particularly evident in older mice; in fact, the treatment essentially made the mice more youthful, restoring the size of their testicles to resemble those of younger mice. The study concluded that since probiotic supplementation can boost sexual function in mice, there is a strong possibility the same could be true in humans.

It has also been shown that mice that are exposed to antibiotics when they are young suffer from a disrupted microbiome that leads to low testosterone and decreased sperm quality.[9]

As for estrogen, in postmenopausal women, it appears that gut microbiota play a key role in regulating levels of estrogen circulating in the blood.[10]

Beyond estrogen and testosterone, gut bacteria control other neurochemicals that change libidinal function. For instance, some strains of gut bacteria can produce gamma-aminobutyric acid (GABA). While GABA is essential for healthy brain function, when GABA receptors are overstimulated, erectile dysfunction (ED), loss of libido, or difficulty achieving an orgasm can result.[11]

When your gut is not functioning properly, it can be difficult to tap into your libido, even when your symptoms aren't expressly related to sexual function. For example, inflammatory bowel disease has been shown to track with depression, arthritis, and poor body image, all of which serve to lower libido.[12]

FOODS AND COMPOUNDS THAT REDUCE DESIRE

In a sense, eating poorly can be a kind of nutritional castration, no matter what your age or gender. Let's take a look at eating patterns and foods that hamper libido and then establish healthier alternatives.

The Western Diet

It should be no surprise that the Western diet is once again a threat to your well-being. High-fat diets have been found to impair testicular function and have been linked with impaired sperm production and function.[13] This is referred to as the GELDING theory, which stands for Gut Endotoxin Leading to a Decline in Gonadal function—a bit of a stretch as an acronym, but a nice play on the word "gelding," which refers to male castration. This theory purports that high-fat and high-calorie diets cause the same kind of "leaky gut" we've seen in other conditions. As a result, gut bacteria pass into the circulation, which allows endotoxins, powerful immune stimulants present in bacteria, to cause low-grade inflammation throughout the body. This impairs testicular function and reproductive performance, providing us with another example of how gut health is essential to sexual health.

In 2017, Justin La and his colleagues reviewed the scientific studies published between 1977 and 2017 on how diet affects men's sexual health.[14] They found that the Western diet was associated with lower semen quality and greater incidence of ED. Obese and overweight men who went on a low-fat, low-calorie diet were able to improve their erections and boost their testosterone.

Another study demonstrated that a high-protein, low-carbohydrate, low-fat diet improved sexual function, with improvement in both erectile function and sexual desire up to one year after the change in diet.[15]

An increase in prevalence of the Western diet correlates with the lower sperm counts in the general male population. Sperm counts have dropped precipitously, by 59 percent in North America, Europe, Australia, and New Zealand.[16] A new Harvard study presented at the 2019 meeting of the European Society of Human Reproduction and Embryology found that the sperm counts for men who typically ate meals of high-fat foods were 25.6 million lower than those of men who ate healthier diets.

I have had several patients of both sexes in my clinic who have switched away from a Western diet and improved their sexual performance. For instance, Joey was a thirty-eight-year-old programmer and football fanatic who lived on the north shore of Massachusetts. He came to see me for depression, which I learned was precipitated by difficulty he and his wife were having in trying to conceive a child.

They had visited an infertility specialist, and to Joey's massive disappointment, he was told that his sperm count was low and that he had poor sperm motility (his sperm were not moving in a healthy way). The doctors could not identify any medical cause for his issues, and he and his wife were devastated. Though they kept trying, they were far less hopeful than they had ever been.

Joey was so depressed that I had to start him on an antidepressant. The trouble is, many common antidepressants like fluoxetine (Prozac) can disturb sexual function. I opted for bupropion (Wellbutrin), which has fewer sexual side effects, but also told him that he had to change his diet. No more game-day hot dogs, nachos, pizza, wings, or any of the usual football food.

I also directed him to eat more nuts. In 2012, Wendie Robbins and her colleagues found that the addition of walnuts to a standard Western diet improves the quality, vitality, and physical form of sperm.[17] A 2018 study confirmed that 60 grams (just over ¼ cup) per day of a mixture of nuts added to a Western diet made a difference in sperm count and sperm quality.[18]

I asked him to try switching to a healthier diet built around daily servings of fruit, vegetables, avocado, olive oil, and healthy nuts and make a serious effort to avoid unhealthy fats and processed carbs. Joey was all in. His new diet was not exactly up his alley, but he was willing to do what it took to have a child. Six months after he started the diet, his wife became pregnant. Now, five years later, they have a beautiful son and daughter. Though Joey has allowed himself to ease back into his weekend football-food rituals, he is much more careful in limiting unhealthy foods.

Though sperm-count studies are obviously geared toward men, kicking the junk-food habit can have reproductive benefits for women as well. A recent study of more than five thousand women found that those who ate fast food more than four times a week (and fruit fewer than three times a month) took longer to get pregnant and had a greater chance of infertility.[19]

This is exactly what happened with my patient Inka. She came to see me because she and her husband had been trying unsuccessfully to conceive a child. Furthermore, she said she was tired of trying, unable to work up excitement and desire to have sex with her husband. When I took a dietary history, I learned that Inka had been working late after a promotion at her law firm. Though she enjoyed her work, she was putting in long hours at the office, which led to an excess of unhealthy take-out food. She admitted that she could not recall the last time she ate at home or even had a fresh piece of fruit. Even when she ate salads, they were covered in bacon and drenched in creamy, rich, unhealthy dressings.

She began by building in a Sunday afternoon of meal prep to help plan out the meals for that week. For breakfasts she added in nutritious, fiber-filled foods like overnight oats, chia pudding (page 255), and scrambled eggs in a mug with vegetables (page 275). She also began to take simple but healthy lunches to work (chopped salad with heaps of tasty mixed lettuces and chopped vegetables, and a side of rotisserie chicken or baked salmon). She stocked her office with fruit and nuts as healthy snacks. Though her meals were simple to put together, she quickly began to feel better about what she was eating. She also noticed that she was more relaxed at home and began to enjoy an intimate relationship with her husband again. Whereas their intimacy had become regimented to match her ovulation schedule, now she looked forward to their Friday and Saturday date nights.

About eighteen months after making these changes to her diet, she and her husband announced they were pregnant. After the birth of a healthy baby girl, she called me to let me know that her healthy eating habits had helped her energy levels during her pregnancy and as a new mother.

Soy Protein

In 2011, clinical neuroscientist Timo Siepmann and his colleagues reported on a case of a nineteen-year-old man who had suddenly lost his libido and developed ED.[20] Though the man did have type 1 diabetes, he was otherwise healthy. When Siepmann's team took a history, they found that he consumed large quantities of soy-based products in a vegan-style diet.

When they first saw him, his blood levels of testosterone were low, and his levels of a testosterone precursor called dehydroepiandrostendione were high—an indicator that this precursor was not being properly made into testosterone. After one year of stopping the vegan diet, these parameters all normalized. As his testosterone came back up, his sexual symptoms disappeared, and he regained full sexual function one year later.

Though Siepmann's research was a single case study, it was an indicator that soy-protein consumption can disrupt normal sex hormone production and libido. Other studies are consistent with this finding, showing that higher intake of soy foods and soy isoflavones is associated with lower sperm concentration.[21]

As we learned in chapter 6, isoflavones are estrogen-like substances found in soy. They are polyphenols, which means that most of the time they are actually good for your brain because of their anti-inflammatory properties. But many researchers believe that the estrogen introduced by isoflavones can impact sex hormones so that men may develop breasts and lose their libido.[22] If you're curious whether the estrogen-boosting properties of soy can help female libido, results are inconclusive—one study did report that soy protein can increase libido in postmenopausal women, but with no greater effect than placebo.[23]

It's worth considering that China and India are the number one and number four, respectively, consumers of soy in the world. Given their population numbers, it would be surprising if soy really had a massive effect on libido and sex-hormone production. Still, if you are a man who consumes lots of soy protein (such as tofu, edamame, and soy-based imitation meat products) and suffers from low libido, it may be worth trying to cut back on the soy to see if your sex drive improves.

Alcohol

I spend lots of time on college campuses, which are often the nexus of discussions about the relationship between sex and alcohol. Pop culture has weighed in on the subject all the way back to Shakespeare, who famously said in *Macbeth* that alcohol "provokes the desire, but it takes away the performance."[24] It turns out the Bard was right.

One study demonstrated that when men are dependent on alcohol, it causes ED, unsatisfying orgasms, and premature ejaculation.[25] Another study showed that intoxicated men take longer than sober men to reach orgasm, without any other sexual side effects.[26] In 2018, Deepak Prabhakaran and his colleagues questioned men with alcohol dependence on their sexual function.[27] They found that sexual dysfunction was reported in 37 percent of their subjects. Twenty-five percent of those reported ED, 20 percent reported "dysfunction in satisfying orgasm," and 15.5 percent reported premature ejaculation. A small percentage of people reported excessive libido. These results were enough to convince the researchers that alcohol plays a role in sexual dysfunction, but they also point out one of the difficulties with gathering this kind of data: since alcohol distorts how people recall their experiences, self-reporting can be inconsistent and unreliable.

Alcohol plays a complex role in women's libido, too. Research has shown that moderate alcohol use enhances desire and makes sexual activity more likely, but high doses of alcohol have the opposite effect.[28] Another study found that alcohol suppresses orgasm in young women, but only at higher dosages.[29] Furthermore, women who have been sexually victimized—for instance, those who have suffered childhood sexual abuse, rape, or attempted rape—are more likely than normal to drink heavily, putting them at risk for further sexual harm.[30]

It's clear that, whether you're a man or a woman, drinking heavily leads to poor sexual performance or—much worse—a greater risk of putting yourself in dangerous sexual situations. However, moderate drinking—no more than 14 drinks per week for men, and no more than 7 drinks per week for women—shouldn't take a toll on your sex life.

Sugar

Sex has long been associated with sweet foods like chocolate-covered strawberries and other candies, especially at Valentine's

Day. However, science has shown that sugar isn't good for the sex lives of those who eat too much of it.

For instance, excessive consumption of sugar-sweetened beverages, especially by those with a high body mass index, is associated with lower testosterone levels.[31] Another study demonstrated that sugary beverages decrease sperm motility too.[32]

Higher-sugar diets also lead to higher leptin levels. Leptin is a hormone made by the body's fat cells that helps you to regulate your energy balance. The higher your leptin levels, the lower your testosterone, especially if you are already overweight.[33] When you are overweight, your fat tissue makes so much leptin that it suppresses the hypothalamic-pituitary-adrenal axis, which in turn stops making testosterone, another possible link between consuming more sugar and lower testosterone.[34]

Just as I do for patients with other conditions, for those with libido issues, I recommend cutting down on sugar as much as possible, particularly sweet drinks and snacks sweetened with high-fructose corn syrup. For desserts, prioritize fresh fruits, medium-glycemic-index natural sweeteners like honey, or lower-sugar treats like dark chocolate. (In fact, as we will soon see, dark chocolate has other helpful properties also. Natural, non-alkalized chocolate is best, as it has higher antioxidant levels.)

Licorice

One particular type of sweet that has been shown to have a negative effect on libido is licorice. Licorice derives its flavor from the roots of the licorice plant and contains the active ingredient glycyrrhizic acid, which several studies have indicated is associated with lower testosterone levels.[35]

Aside from licorice candy, licorice can be found in teas and certain chewing gums. It's important to note that only black licorice contains the harmful chemicals (look for "licorice extract" on the label); red licorice is licorice in name only. But, as we just discussed, eating less candy of any sort is the right thing to do.

Perfluorooctanoic Acid

Perfluorooctanoic acid (PFOA) is a chemical with many applications, most notably in certain kinds of nonstick cookware and food packaging. Studies have suggested the potential of PFOA and similar chemicals to disrupt the endocrine system, increasing the risk of adverse health effects.

PFOA has been shown to turn the hormone receptors (e.g., androgen) off, leading to a reduction of testosterone.[36] The more PFOA you consume, the greater this effect. There is also evidence that PFOA may be associated with infertility, and animal studies have shown that it affects ovaries as well.[37] Furthermore, PFOA can change gut bacteria, causing inflammation.[38]

Thankfully, there has been some response from manufacturers in the face of the growing body of evidence that such chemicals are harmful. A 2019 study showed that between 2005 and 2018, there was a downward trend in using PFOA.[39] However, some microwave popcorn bags and some plastic bags still contain PFOA, and it is also used to make Teflon and other stain- and stick-resistant materials. Jolly Time Popcorn, Snappy Popcorn, and Newman's Own Organics Popcorn are PFOA-free. Or make easy air-popped corn or old-fashioned stovetop popped corn. Use stainless-steel or cast-iron cookware, avoiding nonstick coatings, and switch to unbleached paper bags for snacks and sandwiches.

APHRODISIACS AND LIBIDO-ENHANCING FOODS

The idea that certain foods can increase sexual desire is as old as human civilization. The word "aphrodisiac" is derived from Aphrodite, the Greek goddess of love, but the Greeks weren't the only ancient culture to believe in the power of food to increase libido, potency, or sexual pleasure.[40] Almost every culture has used foods and substances derived from plants, animals, and minerals to enhance sexual desire. And though modern science hasn't fully investigated the claims of every single one of these foods, we know enough to understand that there are genuine connections between certain foods and libido.

Interestingly, some of the most well-known aphrodisiacs are the ones that have been most thoroughly debunked. Take, for example, the cautionary tale of the oyster. You've probably heard that slurping raw oysters can amp up sexual desire. The legendary Casanova swore by them as a way to sustain his sexual appetite. Though the idea that oysters are an aphrodisiac isn't new, the legend grew in the mid-2000s when news outlets reported on a study that attributed the oysters' effects to the presence of an amino acid called D-aspartic. The findings turned out to be all hype, the result of a misunderstanding at a scientific conference.[41]

The same is true for strawberries, another food commonly mentioned as having aphrodisiac properties. Though strawberries do contain phytoestrogens, which could possibly help symptoms in postmenopausal women, there are no other indicators that they enhance sexual performance.

In this section, we'll look at other foods and supplements that are both well-known and more obscure, measuring up the evidence that they can enhance libido.

Oxytocin-Boosting Foods

Oxytocin is known as the "bonding hormone" because of its wide range of functions in sex, love, and child-rearing.[42] It is involved with libido in several ways, eliciting sexual arousal and contributing to the culmination of pleasure, as it's released during orgasm for both men and women. Giving both men and women extra oxytocin has been shown to heighten arousal while watching erotic films.[43]

The brain effects of oxytocin are complex. Many of them occur via the brain's "reward" pathway.[44] Oxytocin receptors are abundant in the mesolimbic system, which links the reward pathway with the brain's limbic system and plays a key role in the registration and expression of emotion.[45] The gut microbiome plays a role in the development and function of this pathway, so gut bacteria can affect the function of neurons that rely on oxytocin.[46]

While you can't get oxytocin directly from food, there are foods that can help you raise oxytocin levels. Chocolate is commonly known as an aphrodisiac, and sure enough, dark chocolate stimulates dopamine in the brain, which in turn increases oxytocin production.[47] However, specific research into chocolate's libido-enhancing properties is not a slam dunk. Although one study demonstrated that chocolate may enhance sexual function in women, when this effect was adjusted for age, it was not significant.[48]

Magnesium has been found to promote the biological activity of oxytocin.[49] While this connection is not robust or well replicated, eating a diet high in magnesium can't hurt. As we covered earlier, make sure to eat lots of green vegetables, nuts, seeds, and unprocessed grains, all of which are rich in magnesium.

Oxytocin is a peptide of nine amino acids. Two of these, isoleucine and leucine, are essential amino acids that must be obtained from the diet as they cannot be produced in your body, so you'll definitely need to eat foods high in them to make sure your body can create oxytocin. You will find them in meat and meat products, grains, milk and dairy products, and, to a lesser degree, vegetables and eggs.

Coffee

In 2015, David Lopez and his colleagues analyzed data from 3,724 men to see if coffee prevented ED.[50] They found that caffeine intake did reduce the odds of ED, especially when subjects drank approximately 2–3 daily cups of coffee (170–375 mg of caffeine/day). Another study demonstrated that 100 mg of caffeine prior to intercourse improved sexual satisfaction.[51]

As we've discussed, it's important not to overdo coffee consumption, but it can be beneficial to your sex life provided you don't exceed 400 mg/day of caffeine.

Red Wine

We've already discussed how heavy drinking can hamper your libido, but moderate consumption of red wine can actually enhance it. In 2009, Nicola Mondaini and his colleagues investigated whether red wine intake affected sexual function in women.[52] They divided a sample of 798 women into three groups: teetotalers, moderate drinkers (1 or 2 glasses of red wine per day), and heavy drinkers (more than 2 glasses of red wine per day and/or other types of alcoholic drinks, including white wine).

They found that women who drank red wine moderately had significantly better overall sexual function, as well as higher sexual desire and lubrication than participants who drank a lot or none at all. No significant differences between the groups were observed concerning sexual arousal, satisfaction, pain, and orgasm.

Other studies have demonstrated that red wine can increase testosterone levels in men.[53] And others have demonstrated that the polyphenols found in red wine may decrease ED.[54]

Of course, while red wine can have benefits, I want to stress that you should always drink in moderation. I ask my patients to stick to 1 glass per day to ensure that their libido doesn't suffer ill effects from too much alcohol.

Pistachios and Other Nuts

In 2011, Mustafa Aldemir and his colleagues studied seventeen married male participants.[55] They gave them 100 grams of pistachios a day for three weeks and tracked erectile function. They found an improvement in erections, as well as an increase in good cholesterol (HDL) and a decrease in bad cholesterol (LDL).

Another study in women in Iran found that a combination of

pistachios and almonds in a traditional Persian dish (made with wild carrots and saffron) enhanced sexual desire, arousal, lubrication, orgasm, and satisfaction.[56]

Given that we've already seen the beneficial effects of walnuts when discussing my patient Joey, I recommend adding pistachios, walnuts, and almonds to your diet. You can overdo it with nuts, so stick to around ¼ cup per day.

Saffron

We have seen that saffron is an effective antidepressant, and it has positive effects on libido as well. Studies have shown that it may increase libido, enhance erectile function, and improve semen quality. A different review of the effects of saffron on sexual function also found that it improved ED.[57]

I recommend adding saffron to your diet, though remember that a little goes a long way—it's very expensive and its flavor can overpower others in dishes. See page 46 for instructions on how to include it in your cooking.

Fenugreek

Fenugreek is a delicious but potent herb. When I mix the fresh or dried herb into a dough to make Indian bread, the aroma can take a week to wear off my hands! However, it might be worth the effort.

In one study, fenugreek was shown to increase testosterone in men.[58] Another double-blind placebo-controlled study confirmed that fenugreek boosts libido in men, with improvements in arousal and orgasm.[59]

A study in men found that taking 600 mg of fenugreek extract per day led to significant improvement in sexual desire and arousal.[60]

Fenugreek has a deep flavor that you might recognize from the butter chicken you can order at an Indian restaurant. The seeds can be crushed, boiled in hot water, and consumed as a flavorful tea with a drop of honey. Fenugreek extract is available as a supplement, but as always I recommend getting it from food instead. Fresh or dried fenugreek leaves can be used to make delicious Indian breads called *methi tepla,* which you can also buy in specialty stores.

Apples

In 2014, a urology research team enrolled 731 women in a study to see if eating an apple a day affected the sex lives of healthy, young, sexually active Italian women.[61] Around half of the women reported regular daily apple intake while the other half did not consume apples regularly. The study determined that women in the apple group had significantly better overall sexual function and lubrication scores than those who didn't eat apples.

Apples are easy to include in your diet, and in addition to improving your libido, they are rich in vitamin C and potassium and have antioxidant and anti-inflammatory properties.

Pomegranate Juice

In one study, pomegranate juice increased sperm quality in rats.[62] In other studies, in men and women, pomegranate juice enhanced testosterone levels by 24 percent.[63]

Rich in polyphenols, pomegranate juice is an effective antioxidant, so it's a great addition to your diet. I always suggest making your own juice from pomegranate seeds, as commercial juices have extremely high sugar content.

Chili Peppers

We saw how chili peppers and their capsaicin can energize you. There is also a long history of belief in capsaicin as a libido enhancer.[64]

In 2015, Laurent Bègue and his colleagues studied 114 males between the ages of eighteen and forty-four years old to see if there was a correlation between eating spicy foods and testosterone levels.[65] The researchers found that the greater the quantity of hot sauce used, the higher the salivary testosterone of the subject.

This study suggests a correlation between preference for spicy food and testosterone levels.

Remember, capsaicin only comes from chili peppers, not from other spicy foods like black pepper or horseradish. To add it to your diet, use red pepper flakes, powdered cayenne pepper, or fresh jalapeño or serrano peppers in your cooking.

Onions

There are promising signs that onions may have beneficial effects on testosterone; they may increase certain key hormones and reduce the formation of free radicals. Onions also increase nitric oxide production in cells found in the testicle, which dilates blood vessels and improves ED. Onions lower blood sugar too, which has a positive effect on the production of testosterone.

In 2019, Saleem Ali Banihani conducted a review of all studies on onions and their effects on testosterone.[66] His review confirmed these factors, but most of the studies were done in animals. Only one human study demonstrated that onions increase testosterone, and none have looked at libido in detail.[67] Still, there are certainly indications that onions are good for libido, and, as we've learned in earlier chapters, they are a great prebiotic too.

Avocados

The Aztecs named the avocado tree *ahuacatl,* meaning "testicle tree," because the fruit hung in pairs like male testicles. There may be more to this comparison than meets the eye.[68]

Avocados are one of the richest dietary sources of the element boron, which is vital for the production of sex hormones. Boron has been shown to increase levels of both testosterone and estradiol in postmenopausal women. In healthy men, it appears that boron helps to make testosterone more available and useful to the body, which can be especially beneficial in older men.[69]

However, in boron-supplementation studies, it appears the

effective dose of boron for a testosterone boost is 10 mg/day. One cup of avocado contains only about 1.67 mg of boron, so you'd need around 6 cups of avocado to get up to that level—in other words, too much. There have been studies that demonstrate that 3 mg/day of boron can boost testosterone levels; that's about 2 cups of avocado. Even for a healthy fat, that's a bit too much on a daily basis, but it's still worth eating avocado in smaller amounts.[70]

Ayurvedic Libido Enhancers

In addition to readily available foods, many traditional herbs and supplements have been thought to enhance libido. While different cultures have their own systems, I will focus on the Ayurvedic tradition.

Ayurveda, a health system that originated in India, uses plants in complex ways.[71] It is one of the most ancient health traditions, but it has many practitioners even today. Ayurveda has numerous approaches to sexual dysfunction. There are more than eighty-two herbs that have been discussed in scientific journals and, under the supervision of Ayurvedic practitioners, popularly used to improve various types of sexual dysfunction.[72]

If you're struggling with libido and aren't satisfied with treatments offered by Western medicine or dietary changes, it's worth learning more about Ayurveda. If you're interested in more information and resources to find a qualified Ayurvedic practitioner, check out the website of the National Ayurvedic Medical Association, which represents Ayurvedic practice in the United States.[73]

JACK'S PRO-LIBIDO DAY

To give you an idea of how I might approach helping a patient with libido issues, consider Jack, a thirty-five-year-old married gay man who felt he'd lost his sex drive. While it was difficult to integrate 5 cups of avocado with fenugreek into his day, I helped him develop a menu that would lead to him getting his groove back.

Since he was stressed out during the week, he generally didn't want to have sex. Over the weekend, he and his husband wanted to be more intimate sexually, so that was a good place to start. I joked that we could maybe start with a meal plan for "Sexy Saturdays," and he liked the idea. We planned a menu for the day so they would be ready to cozy up in the evening.

For breakfast, the choice was avocado toast on healthy whole grain bread, along with coffee and a glass of fresh-squeezed pomegranate juice—cleaning and juicing fresh pomegranates is a fun and sensual activity itself.

Jack made a delicious salad for lunch with romaine lettuce and diced chicken breast. The chicken was made with a cayenne-based rub, which brought a dose of capsaicin to the table. The salad included apples and walnuts.

At dinnertime, he poured on the love with a dish of San Franciscan Seafood Stew (page 289) spiked with chili so that the broth was spicy and delicious. He also made a risotto with cauliflower rice. Dinner was paired with an expertly chosen red wine.

For dessert, he dumped the cake and ice cream and went for dark-chocolate-covered strawberries (page 290)—dark chocolate for the oxytocin boost, and even though strawberries aren't necessarily aphrodisiacs, there's nothing wrong with sticking to the classics.

While you don't need to plan out an elaborate day of libido-enhancing foods every time you want to have sex, I hope this shows that integrating brain-healthy foods into your diet can be fun and physiologically helpful all at the same time. Jack told me that after dinner, he and his husband were ready for the main event, and in the weeks and months afterward he found his libido hit a new groove with the right blend of good attitude and good food.

LIBIDO CHEAT SHEET

Foods to Embrace:

- Foods that boost oxytocin: Dark chocolate, magnesium, and essential amino acids (found in meat, grains, milk, dairy, and, to a lesser degree, vegetables and eggs).
- Coffee: Keep total caffeine consumption under 400 mg/day.
- Red wine: No more than 1 glass/day.
- Nuts: Pistachios, almonds, and walnuts.
- Apples.
- Pomegranate juice.
- Onions.
- Avocados.
- Herbs and spices: Saffron, fenugreek.

Foods and Compounds to Avoid:

- The components of the Western diet: Foods high in bad fats (red meat, fried foods) and high-glycemic-index carbs (white bread, white rice, potatoes, pasta, and anything else made from refined flour).
- Soy protein: For men suffering from low libido, it's worth cutting down on tofu and soy proteins such as those found in vegetarian and vegan imitation-meat products.
- Alcohol: For men, stay under 14 drinks per week and have no more than 4 drinks in any single day. For women, stay under 7 drinks per week and have no more than 3 drinks in any single day.

- Sugar: Baked goods, candy, soda, or anything sweetened with sugar or high-fructose corn syrup.
- Licorice: Avoid candies and other products that contain licorice extract.
- PFOA: Beware of nonstick cookware and food packaging that contains PFOA. Use stainless-steel or cast-iron cookware, eat PFOA-free microwave popcorn, and use unbleached paper snack bags.

CHAPTER ELEVEN

Cooking and Eating for Your Brain

These days, most of my patients come to me expecting food advice. Either they've heard of my clinic and my practice in nutritional psychiatry somewhere out in the world, or they've been referred specifically to me by a colleague who knows the work I do. That wasn't always the case, though. Although I have always been fascinated by the intersection of food and mental health, as you know, nutritional psychiatry is a nascent field, and it wasn't all that long ago that patients who came to see me for problems with their minds were probably confused that I kept talking about their stomachs. When working with those patients, I quickly became aware of how little experience many people have with food prep. I'm not judging—after all, you'll recall that I barely cooked myself until I was an adult living out on my own, and I'm sure my culinary school instructors were similarly struck by me when I showed up barely knowing my mise en place from my miso soup.

In fact, I came to enjoy walking those patients through the baby steps of how to think about ingredients, orient themselves in a kitchen, and dip a toe into the not-so-choppy waters of feeding themselves. Though patients now tend to be at least a bit savvier—which may be a reflection of the population at large in our food-obsessed internet age—I still find that many of them benefit from basic instruction in not only what to eat but how to prepare it.

In this chapter, I want to give you similar basic information about how to grocery shop and set up your kitchen, along with recipes that are good jumping-off points for you to integrate into your routine during your journey toward eating for a healthy brain.

STOCKING YOUR PANTRY WITH BRAIN FOODS

When it comes to grocery shopping, at least one old cliché is true: don't shop when you are hungry. That's never a recipe for being mindful about your choices and is more likely to find you buying unhealthy comfort food rather than whole, nutritious, satisfying foods.

As for what to buy, I'm sure you already have a fairly solid idea of that from the foods we've talked about in these pages. As a bit of a refresher, I've put my central recommendations into the acronym BRAIN FOODS:

B: Berries and beans

R: Rainbow colors of fruits and vegetables

A: Antioxidants

I: Include lean proteins and plant-based proteins

N: Nuts (almonds, walnuts, Brazil nuts, and cashews)

F: Fiber-rich foods, fish, and fermented foods

O: Oils

O: Omega-3-rich foods

D: Dairy (yogurt and kefir, certain cheeses)

S: Spices

Berries and Beans

- Blueberries, blackberries, raspberries, and strawberries all make great additions to your day and double as a dessert.
- Eat berries that are in season. When you buy fresh berries, make sure to eat them soon—good ripe ones won't last long, even in the fridge. At times of the year when fresh, ripe berries aren't available, frozen berries are fine to use as long as you make sure they do not have added sugar or other additives.
- Beans, legumes, and lentils are important staples for your brain.
- A healthy source of nutrients, vitamins, and fiber, beans, legumes, and lentils are easy to prepare and can be a main course or an appetizer, can be added to a salad, or can even be made into a dessert.

Rainbow Colors of Fruits and Vegetables

- I always encourage my patients to eat as many different colorful vegetables as possible. From red cabbage to radicchio to green and yellow bell peppers, expand your palate and maximize the range of nutrients that are beneficial to your brain. This is particularly true of micronutrients, like vitamins, polyphenols, phytonutrients, and flavonoids.
- The same applies to fruits! Berries, apples, and citrus all come in a wide variety of colors. Just be careful not to overdo it with sweet fruits like grapes and cherries.
- Even though I want you to chase color, don't forget the most important color: green. Though eating a broad range of colors is great, you have to make sure you're getting enough dark, leafy greens. My favorites are arugula, romaine, Bibb lettuce, endive, and bok choy. I also love to add microgreens when I

can find them; they add a flavorful nutrient-dense punch to my meals.

Antioxidants

- We've covered many kinds of antioxidants throughout the book, including berries and the polyphenols in colorful vegetables we've just discussed.
- Dark chocolate is a great source of antioxidants, as long as you stick to the dark stuff and make sure that it doesn't include too much sugar. While cocoa and chocolate are delicious—and as a chef I was trained to use Dutch-process (alkalized) for flavor—as a nutritional psychiatrist I know that natural or non-alkalized is best for the highest antioxidant levels, and that's what I've specified in the recipes in this chapter.
- Many vitamins are crucial antioxidants. You can get vitamins from a broad range of dietary sources. This is one of the most important reasons to eat a diverse diet. But get a recommendation for a multivitamin supplement from your doctor; this is a great way to make sure you're not missing anything.

Include Lean Proteins and Plant-Based Proteins

- Well-sourced lean poultry, seafood, and occasional grass-fed beef are good choices to ensure you are getting plenty of protein and the essential amino acids that your brain needs to function.
- For plant-based sources of protein, organic tofu and tempeh can be enhanced with spices for flavor.

Nuts

- Nuts have healthy fats and oils that our brains need to function well, along with vitamins and minerals, for example, selenium in Brazil nuts.

- Eat ¼ cup a day (not more—it's easy to overdo it with nuts!) as a snack or added to your salad or vegetable side dish. Nuts can even be combined into a homemade granola or trail mix that contains much less sugar and salt than store-bought versions.

Fiber-Rich Foods, Fish, and Fermented Foods

- Beans, legumes, lentils, fruit, and vegetables are great sources of fiber. Fiber is important as a prebiotic, can help keep your weight down, and decreases inflammation in the entire body.
- As we discussed earlier, in chapter 2, fish such as salmon add healthy omega-3s to your nutrition plan.
- Fermented foods like kefir, miso, and kimchee are great for your brain and gut since they're a natural source of active-culture bacteria.

Oils

- While you want to avoid an excess of saturated fats and other unhealthy oils like the omega-6 oils used for frying, you want to ensure you're getting enough healthy fats from sources like olive oil, avocados, and oily fish.
- Even with healthy fats, be aware of portion size and try not to eat too much. All fats are calorie dense.

Omega-3-Rich Foods

- We've talked about omega-3s at length throughout the book, so you know well by now to ensure you're getting plenty of them. The most important source of omega-3s (especially docosahexaenoic acid and eicosapentaenoic acid) is oily fish, like salmon, mackerel, and tuna.
- Omega-3s (largely alpha-linolenic acid) can also be found in plant-based sources—chia seeds, Brussels sprouts, walnuts, and flaxseeds to name a few.

Dairy (Yogurt and Kefir, Certain Cheeses)

- Yogurts and kefir with probiotic cultures are great for your gut, providing you with helpful bacteria and protein.
- Grass-fed dairy products are better options for you and your brain.
- Remember that certain conditions, like ADHD, can be aggravated by dairy, so be aware of its negative effects.

Spices

- Spices are a no-calorie, guilt-free way to boost flavor in all your food while adding beneficial brain effects as well.
- In particular, spices like turmeric, black pepper, saffron, red pepper flakes, oregano, and rosemary should be part of your brain armor.

Beyond sticking to these foods, the rules thin out a bit, but there are still useful guidelines. The most important is that you never be afraid to push yourself. I have had many patients with fairly narrow diets, out of either comfort or convenience, who learned they had been missing broad swaths of nutrients and eating pleasures once I gave them a prescription to branch out. If you see new and interesting vegetables and fruits at the grocery store that you've never tried, don't be afraid to buy them. Commit yourself to making sure they don't turn moldy, forgotten in a crisper drawer, and search through recipes in cookbooks and on the internet to find a way to integrate them into your diet, even if just once. As long as you stick to the principles of healthy eating we've been discussing throughout the book, you really can't go wrong, and you may end up discovering a new favorite food!

SET UP YOUR KITCHEN LIKE A CHEF!

Just as your brain and gut need certain nutritional building blocks in order to operate at peak efficiency, your kitchen also needs certain equipment before you can cook a great meal. You don't need a whole lot of fancy equipment—no need for single-use tools like avocado cutters or mango pitters—but you do need some decent-quality basics. Here is a quick list of the tools you'll want to have before tackling the recipes that follow.

Large knife and small utility knife

The large knife should be a chef-style knife that you feel comfortable using. The smaller knife is for smaller jobs in the kitchen. Once you find knives you're comfortable with, make sure to keep them sharp. A sharp knife is less likely to slip and cut you.

Knife sharpener

I prefer the countertop sharpeners, where you just guide the blade through a slot, rather than the large handheld sharpening steel used in professional kitchens.

Vegetable peeler

I use a vegetable peeler both to remove the skins from vegetables and to create easy ribbons for salads. Try this on an English cucumber, zucchini, or carrot—it adds a colorful, phytonutrient-packed element to any salad or vegetable side dish.

Chopping board

You'll need a chopping board, either wood or synthetic. The board can be used for all your prep. Start with vegetables on one side, then flip it for your meat prep. Be sure to keep it clean and sanitized.

Instant-read thermometer

In the recipes, I will refer many times to the internal temperature of cooked food, especially meat. Eyeballing the doneness of your meat can easily lead to it being undercooked and dangerous, or overcooked and dry. With the ease and accuracy of modern instant-read digital thermometers, there's no reason to guess!

Lemon or lime zester

An easy, inexpensive way to add the vibrant bold flavors of citrus rind from lemons, limes, oranges, and clementines to salads, side dishes, and even baking.

Measuring cups

These are used for measuring dry ingredients and are helpful to measure out portions for meal planning.

Measuring pitcher and measuring spoons

The measuring pitcher is for liquids and the measuring spoons are useful in both cooking and baking.

Medium and large stainless-steel or glass bowls

Having plenty of bowls in a range of sizes allows you to be flexible and efficient during food prep.

Mini mise set

This mini prep bowl set helps to organize and set up your ingredients—see more about the importance of mise en place in the next section.

Kitchen towels and paper towels

These are useful for drying dishes and for drying vegetables or fruit after washing. Moisture can breed bacteria, so keeping your workspace and equipment dry is key to a clean kitchen.

Sanitizer spray

I use cleaning and home-care products for my kitchen that get an A rating on the Environmental Working Group testing scale (https://www.ewg.org/guides/cleaners).

Mason jars

These are handy for mixing salad dressings, storing foods, and building salads for meals or snacks.

Half sheet pan/baking pan and glass casserole dish for oven-baked dishes

I love oven-baked meals because they are easy and delicious. A simple aluminum sheet pan is an inexpensive workhorse in the kitchen. No need for nonstick coatings. For recipes that need a higher-walled vessel, use a glass casserole dish.

Parchment paper

Parchment paper makes baking on a sheet pan very easy, as it provides a nonstick surface and allows for browning. It also makes cleanup much easier, since you can throw out the parchment paper and the sheet pan won't require scrubbing.

Stainless-steel pots and pans

If you have not invested in a set of pots and pans, I'd recommend looking at a good-quality stainless-steel set at your local kitchen store. If a whole set is too pricey, the most important components are a large stock pot, a medium-size saucepan, and a 10- to 12-inch sauté pan.

Cast-iron skillet

Cast iron is cheaper than stainless steel, and often its heat retention and superior browning make it the right choice whether on the stovetop or in the oven. I recommend a 10- to 12-inch skillet. A cast-iron skillet can last a lifetime as long as it's properly cleaned and seasoned. You can find instructions for proper cast-iron care online.

Dutch oven

A Dutch oven is a large cast-iron pot with a tight-fitting lid used for soups and stews. Dutch ovens are often enameled (like the classic Dutch ovens from French brand Le Creuset).

Food processor

Food processors take a lot of the labor out of mixing, chopping, and blending food. An 11-cup food processor is a good basic size for any kitchen. Mini food processors (sometimes called mini food choppers) are best for chopping small herbs or pulverizing foods like garlic or ginger.

Blender

Blenders are similar to food processors but are intended to blend liquids rather than solid foods. They are perfect for pureeing wet ingredients or making smoothies.

Immersion blender

An immersion blender is a handheld blender that allows you to blend food in the pot you're cooking in — much more convenient than pouring everything into the bowl of a traditional blender. They're great for smoothing out soups or giving lentils a more even consistency.

Ice-pop molds

Ice pops are a great way to make your own healthy frozen treats for dessert. I prefer stainless-steel molds, which are usually dishwasher safe, making cleanup easier.

Salad spinner

This is a very useful item if you eat lots of leafy greens (as you should!), because you can wash your greens properly without worrying about waiting for them to dry. It's helpful to prepare a large quantity of lettuce, spinach, or kale for a few days at a time, and store the extra in a tightly sealed container.

Mise en Place

Mise en place is a French culinary term that means "everything in its place." When you are organized in the kitchen, it will make your tasks easy and quick. The basic idea is to get all your ingredients ready to go, measured out, and accessible before you start cooking. If you've ever watched cooking shows, you've probably seen the chefs with their ingredients already parceled out into small bowls, ready to be added to the dish. That's not just for TV! I encourage you to use this same principle.

In addition to small prep bowls with ingredients and spices, it's also useful to have two larger bowls for scraps — one for meat scraps, which you can freeze and use later for making stock, and one for vegetable scraps to compost.

Remember Food-Safety Principles!

While your kitchen won't be receiving a letter grade judging its cleanliness, that doesn't mean that food safety is any less important at home than in a restaurant. Make sure to follow these simple guidelines:

1. Wash your hands.
2. Wear an apron (or a chef's coat!).
3. Secure your hair, and remove your rings and jewelry.
4. If you are wearing nail polish, make sure flecks of polish are not falling into your food.
5. Use a tasting spoon and wash between uses if needed.
6. Use your thermometer to check the temperature of your proteins.
7. Keep your prep area clean.
8. Change, flip, or wash your cutting board when working with proteins and vegetables.
9. Do not thaw proteins on your countertop overnight—always leave them in the fridge.
10. Always store poultry on the bottom shelf of your fridge, making sure it does not drip onto other foods or surfaces in your fridge.
11. If family members or friends are in the kitchen with you, respect the kitchen space and be careful when opening the oven or carrying a hot dish. If you absolutely have to walk with a knife, always point it down. You will hear chefs on TV cooking competitions yell "behind" when walking behind another chef for this reason.

Respect All Ingredients

In addition to all the practical considerations, it's important to be in the right mental space for cooking. Eating is a basic human drive and the food you prepare will nourish you and your loved ones.

- Avoid waste; use all parts of the fruit, vegetable, or protein that are food safe. If you can't use all the food for the recipe you are currently making, save it for later, whether that means simply putting it in the fridge or making a stock from it that you can freeze and use in further recipes.
- Be respectful of your ingredient, whether it is a white truffle, a chicken breast, or a simple piece of lettuce.
- Be grateful and mindful of the moment when you handle your ingredients and combine them into a meal. Cooking and eating are a privilege.

Cleanup Practices

Finally, though I know it's not the most thrilling aspect of cooking, it's extremely important to keep a tidy workspace in the kitchen, not just for sanitary reasons, but so that you can be productive and stay motivated to cook. Clean up between steps of a recipe to ease the burden after dinner. And make sure that you do a good job of that post-meal cleanup—if you wake up to a messy kitchen, you'll be much less likely to feel motivated to make yourself a healthy breakfast.

Menus

Now that we've covered the basics for selecting ingredients and setting up your kitchen, it's time to explore what a full brain-healthy menu might look like. For each condition we've covered in the book, I'm going to give you a sample menu that includes all three major meals and snacks in between.

While these menus are geared toward an individual condition, bear in mind that there is enough overlap between the different eating patterns we've examined that all recipes are worth considering for general brain health—as long as you eat in an overall healthy way, you don't need to prioritize any single ingredient at every single meal.

My hope is that through reading these sample menus and trying some of the recipes, you will feel more comfortable in the kitchen, making your own food and relying less on store-bought ready-made or processed foods. Just this in itself is almost guaranteed to lead to a healthier lifestyle; the National Health and Nutrition Examination Survey, the most important research study about home cooking, showed that consumers who eat home-cooked meals also eat fewer calories.

There are times when it's okay to cut corners, though: when a recipe calls for vegetables like artichokes or cauliflower, it's okay to use a healthy frozen version with no added salt or sauce. Since foods are flash-frozen in the United States, frozen fruits and vegetables are healthy alternatives to fresh. For frozen fruit, always check that there's no added syrup or sugar. Of course, if you have the time and kitchen skills, working with fresh vegetables can be even more delicious and rewarding, so don't hold back!

Similarly, while it's great to make your own stock as we discussed earlier, it's not strictly necessary. Store-bought stock will work just fine, but make sure you are using an organic, low-sodium version. That way you can add the salt needed according to your taste.

Without further ado, on to the recipes!

RECIPES

Menu to Help Depression

Breakfast: Mung Bean Tofu Scramble

Snack: 1 tablespoon extra-dark chocolate chips

Lunch: Hearty Vegetable Soup

Snack: Spiced Nut Mix

Dinner: Baked Salmon with Walnut Kale Pesto

Dessert: A fresh orange and a glass of red wine

Mung Bean Tofu Scramble

(vegetarian/vegan/gluten-free/dairy-free)

Sprouted mung beans are a great way to add vitamin B_{12} and folate to your diet. Garlic, onions, and asparagus are rich in prebiotics. The turmeric brings all the beneficial effects of curcumin and gives the tofu a vibrant yellow color to make it look like scrambled eggs. Citrus fruit adds vitamin C easily to your meal.

Servings: 4
Prep Time: 10 minutes
Cooking Time: 10 minutes

1 (14-ounce) block organic soft tofu

1 tablespoon canola oil

¼ medium onion, finely diced

½ clove garlic, finely chopped

2 stalks asparagus, cleaned, peeled, and cut into 1-inch pieces

1 teaspoon ground turmeric

1½ teaspoons kosher salt

¼ teaspoon black pepper

1 (12-ounce) bag mung bean sprouts

Juice of ½ lemon

Roughly chop the block of tofu and then pulse to a chunky size in a food processor. (Use the pulse mode so that you do not turn the tofu into a liquid.) Heat the canola oil in a cast-iron skillet over medium heat. Add the onion, garlic, asparagus, turmeric, salt, and pepper and sauté for 2–3 minutes. Add the tofu and sprouted mung beans and sauté for 3–5 minutes, until the tofu begins to look like scrambled eggs. Add a squeeze of fresh lemon before serving.

Hearty Vegetable Soup

(vegetarian/vegan/gluten-free/dairy-free)

This soup has peas for magnesium, broccoli for iron, and sweet potatoes for vitamin A. It is low in saturated fat and high in fiber and antioxidants.

Servings: 4
Prep Time: 15 minutes
Cooking Time: 30 minutes

2 tablespoons olive oil

1 leek, sliced

1 clove garlic, finely chopped

1 cup fresh or frozen peas

2 cups fresh or frozen broccoli florets

1 sweet potato, unpeeled, cut into ½-inch dice

1 tablespoon kosher salt, plus more if needed

1 teaspoon black pepper, plus more if needed

½ teaspoon dried thyme

½ teaspoon dried parsley

4–6 cups hot vegetable stock or filtered water

Fresh parsley, chopped (optional)

Heat the oil in a cast-iron Dutch oven on medium heat. Add the leek and garlic and sauté for 3–5 minutes, until the leek is soft and almost translucent.

Add the peas, broccoli florets, sweet potato, salt, pepper, thyme, and dried parsley and allow to cook, stirring the mixture once or twice, for 3–5 minutes. Once the vegetables appear partly cooked, add the vegetable stock. Partially cover, and allow the soup to simmer on medium for about 20 minutes.

Season to taste with additional salt and pepper if desired, and garnish with fresh parsley, if desired.

Spiced Nut Mix

(vegetarian/vegan/gluten-free/dairy-free)

This nut mix includes pumpkin seeds for iron, Brazil nuts for selenium, cayenne pepper, and turmeric.

Servings: 8
Prep Time: 10 minutes
Cooking Time: 10 minutes

1 teaspoon ground turmeric

¼ teaspoon black pepper

¼ teaspoon garlic powder

¼ teaspoon cayenne pepper

2 teaspoons kosher salt

1 tablespoon olive oil

1½ cups plain roasted pumpkin seeds

1 cup Brazil nuts

Preheat the oven to 300°F and line a half-sheet baking pan with parchment paper.

Mix the turmeric, black pepper, garlic powder, cayenne pepper, salt, and olive oil in a medium stainless-steel bowl. Toss in the pumpkin seeds and nuts. Spread the seeds and nuts in a single layer on the lined baking pan. Roast for about 10 minutes. Cool and serve. Store in an airtight glass jar at room temperature for up to 2 weeks.

Baked Salmon with Walnut Kale Pesto

(gluten-free)

This is a great way to get omega-3s. It also provides folate from kale and the mood benefits of walnuts.

Servings: 1 (8 servings of pesto)
Prep Time: 5 minutes
Cooking Time: 15 minutes

For the fish:

1 (4–6-ounce) salmon fillet, boneless and skinless

2 tablespoons olive oil

½ teaspoon kosher salt

¼ teaspoon black pepper

For the pesto:

¼ cup olive oil

¼ cup grated Parmesan cheese

1 clove garlic, peeled and microwaved for 30 seconds

2 cups baby kale, washed and chopped

¼ cup walnuts

1 teaspoon lemon juice

½ teaspoon salt

Prepare the fish:

Preheat the oven to 350°F and line a baking sheet with parchment paper. Brush the salmon with the oil and then season with salt and pepper. Place on the baking sheet and bake for 8–12 minutes, or until the salmon is cooked through. A thermometer should read an internal temperature of 145°F.

Prepare the pesto:

Blend the pesto ingredients in a blender or food processor on medium speed. Add cold water to loosen the mixture if needed. Taste for salt, as you may need to add more.

Serve the oven-baked salmon with 1–2 tablespoons of the pesto.

Chef Tips:

- Pesto will last up to a week in the fridge stored in a mason jar.
- Try pesto on a whole wheat pasta salad or a gluten-free buckwheat noodle salad with vegetables.
- Pesto can also be used on oven-baked chicken breast.

Menu to Aid Anxiety

Breakfast: Avocado Hummus

Snack: Green tea

Lunch: Mushroom and Spinach Frittata

Snack: Kimchee with celery sticks

Dinner: Turkey Gumbo with Brown Rice

Dessert: Watermelon and Blueberry Pops

Avocado Hummus

(vegetarian, vegan, gluten-free, dairy-free)

Chickpeas are a source of tryptophan, and avocados and olive oil are great sources of healthy fats, including omega-3s (avocados are rich in fiber and various vitamins too). You can eat this tasty spread on a low-GI toast like pumpernickel, or as a dip for fresh-cut vegetables.

Servings: 6
Prep Time: 10 minutes

½ large ripe avocado, skin and seed removed

2 cups cooked or canned chickpeas

⅓ cup tahini paste

¼ cup fresh lime juice

1 clove garlic

1 teaspoon kosher salt, plus more if needed

¼ teaspoon black pepper

½ teaspoon ground cumin

¼ teaspoon smoked paprika

½ cup fresh cilantro

3 tablespoons olive oil, plus more for drizzling

1 tablespoon sliced, toasted almonds

¼ cup chopped fresh flat-leaf parsley

Using a food processor, combine all the ingredients except the olive oil, almonds, and parsley for about 1 minute.

With the motor running on medium speed, drizzle in the olive oil and continue to process until the hummus is very light and creamy, about 1 more minute. Season with additional salt, if needed.

Transfer the hummus to a shallow bowl.

Top with toasted almonds and chopped parsley and drizzle with additional olive oil.

If you are not eating immediately, cover the hummus with plastic so that the avocado does not turn brown. The hummus can be stored in the fridge for up to 1 day.

Mushroom and Spinach Frittata

(gluten-free, dairy-free)

This easy-to-make frittata has mushrooms for a vitamin D boost and spinach for magnesium. You could save pieces for lunch for the next 2 days or save for up to 1 month in the freezer.

Servings: 6
Prep Time: 10 minutes
Cooking Time: 18 minutes

5 whole eggs

1 cup almond milk

½ teaspoon kosher salt

¼ teaspoon black pepper

1½ teaspoons dried parsley

1 tablespoon olive oil

1 cup spinach (fresh or frozen and thawed)

1 cup mushrooms, chopped

Preheat the oven to 300°F. Line a 9-inch round casserole dish with parchment paper.

In a medium bowl whisk the eggs with the milk, salt, pepper, and parsley and set aside.

Heat the oil in a medium cast-iron pan over medium heat.

If using frozen spinach, wrap in cheesecloth (or a clean dish towel or paper towel) and squeeze to remove the excess water.

Sauté the spinach and mushrooms in the oil until the mushrooms are lightly brown, about 3 minutes. Allow to cool.

Place the cooled mushroom-spinach mixture in the casserole dish. Pour the egg mixture over the vegetables, cover with foil, and bake until the eggs are just set, 15–18 minutes. Ovens vary, so make sure the eggs are set before removing the frittata from the oven. Cut into 6 even pieces and serve.

Turkey Gumbo with Brown Rice

(gluten-free, dairy-free)

Though we've learned about the difficulty of dietary tryptophan absorption, turkey is still a good source of tryptophan. Instead of a high-GI carb like mashed potatoes, serve it over lower-GI brown rice to help as much tryptophan as possible reach the brain while not overdoing it with less nutritious calories.

Servings: 4
Prep Time: 20 minutes
Cooking Time: 25 minutes

1 tablespoon canola oil

¼ cup chopped leeks

¾ cup diced celery

1 carrot, grated

2 cloves garlic, grated

1 pound ground turkey

1½ teaspoons kosher salt

½ cup trimmed and chopped okra (1-inch pieces)

3 cups low-sodium chicken broth or water

1 teaspoon hot sauce

2 cups cooked brown rice

Heat the oil in a cast-iron Dutch oven over medium-high heat. Add the leeks, celery, carrot, and garlic, and sauté about 6 minutes, or until tender.

Add the turkey and salt and simmer for about 5 minutes, or until the turkey is lightly browned, stirring and chopping up the turkey while cooking. Add the okra. Stir in the broth. Bring to a boil, then reduce the heat and simmer uncovered for about 10 minutes. Add the hot sauce and serve over brown rice.

Watermelon and Blueberry Pops

(vegetarian, gluten-free, dairy-free)

These simple homemade ice pops are soothing because of their cool, lightly sweet taste. Watermelons are rich in antioxidants and vitamins A, B_6, and C. These treats can be made with almond milk for a creamier texture or coconut milk for added flavor.

Servings: 6 to 8 pops
Prep Time: 10 minutes

2 cups seeded, chopped watermelon

1 cup almond or coconut milk (optional)

½ teaspoon fresh lime juice

1 tablespoon lime zest

¼ teaspoon honey

½ cup fresh or frozen blueberries

Puree the watermelon with the milk, if using, in a blender. Stir in the lime juice, lime zest, and honey. Pour into stainless-steel ice-pop molds until each mold is two-thirds full, leaving room for the blueberries. Use 2–3 blueberries per mold.

Seal the molds and freeze for 3 hours or overnight.

Healing Trauma Menu

Breakfast: Chia Pudding Topped with Nuts and Berries

Snack: Sardine Snack

Lunch: Spice-Roasted Chicken Breast; Steamed Broccoli with Lemon

Snack: Celery sticks with almond butter

Dinner: Pepper-Crusted Filet Mignon with Baby Spinach Chimichurri

Dessert: Blueberries with lemon zest, a squeeze of fresh lemon, and chopped hazelnuts

Chia Pudding Topped with Nuts and Berries

(vegetarian, gluten-free, dairy-free)

Chia pudding is a great way to start the day and doesn't require any early-morning prep. Since it has to set in the fridge overnight, you can prepare it the night before and then eat on the go.

Servings: 2
Prep Time: 10 minutes

½ cup organic canned light coconut milk

½ teaspoon honey

½ teaspoon vanilla extract

¼ teaspoon ground cinnamon

2 tablespoons chia seeds

Raspberries, blueberries, walnuts, or other fruit or nut toppings

Pour the coconut milk into a mason jar and stir in the honey, vanilla, and cinnamon. Sprinkle the chia seeds on top.

Screw the lid of the mason jar on and shake well so that the seeds mix with the milk.

Chill overnight in the fridge.

Serve topped with nuts and berries.

Sardine Snack

(gluten-free, dairy-free)

Sardines are a great source of nutrients, especially omega-3s. Always buy sardines packed in olive oil and eat no more than half a can for a snack (the rest can be put into a mason jar and eaten the next day).

Servings: 2
Prep Time: 10 minutes

1 (4-ounce) can sardines packed in olive oil

½ tomato, diced

¼ teaspoon kosher salt

½ teaspoon black pepper

Juice of ½ lemon

1 large romaine lettuce leaf, cut in half

Drain some of the oil from the sardines. In a small bowl, mix the sardines with the tomato, salt, pepper, and lemon juice. Serve in a piece of romaine lettuce, letting the leaf act as an edible serving cup.

Spice-Roasted Chicken Breast

(gluten-free, dairy-free)

While chicken breast is a healthy lean protein, it can lack flavor, so the addition of spices here benefits both the brain and the flavor. Leftovers can be used to top a healthy green salad.

Servings: 2
Prep Time: 5 minutes
Cooking Time: 40 minutes

1 teaspoon cayenne pepper

1 teaspoon ground turmeric

¼ teaspoon ground black pepper

½ teaspoon ground coriander

½ teaspoon ground cumin

1 teaspoon kosher salt

½ teaspoon garlic powder

¼ cup olive oil

2 (6-ounce) boneless, skinless chicken breasts

Combine the spices in a small bowl and add them and the olive oil to a large bowl. Allow the spices to blend into the oil for a few minutes. Apply this marinade to the chicken breasts. You can marinate the chicken for as little as 30 minutes or overnight in the fridge.

When ready to cook, preheat the oven to 400°F and position a rack in the middle of the oven. Line a sheet pan with parchment paper.

Place the chicken breasts on the sheet pan and bake for about 30 minutes, or until the internal temperature at the thickest part of the breast reads 165–170°F.

Rest the roasted chicken for 10 minutes before serving.

Steamed Broccoli with Lemon

(vegetarian, vegan, gluten-free, dairy-free)

Whether using fresh or frozen broccoli florets, this is an extremely easy, no-fuss way to make a great vegetable side. You can use the same recipe for green beans, cauliflower florets, sugar snap peas, carrots, asparagus, and green peas.

Servings: 2
Prep Time: 2 minutes
Cooking Time: 5–8 minutes

2 cups fresh or frozen broccoli florets

1 lemon

½–1 teaspoon kosher salt

Place the broccoli in a glass baking dish, adding a few tablespoons of water. Steam uncovered in the microwave for up to 4 minutes. The broccoli should be cooked through with no cold or frozen bits. Drain any excess water.

Grate lemon zest over the broccoli and add a squeeze of fresh lemon juice. Season with salt before serving.

Pepper-Crusted Filet Mignon with Baby Spinach Chimichurri

(gluten-free, dairy-free)

Since you shouldn't eat too much beef, a filet is a great way to get the maximum deliciousness in a small cut. Searing first and then finishing in the oven allows you to get a browned exterior with a smooth, evenly colored interior. Serve this steak with a simple salad of leafy greens for a dinner worthy of a special celebration.

Servings: 1 (6 servings of sauce)
Prep Time: 20 minutes
Cooking Time: 40 minutes

For the steak:

1 (6-ounce, 2-inch-thick) filet mignon steak

1 teaspoon kosher salt

1 teaspoon black pepper

1 tablespoon canola oil

For the sauce:

1 cup fresh flat-leaf parsley

1 cup tightly packed fresh baby spinach

½ cup fresh oregano

2 cloves garlic

Zest of 1 lime

1 tablespoon fresh lime juice

1 tablespoon white wine vinegar

½ cup olive oil

¾ teaspoon kosher salt, plus more as needed

¼ teaspoon black pepper, plus more as needed

Prepare the steak:

Allow the steak to come to room temperature, covered, for 30 minutes. Add the salt and pepper to all sides. Preheat the oven to 425°F.

Heat the oil in a medium cast-iron skillet over medium heat. Place the steak in the hot pan, searing for about 2 minutes per side.

Put the pan in the oven. For medium-rare, roast for about 7 minutes, until the internal temperature reaches 135°F. For medium, roast for about 10 minutes, until the internal temperature reaches 145°F.

Prepare the sauce:

Add the parsley, spinach, oregano, garlic, lime zest, lime juice, and vinegar to a blender. Blend on low to medium until you have chunky consistency. Drizzle in the olive oil and blend on medium speed. Season with salt and pepper, adding more if desired.

Once the steak has reached the desired temperature, remove from the oven and rest for 10–15 minutes. Top with 2 tablespoons of the sauce and serve.

Chef Tips:

- The chimichurri sauce will last for at least a week in the fridge if stored in a sealed glass jar.
- Use the chimichurri sauce over grilled chicken or a pork chop.
- The sauce can also be added to oven-roasted vegetables.

Focus Menu

Breakfast: Chocolate Protein Smoothie

Snack: Small piece of extra-dark chocolate

Lunch: Creamy Artichoke and Leek Soup

Snack: ¼ cup blueberries with 1 tablespoon cashew nut butter

Dinner: Oven-Roasted Chicken Drumsticks; Mushroom Salad

Chocolate Protein Smoothie

(vegetarian, gluten-free)

In chapter 5, we talked about a study that tested a specially formulated breakfast bar that aimed to improve the symptoms of ADHD. Here, I've adapted that formula into a delicious smoothie, providing many of the same benefits.

Servings: 1
Prep Time: 10 minutes

1 cup unsweetened almond milk

1 tablespoon walnuts

1 scoop vanilla whey protein

1 tablespoon ground flaxseeds

1 teaspoon organic ground instant coffee powder

1 teaspoon natural (non-alkalized) cocoa powder

1 tablespoon coconut flakes

½ teaspoon honey

¼ ripe avocado

Place the ingredients in a blender with ¼ cup of ice cubes, and blend. Add more water or ice if the smoothie is too thick for your liking. Sip and enjoy!

Creamy Artichoke and Leek Soup

(vegetarian, vegan, gluten-free, dairy-free)

This gluten-free, dairy-free soup is naturally rich in healthy fiber and prebiotics from the leeks. The addition of a nut milk makes it creamy, but much healthier than using heavy cream.

Servings: 4
Prep Time: 10 minutes
Cooking Time: 20 minutes

1 tablespoon olive oil

½ cup chopped leeks

1½ teaspoons kosher salt, plus more if needed

½ teaspoon black pepper, plus more if needed

1 tablespoon sweet paprika

1 teaspoon garlic powder

½ teaspoon fresh thyme

½ teaspoon fresh chopped parsley

1½ cups frozen artichoke hearts

2 cups low-sodium vegetable stock

2 cups almond or cashew milk

Juice of ½ lemon

1 tablespoon chopped fresh flat-leaf parsley

1 tablespoon toasted pumpkin seeds

Heat the oil in a large stainless-steel pot over medium heat, and sauté the leeks with the salt, pepper, paprika, garlic powder, thyme, and fresh chopped parsley for about 5 minutes, or until the leeks are soft. Add the artichoke hearts and allow them to soften for another 3 minutes.

Add the stock and cover, bringing to a boil over medium heat. Add the almond milk and reduce the heat. Simmer, uncovered, until the artichokes are tender, about 10 minutes.

Allow the soup to cool for a few minutes. Using an immersion blender, puree the soup to a smooth texture (you can also leave it chunky if you prefer).

Season to taste with additional salt and pepper, if needed. Stir in the lemon juice and serve hot, garnished with flat-leaf parsley and toasted pumpkin seeds.

Oven-Roasted Chicken Drumsticks

(gluten-free, dairy-free)

This is a time-saving sheet-pan meal that can easily be scaled up for more people—just add drumsticks and balance the spice blend accordingly.

Servings: 1
Prep Time: 10 minutes
Cooking Time: 40 minutes

1 tablespoon olive oil

1 tablespoon sweet paprika

½ teaspoon ground turmeric

¼ teaspoon black pepper

½ teaspoon kosher salt

2 skinless chicken drumsticks

Preheat the oven to 400°F. Line a sheet pan with parchment paper.

In a medium bowl, mix together the olive oil, paprika, turmeric, pepper, and salt. Coat the chicken with the marinade. With clean hands, massage the marinade into the drumsticks.

Transfer the chicken to the sheet pan and bake for 30 minutes, or until the internal temperature reaches 165°F. The chicken should not have any pink color when you cut into it. If it does, return it to oven for at least another 10 minutes and recheck the temperature. Allow the chicken to rest for 10 minutes on the sheet pan before serving.

Mushroom Salad

(vegetarian, gluten-free, dairy-free)

In recipes that include soy sauce you can omit the salt if you desire. Mushrooms sometimes need more seasoning, so if they need a pinch of salt later, you can sprinkle some on at the end.

Servings: 4
Prep Time: 15 minutes
Cooking Time: 5 minutes

1 tablespoon sesame seeds (optional)

1 tablespoon plus 1½ teaspoons rice wine vinegar

1½ teaspoons almond butter

¼ teaspoon ground ginger

Pinch of crushed red pepper

¼ teaspoon garlic powder

¼ teaspoon honey

¾ teaspoon gluten-free soy sauce

¾ teaspoon sesame oil

2 cups white button mushrooms, cut into bite-size pieces

Toast the sesame seeds, if using, in a medium sauté pan over low heat until lightly browned. Set the toasted seeds aside in glass bowl to cool.

Using the same pan, whisk together the vinegar, almond butter, ginger, red pepper, garlic powder, honey, and soy sauce over medium-high heat. Stir until warmed through. Stir in the sesame oil. Pour the warm dressing over the cut mushrooms in a medium bowl and stir to combine. Sprinkle on the toasted sesame seeds. Allow to cool and serve.

Memory-Boosting Menu

Breakfast: Cup of coffee; 1 cup gluten-free oatmeal with cinnamon and ½ cup chopped fresh strawberries

Snack: 1 chopped hard-boiled egg seasoned with salt and black pepper and served with 5 medium-size whole-grain crackers

Lunch: Cauliflower and Chickpea Stir-Fry served with microgreens

Snack: Steamed edamame with flaked sea salt

Dinner: Southern French–Style Scallops; Turmeric-Infused Cauliflower Rice

Dessert: Cinnamon–Black Pepper Hot Chocolate

Cauliflower and Chickpea Stir-Fry

(vegetarian, vegan, gluten-free, dairy-free)

This simple stir-fry follows the principles of the MIND diet.

Servings: 8
Prep Time: 10 minutes
Cooking Time: 10 minutes

2 tablespoons olive oil

1 teaspoon cayenne pepper

1 teaspoon ground coriander

1 teaspoon ground turmeric

¼ teaspoon black pepper

4 cups frozen cauliflower florets

2 cups cooked chickpeas

1½ teaspoons kosher salt, plus more if needed

1 tablespoon fresh lemon juice

1 tablespoon chopped fresh cilantro (optional)

½ cup microgreens (e.g., pea shoots or radish sprouts)

Heat the oil in a medium cast-iron pan over medium heat. Add the cayenne pepper, coriander, turmeric, and black pepper to the hot oil and let them infuse for a few seconds. Add the cauliflower and chickpeas and stir to combine with the spices. Sauté for about 1 minute and cover to cook for 3 more minutes. If the vegetables are sticking to the pan, add ¼ cup water. Season with salt, adding more if desired. Add lemon juice and a garnish of chopped cilantro, if desired. Sprinkle microgreens on top and serve hot.

Chef Tips:

- This dish can also be served cold as a salad.
- Organic canned chickpeas, rinsed and drained, can be used.

Southern French–Style Scallops

(gluten-free, dairy-free)

Scallops are delicious and easy to cook. They are a great way to impress friends with your chef skills. This gluten-free recipe highlights the memory-boosting benefits of rosemary and omega-3s.

Servings: 6
Prep Time: 10 minutes
Cooking Time: 15 minutes

1 pound bay scallops (or sea scallops, halved horizontally)

1½ teaspoons kosher salt, plus more if desired

1 teaspoon black pepper, plus more if desired

2 tablespoons organic gluten-free flour

2 tablespoons olive oil

2 medium shallots, finely diced

1 clove garlic, finely chopped

1½ teaspoons fresh rosemary (or ¾ teaspoon dried)

2 tablespoons chopped fresh flat-leaf parsley

⅓ cup white wine

1 lemon

Sprinkle the scallops with salt and pepper and then toss them in the flour, shaking off the excess. Heat the olive oil in a large stainless-steel sauté pan on high heat. Add the scallops in a single layer. Lower the heat to medium and allow the scallops to brown lightly on one side. They will release from the pan when ready; turn them over and let them brown lightly on the other side. The scallops should cook for about 4 minutes in total. Remove the scallops and set aside in a medium bowl.

Add the shallots, garlic, rosemary, and 1 tablespoon of the parsley to the pan and sauté for a few minutes. Return the scallops to the pan and add the wine and cook for 1 minute. Zest the lemon over the scallops and sprinkle on the remaining 1 tablespoon parsley. Season with additional salt and black pepper. Serve hot with a squeeze of lemon juice.

Turmeric-Infused Cauliflower Rice

(vegetarian, vegan, gluten-free, dairy-free)

Cauliflower rice is a great way to enjoy the texture of rice without the high glycemic load by providing a serving of vegetables as well as the fiber and nutrients from cauliflower.

Servings: 4
Prep Time: 10 minutes
Cooking Time: 5–8 minutes

1 tablespoon olive oil

2 cups frozen plain cauliflower rice (see Chef Tips for details on ricing fresh cauliflower)

1 tablespoon kosher salt

1 teaspoon ground turmeric

½ teaspoon black pepper

1 teaspoon garlic powder

Zest of 1 lemon

Heat the oil in a medium cast-iron pan over medium heat. Add the rest of the ingredients except the lemon zest to the pan and stir to combine. Cook for 5–8 minutes, until the cauliflower is slightly browned.

Sprinkle on the lemon zest and serve.

Chef Tips:

If you'd like to use fresh cauliflower, remove the outside leaves from a head of cauliflower. Wash the head and pat dry. Break the florets off the cauliflower and, working in small batches, place them in a large food processor with the steel blade attachment. Pulse until the cauliflower is in small rice-size pieces. If there are large chunks of cauliflower remaining, these can be removed and used for another recipe.

Cinnamon–Black Pepper Hot Chocolate

(vegetarian, vegan, dairy-free)

This delicious and rich chocolate treat doesn't need to be too sweet. The complexity of dark chocolate (use natural, non-alkalized) really shines through, and the black pepper gives it a bit of a contrasting bite. Cinnamon and black pepper also help boost your memory.

Servings: 2
Prep Time: 5 minutes
Cooking Time: 10 minutes

¼ cup dark chocolate chips (65 percent cacao or darker)

2 cups coconut, almond, oat, or cashew milk

1 teaspoon vanilla extract

½ teaspoon ground cinnamon

Pinch of black pepper

Place the chocolate chips in a medium heatproof bowl. Warm the milk, vanilla, cinnamon, and pepper in a saucepan over medium heat. When bubbles form around the edges of the milk, remove from the heat and pour it over the chocolate chips.

Allow the warmed milk to begin to melt the chocolate. Wait 2 minutes, then use a whisk to gently mix the milk and chocolate together. If the mixture is too thick, add a little more warmed milk.

Beating OCD Menu

Breakfast: Homemade Cereal

Snack: Cottage cheese with blueberries

Lunch: Lentil Soup with Spinach (Dal)

Snack: 1 small to medium kiwi

Dinner: Paprika-Roasted Turkey Breast with Red Onions and Cherry Tomatoes

Dessert: Banana "Ice Cream"

Homemade Cereal

(vegetarian, vegan, gluten-free, dairy-free)

Even "healthy" store-bought cereals may be high in sugar. It's easy to make a delicious cereal out of whole grains and other brain-healthy ingredients.

Servings: 2
Prep Time: 10 minutes

½ cup rolled oats

¼ cup bran flakes

¼ cup unsweetened coconut flakes

1 tablespoon chopped walnuts

½ teaspoon flaxseeds

Pinch of cinnamon

Pinch of ground nutmeg

Combine all the ingredients in a medium bowl. Store in an airtight mason jar for up to 2 weeks.

You can serve the cereal in a variety of ways—with almond milk or another milk of your choice, with 1 tablespoon of organic dark chocolate chips for a twist, topped with fresh berries, or all of the above! If you need a little sweetness, add a touch of honey.

Lentil Soup with Spinach (Dal)

(vegetarian, vegan, gluten-free, dairy-free)

Dal is one of my favorite comfort foods, but even if you didn't grow up eating it, I'm sure you'll find it filling and soothing. The turmeric is an added bonus. Asafetida powder is used in Indian cooking as a digestive, helping to lower the effects of gas and bloating from foods like beans and lentils. While it has a pungent aroma, it is very flavorful once added to a dish.

Servings: 8
Prep Time: 30 minutes (plus overnight soaking)
Cooking Time: 20 minutes

2 cups yellow split pea lentils

2 tablespoons canola oil

1 teaspoon black mustard seeds (optional)

1 teaspoon cumin seeds

2 cloves garlic, peeled and sliced in half lengthwise

1 dried whole red chili (optional)

1 medium onion, finely chopped

1 medium tomato, finely chopped

1 teaspoon ground turmeric

¼ teaspoon black pepper

2 cups spinach leaves

1 tablespoon kosher salt

½ lemon

1 teaspoon asafetida powder (optional)

Chopped fresh cilantro for garnish

Rinse and soak the lentils in a covered glass bowl in the fridge overnight. Make sure the water covers the lentils by about a half inch. Rinse out the lentils the next day, transfer to a large saucepan, and add 4 cups water. Boil the lentils for about 30 minutes, until soft. The texture should be smooth, like a paste. Alternatively, you can cook the lentils in a pressure cooker—follow the directions supplied by your pressure cooker's manufacturer.

Heat the oil in a medium stainless-steel pot over medium heat. Add the black mustard seeds, if using, and cook until they pop. Add the cumin seeds, garlic, dried red chili, if using, and chopped onion. Cook for 3–5 minutes, or until the onion is translucent. Add the tomato, turmeric, and black pepper, and stir to combine. Add the spinach and allow to wilt for just 1 minute.

Add the lentils, lower the heat, and allow to cook for about 2 minutes. Add 2 cups water, as the mixture will be thick and you want to prevent the lentils from sticking.

Season with the salt, a squeeze of fresh lemon, and the asafetida powder, if using. Serve hot, garnished with chopped cilantro.

Paprika-Roasted Turkey Breast with Red Onions and Cherry Tomatoes

(gluten-free, dairy-free)

For a plant-based option, this recipe works with 1 block of firm tofu cut into slices or cubes. A chicken breast is another option. Turkey is a rich source of B vitamins, and vitamin B_{12} may have a positive impact on OCD.

Servings: 4
Prep Time: 10 minutes
Cooking Time: 20 minutes

2 tablespoons olive oil

2 tablespoons paprika

1 teaspoon ground turmeric

1½ teaspoons kosher salt

¼ teaspoon black pepper

4 (4-ounce) pieces boneless, skinless turkey breast

2 cups cherry tomatoes, pierced

½ red onion, thickly sliced

Preheat the oven to 400°F and line a sheet pan with parchment paper.

In a medium bowl combine the olive oil, paprika, turmeric, salt, and pepper. Put the turkey breasts, tomatoes, and onion in the bowl and stir till well combined and the turkey is coated.

Transfer the turkey, tomatoes, and onions to the sheet pan and bake for 15 minutes, or until the turkey reaches an internal temperature of 165°F. If you'd like to brown the turkey, broil for 3 minutes, or until browned. You may wish to remove the tomatoes and onions before broiling, as they may burn.

Banana "Ice Cream"

(vegetarian, gluten-free, dairy-free)

This is another way to get your fix for a frozen, slightly sweet treat without going overboard on dairy and sugar.

Servings: 6
Prep Time: 12 hours

8 extremely ripe bananas, peeled and diced

1 tablespoon honey

½ cup unsweetened almond, cashew, oat, or coconut milk, as needed to achieve desired consistency

Place the banana pieces on a sheet pan and freeze overnight.

Place the frozen banana pieces in a blender or food processor with the honey. Blend while slowly adding milk to thin the mixture. Watch carefully, as you may need more or less than the ½ cup of milk. You are looking for the texture of soft-serve ice cream. Once this texture is achieved, transfer to a bowl and place in the freezer for at least 3 hours or overnight.

Before serving, add mix-ins, if desired, like chopped nuts, dark chocolate chips, or peanut butter. Top with fresh berries.

Chef Tips:

- For chocolate ice cream, add 2 tablespoons of natural (non-alkalized) cocoa powder at the end before you chill the "ice cream." As you blend the mixture, make sure there are no lumps. You may have to first pass the cocoa powder through a sieve or strainer, so it blends evenly into the mixture.

Menu for Ideal Sleep Patterns and Lower Fatigue

Breakfast: On-the-Go Scrambled Eggs in a Mug

Snack: Banana and almond butter over cottage cheese

Lunch: Spicy Shrimp; mixed green salad

Snack: Pickled Okra

Dinner: Oven-Roasted Turkey Breast; Oven-Roasted Miso-Glazed Sweet Potatoes

Dessert: Golden Milk

On-the-Go Scrambled Eggs in a Mug

(gluten-free, dairy-free)

It's important to have a nutritious and energy-filled start to the day when you're fighting fatigue. This twist on classic scrambled eggs is a great way to enjoy an omega-3-rich meal without having to take the time to sit down and eat. For an extra dose of vitamins, you can add spinach or kale to the eggs, which will wilt easily into the mix.

Servings: 1
Prep Time: 2 minutes
Cooking Time: 3–5 minutes

Organic olive oil spray

2 large omega-3-fortified eggs

1 tablespoon nondairy milk of choice

¼ teaspoon kosher salt

Pinch of black pepper

¼ cup chopped spinach or kale

Spray a coffee mug with the olive oil spray. Crack the eggs into the mug and use a fork to beat them together with the milk, salt, and pepper. Heat in the microwave for 30 seconds to 1 minute. Stir the egg mixture with a fork. Return to the microwave and cook until the eggs appear scrambled, about another minute. Use the fork to fluff up the eggs. Stir in the spinach or kale and allow to wilt.

Spicy Shrimp

(gluten-free, dairy-free)

These shrimp are a great way to get a dose of seafood and capsaicin in your diet. You can add a bit more cayenne pepper if you prefer your food spicier.

Servings: 1
Prep Time: 20 minutes
Cooking Time: 5 minutes

8 medium shrimp, peeled and deveined, tails left on

½ teaspoon ground cumin

½ teaspoon cayenne pepper

½ teaspoon ground turmeric

¼ teaspoon black pepper

¼ teaspoon garlic powder

1 teaspoon kosher salt

2 tablespoons olive oil

In a medium bowl, toss the shrimp with the cumin, cayenne pepper, turmeric, black pepper, garlic powder, and salt.

Heat the oil in a cast-iron skillet over medium heat. Add the shrimp and stir-fry until they are cooked through and pink on the outside, about 3 minutes.

Pickled Okra

(vegetarian, vegan, gluten-free, dairy-free)

Like most pickled vegetables, this okra must be made ahead of time, but once it's made, it keeps very well in the fridge for at least a month if stored in a glass mason jar with a tight-fitting lid. This is another great way to get nigella seeds, capsaicin, and other spices into your diet.

Serving Size: 8
Prep Time: 15 minutes
Cooking Time: 10 minutes

2 cups fresh okra

Juice of ½ lemon

¾ teaspoon sugar

2 cups white vinegar

2 cups filtered water

2 tablespoons kosher salt

2 tablespoons nigella seeds

1 tablespoon coriander seeds

1 tablespoon chili pepper flakes

1 teaspoon celery seeds

1 teaspoon black pepper

3 large cloves garlic, peeled and sliced

4 thick slices lemon

Place the okra in an extra-large mason jar.

In a medium stainless-steel pot, heat the lemon juice, sugar, vinegar, water, and salt over medium heat. When the liquid is warmed through, add the remaining spices, garlic, and lemon. Allow to simmer over low heat for 3 minutes. Remove from the heat and cool slightly before pouring over the okra. Cover tightly and chill in the fridge for at least 3 hours or overnight.

Oven-Roasted Turkey Breast

(gluten-free, dairy-free)

As we mentioned for the Paprika-Roasted Turkey Breast (page 273), if you prefer a plant-based option, this recipe works with 1 block of firm tofu cut into slices or cubes. A chicken breast is another option. Turkey is a rich source of B vitamins, including vitamin B_{12}.

Servings: 4
Prep Time: 10 minutes
Cooking Time: 20 minutes

2 tablespoons olive oil

1 teaspoon garlic powder

1½ teaspoons dried oregano

1 teaspoon fresh thyme leaves, chopped fine

1½ teaspoons kosher salt

¼ teaspoon black pepper

4 (4-ounce) pieces boneless, skinless turkey breast

1 tablespoon lemon zest

Preheat the oven to 400°F and line a sheet pan with parchment paper.

In a medium bowl combine the olive oil, garlic powder, oregano, thyme, salt, and pepper. Put the turkey breasts in the bowl and stir till well combined and the turkey is coated.

Transfer the turkey to the sheet pan and bake for 15 minutes, or until the turkey reaches an internal temperature of 165°F. If you'd like to brown the turkey, broil for 3 minutes or until browned. Sprinkle with lemon zest and serve.

Oven-Roasted Miso-Glazed Sweet Potatoes

(vegetarian, vegan, gluten-free, dairy-free)

This is one of my favorite recipes to share and teach. Fermented miso paste gives both a great probiotic benefit and wonderful depth of flavor to the richness of the sweet potatoes. Once you taste the umami from the miso paste, you may enjoy using it to brighten other roasted vegetable dishes too.

Servings: 8
Prep Time: 20 minutes
Cooking Time: 25 minutes

½ cup white miso paste

¼ cup olive oil

¼ tablespoon kosher salt

¼ teaspoon black pepper

4 medium sweet potatoes, unpeeled, sliced into discs

Preheat the oven to 425°F and line a sheet pan with parchment paper.

Mix the miso paste, olive oil, salt, and pepper in a large bowl. Toss in the sweet potatoes and combine. Place the sweet potatoes on a sheet pan, making sure they are arranged in a single layer. Roast in the oven for 20–25 minutes, until the potatoes are tender (a sharp knife should cut through easily).

Golden Milk

(vegetarian, gluten-free, dairy-free)

This turmeric drink is a treat after dinner. It is especially warming and soothing to help you to sleep.

Servings: 1
Prep Time: 5 minutes
Cooking Time: 5 minutes

1 cup almond milk

1 teaspoon ground turmeric

¼ teaspoon black pepper

½ teaspoon honey

¼ teaspoon grated nutmeg

Heat all the ingredients except the nutmeg in a medium saucepan over medium heat for about 5 minutes. Pour into a mug, sprinkle with nutmeg, and serve.

Menu for Bipolar Disorder and Schizophrenia

Breakfast: Peanut Butter Matcha Smoothie

Snack: Steamed Edamame with Flakes of Sea Salt

Lunch: Oven-Roasted Rosemary Chicken Breast; Romaine Lettuce Salad with Mustard Vinaigrette; green tea

Snack: Macerated Strawberries with Black Pepper

Dinner: Salmon Patties with Ginger and Scallion Sauce

Dessert: Clementines and oranges served with shavings of dark chocolate

Peanut Butter Matcha Smoothie

(dairy-free)

Matcha powder is powdered green tea that is easy to add to smoothies or other foods and drinks — there's no need to steep as you would traditional tea leaves.

Servings: 1
Prep Time: 10 minutes

½ cup almond milk or other nondairy milk

1 scoop organic protein powder

1 pitted date

1 teaspoon matcha powder

1 tablespoon peanut butter

½ banana

Combine all the ingredients in a blender with ½ cup ice cubes; blend until smooth and frothy. Serve immediately.

Steamed Edamame with Flakes of Sea Salt

(vegetarian, vegan, gluten-free, dairy-free)

I prefer edamame in the shell for this snack, as it takes more time to eat and one tends to feel more satiated. Shelled edamame are delicious to add to salads or soups or even steamed as a vegetable side dish.

Servings: 2
Prep Time: 5 minutes
Cooking Time: 2 minutes

1 cup frozen edamame in the shell

¼ teaspoon flaked sea salt

Place the edamame in a glass bowl. Heat in the microwave on medium heat for about 2 minutes. If still frozen or hard, heat for another minute. Sprinkle with salt and eat hot.

Oven-Roasted Rosemary Chicken Breast

(gluten-free, dairy-free)

This recipe uses chicken breasts, but you could use a whole chicken as well, with the seasoning mixture rubbed on the skin. Cooking time will increase, but roast until the deepest part of the thigh registers 165°F.

Servings: 4
Prep Time: 10 minutes
Cooking Time: 20 minutes

2 tablespoons olive oil

1 teaspoon garlic powder

2 tablespoons chopped fresh rosemary leaves

1½ teaspoons kosher salt

¼ teaspoon black pepper

4 (4-ounce) pieces boneless, skinless chicken breast

Preheat the oven to 400°F and line a sheet pan with parchment paper.

In a medium bowl combine the olive oil, garlic powder, rosemary, salt, and pepper. Put the chicken breasts in the bowl and stir till well combined and the chicken is coated.

Transfer the chicken to the sheet pan and bake for 15 minutes, or until the chicken reaches an internal temperature of 165°F. If you slice the chicken breast and there is any pink color, return to the oven for another 5 minutes and check the color again.

Romaine Lettuce Salad with Mustard Vinaigrette

(vegetarian, vegan, gluten-free, dairy-free)

Romaine lettuce is delicious, crunchy, and nutritious. You're much better off making your own dressing rather than buying one, as store-bought dressings tend to be high in sugar, sodium, and preservatives. The classic dressing is a vinaigrette. A vinaigrette is an emulsion, meaning an acid comes together with a fat. One part acid to three parts fat is a good guideline.

Servings: 4
Prep Time: 10 minutes

For the salad:

1 head romaine lettuce

For the dressing:

2 tablespoons red wine vinegar

½ teaspoon kosher salt

¼ teaspoon black pepper

1 teaspoon whole-grain or Dijon mustard

6 tablespoons olive oil

Prepare the salad:

Prepare a head of romaine lettuce by chopping off the end and separating the leaves. Rinse under cool water, then place in a salad spinner to drain off excess water. If you don't have a salad spinner, simply pat dry the leaves with clean paper towels. Once the lettuce is dry, tear or chop the leaves into bite-size pieces.

Prepare the vinaigrette:

Combine all the ingredients in a mason jar. Cover the jar and shake until the dressing is emulsified.

Place the lettuce in a serving bowl and add the vinaigrette. Toss to combine.

Chef Tips:

- You can prepare a whole head of lettuce and use it over 2–3 days for salad as long as the dressing is not added (which would make the lettuce soggy). Store extra romaine lettuce in an airtight container in the fridge for up to 4 days.
- Store your vinaigrette in the mason jar you mixed it in. If you make a larger batch of dressing, it will keep for up to 2 weeks in the fridge. Shake before use to mix up the dressing again.
- You can use a variety of vinegars and add chopped shallots, garlic, or fresh herbs for different flavors.

Macerated Strawberries with Black Pepper

(vegetarian, gluten-free, dairy-free)

I first discovered this unusual combination in culinary school. The benefits of black pepper and the strawberries with their antioxidants, vitamin C, and folate make these a perfect snack.

Servings: 2
Prep Time: 10 minutes

Juice of ½ lemon

½ teaspoon honey

1 cup sliced fresh strawberries

Pinch of black pepper

In a small bowl, combine the lemon juice and honey. Stir. Add the strawberries and toss to combine. Sprinkle with the black pepper. Allow the strawberries to macerate for 10 minutes before serving.

Salmon Patties with Ginger and Scallion Sauce

(gluten-free, dairy-free)

Once again, salmon is a great source of omega-3s, and patties are a great way to eat them. The ginger-scallion sauce has a wonderful flavor while also providing a nutritious boost. Salmon patties are an easy way to eat a protein-rich meal with no additional carbohydrates.

Servings: 2
Prep Time: 10 minutes
Cooking Time: 10 minutes

For the sauce:

1 teaspoon olive oil

½ cup thinly sliced scallions

2 teaspoons grated fresh gingerroot

1 clove garlic, grated

1 tablespoon gluten-free soy sauce

For the patties:

2 tablespoons olive oil

2 fresh salmon patties

1 teaspoon kosher salt

½ teaspoon black pepper

2 large romaine lettuce leaves

Prepare the sauce:

Heat the olive oil in a small saucepan over medium heat. Add the scallions and allow them to sizzle for 1 minute. Add the ginger, garlic, and soy sauce and simmer for 5–10 minutes. If the sauce appears too thick, add up to ¼ cup water.

Prepare the salmon patties:

In a stainless-steel frying pan, heat the olive oil. Season the salmon patties with salt and pepper.

Pan-fry the patties in the oil for 3–5 minutes on each side, until the center is cooked and the internal temperature reaches 145°F.

Serve each salmon patty in a romaine lettuce leaf and drizzle with the ginger-scallion sauce.

Libido-Lifting Menu

Breakfast: Lox, sliced red onions, capers, and lemon juice on whole-grain toast

Snack: Fresh pomegranate juice

Lunch: Oven-Baked Cajun Chicken

Snack: Sliced avocado with ¼ cup unsalted pistachios

Dinner: San Franciscan Seafood Stew

Dessert: Chocolate-Dipped Strawberries

Oven-Baked Cajun Chicken

(gluten-free, dairy-free)

Cajun spice is a great and easy way to get the libido-boosting benefits of capsaicin and garlic. These spices delight the senses.

Servings: 2
Prep Time: 10 minutes
Cooking Time: 25 minutes

2 tablespoons olive oil

2 tablespoons salt-free Cajun seasoning

2 (4–6-ounce) boneless, skinless chicken breasts

1 tablespoon kosher salt

½ teaspoon cracked black pepper

Preheat the oven to 425°F and line a sheet pan with parchment paper.

Combine the olive oil and Cajun seasoning in a small bowl. Season the chicken with salt and pepper, then brush the chicken with the Cajun marinade.

Place the chicken on the sheet pan and bake until it is golden brown and cooked through, 20–25 minutes, or until the thickest part of the chicken reaches an internal temperature of 165°F.

San Franciscan Seafood Stew

(gluten-free, dairy-free)

Roasted or oven-baked salmon can become repetitive. This stew uses both salmon and shellfish, which are rich and healthy brain foods.

Servings: 8
Prep Time: 15 minutes
Cooking Time: 20 minutes

1/4 teaspoon saffron threads

2 tablespoons olive oil

1 medium fennel bulb, thinly sliced

1 medium onion, chopped

1/2 teaspoon Italian seasoning

2 tablespoons kosher salt

2 cloves garlic, grated

3/4 teaspoon cayenne powder or crushed red pepper flakes

2 tablespoons tomato paste

1 1/2 cups chopped tomatoes

1 cup dry white wine

4 cups low-sodium seafood stock

8 mussels, scrubbed and debearded

2 (4-ounce) pieces boneless, skinless salmon, cut into 2-inch chunks

1 lemon

Place the saffron threads in 1/4 cup boiling water, set aside for about 5 minutes, and allow to bloom. Heat the oil in a large cast-iron soup pot over medium heat. Add the fennel, onion, Italian seasoning, and salt and sauté until the onion is translucent, about 10 minutes. Add the garlic and cayenne pepper and cook for 3 minutes. Add the tomato paste and stir gently, followed by the chopped tomatoes, wine, and seafood stock. Add the mussels, cover, and cook for 3 minutes. Add the salmon pieces, cover, reduce the heat to low, and simmer until the seafood is cooked through, about 3 minutes. The salmon should no longer be pink, and the mussels should have opened up. Discard any mussels that do not open, as they are considered unsafe to eat.

Add the saffron with its liquid. Allow the fish stew to simmer for at least 10 minutes for the flavors to meld. Make sure the seafood is cooked; cooking times on your stove may vary.

Squeeze fresh lemon juice over the stew and serve in individual soup bowls.

Chef Tips:

- Your seafood market or seafood counter can help you prepare the salmon pieces and mussels if you are not sure how to work with them.
- Italian seasoning is a salt-free spice blend found in most supermarkets.
- Saffron is a costly spice and should be used sparingly.

Chocolate-Dipped Strawberries

(vegetarian, vegan)

Use natural, non-alkalized extra-dark chocolate chips for better antioxidant levels.

Servings: 15
Prep Time: 5 minutes
Cooking Time: 20 minutes

1 cup extra-dark chocolate chips

2 tablespoons coconut oil

1 pint fresh whole strawberries with stems

Line a sheet pan with parchment paper and chill in the freezer for up to ½ hour. Using a double boiler, melt the chocolate chips with the coconut oil (see Chef Tips) and remove from the heat.

Quickly dip the strawberries in the melted chocolate and allow to dry on the cold sheet pan.

Allow to set in the fridge for 5–10 minutes.

Chef Tips:

To melt chocolate in a double boiler (bain-marie method), fill a stainless-steel saucepan one-third full of water. Put the chocolate in a heatproof glass bowl and place over the saucepan so that its base does not touch the water. Heat the water over medium heat. Once the chocolate starts to melt, remove from the heat using an oven mitt, then gently stir until fully melted.

You can also melt the chocolate in the microwave on medium heat in 30-second bursts until melted. The time depends on the power of your microwave.

Appendix A: Glycemic Load of Carbohydrates

Low Glycemic Load (10 or under): "BOB CATS"

Bran Cereal
Oranges
Beans, kidney and black, and lentils
Carrots, cashews, and peanuts
Apples
Tortilla, wheat
Skim milk

Medium Glycemic Load (11–19): "$B^2R^2OW^2$"

Barley, pearl type (1 cup cooked) *or*
Bulgur (¾ cup cooked)
Rice (¾ cup cooked brown) *or*
Rice cakes (3) Oatmeal (1 cup cooked) Whole grain: pasta (1¼ cups cooked) *or* 1 slice bread

High Glycemic Load (20+):

French fries and baked potato
Soda and other sugar-sweetened drinks
Candy and candy bars
Refined breakfast cereals
Couscous
White basmati rice and pasta (white flour)

Appendix B: Common Sources of Vitamins and Select Minerals

Vitamin	**Mental Condition**	**Dietary Sources**
Vitamin A	Mood Anxiety	Liver: Beef Cod-liver oil Lamb Fish: Bluefin tuna Mackerel Salmon Trout Cheeses: Blue Camembert Cheddar Feta Goat Roquefort Caviar Hard-boiled egg
Vitamin B_1 (thiamine)	Mood Anxiety Focus Sleep	Acorn squash Asparagus Barley Beef Black beans Cauliflower Eggs

Vitamin B_1 (cont.)		Kale Lentils Nuts Oatmeal Oranges Pork Salmon Sunflower seeds Tuna Whole grains
Vitamin B_6 (pyridoxine)	Mood Anxiety Memory Sleep	Eggs Fish Milk Peanuts Pork Poultry: chicken and turkey Whole-grain cereals: oatmeal and wheat germ
Vitamin B_9 (folate)	Mood Memory Sleep Bipolar Depression Schizophrenia	Asparagus Beans Beets Cauliflower Citrus Leafy green vegetables Lettuce Whole grains
Vitamin B_{12} (cobalamin)	Mood OCD Sleep Schizophrenia	Beef Clams Fortified cereal Milk, yogurt, Swiss cheese Nutritional yeast Organ meats Salmon Sardines Trout Tuna

Appendix B: Common Sources of Vitamins and Select Minerals

Vitamin C	Mood Anxiety Focus Memory Sleep Schizophrenia	Black currants Broccoli Brussels sprouts Chili peppers Guavas Kale Kiwifruit Lemons Lychee fruit Oranges Papaya Parsley Persimmons Strawberries Sweet yellow peppers Thyme
Vitamin D	Anxiety Sleep	Canned light tuna Cod-liver oil Egg yolks Herring Mushrooms Oysters Salmon Sardines Shrimp
Vitamin E (alpha-tocopherol)	Anxiety Healing Memory Sleep Schizophrenia (in moderation)	Almonds Avocado Beet greens Butternut squash Peanuts Spinach Sunflower seeds Swiss chard Trout

Vitamin K	Memory	Avocado Beef liver Broccoli Brussels sprouts Chicken Cooked collard greens Cooked green beans Cooked green peas Cooked kale Cooked mustard greens Hard cheeses Kiwifruit Natto Pork chops Prunes Raw spinach Raw Swiss chard Soft cheeses
Iron	Mood ADHD	Broccoli Dark chocolate Lean red meats Legumes Pumpkin seeds Shellfish
Magnesium	Mood Anxiety ADHD Fatigue Bipolar disorder	Avocados Fish such as salmon and mackerel Legumes Nuts Whole grains
Potassium	Mood Anxiety ADHD	Bananas Cucumbers Mushrooms Oranges Peas Sweet potatoes

Selenium	Mood Anxiety	Brazil nuts
Zinc	Mood ADHD Fatigue Bipolar disorder	Beans Nuts Poultry Seafood Whole grains

Appendix C: Antioxidants and ORAC

Certain spices offer distinct cognitive advantages due to their antioxidant potential, as summarized in this table.

ORAC stands for oxygen radical absorbance capacity. It is used to measure the antioxidant capacity of foods or dietary supplements. Although ORAC applies to single food constituents, the actual ORAC value of different constituents may be synergistic. Hence the reported ORAC value may be lower than the actual value.

The next time you choose a recipe, make a note of the ORAC so that you can start to think about this as you cook.

Spice	Measure	ORAC
Dried oregano	1 tsp	3,602
Ground turmeric	1 tsp	3,504
Cumin seed	1 tsp	1,613
Curry powder	1 tsp	970
Chili powder	1 tsp	615
Black pepper	1 tsp	580
Thyme	1 tsp	407
Paprika	1 tsp	376

Acknowledgments

Kuthatha emzaneni. This African proverb, translated from Zulu as "It takes a village," comes to mind when I think about my journey to write this book.

While there were many moments alone with my trusty laptop, there were many more shared with family, colleagues, and trusted advisors about the evolution of my message and my voice.

With gratitude to my patients for trusting me with their health and supporting my work and mission at the clinic. My sincere thanks to the veterans at the MGH Home Base Program, for whom I designed the cooking program in 2017 and where I first tested some of my recipes for this book.

My oncology and surgery team: Dr. Eric Winer, for your strength and compassion and for being a rock; Drs. Tari King and Adrienne Gropper Waks, Jennifer Lowell RN, Angela Kigathi RN, Kathryn Anderson PA-C, Jennifer McKenna NP, and the many staff at Dana-Farber who helped me.

My girlfriends: Denise, Irina, and Kathy, I could not have gotten through without you.

My agents: Celeste Fine and John Maas, along with their team (Anna Petkovich, Emily Sweet, Jaidree Braddix, Amanda Orozco) and the other staff at Park Fine Literary and Media. Celeste and John embodied an inspired direction for this book which was unmatched. My editor, Tracy Behar, for her vision and brilliant guidance, and the entire team at Little Brown, Spark/Hachette, including Jessica Chun, Juliana Horbachevsky, and Ian Straus. Their combined expertise helped me navigate the publishing process. Tracy, I am also eternally grateful for your belief in me.

A very big thank-you to William Boggess for his sincerity and expertise in helping my academic writing evolve into a much more interesting book — thanks for being part of my journey!

My mentors and colleagues in the culinary arts: Chef David Bouley, the late Chef Roberta Dowling, Chef D at the CIA (Hyde Park), who inspired me to "slay" in the kitchen and not apologize for wanting to excel; and my inspiring chef mentor, Jan Isaac, who reminds me to take it to the next level and to the very best version of myself.

To my mentors in science, medicine, and nutrition: You have each encouraged me on this path with great kindness, mentorship, and patience. While sharing the vast depths of your knowledge you steered me forward with encouraging words and actions. Thank you, Maurizio Fava, Walter Willett, David Eisenberg, John Matthews, Donald Goff, Isaac Schiff, Philip Muskin, Jerry Rosenbaum, Carl Salzman, Carol Nadelson, Jonathan Borus, David Mischoulon, Jonathan Alpert, David Rubin, and John Herman.

Finally, I could not have written this book without Srini and Rajiv, part of the famous three, who can always make me smile... thank you for who you each are in my life. A big thank-you to my siblings, Drs. Vahini Naidoo, Maheshwar Naidoo, and Vishal Naidoo for helping keep me steady through these many years; also Kamil, Laura, Namitha, Nag, Sashen, and Sayuri. To Oisín, who is the most delightful reminder that food is joy even when it's healthy.

To Raj and Roshnee Kaul; Shyam Akula, the late Mrs. Raz Pillay (my beautiful mother-in-law who also helped teach me cooking), Aunty Vimala, and Uncle Shunna; and to Mano, Babes, Jaya, and Shan — for your enduring love, sage advice, and encouragement, always.

Notes

Chapter 1. The Gut-Brain Romance

1. If you'd like to learn more about how mental health was viewed before 1800, I recommend reading *Madness and Civilization: A History of Insanity in the Age of Reason* (New York: Vintage, 1988) by Michel Foucault.
2. Miller I. The gut-brain axis: historical reflections. *Microbial Ecology in Health and Disease*. 2018;29(2):1542921. doi:10.1080/16512235.2018.1542921.
3. Ibid.
4. Carabotti M, Scirocco A, Maselli MA, Severi C. The gut-brain axis: interactions between enteric microbiota, central and enteric nervous systems. *Annals of Gastroenterology*. 2015;28(2):203–9.
5. Simrén M, Barbara G, Flint HJ, et al. Intestinal microbiota in functional bowel disorders: a Rome foundation report. *Gut*. 2012;62(1):159–76. doi:10.1136/gutjnl-2012-302167.
6. Giau V, Wu S, Jamerlan A, An S, Kim S, Hulme J. Gut microbiota and their neuroinflammatory implications in Alzheimer's disease. *Nutrients*. 2018;10(11):1765. doi:10.3390/nu10111765; Shishov VA, Kirovskaia TA, Kudrin VS, Oleskin AV. Amine neuromediators, their precursors, and oxidation products in the culture of Escherichia coli K-12 [in Russian]. *Prikladnaia Biokhimiia i Mikrobiologiia*. 2009;45(5):550–54.
7. Galley JD, Nelson MC, Yu Z, et al. Exposure to a social stressor disrupts the community structure of the colonic mucosa-associated microbiota. *BMC Microbiology*. 2014;14(1):189. doi:10.1186/1471-2180-14-189.
8. Valles-Colomer M, Falony G, Darzi Y, et al. The neuroactive potential of the human gut microbiota in quality of life and depression. *Nature Microbiology*. 2019;4(4):623–32. doi:10.1038/s41564-018-0337-x.

9. Ercolini D, Fogliano V. Food design to feed the human gut microbiota. *Journal of Agricultural and Food Chemistry*. 2018;66(15):3754–58. doi:10.1021/acs.jafc.8b00456.
10. New State Rankings Shines Light on Mental Health Crisis, Show Differences in Blue, Red States. Mental Health America website, October 18, 2016, https://www.mhanational.org/new-state-rankings-shines-light-mental-health-crisis-show-differences-blue-red-states. Accessed September 29, 2019.
11. Mental Health and Mental Disorders. HealthyPeople.gov website, https://www.healthypeople.gov/2020/topics-objectives/topic/mental-health-and-mental-disorders. Accessed September 29, 2019.
12. Liang S, Wu X, Jin F. Gut-brain psychology: rethinking psychology from the microbiota–gut–brain axis. *Frontiers in Integrative Neuroscience*. 2018;12. doi:10.3389/fnint.2018.00033.
13. Sarris J, Logan AC, Akbaraly TN, et al. Nutritional medicine as mainstream in psychiatry. *Lancet Psychiatry*. 2015;2(3):271–74. doi:10.1016/s2215-0366(14)00051-0.

Chapter 2. Depression

1. Lazarevich I, Irigoyen Camacho ME, Velázquez-Alva MC, Flores NL, Nájera Medina O, Zepeda Zepeda MA. Depression and food consumption in Mexican college students. *Nutrición Hospitalaria*. 2018;35(3):620–26.
2. Rao TS, Asha MR, Ramesh BN, Rao KS. Understanding nutrition, depression and mental illnesses. *Indian Journal of Psychiatry*. 2008;50(2):77–82.
3. Cheung SG, Goldenthal AR, Uhlemann A-C, Mann JJ, Miller JM, Sublette ME. Systematic review of gut microbiota and major depression. *Frontiers in Psychiatry*. 2019;10:34. doi:10.3389/fpsyt.2019.00034.
4. Messaoudi M, Lalonde R, Violle N, et al. Assessment of psychotropic-like properties of a probiotic formulation (*Lactobacillus helveticus* R0052 and *Bifidobacterium longum* R0175) in rats and human subjects. *British Journal of Nutrition*. 2010;105(5):755–64. doi:10.1017/s0007114510004319.
5. Clapp M, Aurora N, Herrera L, Bhatia M, Wilen E, Wakefield S. Gut microbiota's effect on mental health: the gut-brain axis. *Clinical Practice*. 2017;7(4):987.
6. Francis HM, Stevenson RJ, Chambers JR, Gupta D, Newey B, Lim CK. A brief diet intervention can reduce symptoms of depression in young adults—a randomised controlled trial. *PLoS One*. 2019;14(10):e0222768.
7. Westover AN, Marangell LB. A cross-national relationship between sugar consumption and major depression? *Depression and Anxiety*. 2002;16:118–20. doi:10.1002/da.10054.

8. Hu D, Cheng L, Jiang W. Sugar-sweetened beverages consumption and the risk of depression: a meta-analysis of observational studies. *Journal of Affective Disorders*. 2019;245:348–55. doi:10.1016/j.jad.2018.11.015.
9. Marosi K, Mattson MP. BDNF mediates adaptive brain and body responses to energetic challenges. *Trends in Endocrinology and Metabolism*. 2014;25(2):89–98.
10. Aydemir C, Yalcin ES, Aksaray S, et al. Brain-derived neurotrophic factor (BDNF) changes in the serum of depressed women. *Progress in Neuro-Psychopharmacology and Biological Psychiatry*. 2006;30(7):1256–60. doi:10.1016/j.pnpbp.2006.03.025.
11. Arumugam V, John V, Augustine N, et al. The impact of antidepressant treatment on brain-derived neurotrophic factor level: an evidence-based approach through systematic review and meta-analysis. *Indian Journal of Pharmacology*. 2017;49(3):236. doi:10.4103/ijp.ijp_700_16.
12. Sánchez-Villegas A, Zazpe I, Santiago S, Perez-Cornago A, Martinez-Gonzalez MA, Lahortiga-Ramos F. Added sugars and sugar-sweetened beverage consumption, dietary carbohydrate index and depression risk in the Seguimiento Universidad de Navarra (SUN) Project. *British Journal of Nutrition*. 2017;119(2):211–21. doi:10.1017/s0007114517003361.
13. Gangwisch JE, Hale L, Garcia L, et al. High glycemic index diet as a risk factor for depression: analyses from the Women's Health Initiative. *American Journal of Clinical Nutrition*. 2015;102(2):454–63. doi:10.3945/ajcn.114.103846; Salari-Moghaddam A, Saneei P, Larijani B, Esmaillzadeh A. Glycemic index, glycemic load, and depression: a systematic review and meta-analysis. *European Journal of Clinical Nutrition*. 2018;73(3):356–65. doi:10.1038/s41430-018-0258-z.
14. Guo X, Park Y, Freedman ND, et al. Sweetened beverages, coffee, and tea and depression risk among older US adults. Matsuoka Y, ed. *PLoS One*. 2014;9(4):e94715. doi:10.1371/journal.pone.0094715.
15. Whitehouse CR, Boullata J, McCauley LA. The potential toxicity of artificial sweeteners. *AAOHN Journal*. 2008;56(6):251–59; quiz, 260–61; Humphries P, Pretorius E, Naudé H. Direct and indirect cellular effects of aspartame on the brain. *European Journal of Clinical Nutrition*. 2007;62(4):451–62. doi:10.1038/sj.ejcn.1602866.
16. Choudhary AK, Lee YY. Neurophysiological symptoms and aspartame: what is the connection? *Nutritional Neuroscience*. 2017;21(5):306–16. doi:10.1080/1028415x.2017.1288340.
17. Lobo V, Patil A, Phatak A, Chandra N. Free radicals, antioxidants and functional foods: impact on human health. *Pharmacognosy Reviews*. 2010;4(8):118. doi:10.4103/0973-7847.70902.

18. Rodriguez-Palacios A, Harding A, Menghini P, et al. The artificial sweetener Splenda promotes gut proteobacteria, dysbiosis, and myeloperoxidase reactivity in Crohn's disease–like ileitis. *Inflammatory Bowel Diseases*. 2018;24(5):1005–20. doi:10.1093/ibd/izy060; Jiang H, Ling Z, Zhang Y, et al. Altered fecal microbiota composition in patients with major depressive disorder. *Brain, Behavior, and Immunity*. 2015;48:186–94. doi:10.1016/j.bbi.2015.03.016.
19. Vaccarino V, Brennan M-L, Miller AH, et al. Association of major depressive disorder with serum myeloperoxidase and other markers of inflammation: a twin study. *Biological Psychiatry*. 2008;64(6):476–83. doi:10.1016/j.biopsych.2008.04.023.
20. Yoshikawa E, Nishi D, Matsuoka YJ. Association between frequency of fried food consumption and resilience to depression in Japanese company workers: a cross-sectional study. *Lipids in Health and Disease*. 2016;15(1). doi:10.1186/s12944-016-0331-3.
21. Sánchez-Villegas A, Verberne L, De Irala J, et al. Dietary fat intake and the risk of depression: the SUN Project. *PLoS One*. 2011;6(1):e16268.
22. Ford PA, Jaceldo-Siegl K, Lee JW, Tonstad S. Trans fatty acid intake is related to emotional affect in the Adventist Health Study-2. *Nutrition Research*. 2016;36(6):509–517. doi:10.1016/j.nutres.2016.01.005; Appleton KM, Rogers PJ, Ness AR. Is there a role for n-3 long-chain polyunsaturated fatty acids in the regulation of mood and behaviour? A review of the evidence to date from epidemiological studies, clinical studies and intervention trials. *Nutrition Research Reviews*. 2008;21(1):13–41. doi:10.1017/s0954422408998620.
23. Suzuki E, Yagi G, Nakaki T, Kanba S, Asai M. Elevated plasma nitrate levels in depressive states. *Journal of Affective Disorders*. 2001;63(1–3):221–24. doi:10.1016/s0165-0327(00)00164-6.
24. Khambadkone SG, Cordner ZA, Dickerson F, et al. Nitrated meat products are associated with mania in humans and altered behavior and brain gene expression in rats. *Molecular Psychiatry*. July 2018. doi:10.1038/s41380-018-0105-6.
25. Park W, Kim J-H, Ju M-G, et al. Enhancing quality characteristics of salami sausages formulated with whole buckwheat flour during storage. *Journal of Food Science and Technology*. 2016;54(2):326–32. doi:10.1007/s13197-016-2465-8.
26. Mocking RJT, Harmsen I, Assies J, Koeter MWJ, Ruhé HG, Schene AH. Meta-analysis and meta-regression of omega-3 polyunsaturated fatty acid supplementation for major depressive disorder. *Translational Psychiatry*. 2016;6(3):e756. doi:10.1038/tp.2016.29.

27. Simopoulos A. The importance of the ratio of omega-6/omega-3 essential fatty acids. *Biomedicine and Pharmacotherapy*. 2002;56(8):365–79. doi:10.1016/s0753-3322(02)00253–6.
28. Alpert JE, Fava M. Nutrition and depression: the role of folate. *Nutrition Reviews*. 2009;55(5):145–49. doi:10.1111/j.1753-4887.1997.tb06468.x.
29. Beydoun MA, Shroff MR, Beydoun HA, Zonderman AB. Serum folate, vitamin B-12, and homocysteine and their association with depressive symptoms among U.S. adults. *Psychosomatic Medicine*. 2010;72(9):862–73. doi:10.1097/psy.0b013e3181f61863.
30. Albert PR, Benkelfat C, Descarries L. The neurobiology of depression—revisiting the serotonin hypothesis. I. Cellular and molecular mechanisms. *Philosophical Transactions of the Royal Society B: Biological Sciences*. 2012;367(1601):2378–81. doi:10.1098/rstb.2012.0190.
31. Olson CR, Mello CV. Significance of vitamin A to brain function, behavior and learning. *Molecular Nutrition and Food Research*. 2010;54(4):489–95. doi:10.1002/mnfr.200900246.
32. Misner DL, Jacobs S, Shimizu Y, et al. Vitamin A deprivation results in reversible loss of hippocampal long-term synaptic plasticity. *Proceedings of the National Academy of Sciences*. 2001;98(20):11714–19. doi:10.1073/pnas.191369798.
33. Bitarafan S, Saboor-Yaraghi A, Sahraian MA, et al. Effect of vitamin A supplementation on fatigue and depression in multiple sclerosis patients: a double-blind placebo-controlled clinical trial. *Iranian Journal of Allergy, Asthma, and Immunology*. 2016;15(1):13–19.
34. Bremner JD, McCaffery P. The neurobiology of retinoic acid in affective disorders. *Progress in Neuro-Psychopharmacology and Biological Psychiatry*. 2008;32(2):315–31. doi:10.1016/j.pnpbp.2007.07.001.
35. Pullar J, Carr A, Bozonet S, Vissers M. High vitamin C status is associated with elevated mood in male tertiary students. *Antioxidants*. 2018;7(7):91. doi:10.3390/antiox7070091.
36. Gariballa S. Poor vitamin C status is associated with increased depression symptoms following acute illness in older people. *International Journal for Vitamin and Nutrition Research*. 2014;84(1–2):12–17. doi:10.1024/0300-9831/a000188.
37. Kim J, Wessling-Resnick M. Iron and mechanisms of emotional behavior. *Journal of Nutritional Biochemistry*. 2014;25(11):1101–7. doi:10.1016/j.jnutbio.2014.07.003.
38. Pillay S. A quantitative magnetic resonance imaging study of caudate and lenticular nucleus gray matter volume in primary unipolar major depression:

relationship to treatment response and clinical severity. *Psychiatry Research: Neuroimaging.* 1998;84(2–3):61–74. doi:10.1016/s0925-4927(98)00048-1.
39. Hidese S, Saito K, Asano S, Kunugi H. Association between iron-deficiency anemia and depression: a web-based Japanese investigation. *Psychiatry and Clinical Neurosciences.* 2018;72(7):513–21. doi:10.1111/pcn.12656.
40. Eby GA, Eby KL, Murk H. Magnesium and major depression. In: Vink R, Nechifor M, eds. *Magnesium in the Central Nervous System* [internet]. Adelaide, Australia: University of Adelaide Press; 2011. Available from https://www.ncbi.nlm.nih.gov/books/NBK507265/.
41. Widmer J, Mouthon D, Raffin Y, et al. Weak association between blood sodium, potassium, and calcium and intensity of symptoms in major depressed patients. *Neuropsychobiology.* 1997;36(4):164–71. doi:10.1159/000119378; Torres SJ, Nowson CA, Worsley A. Dietary electrolytes are related to mood. *British Journal of Nutrition.* 2008;100(5):1038–45. doi:10.1017/s0007114508959201.
42. Wang J, Um P, Dickerman B, Liu J. Zinc, magnesium, selenium and depression: a review of the evidence, potential mechanisms and implications. *Nutrients.* 2018;10(5):584. doi:10.3390/nu10050584.
43. Swardfager W, Herrmann N, Mazereeuw G, Goldberger K, Harimoto T, Lanctôt KL. Zinc in depression: a meta-analysis. *Biological Psychiatry.* 2013;74(12):872–78. doi:10.1016/j.biopsych.2013.05.008.
44. Szewczyk B, Kubera M, Nowak G. The role of zinc in neurodegenerative inflammatory pathways in depression. *Progress in Neuro-Psychopharmacology and Biological Psychiatry.* 2011;35(3):693–701. doi:10.1016/j.pnpbp.2010.02.010.
45. Finley JW, Penland JG. Adequacy or deprivation of dietary selenium in healthy men: clinical and psychological findings. *Journal of Trace Elements in Experimental Medicine.* 1998;11(1):11–27. doi:10.1002/(sici)1520-670x(1998)11:1<11::aid-jtra3>3.0.co;2-6.
46. Hausenblas HA, Saha D, Dubyak PJ, Anton SD. Saffron (*Crocus sativus* L.) and major depressive disorder: a meta-analysis of randomized clinical trials. *Journal of Integrative Medicine.* 2013;11(6):377–83. doi:10.3736/jintegrmed2013056.
47. Saffron. Uses of Herbs website. https://usesofherbs.com/saffron. Accessed November 18, 2019.
48. Khazdair MR, Boskabady MH, Hosseini M, Rezaee R, Tsatsakis AM. The effects of *Crocus sativus* (saffron) and its constituents on nervous system: a review. *Avicenna Journal of Phytomedicine.* 2015;5(5):376–91.
49. Ng QX, Koh SSH, Chan HW, Ho CYX. Clinical use of curcumin in depression: a meta-analysis. *Journal of the American Medical Directors Association.* 2017;18(6):503–8. doi:10.1016/j.jamda.2016.12.071.

50. Hewlings S, Kalman D. Curcumin: a review of its effects on human health. *Foods*. 2017;6(10):92. doi:10.3390/foods6100092.
51. Melo FHC, Moura BA, de Sousa DP, et al. Antidepressant-like effect of carvacrol (5-isopropyl-2-methylphenol) in mice: involvement of dopaminergic system. *Fundamental and Clinical Pharmacology*. 2011;25(3):362–67. doi:10.1111/j.1472-8206.2010.00850.x.
52. Yeung KS, Hernandez M, Mao JJ, Haviland I, Gubili J. Herbal medicine for depression and anxiety: a systematic review with assessment of potential psycho-oncologic relevance. *Phytotherapy Research*. 2018;32(5):865–91. doi:10.1002/ptr.6033.
53. Keys A, Grande F. Role of dietary fat in human nutrition. III. Diet and the epidemiology of coronary heart disease. *American Journal of Public Health and the Nation's Health*. 1957;47(12):1520–30.
54. Boucher JL. Mediterranean eating pattern. *Diabetes Spectrum*. 2017;30(2): 72–76. doi:10.2337/ds16-0074.
55. Hoffman R, Gerber M. Evaluating and adapting the Mediterranean diet for non-Mediterranean populations: a critical appraisal. *Nutrition Reviews*. 2013;71(9):573–84. doi:10.1111/nure.12040.
56. Harasym J, Oledzki R. Effect of fruit and vegetable antioxidants on total antioxidant capacity of blood plasma. *Nutrition*. 2014;30(5):511–17. doi:10.1016/j.nut.2013.08.019; Battino M, Ferreiro MS. Ageing and the Mediterranean diet: a review of the role of dietary fats. *Public Health Nutrition*. 2004;7(7):953–58.
57. Fresán U, Bes-Rastrollo M, Segovia-Siapco G, et al. Does the MIND diet decrease depression risk? A comparison with Mediterranean diet in the SUN cohort. *European Journal of Nutrition*. 2018;58(3):1271–82. doi:10.1007/s00394-018-1653-x.
58. Sánchez-Villegas A, Cabrera-Suárez B, Molero P, et al. Preventing the recurrence of depression with a Mediterranean diet supplemented with extra-virgin olive oil. The PREDI-DEP trial: study protocol. *BMC Psychiatry*. 2019;19. doi:10.1186/s12888-019-2036-4.
59. Mithril C, Dragsted LO, Meyer C, Blauert E, Holt MK, Astrup A. Guidelines for the new Nordic diet. *Public Health Nutrition*. 2012;15(10):1941–47. doi:10.1017/s136898001100351x.
60. Quirk SE, Williams LJ, O'Neil A, et al. The association between diet quality, dietary patterns and depression in adults: a systematic review. *BMC Psychiatry*. 2013;13(1). doi:10.1186/1471-244x-13-175.

Chapter 3. Anxiety

1. Bandelow B, Michaelis S. Epidemiology of anxiety disorders in the 21st century. *Dialogues in Clinical Neuroscience*. 2015;17(3):327–35.
2. Lach G, Schellekens H, Dinan TG, Cryan JF. Anxiety, depression, and the microbiome: a role for gut peptides. *Neurotherapeutics*. 2017;15(1):36–59. doi:10.1007/s13311-017-0585-0.
3. Dockray GJ. Gastrointestinal hormones and the dialogue between gut and brain. *Journal of Physiology*. 2014;592(14):2927–41. doi:10.1113/jphysiol.2014.270850.
4. Liberzon I, Duval E, Javanbakht A. Neural circuits in anxiety and stress disorders: a focused review. *Therapeutics and Clinical Risk Management*. January 2015:115. doi:10.2147/tcrm.s48528.
5. Luczynski P, Whelan SO, O'Sullivan C, et al. Adult microbiota-deficient mice have distinct dendritic morphological changes: differential effects in the amygdala and hippocampus. Gaspar P, ed. *European Journal of Neuroscience*. 2016;44(9):2654–66. doi:10.1111/ejn.13291.
6. Hoban AE, Stilling RM, Moloney G, et al. The microbiome regulates amygdala-dependent fear recall. *Molecular Psychiatry*. 2017;23(5):1134–44. doi:10.1038/mp.2017.100.
7. Cowan CSM, Hoban AE, Ventura-Silva AP, Dinan TG, Clarke G, Cryan JF. Gutsy moves: the amygdala as a critical node in microbiota to brain signaling. *BioEssays*. 2017;40(1):170–72. doi:10.1002/bies.201700172.
8. Sudo N, Chida Y, Aiba Y, et al. Postnatal microbial colonization programs the hypothalamic-pituitary-adrenal system for stress response in mice. *Journal of Physiology*. 2004;558(1):263–75. doi:10.1113/jphysiol.2004.063388.
9. Jiang H, Zhang X, Yu Z, et al. Altered gut microbiota profile in patients with generalized anxiety disorder. *Journal of Psychiatric Research*. 2018;104:130–36. doi:10.1016/j.jpsychires.2018.07.007.
10. Clapp M, Aurora N, Herrera L, Bhatia M, Wilen E, Wakefield S. Gut microbiota's effect on mental health: the gut-brain axis. *Clinics and Practice*. 2017;7(4). doi:10.4081/cp.2017.987.
11. Perna G, Iannone G, Alciati A, Caldirola D. Are anxiety disorders associated with accelerated aging? A focus on neuroprogression. *Neural Plasticity*. 2016;2016:1–19. doi:10.1155/2016/8457612.
12. Liu L, Zhu G. Gut–brain axis and mood disorder. *Frontiers in Psychiatry*. 2018;9. doi:10.3389/fpsyt.2018.00223.
13. Sarkhel S, Banerjee A, Sarkar R, Dhali G. Anxiety and depression in irritable bowel syndrome. *Indian Journal of Psychological Medicine*. 2017;39(6):741. doi:10.4103/ijpsym.ijpsym_46_17.

14. Fadgyas-Stanculete M, Buga A-M, Popa-Wagner A, Dumitrascu DL. The relationship between irritable bowel syndrome and psychiatric disorders: from molecular changes to clinical manifestations. *Journal of Molecular Psychiatry*. 2014;2(1):4. doi:10.1186/2049-9256-2-4.
15. Dutheil S, Ota KT, Wohleb ES, Rasmussen K, Duman RS. High-fat diet induced anxiety and anhedonia: impact on brain homeostasis and inflammation. *Neuropsychopharmacology*. 2015;41(7):1874–87. doi:10.1038/npp.2015.357.
16. Gancheva S, Galunska B, Zhelyazkova-Savova M. Diets rich in saturated fat and fructose induce anxiety and depression-like behaviours in the rat: is there a role for lipid peroxidation? *International Journal of Experimental Pathology*. 2017;98(5):296–306. doi:10.1111/iep.12254.
17. Parikh I, Guo J, Chuang KH, et al. Caloric restriction preserves memory and reduces anxiety of aging mice with early enhancement of neurovascular functions. *Aging*. 2016;8(11):2814–26.
18. Bray GA, Popkin BM. Dietary sugar and body weight: have we reached a crisis in the epidemic of obesity and diabetes? *Diabetes Care*. 2014;37(4):950–56. doi:10.2337/dc13-2085.
19. Haleem DJ, Mahmood K. Brain serotonin in high-fat diet-induced weight gain, anxiety and spatial memory in rats. *Nutritional Neuroscience*. May 2019:1–10. doi:10.1080/1028415x.2019.1619983.
20. Xu L, Xu S, Lin L, et al. High-fat diet mediates anxiolytic-like behaviors in a time-dependent manner through the regulation of SIRT1 in the brain. *Neuroscience*. 2018;372:237–45. doi:10.1016/j.neuroscience.2018.01.001; Gainey SJ, Kwakwa KA, Bray JK, et al. Short-term high-fat diet (HFD) induced anxiety-like behaviors and cognitive impairment are improved with treatment by glyburide. *Frontiers in Behavioral Neuroscience*. 2016;10. doi:10.3389/fnbeh.2016.00156.
21. Simon GE, Von Korff M, Saunders K, et al. Association between obesity and psychiatric disorders in the US adult population. *Archives of General Psychiatry*. 2006;63(7):824. doi:10.1001/archpsyc.63.7.824.
22. Kyrou I, Tsigos C. Stress hormones: physiological stress and regulation of metabolism. *Current Opinion in Pharmacology*. 2009;9(6):787–93. doi:10.1016/j.coph.2009.08.007.
23. Bruce-Keller AJ, Salbaum JM, Luo M, et al. Obese-type gut microbiota induce neurobehavioral changes in the absence of obesity. *Biological Psychiatry*. 2015;77(7):607–15. doi:10.1016/j.biopsych.2014.07.012.
24. Peleg-Raibstein D, Luca E, Wolfrum C. Maternal high-fat diet in mice programs emotional behavior in adulthood. *Behavioural Brain Research*. 2012 Aug 1;233(2):398–404. doi:10.1016/j.bbr.2012.05.027.

25. Smith JE, Lawrence AD, Diukova A, Wise RG, Rogers PJ. Storm in a coffee cup: caffeine modifies brain activation to social signals of threat. *Social Cognitive and Affective Neuroscience*. 2011;7(7):831–40. doi:10.1093/scan/nsr058.
26. Mobbs D, Petrovic P, Marchant JL, et al. When fear is near: threat imminence elicits prefrontal-periaqueductal gray shifts in humans. *Science*. 2007;317(5841):1079–83. doi:10.1126/science.1144298.
27. Wikoff D, Welsh BT, Henderson R, et al. Systematic review of the potential adverse effects of caffeine consumption in healthy adults, pregnant women, adolescents, and children. *Food and Chemical Toxicology*. 2017;109:585–648. doi:10.1016/j.fct.2017.04.002.
28. For an extended chart of caffeine quantities in various popular beverages, visit: Caffeine Chart. Center for Science in the Public Interest website. https://cspinet.org/eating-healthy/ingredients-of-concern/caffeine-chart. Accessed February 25, 2016.
29. Becker HC. Effects of alcohol dependence and withdrawal on stress responsiveness and alcohol consumption. *Alcohol Research*. 2012;34(4):448–58; Chueh K-H, Guilleminault C, Lin C-M. Alcohol consumption as a moderator of anxiety and sleep quality. *Journal of Nursing Research*. 2019;27(3):e23. doi:10.1097/jnr.0000000000000300.
30. Danaei G, Ding EL, Mozaffarian D, et al. The preventable causes of death in the United States: comparative risk assessment of dietary, lifestyle, and metabolic risk factors. Hales S, ed. *PLoS Medicine*. 2009;6(4):e1000058. doi:10.1371/journal.pmed.1000058; Chikritzhs TN, Jonas HA, Stockwell TR, Heale PF, Dietze PM. Mortality and life-years lost due to alcohol: a comparison of acute and chronic causes. *Medical Journal of Australia*. 2001;174(6):281–84.
31. Terlecki MA, Ecker AH, Buckner JD. College drinking problems and social anxiety: the importance of drinking context. *Psychology of Addictive Behaviors*. 2014;28(2):545–52. doi:10.1037/a0035770.
32. Dawson DA. Defining risk drinking. *Alcohol Research and Health*. 2011;34(2):144–56.
33. Smith DF, Gerdes LU. Meta-analysis on anxiety and depression in adult celiac disease. *Acta Psychiatrica Scandinavica*. 2011;125(3):189–93. doi:10.1111/j.1600-0447.2011.01795.
34. Addolorato G. Anxiety but not depression decreases in coeliac patients after one-year gluten-free diet: a longitudinal study. *Scandinavian Journal of Gastroenterology*. 2001;36(5):502–6. doi:10.1080/00365520119754.
35. Häuser W. Anxiety and depression in adult patients with celiac disease on a gluten-free diet. *World Journal of Gastroenterology*. 2010;16(22):2780. doi:10.3748/wjg.v16.i22.2780.

36. Pennisi M, Bramanti A, Cantone M, Pennisi G, Bella R, Lanza G. Neurophysiology of the "celiac brain": disentangling gut-brain connections. *Frontiers in Neuroscience*. 2017;11. doi:10.3389/fnins.2017.00498.
37. Choudhary AK, Lee YY. Neurophysiological symptoms and aspartame: what is the connection? *Nutritional Neuroscience*. 2017;21(5):306–16. doi:10.1080/1028415x.2017.1288340.
38. Taylor AM, Holscher HD. A review of dietary and microbial connections to depression, anxiety, and stress. *Nutritional Neuroscience*. July 2018:1–14. doi:10.1080/1028415x.2018.1493808.
39. Foster JA, McVey Neufeld K-A. Gut–brain axis: how the microbiome influences anxiety and depression. *Trends in Neurosciences*. 2013;36(5):305–12. doi:10.1016/j.tins.2013.01.005.
40. Howarth NC, Saltzman E, Roberts SB. Dietary fiber and weight regulation. *Nutrition Reviews*. 2009;59(5):129–39. doi:10.1111/j.1753-4887.2001.tb07001.x.
41. Salim S, Chugh G, Asghar M. Inflammation in anxiety. In: *Advances in Protein Chemistry and Structural Biology*. Vol. 88. Oxford: Elsevier; 2012:-1–25. doi:10.1016/b978-0-12-398314-5.00001-5.
42. Michopoulos V, Powers A, Gillespie CF, Ressler KJ, Jovanovic T. Inflammation in fear- and anxiety-based disorders: PTSD, GAD, and beyond. *Neuropsychopharmacology*. 2016;42(1):254–70. doi:10.1038/npp.2016.146.
43. Felger JC. Imaging the role of inflammation in mood and anxiety-related disorders. *Current Neuropharmacology*. 2018;16(5):533–58. doi:10.2174/1570159x15666171123201142.
44. Kiecolt-Glaser JK, Belury MA, Andridge R, Malarkey WB, Glaser R. Omega-3 supplementation lowers inflammation and anxiety in medical students: a randomized controlled trial. *Brain, Behavior, and Immunity*. 2011;25(8):1725–34. doi:10.1016/j.bbi.2011.07.229.
45. Su K-P, Tseng P-T, Lin P-Y, et al. Association of use of omega-3 polyunsaturated fatty acids with changes in severity of anxiety symptoms. *JAMA Network Open*. 2018;1(5):e182327. doi:10.1001/jamanetworkopen.2018.2327.
46. Su K-P, Matsuoka Y, Pae C-U. Omega-3 polyunsaturated fatty acids in prevention of mood and anxiety disorders. *Clinical Psychopharmacology and Neuroscience*. 2015;13(2):129–37. doi:10.9758/cpn.2015.13.2.129.
47. Song C, Li X, Kang Z, Kadotomi Y. Omega-3 fatty acid ethyl-eicosapentaenoate attenuates IL-1β-induced changes in dopamine and metabolites in the shell of the nucleus accumbens: involved with PLA2 activity and corticosterone secretion. *Neuropsychopharmacology*. 2006;32(3):736–44. doi:10.1038/sj.npp.1301117; Healy-Stoffel M, Levant B. N-3 (omega-3) fatty acids:

effects on brain dopamine systems and potential role in the etiology and treatment of neuropsychiatric disorders. *CNS and Neurological Disorders—Drug Targets*. 2018;17(3):216–32. doi:10.2174/1871527317666180412153612.

48. Selhub EM, Logan AC, Bested AC. Fermented foods, microbiota, and mental health: ancient practice meets nutritional psychiatry. *Journal of Physiological Anthropology*. 2014;33(1). doi:10.1186/1880-6805-33-2.
49. Sivamaruthi B, Kesika P, Chaiyasut C. Impact of fermented foods on human cognitive function—a review of outcome of clinical trials. *Scientia Pharmaceutica*. 2018;86(2):22. doi:10.3390/scipharm86020022.
50. Kim B, Hong VM, Yang J, et al. A review of fermented foods with beneficial effects on brain and cognitive function. *Preventive Nutrition and Food Science*. 2016;21(4):297–309. doi:10.3746/pnf.2016.21.4.297.
51. Hilimire MR, DeVylder JE, Forestell CA. Fermented foods, neuroticism, and social anxiety: an interaction model. *Psychiatry Research*. 2015;228(2): 203–8. doi:10.1016/j.psychres.2015.04.023.
52. Widiger TA, Oltmanns JR. Neuroticism is a fundamental domain of personality with enormous public health implications. *World Psychiatry*. 2017;16(2):144–45. doi:10.1002/wps.20411.
53. Silva LCA, Viana MB, Andrade JS, Souza MA, Céspedes IC, D'Almeida V. Tryptophan overloading activates brain regions involved with cognition, mood and anxiety. *Anais da Academia Brasileira de Ciências*. 2017;89(1): 273–83. doi:10.1590/0001-3765201720160177.
54. Young SN. How to increase serotonin in the human brain without drugs. *Journal of Psychiatry and Neuroscience*. 2007;32(6):394–99.
55. Lindseth G, Helland B, Caspers J. The effects of dietary tryptophan on affective disorders. *Archives of Psychiatric Nursing*. 2015;29(2):102–7. doi:10.1016/j.apnu.2014.11.008.
56. Wurtman RJ, Hefti F, Melamed E. Precursor control of neurotransmitter synthesis. *Pharmacological Reviews*. 1980;32(4):315–35.
57. Spring B. Recent research on the behavioral effects of tryptophan and carbohydrate. *Nutrition and Health*. 1984;3(1–2):55–67. doi:10.1177/026010608400300204.
58. Aan het Rot M, Moskowitz DS, Pinard G, Young SN. Social behaviour and mood in everyday life: the effects of tryptophan in quarrelsome individuals. *Journal of Psychiatry and Neuroscience*. 2006;31(4):253–62.
59. Fazelian S, Amani R, Paknahad Z, Kheiri S, Khajehali L. Effect of vitamin D supplement on mood status and inflammation in vitamin D deficient type 2 diabetic women with anxiety: a randomized clinical trial. *International Journal of Preventive Medicine*. 2019;10:17.

60. Anjum I, Jaffery SS, Fayyaz M, Samoo Z, Anjum S. The role of vitamin D in brain health: a mini literature review. *Cureus*. July 2018. doi:10.7759/cureus.2960.
61. Martin EI, Ressler KJ, Binder E, Nemeroff CB. The neurobiology of anxiety disorders: brain imaging, genetics, and psychoneuroendocrinology. *Psychiatric Clinics of North America*. 2009;32(3):549–75. doi:10.1016/j.psc.2009.05.004; Shin LM, Liberzon I. The neurocircuitry of fear, stress, and anxiety disorders. *Neuropsychopharmacology*. 2009;35(1):169–91. doi:10.1038/npp.2009.83.
62. Naeem Z. Vitamin D deficiency—an ignored epidemic. *International Journal of Health Sciences*. 2010;4(1):v–vi.
63. Kennedy D. B vitamins and the brain: mechanisms, dose and efficacy—a review. *Nutrients*. 2016;8(2):68. doi:10.3390/nu8020068.
64. Cornish S, Mehl-Madrona L. The role of vitamins and minerals in psychiatry. *Integrative Medicine Insights*. 2008;3:33–42.
65. Markova N, Bazhenova N, Anthony DC, et al. Thiamine and benfotiamine improve cognition and ameliorate GSK-3β-associated stress-induced behaviours in mice. *Progress in Neuro-Psychopharmacology and Biological Psychiatry*. 2017;75:148–56. doi:10.1016/j.pnpbp.2016.11.001; Vignisse J, Sambon M, Gorlova A, et al. Thiamine and benfotiamine prevent stress-induced suppression of hippocampal neurogenesis in mice exposed to predation without affecting brain thiamine diphosphate levels. *Molecular and Cellular Neuroscience*. 2017;82:126–36. doi:10.1016/j.mcn.2017.05.005.
66. McCabe D, Lisy K, Lockwood C, Colbeck M. The impact of essential fatty acid, B vitamins, vitamin C, magnesium and zinc supplementation on stress levels in women: a systematic review. *JBI Database of Systematic Reviews and Implementation Reports*. 2017;15(2):402–53.
67. Lewis JE, Tiozzo E, Melillo AB, et al. The effect of methylated vitamin B complex on depressive and anxiety symptoms and quality of life in adults with depression. *ISRN Psychiatry*. 2013;2013:1–7. doi:10.1155/2013/621453.
68. Gautam M, Agrawal M, Gautam M, Sharma P, Gautam A, Gautam S. Role of antioxidants in generalised anxiety disorder and depression. *Indian Journal of Psychiatry*. 2012;54(3):244. doi:10.4103/0019-5545.102424.
69. Carroll D, Ring C, Suter M, Willemsen G. The effects of an oral multivitamin combination with calcium, magnesium, and zinc on psychological well-being in healthy young male volunteers: a double-blind placebo-controlled trial. *Psychopharmacology*. 2000;150(2):220–25. doi:10.1007/s002130000406; Schlebusch L, Bosch BA, Polglase G, Kleinschmidt I, Pillay BJ, Cassimjee MH. A double-blind, placebo-controlled, double-centre

study of the effects of an oral multivitamin-mineral combination on stress. *South African Medical Journal.* 2000;90(12):1216–23.

70. Long S-J, Benton D. Effects of vitamin and mineral supplementation on stress, mild psychiatric symptoms, and mood in nonclinical samples. *Psychosomatic Medicine.* 2013;75(2):144–53. doi:10.1097/psy.0b013e31827d5fbd.
71. Grases G, Pérez-Castelló JA, Sanchis P, et al. Anxiety and stress among science students. Study of calcium and magnesium alterations. *Magnesium Research.* 2006;19(2):102–6.
72. Boyle NB, Lawton C, Dye L. The effects of magnesium supplementation on subjective anxiety and stress—a systematic review. *Nutrients.* 2017;9(5):429. doi:10.3390/nu9050429.
73. Murck H, Steiger A. Mg 2+ reduces ACTH secretion and enhances spindle power without changing delta power during sleep in men—possible therapeutic implications. *Psychopharmacology.* 1998;137(3):247–52. doi:10.1007/s002130050617.
74. Boyle NB, Lawton C, Dye L. The effects of magnesium supplementation on subjective anxiety and stress—a systematic review. *Nutrients.* 2017;9(5):429. doi:10.3390/nu9050429.
75. Lakhan SE, Vieira KF. Nutritional and herbal supplements for anxiety and anxiety-related disorders: systematic review. *Nutrition Journal.* 2010;9(1). doi:10.1186/1475-2891-9-42.
76. Crichton-Stuart, C. "What are some foods to ease your anxiety?" *Medical News Today.* August 1, 2018. Retrieved from https://www.medicalnewstoday.com/articles/322652.php.
77. Noorafshan A, Vafabin M, Karbalay-Doust S, Asadi-Golshan R. Efficacy of curcumin in the modulation of anxiety provoked by sulfite, a food preservative, in rats. *Preventive Nutrition and Food Science.* 2017;22(2):144–48; Ng QX, Koh SSH, Chan HW, Ho CYX. Clinical use of curcumin in depression: a meta-analysis. *Journal of the American Medical Directors Association.* 2017;18(6):503–8. doi:10.1016/j.jamda.2016.12.071.
78. Mao JJ, Xie SX, Keefe JR, Soeller I, Li QS, Amsterdam JD. Long-term chamomile (*Matricaria chamomilla* L.) treatment for generalized anxiety disorder: a randomized clinical trial. *Phytomedicine.* 2016;23(14):1735–42. doi:10.1016/j.phymed.2016.10.012.
79. Koulivand PH, Khaleghi Ghadiri M, Gorji A. Lavender and the nervous system. *Evidence-Based Complementary and Alternative Medicine.* 2013;2013:1–10. doi:10.1155/2013/681304.

Chapter 4. PTSD

1. Bisson JI, Cosgrove S, Lewis C, Roberts NP. Post-traumatic stress disorder. *BMJ*. November 2015:h6161. doi:10.1136/bmj.h6161.
2. Lancaster C, Teeters J, Gros D, Back S. Posttraumatic stress disorder: overview of evidence-based assessment and treatment. *Journal of Clinical Medicine*. 2016;5(11):105. doi:10.3390/jcm5110105.
3. Chapman C, Mills K, Slade T, et al. Remission from post-traumatic stress disorder in the general population. *Psychological Medicine*. 2011;42(8):1695–1703. doi:10.1017/s0033291711002856.
4. Rauch SL, Shin LM, Phelps EA. Neurocircuitry models of posttraumatic stress disorder and extinction: human neuroimaging research—past, present, and future. *Biological Psychiatry*. 2006;60(4):376–82. doi:10.1016/j.biopsych.2006.06.004.
5. Sherin JE, Nemeroff CB. Post-traumatic stress disorder: the neurobiological impact of psychological trauma. *Dialogues in Clinical Neuroscience*. 2011;13(3):263–78.
6. Andreski P, Chilcoat H, Breslau N. Post-traumatic stress disorder and somatization symptoms: a prospective study. *Psychiatry Research*. 1998;79(2):131–138. doi:10.1016/s0165-1781(98)00026-2.
7. Ng QX, Soh AYS, Loke W, Venkatanarayanan N, Lim DY, Yeo W-S. Systematic review with meta-analysis: the association between post-traumatic stress disorder and irritable bowel syndrome. *Journal of Gastroenterology and Hepatology*. 2018;34(1):68–73. doi:10.1111/jgh.14446.
8. Bravo JA, Forsythe P, Chew MV, et al. Ingestion of *Lactobacillus* strain regulates emotional behavior and central GABA receptor expression in a mouse via the vagus nerve. *Proceedings of the National Academy of Sciences*. 2011;108(38):-16050–55. doi:10.1073/pnas.1102999108; Bercik P, Park AJ, Sinclair D, et al. The anxiolytic effect of *Bifidobacterium longum* NCC3001 involves vagal pathways for gut-brain communication. *Neurogastroenterology and Motility*. 2011;23(12):1132–39. doi:10.1111/j.1365-2982.2011.01796.x.
9. Hemmings SMJ, Malan-Müller S, van den Heuvel LL, et al. The microbiome in posttraumatic stress disorder and trauma-exposed controls. *Psychosomatic Medicine*. 2017;79(8):936–46. doi:10.1097/psy.0000000000000512.
10. Lowry CA, Smith DG, Siebler PH, et al. The microbiota, immunoregulation, and mental health: implications for public health. *Current Environmental Health Reports*. 2016;3(3):270–86. doi:10.1007/s40572-016-0100-5.

11. Stiemsma L, Reynolds L, Turvey S, Finlay B. The hygiene hypothesis: current perspectives and future therapies. *ImmunoTargets and Therapy*. July 2015:143. doi:10.2147/itt.s61528.
12. Eraly SA, Nievergelt CM, Maihofer AX, et al. Assessment of plasma C-reactive protein as a biomarker of posttraumatic stress disorder risk. *JAMA Psychiatry*. 2014;71(4):423. doi:10.1001/jamapsychiatry.2013.4374.
13. Karl JP, Margolis LM, Madslien EH, et al. Changes in intestinal microbiota composition and metabolism coincide with increased intestinal permeability in young adults under prolonged physiological stress. *American Journal of Physiology-Gastrointestinal and Liver Physiology*. 2017;312(6):G559–G571. doi:10.1152/ajpgi.00066.2017.
14. Kalyan-Masih P, Vega-Torres JD, Miles C, et al. Western high-fat diet consumption during adolescence increases susceptibility to traumatic stress while selectively disrupting hippocampal and ventricular volumes. *eNeuro*. 2016;3(5):ENEURO.0125-16.2016. doi:10.1523/eneuro.0125-16.2016.
15. Logue MW, van Rooij SJH, Dennis EL, et al. Smaller hippocampal volume in posttraumatic stress disorder: a multisite ENIGMA-PGC study: subcortical volumetry results from posttraumatic stress disorder consortia. *Biological Psychiatry*. 2018;83(3):244–53. doi:10.1016/j.biopsych.2017.09.006.
16. Masodkar K, Johnson J, Peterson MJ. A review of posttraumatic stress disorder and obesity. *Primary Care Companion for CNS Disorders*. January 2016. doi:10.4088/pcc.15r01848.
17. Michopoulos V, Vester A, Neigh G. Posttraumatic stress disorder: a metabolic disorder in disguise? *Experimental Neurology*. 2016;284:220–29. doi:10.1016/j.expneurol.2016.05.038.
18. Vieweg WV, Fernandez A, Julius DA, et al. Body mass index relates to males with posttraumatic stress disorder. *Journal of the National Medical Association*. 2006;98(4):580–86.
19. Violanti JM, Fekedulegn D, Hartley TA, et al. Police trauma and cardiovascular disease: association between PTSD symptoms and metabolic syndrome. *International Journal of Emergency Mental Health*. 2006;8(4):227–37.
20. Vieweg WVR, Julius DA, Bates J, Quinn III JF, Fernandez A, Hasnain M, Pandurangi AK. Posttraumatic stress disorder as a risk factor for obesity among male military veterans. *Acta Psychiatrica Scandinavica*. 2007;116(6): 483–87. doi:10.1111/j.1600-0447.2007.01071.x.
21. Wolf EJ, Sadeh N, Leritz EC, et al. Posttraumatic stress disorder as a catalyst for the association between metabolic syndrome and reduced cortical thickness. *Biological Psychiatry*. 2016;80(5):363–71. doi:10.1016/j.biopsych.2015.11.023.

22. Nowotny B, Cavka M, Herder C, et al. Effects of acute psychological stress on glucose metabolism and subclinical inflammation in patients with posttraumatic stress disorder. *Hormone and Metabolic Research*. 2010;42(10):746–53. doi:10.1055/s-0030-1261924.
23. Roberts AL, Agnew-Blais JC, Spiegelman D, et al. Posttraumatic stress disorder and incidence of type 2 diabetes mellitus in a sample of women. *JAMA Psychiatry*. 2015;72(3):203. doi:10.1001/jamapsychiatry.2014.2632.
24. Vaccarino V, Goldberg J, Magruder KM, et al. Posttraumatic stress disorder and incidence of type-2 diabetes: a prospective twin study. *Journal of Psychiatric Research*. 2014;56:158–64. doi:10.1016/j.jpsychires.2014.05.019.
25. Hirth JM, Rahman M, Berenson AB. The association of posttraumatic stress disorder with fast food and soda consumption and unhealthy weight loss behaviors among young women. *Journal of Women's Health*. 2011;20(8):1141–49. doi:10.1089/jwh.2010.2675.
26. Ho N, Sommers MS, Lucki I. Effects of diabetes on hippocampal neurogenesis: links to cognition and depression. *Neuroscience and Biobehavioral Reviews*. 2013;37(8):1346–62. doi:10.1016/j.neubiorev.2013.03.010.
27. Hettiaratchi UP, Ekanayake S, Welihinda J. Sri Lankan rice mixed meals: effect on glycaemic index and contribution to daily dietary fibre requirement. *Malaysian Journal of Nutrition*. 2011;17(1):97–104.
28. Sugiyama M, Tang AC, Wakaki Y, Koyama W. Glycemic index of single and mixed meal foods among common Japanese foods with white rice as a reference food. *European Journal of Clinical Nutrition*. 2003;57(6):743–52. doi:10.1038/sj.ejcn.1601606.
29. Mallick HN. Understanding safety of glutamate in food and brain. *Indian Journal of Physiology and Pharmacology*. 2007;51(3):216–34.
30. Uneyama H, Niijima A, San Gabriel A, Torii K. Luminal amino acid sensing in the rat gastric mucosa. *American Journal of Physiology-Gastrointestinal and Liver Physiology*. 2006;291(6):G1163–G1170. doi:10.1152/ajpgi.00587.2005; Kondoh T, Mallick HN, Torii K. Activation of the gut-brain axis by dietary glutamate and physiologic significance in energy homeostasis. *American Journal of Clinical Nutrition*. 2009;90(3):832S–837S. doi:10.3945/ajcn.2009.27462v.
31. Lee M. MSG: can an amino acid really be harmful? *Clinical Correlations*. April 30, 2014. https://www.clinicalcorrelations.org/2014/04/30/msg-can-an-amino-acid-really-be-harmful/. Accessed September 30, 2019.
32. Averill LA, Purohit P, Averill CL, Boesl MA, Krystal JH, Abdallah CG. Glutamate dysregulation and glutamatergic therapeutics for PTSD: evidence from human studies. *Neuroscience Letters*. 2017;649:147–55. doi:10.1016/j.neulet.2016.11.064.

33. Brandley E, Kirkland A, Sarlo G, VanMeter J, Baraniuk J, Holton K. The effects of a low glutamate dietary intervention on anxiety and PTSD in veterans with Gulf War illness (FS15-08-19). *Current Developments in Nutrition*. 2019;3(suppl 1). doi:10.1093/cdn/nzz031.fs15-08-19.

34. Ebenezer PJ, Wilson CB, Wilson LD, Nair AR, J F. The anti-inflammatory effects of blueberries in an animal model of post-traumatic stress disorder (PTSD). Scavone C, ed. *PLoS One*. 2016;11(9):e0160923. doi:10.1371/journal.pone.0160923.

35. Alquraan L, Alzoubi KH, Hammad H, Rababa'h SY, Mayyas F. Omega-3 fatty acids prevent post-traumatic stress disorder-induced memory impairment. *Biomolecules*. 2019;9(3):100. doi:10.3390/biom9030100.

36. Nishi D, Koido Y, Nakaya N, et al. Fish oil for attenuating posttraumatic stress symptoms among rescue workers after the Great East Japan Earthquake: a randomized controlled trial. *Psychotherapy and Psychosomatics*. 2012;81(5):315–17. doi:10.1159/000336811.

37. Matsuoka Y, Nishi D, Hamazaki K. Serum levels of polyunsaturated fatty acids and the risk of posttraumatic stress disorder. *Psychotherapy and Psychosomatics*. 2013;82(6):408–10. doi:10.1159/000351993.

38. Barth J, Bermetz L, Heim E, Trelle S, Tonia T. The current prevalence of child sexual abuse worldwide: a systematic review and meta-analysis. *International Journal of Public Health*. 2012;58(3):469–83. doi:10.1007/s00038-012-0426-1.

39. Miller MW, Sadeh N. Traumatic stress, oxidative stress and post-traumatic stress disorder: neurodegeneration and the accelerated-aging hypothesis. *Molecular Psychiatry*. 2014;19(11):1156–62. doi:10.1038/mp.2014.111.

40. De Souza CP, Gambeta E, Stern CAJ, Zanoveli JM. Posttraumatic stress disorder-type behaviors in streptozotocin-induced diabetic rats can be prevented by prolonged treatment with vitamin E. *Behavioural Brain Research*. 2019;359:749–54. doi:10.1016/j.bbr.2018.09.008.

41. Parker R, Rice MJ. Benefits of antioxidant supplementation in multi-trauma patients. *Romanian Journal of Anaesthesia and Intensive Care*. 2015;22(2):77–78; Dobrovolny J, Smrcka M, Bienertova-Vasku J. Therapeutic potential of vitamin E and its derivatives in traumatic brain injury-associated dementia. *Neurological Sciences*. 2018;39(6):989–98. doi:10.1007/s10072-018-3398-y.

42. Henderson TA, Morries L, Cassano P. Treatments for traumatic brain injury with emphasis on transcranial near-infrared laser phototherapy. *Neuropsychiatric Disease and Treatment*. August 2015:2159. doi:10.2147/ndt.s65809.

43. Habibi L, Ghorbani B, Norouzi AR, Gudarzi SS, Shams J, Yasami M. The efficacy and safety of add-on ginko TD (ginkgo biloba) treatment for PTSD:

results of a 12-week double-blind placebo-controlled study. *Iranian Journal of Psychiatry*. 2007;2(2):58–64.

44. Lee B, Lee H. Systemic administration of curcumin affect anxiety-related behaviors in a rat model of posttraumatic stress disorder via activation of serotonergic systems. *Evidence-Based Complementary and Alternative Medicine*. 2018;2018:1–12. doi:10.1155/2018/9041309; Monsey MS, Gerhard DM, Boyle LM, Briones MA, Seligsohn M, Schafe GE. A diet enriched with curcumin impairs newly acquired and reactivated fear memories. *Neuropsychopharmacology*. 2014;40(5):1278–88. doi:10.1038/npp.2014.315.

Chapter 5. ADHD

1. Luo Y, Weibman D, Halperin JM, Li X. A review of heterogeneity in attention deficit/hyperactivity disorder (ADHD). *Frontiers in Human Neuroscience*. 2019;13:42. doi:10.3390/jcm5110105.
2. Reale L, Bartoli B, Cartabia M, et al. Comorbidity prevalence and treatment outcome in children and adolescents with ADHD. *European Child and Adolescent Psychiatry*. 2017;26(12):1443–57. doi:10.1007/s00787-017-1005-z.
3. Geffen J, Forster K. Treatment of adult ADHD: a clinical perspective. *Therapeutic Advances in Psychopharmacology*. 2018;8(1):25–32. doi:10.1177/2045125317734977; Culpepper L, Mattingly G. Challenges in identifying and managing attention-deficit/hyperactivity disorder in adults in the primary care setting: a review of the literature. *Primary Care Companion to the Journal of Clinical Psychiatry*. 2010;12(6). doi:10.4088/PCC.10r00951pur.
4. For more information about various ways ADHD can negatively affect patients, see Fredriksen M, Dahl AA, Martinsen EW, Klungsoyr O, Faraone SV, Peleikis DE. Childhood and persistent ADHD symptoms associated with educational failure and long-term occupational disability in adult ADHD. *Attention Deficit and Hyperactivity Disorders*. 2014;6(2):87–99. doi:10.1007/s12402-014-0126-1; Agarwal R, Goldenberg M, Perry R, Ishak WW. The quality of life of adults with attention deficit hyperactivity disorder: a systematic review. *Innovations in Clinical Neuroscience*. 2012;9(5–6):10–21; Minde K, Eakin L, Hechtman L, et al. The psychosocial functioning of children and spouses of adults with ADHD. *Journal of Child Psychology and Psychiatry, and Allied Disciplines*. 2003;44(4):637–46.
5. Epstein JN, Weiss MD. Assessing treatment outcomes in attention-deficit/hyperactivity disorder: a narrative review. *Primary Care Companion for CNS Disorders*. 2012;14(6) doi:10.4088/PCC.11r01336.

6. Curatolo P, D'Agati E, Moavero R. The neurobiological basis of ADHD. *Italian Journal of Pediatrics*. 2010;36(1):79. doi:10.1186/1824-7288-36-79.
7. Lyte M. Microbial endocrinology in the microbiome-gut-brain axis: how bacterial production and utilization of neurochemicals influence behavior. Miller V, ed. *PLoS Pathogens*. 2013;9(11):e1003726. doi:10.1371/journal.ppat.1003726.
8. Desbonnet L, Garrett L, Clarke G, Bienenstock J, Dinan TG. The probiotic *Bifidobacteria infantis:* An assessment of potential antidepressant properties in the rat. *Journal of Psychiatric Research*. 2008;43(2):164–74. doi:10.1016/j.jpsychires.2008.03.009; Clayton TA. Metabolic differences underlying two distinct rat urinary phenotypes, a suggested role for gut microbial metabolism of phenylalanine and a possible connection to autism. *FEBS Letters*. 2012;586(7):956–61. doi:10.1016/j.febslet.2012.01.049; Gertsman I, Gangoiti JA, Nyhan WL, Barshop BA. Perturbations of tyrosine metabolism promote the indolepyruvate pathway via tryptophan in host and microbiome. *Molecular Genetics and Metabolism*. 2015;114(3):431–37. doi:10.1016/j.ymgme.2015.01.005.
9. Sandgren AM, Brummer RJM. ADHD-originating in the gut? The emergence of a new explanatory model. *Medical Hypotheses*. 2018;120:135–45. doi:10.1016/j.mehy.2018.08.022.
10. Aarts E, Ederveen THA, Naaijen J, et al. Gut microbiome in ADHD and its relation to neural reward anticipation. Hashimoto K, ed. *PLoS One*. 2017;12(9):e0183509. doi:10.1371/journal.pone.0183509.
11. Volkow ND, Wang G-J, Newcorn JH, et al. Motivation deficit in ADHD is associated with dysfunction of the dopamine reward pathway. *Molecular Psychiatry*. 2010;16(11):1147–54. doi:10.1038/mp.2010.97.
12. Ming X, Chen N, Ray C, Brewer G, Kornitzer J, Steer RA. A gut feeling. *Child Neurology Open*. 2018;5:2329048X1878679. doi:10.1177/2329048x18786799.
13. Niederhofer H, Pittschieler K. A preliminary investigation of ADHD symptoms in persons with celiac disease. *Journal of Attention Disorders*. 2006;10(2):200–204. doi:10.1177/1087054706292109.
14. Cruchet S, Lucero Y, Cornejo V. Truths, myths and needs of special diets: attention-deficit/hyperactivity disorder, autism, non-celiac gluten sensitivity, and vegetarianism. *Annals of Nutrition and Metabolism*. 2016;68(1):43–50. doi:10.1159/000445393.
15. Jackson JR, Eaton WW, Cascella NG, Fasano A, Kelly DL. Neurologic and psychiatric manifestations of celiac disease and gluten sensitivity. *Psychiatric Quarterly*. 2011;83(1):91–102. doi:10.1007/s11126-011-9186-y.

16. Pynnönen PA, Isometsä ET, Verkasalo MA, et al. Gluten-free diet may alleviate depressive and behavioural symptoms in adolescents with coeliac disease: a prospective follow-up case-series study. *BMC Psychiatry*. 2005;5(1). doi:10.1186/1471-244x-5-14.
17. Ly V, Bottelier M, Hoekstra PJ, Arias Vasquez A, Buitelaar JK, Rommelse NN. Elimination diets' efficacy and mechanisms in attention deficit hyperactivity disorder and autism spectrum disorder. *European Child and Adolescent Psychiatry*. 2017;26(9):1067–79. doi:10.1007/s00787-017-0959-1.
18. Jianqin S, Leiming X, Lu X, Yelland GW, Ni J, Clarke AJ. Effects of milk containing only A2 beta casein versus milk containing both A1 and A2 beta casein proteins on gastrointestinal physiology, symptoms of discomfort, and cognitive behavior of people with self-reported intolerance to traditional cows' milk. *Nutrition Journal*. 2015;15(1). doi:10.1186/s12937-016-0147-z.
19. Küllenberg de Gaudry D, Lohner S, Schmucker C, et al. Milk A1 β-casein and health-related outcomes in humans: a systematic review. *Nutrition Reviews*. 2019;77(5):278–306. doi:10.1093/nutrit/nuy063.
20. Truswell AS. The A2 milk case: a critical review. *European Journal of Clinical Nutrition*. 2005;59(5):623–631. doi:10.1038/sj.ejcn.1602104; Farrell HM Jr, Jimenez-Flores R, Bleck GT, et al. Nomenclature of the proteins of cows' milk—sixth revision. *Journal of Dairy Science*. 2004;87(6):1641–74. doi:10.3168/jds.s0022-0302(04)73319-6.
21. Dykman KD, Dykman RA. Effect of nutritional supplements on attentional-deficit hyperactivity disorder. *Integrative Physiological and Behavioral Science*. 1998;33(1):49–60.
22. Johnson RJ, Gold MS, Johnson DR, et al. Attention-deficit/hyperactivity disorder: is it time to reappraise the role of sugar consumption? *Postgraduate Medicine*. 2011;123(5):39–49. doi:10.3810/pgm.2011.09.2458.
23. Del-Ponte B, Anselmi L, Assunção MCF, et al. Sugar consumption and attention-deficit/hyperactivity disorder (ADHD): a birth cohort study. *Journal of Affective Disorders*. 2019;243:290–96. doi:10.1016/j.jad.2018.09.051.
24. Yu C-J, Du J-C, Chiou H-C, et al. Sugar-sweetened beverage consumption is adversely associated with childhood attention deficit/hyperactivity disorder. *International Journal of Environmental Research and Public Health*. 2016;13(7):678. doi:10.3390/ijerph13070678.
25. Feingold BF. Hyperkinesis and learning disabilities linked to artificial food flavors and colors. *American Journal of Nursing*. 1975;75(5):797–803.
26. Spitler DK. Elimination diets and patient's allergies. A handbook of allergy. *Bulletin of the Medical Library Association*. 1944;32(4):534.

27. Kavale KA, Forness SR. Hyperactivity and diet treatment. *Journal of Learning Disabilities*. 1983;16(6):324–30. doi:10.1177/002221948301600604.
28. Schab DW, Trinh NH. Do artificial food colors promote hyperactivity in children with hyperactive syndromes? A meta-analysis of double-blind placebo-controlled trials. *Journal of Developmental and Behavioral Pediatrics*. 2004;25(6):423–34.
29. Nigg JT, Lewis K, Edinger T, Falk M. Meta-analysis of attention-deficit/hyperactivity disorder or attention-deficit/hyperactivity disorder symptoms, restriction diet, and synthetic food color additives. *Journal of the American Academy of Child and Adolescent Psychiatry*. 2012;51(1):86–97.e8. doi:10.1016/j.jaac.2011.10.015; Nigg JT, Holton K. Restriction and elimination diets in ADHD treatment. *Child and Adolescent Psychiatric Clinics of North America*. 2014;23(4):937–53. doi:10.1016/j.chc.2014.05.010; Pelsser LM, Frankena K, Toorman J, Rodrigues Pereira R. Diet and ADHD, reviewing the evidence: a systematic review of meta-analyses of double-blind placebo-controlled trials evaluating the efficacy of diet interventions on the behavior of children with ADHD. *PLoS One*. 2017 Jan 25;12(1):e0169277. doi:10.1371/journal.pone.0169277.
30. Ghanizadeh A, Haddad B. The effect of dietary education on ADHD, a randomized controlled clinical trial. *Annals of General Psychiatry*. 2015;14:12.
31. Ríos-Hernández A, Alda JA, Farran-Codina A, Ferreira-García E, Izquierdo-Pulido M. The Mediterranean diet and ADHD in children and adolescents. *Pediatrics*. 2017;139(2):e20162027. doi:10.1542/peds.2016–2027.
32. San Mauro Martín I, Blumenfeld Olivares JA, Garicano Vilar E, et al. Nutritional and environmental factors in attention-deficit hyperactivity disorder (ADHD): a cross-sectional study. *Nutritional Neuroscience*. 2017;21(9):641–47. doi:10.1080/1028415x.2017.1331952.
33. Durá-Travé T, Gallinas-Victoriano F. Caloric and nutrient intake in children with attention deficit hyperactivity disorder treated with extended-release methylphenidate: analysis of a cross-sectional nutrition survey. *JRSM Open*. 2014;5(2):204253331351769. doi:10.1177/2042533313517690.
34. Kennedy DO, Wightman EL, Forster J, Khan J, Haskell-Ramsay CF, Jackson PA. Cognitive and mood effects of a nutrient enriched breakfast bar in healthy adults: a randomised, double-blind, placebo-controlled, parallel groups study. *Nutrients*. 2017;9(12):1332. doi:10.3390/nu9121332.
35. Bidwell LC, McClernon FJ, Kollins SH. Cognitive enhancers for the treatment of ADHD. *Pharmacology Biochemistry and Behavior*. 2011;99(2):262–74. doi:10.1016/j.pbb.2011.05.002; Liu K, Liang X, Kuang W. Tea consumption may be an effective active treatment for adult attention deficit hyperactivity

disorder (ADHD). *Medical Hypotheses*. 2011;76(4):461–63. doi:10.1016/j.mehy.2010.08.049.

36. Ioannidis K, Chamberlain SR, Müller U. Ostracising caffeine from the pharmacological arsenal for attention-deficit hyperactivity disorder—was this a correct decision? A literature review. *Journal of Psychopharmacology*. 2014;28(9):830–36. doi:10.1177/0269881114541014.
37. Verlaet A, Maasakkers C, Hermans N, Savelkoul H. Rationale for dietary antioxidant treatment of ADHD. *Nutrients*. 2018;10(4):405. doi:10.3390/nu10040405.
38. Joseph N, Zhang-James Y, Perl A, Faraone SV. Oxidative stress and ADHD. *Journal of Attention Disorders*. 2013;19(11):915–24. doi:10.1177/1087054713510354.
39. Golub MS, Takeuchi PT, Keen CL, Hendrick AG, Gershwin ME. Activity and attention in zinc-deprived adolescent monkeys. *American Journal of Clinical Nutrition*. 1996;64(6):908–15. doi:10.1093/ajcn/64.6.908.
40. Gao Q, Liu L, Qian Q, Wang Y. Advances in molecular genetic studies of attention deficit hyperactivity disorder in China. *Shanghai Archives of Psychiatry*. 2014;26(4):194–206; Lepping P, Huber M. Role of zinc in the pathogenesis of attention-deficit hyperactivity disorder: implications for research and treatment. *CNS Drugs*. 2010;24(9):721–28.
41. Cortese S, Angriman M, Lecendreux M, Konofal E. Iron and attention deficit/hyperactivity disorder: what is the empirical evidence so far? A systematic review of the literature. *Expert Review of Neurotherapeutics*. 2012;12(10):1227–40; Curtis LT, Patel K. Nutritional and environmental approaches to preventing and treating autism and attention deficit hyperactivity disorder (ADHD): a review. *Journal of Alternative and Complementary Medicine*. 2008;14(1):79–85.
42. Kim JY, Kang HL, Kim DK, Kang SW, Park YK. Eating habits and food additive intakes are associated with emotional states based on EEG and HRV in healthy Korean children and adolescents. *Journal of the American College of Nutrition*. 2017;36(5):335–41.
43. Weyandt LL, Oster DR, Marraccini ME, et al. Prescription stimulant medication misuse: where are we and where do we go from here? *Experimental and Clinical Psychopharmacology*. 2016;24(5):400–414.

Chapter 6. Dementia and Brain Fog

1. Farzi A, Fröhlich EE, Holzer P. Gut microbiota and the neuroendocrine system. *Neurotherapeutics*. 2018;15(1):5–22. doi:10.1007/s13311-017-0600-5.

2. Alkasir R, Li J, Li X, Jin M, Zhu B. Human gut microbiota: the links with dementia development. *Protein and Cell.* 2017;8(2):90–102. doi:10.1007/s13238-016-0338-6.
3. Tully K, Bolshakov VY. Emotional enhancement of memory: how norepinephrine enables synaptic plasticity. *Molecular Brain.* 2010;3:15. doi:10.1186/1756-6606-3-15.
4. Ghacibeh GA, Shenker JI, Shenal B, Uthman BM, Heilman KM. The influence of vagus nerve stimulation on memory. *Cognitive and Behavioral Neurology.* 2006;19(3):119–22. doi:10.1097/01.wnn.0000213908.34278.7d.
5. Cawthon CR, de La Serre CB. Gut bacteria interaction with vagal afferents. *Brain Research.* 2018;1693(Pt B):134–39. doi:10.1016/j.brainres.2018.01.012.
6. Scheperjans F, Aho V, Pereira PA, et al. Gut microbiota are related to Parkinson's disease and clinical phenotype. *Movement Disorders.* 2015;30(3):350–58.
7. Evidence suggests rosacea may be linked to Parkinson's and Alzheimer's disease. *Nursing Standard.* 2016;30(39):14. doi:10.7748/ns.30.39.14.s16.
8. Parodi A, Paolino S, Greco A, et al. Small intestinal bacterial overgrowth in rosacea: clinical effectiveness of its eradication. *Clinical Gastroenterology Hepatology.* 2008;6(7):759–64. doi:10.1016/j.cgh.2008.02.054.
9. Alkasir R, Li J, Li X, Jin M, Zhu B. Human gut microbiota: the links with dementia development. *Protein and Cell.* 2017;8(2):90–102. doi:10.1007/s13238-016-0338-6.
10. Yamashita T, Kasahara K, Emoto T, et al. Intestinal immunity and gut microbiota as therapeutic targets for preventing atherosclerotic cardiovascular diseases. *Circulation Journal.* 2015;79(9):1882–90. doi:10.1253/circj.CJ-15-0526.
11. Morris MJ, Beilharz JE, Maniam J, Reichelt AC, Westbrook RF. Why is obesity such a problem in the 21st century? The intersection of palatable food, cues and reward pathways, stress, and cognition. *Neuroscience and Biobehavorial Reviews.* 2015;58:36-45. doi:10.1016/j.neubiorev.2014.12.002.
12. Morin JP, Rodríguez-Durán LF, Guzmán-Ramos K, et al. Palatable hyper-caloric foods impact on neuronal plasticity. *Frontiers in Behavioral Neuroscience.* 2017;11:19. doi:10.3389/fnbeh.2017.00019.
13. Woollett K, Maguire EA. Acquiring "the Knowledge" of London's layout drives structural brain changes. *Current Biology.* 2011;21(24):2109-14. doi:10.1016/j.cub.2011.11.018; Noble KG, Grieve SM, Korgaonkar MS, et al. Hippocampal volume varies with educational attainment across the life-span. *Frontiers in Human Neuroscience.* 2012;6:307. doi:10.3389/fnhum.2012.00307.

14. Stevenson RJ, Francis HM. The hippocampus and the regulation of human food intake. *Psychological Bulletin*. 2017;143(10):1011–32. doi:10.1037/bul0000109.
15. Gomez-Pinilla F. The combined effects of exercise and foods in preventing neurological and cognitive disorders. *Preventive Medicine*. 2011;52(suppl 1):S75–80.
16. Mcnay EC, Ong CT, Mccrimmon RJ, Cresswell J, Bogan JS, Sherwin RS. Hippocampal memory processes are modulated by insulin and high-fat-induced insulin resistance. *Neurobiology of Learning and Memory*. 2010;93(4):546–53. doi:10.1016/j.nlm.2010.02.002.
17. Wu A, Ying Z, Gomez-Pinilla F. The interplay between oxidative stress and brain-derived neurotrophic factor modulates the outcome of a saturated fat diet on synaptic plasticity and cognition. *European Journal of Neuroscience*. 2004;19(7):1699–707. doi:10.1111/j.1460-9568.2004.03246.x.
18. Lowe CJ, Reichelt AC, Hall PA. The prefrontal cortex and obesity: a health neuroscience perspective. *Trends in Cognitive Sciences*. 2019;23(4):349–61. doi:10.1016/j.tics.2019.01.005.
19. Hsu TM, Kanoski SE. Blood-brain barrier disruption: mechanistic links between Western diet consumption and dementia. *Frontiers in Aging Neuroscience*. 2014;6:88. doi:10.3389/fnagi.2014.00088.
20. Pistell PJ, Morrison CD, Gupta S, et al. Cognitive impairment following high fat diet consumption is associated with brain inflammation. *Journal of Neuroimmunology*. 2010;219(1–2):25–32. doi:10.1016/j.jneuroim.2009.11.010.
21. Naneix F, Tantot F, Glangetas C, et al. Impact of early consumption of high-fat diet on the mesolimbic dopaminergic system. *eNeuro*. 2017;4(3). doi:10.1523/ENEURO.0120-17.2017; Valladolid-Acebes I, Merino B, Principato A, et al. High-fat diets induce changes in hippocampal glutamate metabolism and neurotransmission. *American Journal of Physiology, Endocrinology and Metabolism*. 2012;302(4):E396–402. doi:10.1152/ajpendo.00343.2011.
22. Boitard C, Etchamendy N, Sauvant J, et al. Juvenile, but not adult exposure to high-fat diet impairs relational memory and hippocampal neurogenesis in mice. *Hippocampus*. 2012;22(11):2095–100. doi:10.1002/hipo.22032.
23. Nilsson LG, Nilsson E. Overweight and cognition. *Scandinavian Journal of Psychology*. 2009;50(6):660–67. doi:10.1111/j.1467-9450.2009.00777.x.
24. Loprinzi PD, Ponce P, Zou L, Li H. The counteracting effects of exercise on high-fat diet-induced memory impairment: a systematic review. *Brain Sciences*. 2019;9(6).
25. Losurdo G, Principi M, Iannone A, et al. Extra-intestinal manifestations of non-celiac gluten sensitivity: an expanding paradigm. *World Journal of Gastroenterology*. 2018;24(14):1521–30. doi:10.3748/wjg.v24.i14.1521.

26. Rashtak S, Murray JA. Celiac disease in the elderly. *Gastroenterology Clinics of North America*. 2009;38(3):433–46. doi:10.1016/j.gtc.2009.06.005.
27. Lichtwark IT, Newnham ED, Robinson SR, et al. Cognitive impairment in coeliac disease improves on a gluten-free diet and correlates with histological and serological indices of disease severity. *Alimentary Pharmacology and Therapeutics*. 2014;40(2):160–70. doi:10.1111/apt.12809; Casella S, Zanini B, Lanzarotto F, et al. Cognitive performance is impaired in coeliac patients on gluten free diet: a case-control study in patients older than 65 years of age. *Digestive and Liver Disease*. 2012;44(9):729–35. doi:10.1016/j.dld.2012.03.008.
28. Witte AV, Fobker M, Gellner R, Knecht S, Flöel A. Caloric restriction improves memory in elderly humans. *Proceedings of the National Academy of Sciences of the United States of America*. 2009;106(4):1255–60. doi:10.1073/pnas.0808587106.
29. Martin B, Mattson MP, Maudsley S. Caloric restriction and intermittent fasting: two potential diets for successful brain aging. *Ageing Research Reviews*. 2006;5(3):332–53. doi:10.1016/j.arr.2006.04.002; Wang J, Ho L, Qin W, et al. Caloric restriction attenuates beta-amyloid neuropathology in a mouse model of Alzheimer's disease. *FASEB Journal*. 2005;19(6):659–61. doi:10.1096/fj.04-3182fje; Srivastava S, Haigis MC. Role of sirtuins and calorie restriction in neuroprotection: implications in Alzheimer's and Parkinson's diseases. *Current Pharmaceutical Design*. 2011;17(31):3418–33. doi:10.2174/138161211798072526.
30. Leclerc E, Trevizol AP, Grigolon RB, et al. The effect of caloric restriction on working memory in healthy non-obese adults. *CNS Spectrums*. 2019:1–7. doi:10.1017/S1092852918001566.
31. Green MW, Rogers PJ. Impairments in working memory associated with spontaneous dieting behaviour. *Psychological Medicine*. 1998;28(5):1063–70. doi:10.1017/s0033291798007016; Kemps E, Tiggemann M, Marshall K. Relationship between dieting to lose weight and the functioning of the central executive. *Appetite*. 2005;45(3):287–94. doi:10.1016/j.appet.2005.07.002.
32. For more information about soy isoflavones, see Soy Isoflavones. Oregon State University website. https://lpi.oregonstate.edu/mic/dietary-factors/phytochemicals/soy-isoflavones. Accessed November 22, 2016.
33. Cheng PF, Chen JJ, Zhou XY, et al. Do soy isoflavones improve cognitive function in postmenopausal women? A meta-analysis. *Menopause*. 2015;22(2):198–206. doi:10.1097/GME.0000000000000290.
34. Gleason CE, Fischer BL, Dowling NM, et al. Cognitive effects of soy isoflavones in patients with Alzheimer's disease. *Journal of Alzheimer's Disease*. 2015;47(4):1009–19. doi:10.3233/JAD-142958.

35. Setchell KD, Clerici C. Equol: pharmacokinetics and biological actions. *Journal of Nutrition*. 2010;140(7):1363S–68S. doi:10.3945/jn.109.119784.
36. Fischer K, Melo van Lent D, Wolfsgruber S, et al. Prospective associations between single foods, Alzheimer's dementia and memory decline in the elderly. *Nutrients*. 2018 Jul;10(7):852.
37. Rehm J, Hasan OSM, Black SE, Shield KD, Schwarzinger M. Alcohol use and dementia: a systematic scoping review. *Alzheimer's Research and Therapy*. 2019;11(1):1. doi:10.1186/s13195-018-0453-0.
38. Sabia S, Fayosse A, Dumurgier J, et al. Alcohol consumption and risk of dementia: 23 year follow-up of Whitehall II cohort study. *BMJ*. 2018;362:k2927. doi:10.1136/bmj.k2927.
39. van Gelder BM, Buijsse B, Tijhuis M, et al. Coffee consumption is inversely associated with cognitive decline in elderly European men: the FINE Study. *European Journal of Clinical Nutrition*. 2007;61(2):226–32. doi:10.1038/sj.ejcn.1602495.
40. Eskelinen MH, Ngandu T, Tuomilehto J, Soininen H, Kivipelto M. Midlife coffee and tea drinking and the risk of late-life dementia: a population-based CAIDE study. *Journal of Alzheimer's Disease*. 2009;16(1):85–91. doi:10.3233/JAD-2009-0920.
41. Wierzejska R. Can coffee consumption lower the risk of Alzheimer's disease and Parkinson's disease? A literature review. *Archives of Medical Science*. 2017;13(3):507–14. doi:10.5114/aoms.2016.63599.
42. Jee SH, He J, Appel LJ, Whelton PK, Suh I, Klag MJ. Coffee consumption and serum lipids: a meta-analysis of randomized controlled clinical trials. *American Journal of Epidemiology*. 2001;153(4):353–62. doi:10.1093/aje/153.4.353.
43. Wierzejska R. Can coffee consumption lower the risk of Alzheimer's disease and Parkinson's disease? A literature review. *Archives of Medical Science*. 2017;13(3):507–14. doi:10.5114/aoms.2016.63599.
44. Rinaldi de Alvarenga JF, Quifer-Rada P, Francetto Juliano F, et al. Using extra virgin olive oil to cook vegetables enhances polyphenol and carotenoid extractability: a study applying the *sofrito* technique. *Molecules*. 2019 Apr;24(8):1555. doi:10.3390/molecules24081555.
45. Kang H, Zhao F, You L, et al. Pseudo-dementia: a neuropsychological review. *Annals of Indian Academy of Neurology*. 2014;17(2):147–54. doi:10.4103/0972-2327.132613.
46. Da Costa IM, Freire MAM, De Paiva Cavalcanti JRL, et al. Supplementation with *Curcuma longa* reverses neurotoxic and behavioral damage in models of Alzheimer's disease: a systematic review. *Current Neuropharmacology*. 2019;17(5):406–21. doi:10.2174/1570159X16666180117112610.

47. Seddon N, D'Cunha NM, Mellor DD, McKune AJ, Georgousopoulou EN, Panagiotakos DB, et al. Effects of curcumin on cognitive function—a systematic review of randomized controlled trials. *Exploratory Research and Hypothesis in Medicine*. 2019;4(1):1. doi:10.14218/ERHM.2018.00024.

48. Shoba G, Joy D, Joseph T, Majeed M, Rajendran R, Srinivas PS. Influence of piperine on the pharmacokinetics of curcumin in animals and human volunteers. *Planta Medica*. 1998;64(4):353–56. doi:10.1055/s-2006-957450.

49. Ng TP, Chiam PC, Lee T, Chua HC, Lim L, Kua EH. Curry consumption and cognitive function in the elderly. *American Journal of Epidemiology*. 2006;164(9):898–906. doi:10.1093/aje/kwj267.

50. Mathuranath PS, George A, Ranjith N, et al. Incidence of Alzheimer's disease in India: a 10 years follow-up study. *Neurology India*. 2012;60(6): 625–30. doi:10.4103/0028-3886.105198.

51. Pandit C, Sai Latha S, Usha Rani T, Anilakumar KR. Pepper and cinnamon improve cold induced cognitive impairment via increasing non-shivering thermogenesis; a study. *International Journal of Hyperthermia*. 2018;35(1): 518–27. doi:10.1080/02656736.2018.1511835.

52. Akhondzadeh S, Sabet MS, Harirchian MH, et al. Saffron in the treatment of patients with mild to moderate Alzheimer's disease: a 16-week, randomized and placebo-controlled trial. *Journal of Clinical Pharmacy and Therapeutics*. 2010;35(5):581–88. doi:10.1111/j.1365-2710.2009.01133.x.

53. Diego MA, Jones NA, Field T, et al. Aromatherapy positively affects mood, EEG patterns of alertness and math computations. *International Journal of Neuroscience*. 1998;96(3–4):217–24. doi:10.3109/00207459808986469.

54. Moss M, Oliver L. Plasma 1,8-cineole correlates with cognitive performance following exposure to rosemary essential oil aroma. *Therapeutic Advances in Psychopharmacology*. 2012;2(3):103–13. doi:10.1177/2045125312436573.

55. Moss M, Cook J, Wesnes K, Duckett P. Aromas of rosemary and lavender essential oils differentially affect cognition and mood in healthy adults. *International Journal of Neuroscience*. 2003;113(1):15–38. doi:10.1080/00207450390161903.

56. Saenghong N, Wattanathorn J, Muchimapura S, et al. *Zingiber officinale* improves cognitive function of the middle-aged healthy women. *Evidence-Based Complementary and Alternative Medicine*. 2012;2012:383062. doi:10.1155/2012/383062.

57. Zeng GF, Zhang ZY, Lu L, Xiao DQ, Zong SH, He JM. Protective effects of ginger root extract on Alzheimer disease-induced behavioral dysfunction in rats. *Rejuvenation Research*. 2013;16(2):124–33. doi:10.1089/rej.2012.1389; Azam F, Amer AM, Abulifa AR, Elzwawi MM. Ginger components as new leads for the design and development of novel multi-targeted

anti-Alzheimer's drugs: a computational investigation. *Drug Design, Development and Therapy*. 2014;8:2045–59. doi:10.2147/DDDT.S67778.

58. Lopresti AL. *Salvia* (sage): a review of its potential cognitive-enhancing and protective effects. *Drugs in R&D*. 2017;17(1):53–64. doi:10.1007/s40268-016-0157-5.
59. Tildesley NT, Kennedy DO, Perry EK, et al. *Salvia lavandulaefolia* (Spanish sage) enhances memory in healthy young volunteers. *Pharmacology, Biochemistry, and Behavior*. 2003;75(3):669–74; Tildesley NT, Kennedy DO, Perry EK, Ballard CG, Wesnes KA, Scholey AB. Positive modulation of mood and cognitive performance following administration of acute doses of *Salvia lavandulaefolia* essential oil to healthy young volunteers. *Physiology and Behavior*. 2005;83(5):699–709.
60. Kennedy DO, Pace S, Haskell C, Okello EJ, Milne A, Scholey AB. Effects of cholinesterase inhibiting sage (*Salvia officinalis*) on mood, anxiety and performance on a psychological stressor battery. *Neuropsychopharmacology*. 2006;31(4):845–52.
61. Morris MC, Tangney CC, Wang Y, Sacks FM, Bennett DA, Aggarwal NT. MIND diet associated with reduced incidence of Alzheimer's disease. *Alzheimer's and Dementia*. 2015;11(9):1007–14. doi:10.1016/j.jalz.2014.11.009.
62. Challa HJ, Tadi P, Uppaluri KR. *DASH Diet (Dietary Approaches to Stop Hypertension)* [updated May 15, 2019]. In: StatPearls [internet]. Treasure Island, FL: StatPearls Publishing; 2019 Jan–. Available from: https://www.ncbi.nlm.nih.gov/books/NBK482514/.
63. Morris MC, Tangney CC, Wang Y, Sacks FM, Bennett DA, Aggarwal NT. MIND diet associated with reduced incidence of Alzheimer's disease. *Alzheimer's and Dementia*. 2015;11(9):1007–14. doi:10.1016/j.jalz.2014.11.009.
64. Hosking DE, Eramudugolla R, Cherbuin N, Anstey KJ. MIND not Mediterranean diet related to 12-year incidence of cognitive impairment in an Australian longitudinal cohort study. *Alzheimer's and Dementia*. 2019;15(4):581–89. doi:10.1016/j.jalz.2018.12.011.
65. Agarwal P, Wang Y, Buchman AS, Holland TM, Bennett DA, Morris MC. MIND diet associated with reduced incidence and delayed progression of Parkinsonism in old age. *Journal of Nutrition, Health and Aging*. 2018;22(10):1211–15. doi:10.1007/s12603-018-1094-5.
66. Morris MC, Tangney CC, Wang Y, et al. MIND diet slows cognitive decline with aging. *Alzheimer's and Dementia*. 2015;11(9):1015–22. doi:10.1016/j.jalz.2015.04.011.
67. Theoharides TC, Stewart JM, Hatziagelaki E, Kolaitis G. Brain "fog," inflammation and obesity: key aspects of neuropsychiatric disorders

improved by luteolin. *Frontiers in Neuroscience*. 2015;9:225. doi:10.3389/fnins.2015.00225.

68. Rao SSC, Rehman A, Yu S, Andino NM. Brain fogginess, gas and bloating: a link between SIBO, probiotics and metabolic acidosis. *Clinical and Translational Gastroenterology*. 2018;9(6):162.
69. Harper L, Bold J. An exploration into the motivation for gluten avoidance in the absence of coeliac disease. *Gastroenterology and Hepatology from Bed to Bench*. 2018;11(3):259–68.
70. Kato-Kataoka A, Sakai M, Ebina R, Nonaka C, Asano T, Miyamori T. Soybean-derived phosphatidylserine improves memory function of the elderly Japanese subjects with memory complaints. *Journal of Clinical Biochemistry and Nutrition*. 2010;47(3):246–55. doi:10.3164/jcbn.10-62.
71. Fioravanti M, Buckley AE. Citicoline (Cognizin) in the treatment of cognitive impairment. *Clinical Interventions in Aging*. 2006;1(3):247–51. doi:10.2147/ciia.2006.1.3.247.

Chapter 7. Obsessive-Compulsive Disorder

1. Goodwin GM. The overlap between anxiety, depression, and obsessive-compulsive disorder. *Dialogues in Clinical Neuroscience*. 2015;17(3):249–60.
2. Pallanti S, Grassi G, Sarrecchia ED, Cantisani A, Pellegrini M. Obsessive-compulsive disorder comorbidity: clinical assessment and therapeutic implications. *Frontiers in Psychiatry*. 2011;2. doi:10.3389/fpsyt.2011.00070.
3. Kantak PA, Bobrow DN, Nyby JG. Obsessive-compulsive-like behaviors in house mice are attenuated by a probiotic (*Lactobacillus rhamnosus* GG). *Behavioural Pharmacology*. 2014;25(1):71–79. doi:10.1097/fbp.0000000000000013.
4. Jung TD, Jung PS, Raveendran L, et al. Changes in gut microbiota during development of compulsive checking and locomotor sensitization induced by chronic treatment with the dopamine agonist quinpirole. *Behavioural Pharmacology*. 2018;29(2–3; special issue):211–24.
5. Turna J, Grosman Kaplan K, Anglin R, Van Ameringen M. "What's bugging the gut in OCD?" A review of the gut microbiome in obsessive-compulsive disorder. *Depression and Anxiety*. 2015;33(3):171–78. doi:10.1002/da.22454.
6. Gustafsson PE, Gustafsson PA, Ivarsson T, Nelson N. Diurnal cortisol levels and cortisol response in youths with obsessive-compulsive disorder. *Neuropsychobiology*. 2008;57(1–2):14–21. doi:10.1159/000123117.
7. Rees JC. Obsessive-compulsive disorder and gut microbiota dysregulation. *Medical Hypotheses*. 2014;82(2):163–66. doi:10.1016/j.mehy.2013.11.026.

8. Real E, Labad J, Alonso P, et al. Stressful life events at onset of obsessive-compulsive disorder are associated with a distinct clinical pattern. *Depression and Anxiety*. 2011;28(5):367–76. doi:10.1002/da.20792.
9. Holton KF, Cotter EW. Could dietary glutamate be contributing to the symptoms of obsessive-compulsive disorder? *Future Science OA*. 2018;4(3):FSO277. doi:10.4155/fsoa-2017-0105.
10. Vlček P, Polák J, Brunovský M, Horáček J. Correction: role of glutamatergic system in obsessive-compulsive disorder with possible therapeutic implications. *Pharmacopsychiatry*. 2017;51(6):e3–e3. doi:10.1055/s-0043-121511.
11. Pittenger C, Bloch MH, Williams K. Glutamate abnormalities in obsessive compulsive disorder: neurobiology, pathophysiology, and treatment. *Pharmacology and Therapeutics*. 2011;132(3):314–32. doi:10.1016/j.pharmthera.2011.09.006.
12. Li Y, Zhang CC, Weidacker K, et al. Investigation of anterior cingulate cortex gamma-aminobutyric acid and glutamate-glutamine levels in obsessive-compulsive disorder using magnetic resonance spectroscopy. *BMC Psychiatry*. 2019;19(1). doi:10.1186/s12888-019-2160-1.
13. Rodrigo L, Álvarez N, Fernández-Bustillo E, Salas-Puig J, Huerta M, Hernández-Lahoz C. Efficacy of a gluten-free diet in the Gilles de la Tourette syndrome: a pilot study. *Nutrients*. 2018;10(5):573. doi:10.3390/nu10050573.
14. Pennisi M, Bramanti A, Cantone M, Pennisi G, Bella R, Lanza G. Neurophysiology of the "celiac brain": disentangling gut-brain connections. *Frontiers in Neuroscience*. 2017;11. doi:10.3389/fnins.2017.00498.
15. Weiss AP, Jenike MA. Late-onset obsessive-compulsive disorder. *Journal of Neuropsychiatry and Clinical Neurosciences*. 2000;12(2):265–68. doi:10.1176/jnp.12.2.265.
16. Wright RA, Arnold MB, Wheeler WJ, Ornstein PL, Schoepp DD. [3H] LY341495 binding to group II metabotropic glutamate receptors in rat brain. *Journal of Pharmacology and Experimental Therapeutics*. 2001;298(2):453–60.
17. Berk M, Ng F, Dean O, Dodd S, Bush AI. Glutathione: a novel treatment target in psychiatry. *Trends in Pharmacological Sciences*. 2008;29(7):346–51. doi:10.1016/j.tips.2008.05.001; Ng F, Berk M, Dean O, Bush AI. Oxidative stress in psychiatric disorders: evidence base and therapeutic implications. *International Journal of Neuropsychopharmacology*. 2008;11(6). doi:10.1017/s1461145707008401.
18. Ghanizadeh A, Mohammadi MR, Bahraini S, Keshavarzi Z, Firoozabadi A, Alavi Shoshtari A. Efficacy of N-acetylcysteine augmentation on obsessive

compulsive disorder: a multicenter randomized double blind placebo controlled clinical trial. *Iranian Journal of Psychiatry.* 2017;12(2):134–41.

19. Lafleur DL, Pittenger C, Kelmendi B, et al. N-acetylcysteine augmentation in serotonin reuptake inhibitor refractory obsessive-compulsive disorder. *Psychopharmacology.* 2005;184(2):254–56. doi:10.1007/s00213-005-0246-6.
20. Grant JE, Odlaug BL, Won Kim S. N-acetylcysteine, a glutamate modulator, in the treatment of trichotillomania. *Archives of General Psychiatry.* 2009;66(7):756. doi:10.1001/archgenpsychiatry.2009.60.
21. Berk M, Jeavons S, Dean OM, et al. Nail-biting stuff? The effect of N-acetyl cysteine on nail-biting. *CNS Spectrums.* 2009;14(7):357–60. doi:10.1017/s1092852900023002; Odlaug BL, Grant JE. N-acetyl cysteine in the treatment of grooming disorders. *Journal of Clinical Psychopharmacology.* 2007;27(2):227–29. doi:10.1097/01.jcp.0000264976.86990.00; Braun TL, Patel V, DeBord LC, Rosen T. A review of N-acetylcysteine in the treatment of grooming disorders. *International Journal of Dermatology.* 2019;58(4):502–10. doi:10.1111/ijd.14371.
22. Frey R, Metzler D, Fischer P, et al. Myo-inositol in depressive and healthy subjects determined by frontal 1H-magnetic resonance spectroscopy at 1.5 tesla. *Journal of Psychiatric Research.* 1998;32(6):411–20. doi:10.1016/s0022-3956(98)00033-8.
23. Fisher SK, Heacock AM, Agranoff BW. Inositol lipids and signal transduction in the nervous system: an update. *Journal of Neurochemistry.* 1992;58(1):18–38. doi:10.1111/j.1471-4159.1992.tb09273.x.
24. Einat H, Belmaker R. The effects of inositol treatment in animal models of psychiatric disorders. *Journal of Affective Disorders.* 2001;62(1–2):113–21. doi:10.1016/s0165-0327(00)00355-4.
25. Fux M, Levine J, Aviv A, Belmaker RH. Inositol treatment of obsessive-compulsive disorder. *American Journal of Psychiatry.* 1996;153(9):1219–21. doi:10.1176/ajp.153.9.1219.
26. Fux M, Benjamin J, Belmaker RH. Inositol versus placebo augmentation of serotonin reuptake inhibitors in the treatment of obsessive-compulsive disorder: a double-blind cross-over study. *International Journal of Neuropsychopharmacology.* 1999;2(3):193–95. doi:10.1017/s1461145799001546.
27. Albelda N, Bar-On N, Joel D. The role of NMDA receptors in the signal attenuation rat model of obsessive-compulsive disorder. *Psychopharmacology.* 2010;210(1):13–24. doi:10.1007/s00213-010-1808-9; Singer HS, Morris C, Grados M. Glutamatergic modulatory therapy for Tourette syndrome. *Medical Hypotheses.* 2010;74(5):862–67. doi:10.1016/j.mehy.2009.11.028.

28. Greenberg WM, Benedict MM, Doerfer J, et al. Adjunctive glycine in the treatment of obsessive-compulsive disorder in adults. *Journal of Psychiatric Research*. 2009;43(6):664–70. doi:10.1016/j.jpsychires.2008.10.007.
29. Cleveland WL, DeLaPaz RL, Fawwaz RA, Challop RS. High-dose glycine treatment of refractory obsessive-compulsive disorder and body dysmorphic disorder in a 5-year period. *Neural Plasticity*. 2009;2009:1–25. doi:10.1155/2009/768398.
30. Mazzio E, Harris N, Soliman K. Food constituents attenuate monoamine oxidase activity and peroxide levels in C6 astrocyte cells. *Planta Medica*. 1998;64(7):603–6. doi:10.1055/s-2006-957530.
31. Sayyah M, Boostani H, Pakseresht S, Malayeri A. Comparison of *Silybum marianum* (L.) Gaertn. with fluoxetine in the treatment of obsessive-compulsive disorder. *Progress in Neuro-Psychopharmacology and Biological Psychiatry*. 2010;34(2):362–65. doi:10.1016/j.pnpbp.2009.12.016.
32. Hermesh H, Weizman A, Shahar A, Munitz H. Vitamin B12 and folic acid serum levels in obsessive compulsive disorder. *Acta Psychiatrica Scandinavica*. 1988;78(1):8–10. doi:10.1111/j.1600-0447.1988.tb06294.x; Ozdemir O, Turksoy N, Bilici R, et al. Vitamin B12, folate, and homocysteine levels in patients with obsessive-compulsive disorder. *Neuropsychiatric Disease and Treatment*. September 2014:1671. doi:10.2147/ndt.s67668.
33. Sharma V, Biswas D. Cobalamin deficiency presenting as obsessive compulsive disorder: case report. *General Hospital Psychiatry*. 2012;34(5):578.e7–578.e8. doi:10.1016/j.genhosppsych.2011.11.006.
34. Watanabe F, Yabuta Y, Bito T, Teng F. Vitamin B12-containing plant food sources for vegetarians. *Nutrients*. 2014;6(5):1861–73. doi:10.3390/nu6051861.
35. Watanabe F, Katsura H, Takenaka S, et al. Pseudovitamin B12 is the predominant cobamide of an algal health food, spirulina tablets. *Journal of Agricultural and Food Chemistry*. 1999;47(11):4736–41. doi:10.1021/jf990541b.
36. Chimakurthy J, Murthy TE. Effect of curcumin on quinpirole induced compulsive checking: an approach to determine the predictive and construct validity of the model. *North American Journal of Medical Sciences*. 2010;2(2):81–86.
37. Depa J, Barrada J, Roncero M. Are the motives for food choices different in orthorexia nervosa and healthy orthorexia? *Nutrients*. 2019;11(3):697. doi:10.3390/nu11030697.
38. Turner PG, Lefevre CE. Instagram use is linked to increased symptoms of orthorexia nervosa. *Eating and Weight Disorders—Studies on Anorexia, Bulimia and Obesity*. 2017;22(2):277–84. doi:10.1007/s40519-017-0364-2.

39. Contesini N, Adami F, Blake M, et al. Nutritional strategies of physically active subjects with muscle dysmorphia. *International Archives of Medicine*. 2013;6(1):25. doi:10.1186/1755-7682-6-25.
40. Position of the American Dietetic Association, Dietitians of Canada, and the American College of Sports Medicine: nutrition and athletic performance. *Journal of the American Dietetic Association*. 2009;109(3):509–27. doi:10.1016/j.jada.2009.01.005.

Chapter 8. Insomnia and Fatigue

1. Bhaskar S, Hemavathy D, Prasad S. Prevalence of chronic insomnia in adult patients and its correlation with medical comorbidities. *Journal of Family Medicine and Primary Care*. 2016;5(4):780. doi:10.4103/2249-4863.201153.
2. Dikeos D, Georgantopoulos G. Medical comorbidity of sleep disorders. *Current Opinion in Psychiatry*. 2011;24(4):346–54. doi:10.1097/yco.0b013e3283473375.
3. Li Y, Hao Y, Fan F, Zhang B. The role of microbiome in insomnia, circadian disturbance and depression. *Frontiers in Psychiatry*. 2018;9. doi:10.3389/fpsyt.2018.00669.
4. Davies SK, Ang JE, Revell VL, et al. Effect of sleep deprivation on the human metabolome. *Proceedings of the National Academy of Sciences of the United States of America*. 2014;111(29):10761–66. doi:10.1073/pnas.1402663111.
5. Johnston JD, Ordovás JM, Scheer FA, Turek FW. Circadian rhythms, metabolism, and chrononutrition in rodents and humans. *Advances in Nutrition*. 2016;7(2):399–406. doi:10.3945/an.115.010777.
6. Thaiss CA, Zeevi D, Levy M, et al. Transkingdom control of microbiota diurnal oscillations promotes metabolic homeostasis. *Cell*. 2014;159(3): 514–29. doi:10.1016/j.cell.2014.09.048.
7. Thaiss CA, Levy M, Korem T, et al. Microbiota diurnal rhythmicity programs host transcriptome oscillations. *Cell*. 2016;167(6):1495–1510.e12. doi:10.1016/j.cell.2016.11.003.
8. Thaiss et al. Transkingdom control of microbiota diurnal oscillations promotes metabolic homeostasis. *Cell*. 2014;159(3):514–29. doi:10.1016/j.cell.2014.09.048.
9. Kunze KN, Hanlon EC, Prachand VN, Brady MJ. Peripheral circadian misalignment: contributor to systemic insulin resistance and potential intervention to improve bariatric surgical outcomes. *American Journal of Physiology. Regulatory, Integrative and Comparative Physiology*. 2016;311(3): R558–R563. doi:10.1152/ajpregu.00175.2016.

10. Poroyko VA, Carreras A, Khalyfa A, et al. Chronic sleep disruption alters gut microbiota, induces systemic and adipose tissue inflammation and insulin resistance in mice. *Scientific Reports*. 2016;6(1). doi:10.1038/srep35405.
11. Vanuytsel T, van Wanrooy S, Vanheel H, et al. Psychological stress and corticotropin-releasing hormone increase intestinal permeability in humans by a mast cell-dependent mechanism. *Gut*. 2013;63(8):1293–99. doi:10.1136/gutjnl-2013-305690.
12. A Demographic Profile of U.S. Workers Around the Clock. Population Reference Bureau website. September 18, 2008. https://www.prb.org/workingaroundtheclock/. Accessed October 3, 2019.
13. Reynolds AC, Paterson JL, Ferguson SA, Stanley D, Wright KP Jr, Dawson D. The shift work and health research agenda: considering changes in gut microbiota as a pathway linking shift work, sleep loss and circadian misalignment, and metabolic disease. *Sleep Medicine Reviews*. 2017;34:3–9. doi:10.1016/j.smrv.2016.06.009.
14. Katagiri R, Asakura K, Kobayashi S, Suga H, Sasaki S. Low intake of vegetables, high intake of confectionary, and unhealthy eating habits are associated with poor sleep quality among middle-aged female Japanese workers. *Journal of Occupational Health*. 2014;56(5):359–68. doi:10.1539/joh.14-0051-oa.
15. Afaghi A, O'Connor H, Chow CM. High-glycemic-index carbohydrate meals shorten sleep onset. *American Journal of Clinical Nutrition*. 2007;85(2):426–30. doi:10.1093/ajcn/85.2.426.
16. St-Onge M-P, Roberts A, Shechter A, Choudhury AR. Fiber and saturated fat are associated with sleep arousals and slow wave sleep. *Journal of Clinical Sleep Medicine*. 2016;12(1):19–24. doi:10.5664/jcsm.5384.
17. Shechter A, O'Keeffe M, Roberts AL, Zammit GK, Choudhury AR, St-Onge M-P. Alterations in sleep architecture in response to experimental sleep curtailment are associated with signs of positive energy balance. *American Journal of Physiology. Regulatory, Integrative and Comparative Physiology*. 2012;303(9):R883–R889. doi:10.1152/ajpregu.00222.2012.
18. Grandner MA, Jackson N, Gerstner JR, Knutson KL. Dietary nutrients associated with short and long sleep duration. Data from a nationally representative sample. *Appetite*. 2013;64:71–80.
19. Sheehan CM, Frochen SE, Walsemann KM, Ailshire JA. Are U.S. adults reporting less sleep? Findings from sleep duration trends in the National Health Interview Survey, 2004–2017. *Sleep*. 2018;42(2). doi:10.1093/sleep/zsy221.

20. Ribeiro JA1, Sebastião AM. Caffeine and adenosine. *Journal of Alzheimer's Disease*. 2010;20(suppl 1):S3–15. doi:10.3233/JAD-2010-1379.
21. Drake C, Roehrs T, Shambroom J, Roth T. Caffeine effects on sleep taken 0, 3, or 6 hours before going to bed. *Journal of Clinical Sleep Medicine*. November 2013. doi:10.5664/jcsm.3170.
22. Poole R, Kennedy OJ, Roderick P, Fallowfield JA, Hayes PC, Parkes J. Coffee consumption and health: umbrella review of meta-analyses of multiple health outcomes. *BMJ*. November 2017:j5024. doi:10.1136/bmj.j5024.
23. Roehrs T. Ethanol as a hypnotic in insomniacs: self administration and effects on sleep and mood. *Neuropsychopharmacology*. 1999;20(3):279–86. doi:10.1016/s0893-133x(98)00068-2.
24. Feige B, Gann H, Brueck R, et al. Effects of alcohol on polysomnographically recorded sleep in healthy subjects. *Alcoholism: Clinical and Experimental Research*. 2006;30(9):1527–37. doi:10.1111/j.1530-0277.2006.00184.x.
25. Chan JKM, Trinder J, Andrewes HE, Colrain IM, Nicholas CL. The acute effects of alcohol on sleep architecture in late adolescence. *Alcoholism: Clinical and Experimental Research*. June 2013:n/a-n/a. doi:10.1111/acer.12141.
26. Rosales-Lagarde A, Armony JL, del Río-Portilla Y, Trejo-Martínez D, Conde R, Corsi-Cabrera M. Enhanced emotional reactivity after selective REM sleep deprivation in humans: an fMRI study. *Frontiers in Behavioral Neuroscience*. 2012;6. doi:10.3389/fnbeh.2012.00025.
27. Lowe PP, Gyongyosi B, Satishchandran A, et al. Reduced gut microbiome protects from alcohol-induced neuroinflammation and alters intestinal and brain inflammasome expression. *Journal of Neuroinflammation*. 2018;15(1). doi:10.1186/s12974-018-1328-9; Gorky J, Schwaber J. The role of the gut-brain axis in alcohol use disorders. *Progress in Neuro-Psychopharmacology and Biological Psychiatry*. 2016;65:234–41. doi:10.1016/j.pnpbp.2015.06.013.
28. Decoeur F, Benmamar-Badel A, Leyrolle Q, Persillet M, Layé S, Nadjar A. Dietary N-3 PUFA deficiency affects sleep-wake activity in basal condition and in response to an inflammatory challenge in mice. *Brain, Behavior, and Immunity*. May 2019. doi:10.1016/j.bbi.2019.05.016; Alzoubi KH, Mayyas F, Abu Zamzam HI. Omega-3 fatty acids protects against chronic sleep-deprivation induced memory impairment. *Life Sciences*. 2019;227:1–7. doi:10.1016/j.lfs.2019.04.028.
29. Jahangard L, Sadeghi A, Ahmadpanah M, et al. Influence of adjuvant omega-3-polyunsaturated fatty acids on depression, sleep, and emotion regulation among outpatients with major depressive disorders—results from a

double-blind, randomized and placebo-controlled clinical trial. *Journal of Psychiatric Research.* 2018;107:48–56. doi:10.1016/j.jpsychires.2018.09.016.

30. Yehuda S, Rabinovitz S, Mostofsk DI. Essential fatty acids and sleep: mini-review and hypothesis. *Medical Hypotheses.* 1998;50(2):139–45. doi:10.1016/s0306-9877(98)90200-6.
31. Urade Y, Hayaishi O. Prostaglandin D2 and sleep/wake regulation. *Sleep Medicine Reviews.* 2011;15(6):411–418. doi:10.1016/j.smrv.2011.08.003; Zhang H, Hamilton JH, Salem N, Kim HY. N-3 fatty acid deficiency in the rat pineal gland: effects on phospholipid molecular species composition and endogenous levels of melatonin and lipoxygenase products. *Journal of Lipid Research.* 1998;39(7):1397–403.
32. Papandreou C. Independent associations between fatty acids and sleep quality among obese patients with obstructive sleep apnoea syndrome. *Journal of Sleep Research.* 2013;22(5):569–72. doi:10.1111/jsr.12043.
33. Hartmann E. Effects of L-tryptophan on sleepiness and on sleep. *Journal of Psychiatric Research.* 1982;17(2):107–13. doi:10.1016/0022-3956(82)90012-7.
34. Esteban S, Nicolaus C, Garmundi A, et al. Effect of orally administered l-tryptophan on serotonin, melatonin, and the innate immune response in the rat. *Molecular and Cellular Biochemistry.* 2004;267(1–2):39–46. doi:10.1023/b:mcbi.0000049363.97713.74.
35. Miyake M, Kirisako T, Kokubo T, et al. Randomised controlled trial of the effects of L-ornithine on stress markers and sleep quality in healthy workers. *Nutrition Journal.* 2014;13(1). doi:10.1186/1475-2891-13-53.
36. Adib-Hajbaghery M, Mousavi SN. The effects of chamomile extract on sleep quality among elderly people: a clinical trial. *Complementary Therapies in Medicine.* 2017;35:109–14. doi:10.1016/j.ctim.2017.09.010.
37. Hieu TH, Dibas M, Surya Dila KA, et al. Therapeutic efficacy and safety of chamomile for state anxiety, generalized anxiety disorder, insomnia, and sleep quality: a systematic review and meta-analysis of randomized trials and quasi-randomized trials. *Phytotherapy Research.* 2019;33(6):1604–15. doi:10.1002/ptr.6349.
38. Avallone R, Zanoli P, Corsi L, Cannazza G, Baraldi M. Benzodiazepine-like compounds and GABA in flower heads of *Matricaria chamomilla. Phytotherapy Research.* 1996;10:S177–S179.
39. Zeng Y, Pu X, Yang J, et al. Preventive and therapeutic role of functional ingredients of barley grass for chronic diseases in human beings. *Oxidative Medicine and Cellular Longevity.* 2018;2018:1–15. doi:10.1155/2018/3232080.

40. Zeng Y, Pu X, Yang J, et al. Preventive and therapeutic role of functional ingredients of barley grass for chronic diseases in human beings. *Oxidative Medicine and Cellular Longevity*. 2018;2018:1–15. doi:10.1155/2018/3232080.
41. Chanana P, Kumar A. GABA-BZD receptor modulating mechanism of *Panax quinquefolius* against 72-h sleep deprivation induced anxiety like behavior: possible roles of oxidative stress, mitochondrial dysfunction and neuroinflammation. *Frontiers in Neuroscience*. 2016;10. doi:10.3389/fnins.2016.00084.
42. Chu Q-P, Wang L-E, Cui X-Y, et al. Extract of *Ganoderma lucidum* potentiates pentobarbital-induced sleep via a GABAergic mechanism. *Pharmacology Biochemistry and Behavior*. 2007;86(4):693–98. doi:10.1016/j.pbb.2007.02.015.
43. Kim HD, Hong K-B, Noh DO, Suh HJ. Sleep-inducing effect of lettuce (*Lactuca sativa*) varieties on pentobarbital-induced sleep. *Food Science and Biotechnology*. 2017;26(3):807–14. doi:10.1007/s10068-017-0107-1.
44. Kelley D, Adkins Y, Laugero K. A review of the health benefits of cherries. *Nutrients*. 2018;10(3):368. doi:10.3390/nu10030368.
45. Pigeon WR, Carr M, Gorman C, Perlis ML. Effects of a tart cherry juice beverage on the sleep of older adults with insomnia: a pilot study. *Journal of Medicinal Food*. 2010;13(3):579–83. doi:10.1089/jmf.2009.0096.
46. Losso JN, Finley JW, Karki N, et al. Pilot study of the tart cherry juice for the treatment of insomnia and investigation of mechanisms. *American Journal of Therapeutics*. 2018;25(2):e194–e201. doi:10.1097/mjt.0000000000000584.
47. Sears B. Anti-inflammatory diets. *Journal of the American College of Nutrition*. 2015;34(suppl 1):14–21. doi:10.1080/07315724.2015.1080105.
48. Pérez-Jiménez J, Neveu V, Vos F, Scalbert A. Identification of the 100 richest dietary sources of polyphenols: an application of the Phenol-Explorer database. *European Journal of Clinical Nutrition*. 2010;64(S3):S112–S120. doi:10.1038/ejcn.2010.221.
49. Mellen PB, Daniel KR, Brosnihan KB, Hansen KJ, Herrington DM. Effect of muscadine grape seed supplementation on vascular function in subjects with or at risk for cardiovascular disease: a randomized crossover trial. *Journal of the American College of Nutrition*. 2010;29(5):469–75.
50. Ricker MA, Haas WC. Anti-inflammatory diet in clinical practice: a review. *Nutrition in Clinical Practice*. 2017;32(3):318–25. doi:10.1177/0884533617700353.
51. Joseph P, Abey S, Henderson W. Emerging role of nutri-epigenetics in inflammation and cancer. *Oncology Nursing Forum*. 2016;43(6):784–88. doi:10.1188/16.onf.784–788.

52. Cox IM, Campbell MJ, Dowson D. Red blood cell magnesium and chronic fatigue syndrome. *Lancet*. 1991;337(8744):757–60. doi:10.1016/0140-6736(91)91371-z.

53. Cheng S-M, Yang D-Y, Lee C-P, et al. Effects of magnesium sulfate on dynamic changes of brain glucose and its metabolites during a short-term forced swimming in gerbils. *European Journal of Applied Physiology*. 2007;99(6):695–99. doi:10.1007/s00421-006-0374-7.

54. Watkins JH, Nakajima H, Hanaoka K, Zhao L, Iwamoto T, Okabe T. Effect of zinc on strength and fatigue resistance of amalgam. *Dental Materials*. 1995;11(1):24–33. doi:10.1016/0109-5641(95)80005-0; Ribeiro SMF, Braga CBM, Peria FM, Martinez EZ, Rocha JJRD, Cunha SFC. Effects of zinc supplementation on fatigue and quality of life in patients with colorectal cancer. *Einstein* (São Paulo). 2017;15(1):24–28. doi:10.1590/s1679-45082017ao3830.

55. Heap LC, Peters TJ, Wessely S. Vitamin B status in patients with chronic fatigue syndrome. *Journal of the Royal Society of Medicine*. 1999;92(4):183–85.

56. Kirksey A, Morré DM, Wasynczuk AZ. Neuronal development in vitamin B6 deficiency. *Annals of the New York Academy of Sciences*. 1990;585(1 Vitamin B6):202–18. doi:10.1111/j.1749-6632.1990.tb28054.x.

57. Jacobson W, Saich T, Borysiewicz LK, Behan WMH, Behan PO, Wreghitt TG. Serum folate and chronic fatigue syndrome. *Neurology*. 1993;43(12): 2645–47. doi:10.1212/wnl.43.12.2645.

58. Mahmood L. The metabolic processes of folic acid and vitamin B12 deficiency. *Journal of Health Research and Reviews*. 2014;1(1):5. doi:10.4103/2394-2010.143318.

59. Tweet MS, Polga KM. 44-year-old man with shortness of breath, fatigue, and paresthesia. *Mayo Clinic Proceedings*. 2010;85(12):1148–51. doi:10.4065/mcp.2009.0662.

60. Huijts M, Duits A, Staals J, van Oostenbrugge RJ. Association of vitamin B12 deficiency with fatigue and depression after lacunar stroke. De Windt LJ, ed. *PLoS One*. 2012;7(1):e30519. doi:10.1371/journal.pone.0030519.

61. Chan CQH, Low LL, Lee KH. Oral vitamin B12 replacement for the treatment of pernicious anemia. *Frontiers in Medicine*. 2016;3. doi:10.3389/fmed.2016.00038.

62. Does vitamin C influence neurodegenerative diseases and psychiatric disorders? *Nutrients*. 2017;9(7):659. doi:10.3390/nu9070659.

63. Anjum I, Jaffery SS, Fayyaz M, Samoo Z, Anjum S. The role of vitamin D in brain health: a mini literature review. *Cureus*. July 2018. doi:10.7759/cureus.2960.

64. Neale RE, Khan SR, Lucas RM, Waterhouse M, Whiteman DC, Olsen CM. The effect of sunscreen on vitamin D: a review. *British Journal of Dermatology*. July 2019. doi:10.1111/bjd.17980.
65. Traber MG. Vitamin E inadequacy in humans: causes and consequences. *Advances in Nutrition*. 2014;5(5):503–14. doi:10.3945/an.114.006254.
66. Hsu Y-J, Huang W-C, Chiu C-C, et al. Capsaicin supplementation reduces physical fatigue and improves exercise performance in mice. *Nutrients*. 2016;8(10):648. doi:10.3390/nu8100648.
67. Janssens PLHR, Hursel R, Martens EAP, Westerterp-Plantenga MS. Acute effects of capsaicin on energy expenditure and fat oxidation in negative energy balance. Tomé D, ed. *PLoS One*. 2013;8(7):e67786. doi:10.1371/journal.pone.0067786.
68. Fattori V, Hohmann M, Rossaneis A, Pinho-Ribeiro F, Verri W. Capsaicin: current understanding of its mechanisms and therapy of pain and other pre-clinical and clinical uses. *Molecules*. 2016;21(7):844. doi:10.3390/molecules21070844.
69. Zheng J, Zheng S, Feng Q, Zhang Q, Xiao X. Dietary capsaicin and its anti-obesity potency: from mechanism to clinical implications. *Bioscience Reports*. 2017;37(3):BSR20170286. doi:10.1042/bsr20170286.
70. Gregersen NT, Belza A, Jensen MG, et al. Acute effects of mustard, horseradish, black pepper and ginger on energy expenditure, appetite, ad libitum energy intake and energy balance in human subjects. *British Journal of Nutrition*. 2012;109(3):556–63. doi:10.1017/s0007114512001201.
71. Rahman M, Yang DK, Kim G-B, Lee S-J, Kim S-J. *Nigella sativa* seed extract attenuates the fatigue induced by exhaustive swimming in rats. *Biomedical Reports*. 2017;6(4):468–74. doi:10.3892/br.2017.866; Yimer EM, Tuem KB, Karim A, Ur-Rehman N, Anwar F. *Nigella sativa* L. (black cumin): a promising natural remedy for wide range of illnesses. *Evidence-Based Complementary and Alternative Medicine*. 2019;2019:1–16. doi:10.1155/2019/1528635.
72. Huang W-C, Chiu W-C, Chuang H-L, et al. Effect of curcumin supplementation on physiological fatigue and physical performance in mice. *Nutrients*. 2015;7(2):905–21. doi:10.3390/nu7020905.

Chapter 9. Bipolar Disorder and Schizophrenia

1. Insel T. Post by Former NIMH Director Thomas Insel: Transforming Diagnosis. National Institute of Mental Health website. April 29, 2013. https://www.nimh.nih.gov/about/directors/thomas-insel/blog/2013/transforming-diagnosis.shtml. Accessed October 4, 2019.

2. Lynham AJ, Hubbard L, Tansey KE, et al. Examining cognition across the bipolar/schizophrenia diagnostic spectrum. *Journal of Psychiatry and Neuroscience*. 2018;43(4):245–53. doi:10.1503/jpn.170076.
3. Leboyer M, Soreca I, Scott J, et al. Can bipolar disorder be viewed as a multi-system inflammatory disease? *Journal of Affective Disorders*. 2012;141(1):1–10. doi:10.1016/j.jad.2011.12.049.
4. Tseng P-T, Zeng B-S, Chen Y-W, Wu M-K, Wu C-K, Lin P-Y. A meta-analysis and systematic review of the comorbidity between irritable bowel syndrome and bipolar disorder. *Medicine*. 2016;95(33):e4617. doi:10.1097/md.0000000000004617.
5. Legendre T, Boudebesse C, Henry C, Etain B. Antibiomania: penser au syndrome maniaque secondaire à une antibiothérapie. *L'Encéphale*. 2017;43(2):183–86. doi:10.1016/j.encep.2015.06.008.
6. Gao J. Correlation between anxiety-depression status and cytokines in diarrhea-predominant irritable bowel syndrome. *Experimental and Therapeutic Medicine*. 2013;6(1):93–96. doi:10.3892/etm.2013.1101.
7. Liu L, Zhu G. Gut-brain axis and mood disorder. *Frontiers in Psychiatry*. 2018;9. doi:10.3389/fpsyt.2018.00223.
8. Evans SJ, Bassis CM, Hein R, et al. The gut microbiome composition associates with bipolar disorder and illness severity. *Journal of Psychiatric Research*. 2017;87:23–29. doi:10.1016/j.jpsychires.2016.12.007.
9. Lyte M. Probiotics function mechanistically as delivery vehicles for neuroactive compounds: microbial endocrinology in the design and use of probiotics. *BioEssays*. 2011;33(8):574–581. doi:10.1002/bies.201100024; Barrett E, Ross RP, O'Toole PW, Fitzgerald GF, Stanton C. γ-Aminobutyric acid production by culturable bacteria from the human intestine. *Journal of Applied Microbiology*. 2012;113(2):411–17. doi:10.1111/j.1365-2672.2012.05344.x.
10. Machado-Vieira R, Manji HK, Zarate Jr CA. The role of lithium in the treatment of bipolar disorder: convergent evidence for neurotrophic effects as a unifying hypothesis. *Bipolar Disorders*. 2009;11:92–109. doi:10.1111/j.1399-5618.2009.00714.x.
11. Jacka FN, Pasco JA, Mykletun A, et al. Diet quality in bipolar disorder in a population-based sample of women. *Journal of Affective Disorders*. 2011;129(1–3):332–37. doi:10.1016/j.jad.2010.09.004.
12. Elmslie JL, Mann JI, Silverstone JT, Williams SM, Romans SE. Determinants of overweight and obesity in patients with bipolar disorder. *Journal of Clinical Psychiatry*. 2001;62(6):486–91. doi:10.4088/jcp.v62n0614.
13. Noguchi R, Hiraoka M, Watanabe Y, Kagawa Y. Relationship between dietary patterns and depressive symptoms: difference by gender, and

unipolar and bipolar depression. *Journal of Nutritional Science and Vitaminology*. 2013;59(2):115–22. doi:10.3177/jnsv.59.115; Noaghiul S, Hibbeln JR. Cross-national comparisons of seafood consumption and rates of bipolar disorders. *American Journal of Psychiatry*. 2003;160(12):2222–27. doi:10.1176/appi.ajp.160.12.2222.

14. Łojko D, Stelmach-Mardas M, Suwalska A. Diet quality and eating patterns in euthymic bipolar patients. *European Review for Medical and Pharmacological Sciences*. 2019;23(3):1221–38. doi:10.26355/eurrev_201902_17016; McElroy SL, Crow S, Biernacka JM, et al. Clinical phenotype of bipolar disorder with comorbid binge eating disorder. *Journal of Affective Disorders*. 2013;150(3):981–86. doi:10.1016/j.jad.2013.05.024.
15. Melo MCA, de Oliveira Ribeiro M, de Araújo CFC, de Mesquita LMF, de Bruin PFC, de Bruin VMS. Night eating in bipolar disorder. *Sleep Medicine*. 2018 Aug;48:49–52. doi:10.1016/j.sleep.2018.03.031.
16. Bauer IE, Gálvez JF, Hamilton JE, et al. Lifestyle interventions targeting dietary habits and exercise in bipolar disorder: a systematic review. *Journal of Psychiatric Research*. 2016;74:1–7. doi:10.1016/j.jpsychires.2015.12.006; Frank E, Wallace ML, Hall M, et al. An integrated risk reduction intervention can reduce body mass index in individuals being treated for bipolar I disorder: results from a randomized trial. *Bipolar Disorders*. 2014;17(4):424–37. doi:10.1111/bdi.12283.
17. Brietzke E, Mansur RB, Subramaniapillai M, et al. Ketogenic diet as a metabolic therapy for mood disorders: evidence and developments. *Neuroscience and Biobehavioral Reviews*. 2018;94:11–16. doi:10.1016/j.neubiorev.2018.07.020; Phelps JR, Siemers SV, El-Mallakh RS. The ketogenic diet for type II bipolar disorder. *Neurocase*. 2013;19(5):423–26. doi:10.1080/13554794.2012.690421.
18. Campbell IH, Campbell H. Ketosis and bipolar disorder: controlled analytic study of online reports. *BJPsych Open*. 2019;5(4). doi:10.1192/bjo.2019.49.
19. Brietzke E, Mansur RB, Subramaniapillai M, et al. Ketogenic diet as a metabolic therapy for mood disorders: evidence and developments. *Neuroscience and Biobehavioral Reviews*. 2018;94:11–16. doi:10.1016/j.neubiorev.2018.07.020.
20. Kim Y, Santos R, Gage FH, Marchetto MC. Molecular mechanisms of bipolar disorder: progress made and future challenges. *Frontiers in Cellular Neuroscience*. 2017;11. doi:10.3389/fncel.2017.00030.
21. Malinauskas BM, Aeby VG, Overton RF, Carpenter-Aeby T, Barber-Heidal K. A survey of energy drink consumption patterns among college students. *Nutrition Journal*. 2007;6(1). doi:10.1186/1475-2891-6-35.

22. Rizkallah É, Bélanger M, Stavro K, et al. Could the use of energy drinks induce manic or depressive relapse among abstinent substance use disorder patients with comorbid bipolar spectrum disorder? *Bipolar Disorders.* 2011;13(5–6):578–80. doi:10.1111/j.1399-5618.2011.00951.x; Kiselev BM, Shebak SS, Milam TR. Manic episode following ingestion of caffeine pills. *Primary Care Companion for CNS Disorders.* June 2015. doi:10.4088/pcc.14l01764.
23. Winston AP, Hardwick E, Jaberi N. Neuropsychiatric effects of caffeine. *Advances in Psychiatric Treatment.* 2005;11(6):432–39. doi:10.1192/apt.11.6.432; Lorist MM, Tops M. Caffeine, fatigue, and cognition. *Brain and Cognition.* 2003;53(1):82–94.
24. Kiselev BM, Shebak SS, Milam TR. Manic episode following ingestion of caffeine pills. *Primary Care Companion for CNS Disorders.* June 2015. doi:10.4088/pcc.14l01764.
25. Johannessen L, Strudsholm U, Foldager L, Munk-Jørgensen P. Increased risk of hypertension in patients with bipolar disorder and patients with anxiety compared to background population and patients with schizophrenia. *Journal of Affective Disorders.* 2006;95(1–3):13–17. doi:10.1016/j.jad.2006.03.027; Rihmer Z, Gonda X, Dome P. Is mania the hypertension of the mood? Discussion of a hypothesis. *Current Neuropharmacology.* 2017;15(3):424–33. doi:10.2174/1570159x14666160902145635.
26. Dickerson F, Stallings C, Origoni A, Vaughan C, Khushalani S, Yolken R. Markers of gluten sensitivity in acute mania: a longitudinal study. *Psychiatry Research.* 2012;196(1):68–71. doi:10.1016/j.psychres.2011.11.007.
27. Severance EG, Gressitt KL, Yang S, et al. Seroreactive marker for inflammatory bowel disease and associations with antibodies to dietary proteins in bipolar disorder. *Bipolar Disorders.* 2013;16(3):230–40. doi:10.1111/bdi.12159.
28. Goldstein BI, Velyvis VP, Parikh SV. The association between moderate alcohol use and illness severity in bipolar disorder. *Journal of Clinical Psychiatry.* 2006;67(1):102–6. doi:10.4088/jcp.v67n0114.
29. Jaffee WB, Griffin ML, Gallop R, et al. Depression precipitated by alcohol use in patients with co-occurring bipolar and substance use disorders. *Journal of Clinical Psychiatry.* 2008;70(2):171–76. doi:10.4088/jcp.08m04011; Manwani SG, Szilagyi KA, Zablotsky B, Hennen J, Griffin ML, Weiss RD. Adherence to pharmacotherapy in bipolar disorder patients with and without co-occurring substance use disorders. *Journal of Clinical Psychiatry.* 2007;68(8):1172–76. doi:10.4088/jcp.v68n0802.
30. van Zaane J, van den Brink W, Draisma S, Smit JH, Nolen WA. The effect of moderate and excessive alcohol use on the course and outcome

of patients with bipolar disorders. *Journal of Clinical Psychiatry*. 2010;71(7): 885–93. doi:10.4088/jcp.09m05079gry; Ostacher MJ, Perlis RH, Nierenberg AA, et al. Impact of substance use disorders on recovery from episodes of depression in bipolar disorder patients: prospective data from the Systematic Treatment Enhancement Program for Bipolar Disorder (STEP-BD). *American Journal of Psychiatry*. 2010;167(3):289–97. doi:10.1176/appi.ajp.2009.09020299.

31. Bailey DG, Dresser G, Arnold JMO. Grapefruit-medication interactions: forbidden fruit or avoidable consequences? *Canadian Medical Association Journal*. 2012;185(4):309–16. doi:10.1503/cmaj.120951.
32. Noaghiul S, Hibbeln JR. Cross-national comparisons of seafood consumption and rates of bipolar disorders. *American Journal of Psychiatry*. 2003;160(12):2222–27. doi:10.1176/appi.ajp.160.12.2222.
33. Sarris J, Mischoulon D, Schweitzer I. Omega-3 for bipolar disorder. *Journal of Clinical Psychiatry*. 2011;73(1):81–86. doi:10.4088/jcp.10r06710.
34. Bauer IE, Green C, Colpo GD, et al. A double-blind, randomized, placebo-controlled study of aspirin and N-acetylcysteine as adjunctive treatments for bipolar depression. *Journal of Clinical Psychiatry*. 2018;80(1). doi:10.4088/jcp.18m12200.
35. Berk M, Turner A, Malhi GS, et al. A randomised controlled trial of a mitochondrial therapeutic target for bipolar depression: mitochondrial agents, N-acetylcysteine, and placebo. *BMC Medicine*. 2019;17(1). doi:10.1186/s12916-019-1257-1.
36. Nierenberg AA, Montana R, Kinrys G, Deckersbach T, Dufour S, Baek JH. L-methylfolate for bipolar I depressive episodes: an open trial proof-of-concept registry. *Journal of Affective Disorders*. 2017;207:429–33. doi:10.1016/j.jad.2016.09.053.
37. Coppen A, Chaudhry S, Swade C. Folic acid enhances lithium prophylaxis. *Journal of Affective Disorders*. 1986;10(1):9–13. doi:10.1016/0165-0327(86)90043-1.
38. Sharpley AL, Hockney R, McPeake L, Geddes JR, Cowen PJ. Folic acid supplementation for prevention of mood disorders in young people at familial risk: a randomised, double blind, placebo controlled trial. *Journal of Affective Disorders*. 2014;167:306–11. doi:10.1016/j.jad.2014.06.011.
39. Behzadi AH, Omrani Z, Chalian M, Asadi S, Ghadiri M. Folic acid efficacy as an alternative drug added to sodium valproate in the treatment of acute phase of mania in bipolar disorder: a double-blind randomized controlled trial. *Acta Psychiatrica Scandinavica*. 2009;120(6):441–45. doi:10.1111/j.1600-0447.2009.01368.x.

40. Heiden A, Frey R, Presslich O, Blasbichler T, Smetana R, Kasper S. Treatment of severe mania with intravenous magnesium sulphate as a supplementary therapy. *Psychiatry Research.* 1999;89(3):239–46. doi:10.1016/s0165-1781(99)00107-9.
41. Chouinard G, Beauclair L, Geiser R, Etienne P. A pilot study of magnesium aspartate hydrochloride (Magnesiocard®) as a mood stabilizer for rapid cycling bipolar affective disorder patients. *Progress in Neuro-Psychopharmacology and Biological Psychiatry.* 1990;14(2):171–80. doi:10.1016/0278-5846(90)90099-3.
42. Siwek M, Sowa-Kućma M, Styczeń K, et al. Decreased serum zinc concentration during depressive episode in patients with bipolar disorder. *Journal of Affective Disorders.* 2016;190:272–77. doi:10.1016/j.jad.2015.10.026.
43. Millett CE, Mukherjee D, Reider A, et al. Peripheral zinc and neopterin concentrations are associated with mood severity in bipolar disorder in a gender-specific manner. *Psychiatry Research.* 2017;255:52–58. doi:10.1016/j.psychres.2017.05.022.
44. Zheng P, Zeng B, Liu M, et al. The gut microbiome from patients with schizophrenia modulates the glutamate-glutamine-GABA cycle and schizophrenia-relevant behaviors in mice. *Science Advances.* 2019;5(2):eaau8317.
45. Severance EG, Prandovszky E, Castiglione J, Yolken RH. Gastroenterology issues in schizophrenia: why the gut matters. *Current Psychiatry Reports.* 2015;17(5). doi:10.1007/s11920-015-0574-0.
46. Benros ME, Mortensen PB, Eaton WW. Autoimmune diseases and infections as risk factors for schizophrenia. *Annals of the New York Academy of Sciences.* 2012;1262(1):56–66. doi:10.1111/j.1749-6632.2012.06638.x; Caso J, Balanzá-Martínez V, Palomo T, García-Bueno B. The microbiota and gut-brain axis: contributions to the immunopathogenesis of schizophrenia. *Current Pharmaceutical Design.* 2016;22(40):6122–33. doi:10.2174/1381612822666160906160911.
47. Dickerson F, Severance E, Yolken R. The microbiome, immunity, and schizophrenia and bipolar disorder. *Brain, Behavior, and Immunity.* 2017;62:-46–52. doi:10.1016/j.bbi.2016.12.010.
48. Tsuruga K, Sugawara N, Sato Y, et al. Dietary patterns and schizophrenia: a comparison with healthy controls. *Neuropsychiatric Disease and Treatment.* April 2015:1115. doi:10.2147/ndt.s74760.
49. Yang X, Sun L, Zhao A, et al. Serum fatty acid patterns in patients with schizophrenia: a targeted metabonomics study. *Translational Psychiatry.* 2017;7(7):e1176–e1176. doi:10.1038/tp.2017.152.
50. Dohan FC. Cereals and schizophrenia data and hypothesis. *Acta Psychiatrica Scandinavica.* 1966;42(2):125–52. doi:10.1111/j.1600-0447.1966.tb01920.x.

51. Čiháková D, Eaton WW, Talor MV, et al. Gliadin-related antibodies in schizophrenia. *Schizophrenia Research.* 2018;195:585–86. doi:10.1016/j.schres.2017.08.051; Kelly DL, Demyanovich HK, Rodriguez KM, et al. Randomized controlled trial of a gluten-free diet in patients with schizophrenia positive for antigliadin antibodies (AGA IgG): a pilot feasibility study. *Journal of Psychiatry and Neuroscience.* 2019;44(4):269–76. doi:10.1503/jpn.180174.
52. Levinta A, Mukovozov I, Tsoutsoulas C. Use of a gluten-free diet in schizophrenia: a systematic review. *Advances in Nutrition.* 2018;9(6):824–32. doi:10.1093/advances/nmy056.
53. Kelly DL, Demyanovich HK, Rodriguez KM, et al. Randomized controlled trial of a gluten-free diet in patients with schizophrenia positive for antigliadin antibodies (AGA IgG): a pilot feasibility study. *Journal of Psychiatry and Neuroscience.* 2019;44(4):269–76. doi:10.1503/jpn.180174.
54. Peet M. Diet, diabetes and schizophrenia: review and hypothesis. *British Journal of Psychiatry.* 2004;184(S47):s102–s105. doi:10.1192/bjp.184.47.s102.
55. Aucoin M, LaChance L, Cooley K, Kidd S. Diet and psychosis: a scoping review. *Neuropsychobiology.* October 2018:1–23. doi:10.1159/000493399.
56. Subramaniam M, Mahesh MV, Peh CX, et al. Hazardous alcohol use among patients with schizophrenia and depression. *Alcohol.* 2017;65:-63–69. doi:10.1016/j.alcohol.2017.07.008; Hambrecht M, Häfner H. Do alcohol or drug abuse induce schizophrenia? [in German]. *Nervenarzt.* 1996;67(1):36–45.
57. Soni SD, Brownlee M. Alcohol abuse in chronic schizophrenics: implications for management in the community. *Acta Psychiatrica Scandinavica.* 1991;84(3):272–76. doi:10.1111/j.1600-0447.1991.tb03143.x.
58. Messias E, Bienvenu OJ. Suspiciousness and alcohol use disorders in schizophrenia. *Journal of Nervous and Mental Disease.* 2003;191(6):387–90. doi:10.1097/01.nmd.0000071587.92959.ba; Pristach CA, Smith CM. Self-reported effects of alcohol use on symptoms of schizophrenia. *Psychiatric Services.* 1996;47(4):421–23. doi:10.1176/ps.47.4.421.
59. Nesvag R, Frigessi A, Jonsson E, Agartz I. Effects of alcohol consumption and antipsychotic medication on brain morphology in schizophrenia. *Schizophrenia Research.* 2007;90(1–3):52–61. doi:10.1016/j.schres.2006.11.008; Smith MJ, Wang L, Cronenwett W, et al. Alcohol use disorders contribute to hippocampal and subcortical shape differences in schizophrenia. *Schizophrenia Research.* 2011;131(1–3):174–83. doi:10.1016/j.schres.2011.05.014.
60. Amminger GP, Schäfer MR, Papageorgiou K, et al. Long-chain ω-3 fatty acids for indicated prevention of psychotic disorders. *Archives of General Psychiatry.* 2010;67(2):146. doi:10.1001/archgenpsychiatry.2009.192.

61. Akter K, Gallo DA, Martin SA, et al. A review of the possible role of the essential fatty acids and fish oils in the aetiology, prevention or pharmacotherapy of schizophrenia. *Journal of Clinical Pharmacy and Therapeutics*. 2011;37(2):132–39. doi:10.1111/j.1365-2710.2011.01265.x.
62. Fendri C, Mechri A, Khiari G, Othman A, Kerkeni A, Gaha L. Oxidative stress involvement in schizophrenia pathophysiology: a review [in French]. *Encephale*. 2006;32(2 Pt 1):244–52.
63. Yao JK, Leonard S, Reddy R. Altered glutathione redox state in schizophrenia. *Disease Markers*. 2006;22(1–2):83–93. doi:10.1155/2006/248387; Lavoie S, Murray MM, Deppen P, et al. Glutathione precursor, N-acetyl-cysteine, improves mismatch negativity in schizophrenia patients. *Neuropsychopharmacology*. 2007;33(9):2187–99. doi:10.1038/sj.npp.1301624; Witschi A, Reddy S, Stofer B, Lauterburg BH. The systemic availability of oral glutathione. *European Journal of Clinical Pharmacology*. 1992;43(6):667–69. doi:10.1007/bf02284971.
64. Arroll MA, Wilder L, Neil J. Nutritional interventions for the adjunctive treatment of schizophrenia: a brief review. *Nutrition Journal*. 2014;13(1). doi:10.1186/1475-2891-13-91.
65. Farokhnia M, Azarkolah A, Adinehfar F, et al. N-acetylcysteine as an adjunct to risperidone for treatment of negative symptoms in patients with chronic schizophrenia. *Clinical Neuropharmacology*. 2013;36(6):185–92. doi:10.1097/wnf.0000000000000001.
66. Berk M, Copolov D, Dean O, et al. N-acetyl cysteine as a glutathione precursor for schizophrenia—a double-blind, randomized, placebo-controlled trial. *Biological Psychiatry*. 2008;64(5):361–68. doi:10.1016/j.biopsych.2008.03.004.
67. Shay KP, Moreau RF, Smith EJ, Smith AR, Hagen TM. Alpha-lipoic acid as a dietary supplement: molecular mechanisms and therapeutic potential. *Biochimica et Biophysica Acta (BBA)—General Subjects*. 2009;1790(10):1149–60. doi:10.1016/j.bbagen.2009.07.026.
68. Ratliff JC, Palmese LB, Reutenauer EL, Tek C. An open-label pilot trial of alpha-lipoic acid for weight loss in patients with schizophrenia without diabetes. *Clinical Schizophrenia and Related Psychoses*. 2015;8(4):196–200. doi:10.3371/csrp.rapa.030113; Sanders LLO, de Souza Menezes CE, Chaves Filho AJM, et al. α-Lipoic acid as adjunctive treatment for schizophrenia. *Journal of Clinical Psychopharmacology*. 2017;37(6):697–701. doi:10.1097/jcp.0000000000000800.
69. Seybolt SEJ. Is it time to reassess alpha lipoic acid and niacinamide therapy in schizophrenia? *Medical Hypotheses*. 2010;75(6):572–75. doi:10.1016/j.mehy.2010.07.034.

70. Arroll MA, Wilder L, Neil J. Nutritional interventions for the adjunctive treatment of schizophrenia: a brief review. *Nutrition Journal.* 2014;13(1). doi:10.1186/1475-2891-13-91.
71. Brown HE, Roffman JL. Vitamin supplementation in the treatment of schizophrenia. *CNS Drugs.* 2014;28(7):611–22. doi:10.1007/s40263-014-0172-4.
72. Brown AS, Bottiglieri T, Schaefer CA, et al. Elevated prenatal homocysteine levels as a risk factor for schizophrenia. *Archives of General Psychiatry.* 2007;64(1):31. doi:10.1001/archpsyc.64.1.31.
73. Kemperman RFJ, Veurink M, van der Wal T, et al. Low essential fatty acid and B-vitamin status in a subgroup of patients with schizophrenia and its response to dietary supplementation. *Prostaglandins, Leukotrienes and Essential Fatty Acids.* 2006;74(2):75–85. doi:10.1016/j.plefa.2005.11.004.
74. Muntjewerff J-W, van der Put N, Eskes T, et al. Homocysteine metabolism and B-vitamins in schizophrenic patients: low plasma folate as a possible independent risk factor for schizophrenia. *Psychiatry Research.* 2003;121(1): 1–9. doi:10.1016/s0165-1781(03)00200-2.
75. Goff DC, Bottiglieri T, Arning E, et al. Folate, homocysteine, and negative symptoms in schizophrenia. *American Journal of Psychiatry.* 2004;161(9): 1705–8. doi:10.1176/appi.ajp.161.9.1705.
76. Godfrey PS, Toone BK, Bottiglieri T, et al. Enhancement of recovery from psychiatric illness by methylfolate. *Lancet.* 1990;336(8712):392–395. doi:10.1016/0140-6736(90)91942-4.
77. Roffman JL, Lamberti JS, Achtyes E, et al. Randomized multicenter investigation of folate plus vitamin B12 supplementation in schizophrenia. *JAMA Psychiatry.* 2013;70(5):481. doi:10.1001/jamapsychiatry.2013.900.
78. Roffman JL, Petruzzi LJ, Tanner AS, et al. Biochemical, physiological and clinical effects of l-methylfolate in schizophrenia: a randomized controlled trial. *Molecular Psychiatry.* 2017;23(2):316–22. doi:10.1038/mp.2017.41.
79. Ritsner MS, Miodownik C, Ratner Y, et al. L-theanine relieves positive, activation, and anxiety symptoms in patients with schizophrenia and schizoaffective disorder. *Journal of Clinical Psychiatry.* 2010;72(1):34–42. doi:10.4088/jcp.09m05324gre; Ota M, Wakabayashi C, Sato N, et al. Effect of l-theanine on glutamatergic function in patients with schizophrenia. *Acta Neuropsychiatrica.* 2015;27(5):291–96. doi:10.1017/neu.2015.22.
80. Shamir E, Laudon M, Barak Y, et al. Melatonin improves sleep quality of patients with chronic schizophrenia. *Journal of Clinical Psychiatry.* 2000;61(5):373–77. doi:10.4088/jcp.v61n0509; Anderson G, Maes M. Melatonin: an overlooked factor in schizophrenia and in the inhibition of anti-psychotic side effects. *Metabolic Brain Disease.* 2012;27(2):113–119. doi:10.1007/s11011-012-9307-9.

Chapter 10. Libido

1. Gunter PAY. Bergson and Jung. *Journal of the History of Ideas*. 1982;43(4):635. doi:10.2307/2709347.
2. Burton ES. Ronald Fairbairn. Institute of Psychoanalysis, British Psychoanalytical Society website. 2016. https://psychoanalysis.org.uk/our-authors-and-theorists/ronald-fairbairn. Accessed October 3, 2019.
3. Graziottin A. Libido: the biologic scenario. *Maturitas*. 2000;34:S9–S16. doi:10.1016/s0378-5122(99)00072-9.
4. Arias-Carrión O, Stamelou M, Murillo-Rodríguez E, Menéndez-González M, Pöppel E. Dopaminergic reward system: a short integrative review. *International Archives of Medicine*. 2010;3(1):24. doi:10.1186/1755-7682-3-24.
5. Schneider JE. Metabolic and hormonal control of the desire for food and sex: implications for obesity and eating disorders. *Hormones and Behavior*. 2006;50(4):562–71. doi:10.1016/j.yhbeh.2006.06.023.
6. Ramasamy R, Schulster M, Bernie A. The role of estradiol in male reproductive function. *Asian Journal of Andrology*. 2016;18(3):435. doi:10.4103/1008-682x.173932.
7. Cappelletti M, Wallen K. Increasing women's sexual desire: the comparative effectiveness of estrogens and androgens. *Hormones and Behavior*. 2016;78:178–93. doi:10.1016/j.yhbeh.2015.11.003.
8. Poutahidis T, Springer A, Levkovich T, et al. Probiotic microbes sustain youthful serum testosterone levels and testicular size in aging mice. Schlatt S, ed. *PLoS One*. 2014;9(1):e84877. doi:10.1371/journal.pone.0084877.
9. Hou X, Zhu L, Zhang X, et al. Testosterone disruptor effect and gut microbiome perturbation in mice: early life exposure to doxycycline. *Chemosphere*. 2019;222:722–31. doi:10.1016/j.chemosphere.2019.01.101.
10. Baker JM, Al-Nakkash L, Herbst-Kralovetz MM. Estrogen-gut microbiome axis: physiological and clinical implications. *Maturitas*. 2017;103:45–53. doi:10.1016/j.maturitas.2017.06.025.
11. Hamed SA. Sexual dysfunctions induced by pregabalin. *Clinical Neuropharmacology*. 2018;41(4):116–22. doi:10.1097/wnf.0000000000000286.
12. Christensen B. Inflammatory bowel disease and sexual dysfunction. *Gastroenterology and Hepatology*. 2014;10(1):53–55.
13. Tremellen K. Gut Endotoxin Leading to a Decline IN Gonadal function (GELDING)—a novel theory for the development of late onset hypogonadism in obese men. *Basic and Clinical Andrology*. 2016;26(1). doi:10.1186/s12610-016-0034-7.
14. La J, Roberts NH, Yafi FA. Diet and men's sexual health. *Sexual Medicine Reviews*. 2018;6(1):54–68. doi:10.1016/j.sxmr.2017.07.004.

15. Khoo J, Piantadosi C, Duncan R, et al. Comparing effects of a low-energy diet and a high-protein low-fat diet on sexual and endothelial function, urinary tract symptoms, and inflammation in obese diabetic men. *Journal of Sexual Medicine*. 2011;8(10):2868–75. doi:10.1111/j.1743-6109.2011.02417.x.
16. Levine H, Jørgensen N, Martino-Andrade A, et al. Temporal trends in sperm count: a systematic review and meta-regression analysis. *Human Reproduction Update*. 2017;23(6):646–59. doi:10.1093/humupd/dmx022.
17. Robbins WA, Xun L, FitzGerald LZ, Esguerra S, Henning SM, Carpenter CL. Walnuts improve semen quality in men consuming a Western-style diet: randomized control dietary intervention trial. *Biology of Reproduction*. 2012;87(4). doi:10.1095/biolreprod.112.101634.
18. Salas-Huetos A, Moraleda R, Giardina S, et al. Effect of nut consumption on semen quality and functionality in healthy men consuming a Western-style diet: a randomized controlled trial. *American Journal of Clinical Nutrition*. 2018;108(5):953–62. doi:10.1093/ajcn/nqy181.
19. Grieger JA, Grzeskowiak LE, Bianco-Miotto T, et al. Pre-pregnancy fast food and fruit intake is associated with time to pregnancy. *Human Reproduction*. 2018;33(6):1063–70. doi:10.1093/humrep/dey079.
20. Siepmann T, Roofeh J, Kiefer FW, Edelson DG. Hypogonadism and erectile dysfunction associated with soy product consumption. *Nutrition*. 2011;27(-7–8):859–62. doi:10.1016/j.nut.2010.10.018.
21. Chavarro JE, Toth TL, Sadio SM, Hauser R. Soy food and isoflavone intake in relation to semen quality parameters among men from an infertility clinic. *Human Reproduction*. 2008;23(11):2584–90. doi:10.1093/humrep/den243.
22. Martinez J, Lewi J. An unusual case of gynecomastia associated with soy product consumption. *Endocrine Practice*. 2008;14(4):415–18. doi:10.4158/ep.14.4.415.
23. Kotsopoulos D, Dalais FS, Liang YL, Mcgrath BP, Teede HJ. The effects of soy protein containing phytoestrogens on menopausal symptoms in postmenopausal women. *Climacteric*. 2000;3(3):161–67.
24. Shakespeare W. *The Tragedy of Macbeth*. The Harvard Classics. 1909–14. Available online at https://www.bartleby.com/46/4/23.html.
25. Prabhakaran D, Nisha A, Varghese PJ. Prevalence and correlates of sexual dysfunction in male patients with alcohol dependence syndrome: a cross-sectional study. *Indian Journal of Psychiatry*. 2018;60(1):71. doi:10.4103/psychiatry.indianjpsychiatry_42_17.
26. George WH, Davis KC, Norris J, et al. Alcohol and erectile response: the effects of high dosage in the context of demands to maximize sexual

arousal. *Experimental and Clinical Psychopharmacology*. 2006;14(4):461–70. doi:10.1037/1064-1297.14.4.461.

27. Prabhakaran D, Nisha A, Varghese PJ. Prevalence and correlates of sexual dysfunction in male patients with alcohol dependence syndrome: a cross-sectional study. *Indian Journal of Psychiatry*. 2018;60(1):71. doi:10.4103/psychiatry.indianjpsychiatry_42_17.
28. Castleman M. The Pros and Cons of Mixing Sex and Alcohol. Psychology Today website. July 1, 2019. https://www.psychologytoday.com/us/blog/all-about-sex/201907/the-pros-and-cons-mixing-sex-and-alcohol. Accessed December 2, 2019.
29. George WH, Davis KC, Heiman JR, et al. Women's sexual arousal: effects of high alcohol dosages and self-control instructions. *Hormones and Behavior*. 2011;59(5):730–38. doi:10.1016/j.yhbeh.2011.03.006.
30. George WH, Davis KC, Masters NT, et al. Sexual victimization, alcohol intoxication, sexual-emotional responding, and sexual risk in heavy episodic drinking women. *Archives of Sexual Behavior*. 2013;43(4):645–58. doi:10.1007/s10508-013-0143-8.
31. Chen L, Xie Y-M, Pei J-H, et al. Sugar-sweetened beverage intake and serum testosterone levels in adult males 20–39 years old in the United States. *Reproductive Biology and Endocrinology*. 2018;16(1). doi:10.1186/s12958-018-0378-2.
32. Chiu YH, Afeiche MC, Gaskins AJ, et al. Sugar-sweetened beverage intake in relation to semen quality and reproductive hormone levels in young men. *Human Reproduction*. 2014;29(7):1575–84. doi:10.1093/humrep/deu102.
33. Behre HM, Simoni M, Nieschlag E. Strong association between serum levels of leptin and testosterone in men. *Clinical Endocrinology*. 1997;47(2): 237–40. doi:10.1046/j.1365-2265.1997.2681067.x.
34. Gautier A, Bonnet F, Dubois S, et al. Associations between visceral adipose tissue, inflammation and sex steroid concentrations in men. *Clinical Endocrinology*. 2013;78(3):373–78. doi:10.1111/j.1365-2265.2012.04401.x; Spruijt-Metz D, Belcher B, Anderson D, et al. A high-sugar/low-fiber meal compared with a low-sugar/high-fiber meal leads to higher leptin and physical activity levels in overweight Latina females. *Journal of the American Dietetic Association*. 2009;109(6):1058–63. doi:10.1016/j.jada.2009.03.013.
35. Fukui M, Kitagawa Y, Nakamura N, Yoshikawa T. Glycyrrhizin and serum testosterone concentrations in male patients with type 2 diabetes. *Diabetes Care*. 2003;26(10):2962–62. doi:10.2337/diacare.26.10.2962; Armanini D, Bonanni G, Palermo M. Reduction of serum testosterone in men by licorice. *New England Journal of Medicine*. 1999;341(15):1158. doi:10.1056/nejm199910073411515.

36. Kjeldsen LS, Bonefeld-Jørgensen EC. Perfluorinated compounds affect the function of sex hormone receptors. *Environmental Science and Pollution Research*. 2013;20(11):8031–44. doi:10.1007/s11356-013-1753-3.
37. La Rocca C, Alessi E, Bergamasco B, et al. Exposure and effective dose biomarkers for perfluorooctane sulfonic acid (PFOS) and perfluorooctanoic acid (PFOA) in infertile subjects: preliminary results of the PREVIENI project. *International Journal of Hygiene and Environmental Health*. 2012;215(2):206–11. doi:10.1016/j.ijheh.2011.10.016.
38. Lai KP, Ng AH-M, Wan HT, et al. Dietary exposure to the environmental chemical, PFOS on the diversity of gut microbiota, associated with the development of metabolic syndrome. *Frontiers in Microbiology*. 2018;9. doi:10.3389/fmicb.2018.02552.
39. Monge Brenes AL, Curtzwiler G, Dixon P, Harrata K, Talbert J, Vorst K. PFOA and PFOS levels in microwave paper packaging between 2005 and 2018. *Food Additives and Contaminants: Part B*. 2019;12(3):191–98. doi:10.1080/19393210.2019.1592238.
40. Ali J, Ansari S, Kotta S. Exploring scientifically proven herbal aphrodisiacs. *Pharmacognosy Reviews*. 2013;7(1):1. doi:10.4103/0973-7847.112832.
41. Chaussee J. The Weird History of Oysters as Aphrodisiacs. *Wired* magazine website. September 30, 2016. https://www.wired.com/2016/09/weird-history-oysters-aphrodisiacs/. Accessed October 3, 2019.
42. Leonti M, Casu L. Ethnopharmacology of love. *Frontiers in Pharmacology*. 2018;9. doi:10.3389/fphar.2018.00567.
43. Rupp HA, James TW, Ketterson ED, Sengelaub DR, Ditzen B, Heiman JR. Lower sexual interest in postpartum women: relationship to amygdala activation and intranasal oxytocin. *Hormones and Behavior*. 2013;63(1):114–21. doi:10.1016/j.yhbeh.2012.10.007.
44. Gregory R, Cheng H, Rupp HA, Sengelaub DR, Heiman JR. Oxytocin increases VTA activation to infant and sexual stimuli in nulliparous and postpartum women. *Hormones and Behavior*. 2015;69:82–88. doi:10.1016/j.yhbeh.2014.12.009.
45. Loup F, Tribollet E, Dubois-Dauphin M, Dreifuss JJ. Localization of high-affinity binding sites for oxytocin and vasopressin in the human brain. An autoradiographic study. *Brain Research*. 1991;555(2):220–32. doi:10.1016/0006-8993(91)90345-v; RajMohan V, Mohandas E. The limbic system. *Indian Journal of Psychiatry*. 2007;49(2):132. doi:10.4103/0019-5545.33264.
46. Agustí A, García-Pardo MP, López-Almela I, et al. Interplay between the gut-brain axis, obesity and cognitive function. *Frontiers in Neuroscience*. 2018;12. doi:10.3389/fnins.2018.00155.

47. Nehlig A. The neuroprotective effects of cocoa flavanol and its influence on cognitive performance. *British Journal of Clinical Pharmacology.* 2013;75(3):716–27. doi:10.1111/j.1365-2125.2012.04378.x; Baskerville T, Douglas A. Interactions between dopamine and oxytocin in the control of sexual behaviour. In: Neumann ID, Landgraf R, eds. *Advances in Vasopressin and Oxytocin—From Genes to Behaviour to Disease.* Amsterdam: Elsevier; 2008:277–90. doi:10.1016/s0079-6123(08)00423-8.
48. Salonia A, Fabbri F, Zanni G, et al. Original research—women's sexual health: chocolate and women's sexual health: an intriguing correlation. *Journal of Sexual Medicine.* 2006;3(3):476–82. doi:10.1111/j.1743-6109.2006.00236.x.
49. Slaninová J, Maletínská L, Vondrášek J, Procházka Z. Magnesium and biological activity of oxytocin analogues modified on aromatic ring of amino acid in position 2. *Journal of Peptide Science.* 2001;7(8):413–24. doi:10.1002/psc.334.
50. Lopez DS, Wang R, Tsilidis KK, et al. Role of caffeine intake on erectile dysfunction in US men: results from NHANES 2001–2004. Walter M, ed. *PLoS One.* 2015;10(4):e0123547. doi:10.1371/journal.pone.0123547.
51. Saadat S, Ahmadi K, Panahi Y. The effect of on-demand caffeine consumption on treating patients with premature ejaculation: a double-blind randomized clinical trial. *Current Pharmaceutical Biotechnology.* 2015;16(3): 281–87. doi:10.2174/1389201016666150118133045.
52. Mondaini N, Cai T, Gontero P, et al. Regular moderate intake of red wine is linked to a better women's sexual health. *Journal of Sexual Medicine.* 2009;6(10):2772–77. doi:10.1111/j.1743-6109.2009.01393.x.
53. Jenkinson C, Petroczi A, Naughton DP. Red wine and component flavonoids inhibit UGT2B17 in vitro. *Nutrition Journal.* 2012;11(1). doi:10.1186/1475-2891-11-67.
54. Cassidy A, Franz M, Rimm EB. Dietary flavonoid intake and incidence of erectile dysfunction. *American Journal of Clinical Nutrition.* 2016;103(2): 534–41. doi:10.3945/ajcn.115.122010.
55. Aldemir M, Okulu E, Neşelioğlu S, Erel O, Kayıgil O. Pistachio diet improves erectile function parameters and serum lipid profiles in patients with erectile dysfunction. *International Journal of Impotence Research.* 2011 Jan–Feb;23(1):32–38. doi:10.1038/ijir.2010.33.
56. Molkara T, Akhlaghi F, Ramezani MA, et al. Effects of a food product (based on *Daucus carota*) and education based on traditional Persian medicine on female sexual dysfunction: a randomized clinical trial. *Electronic Physician.* 2018;10(4):6577–87. doi:10.19082/6577.
57. Maleki-Saghooni N, Mirzaeii K, Hosseinzadeh H, Sadeghi R, Irani M. A systematic review and meta-analysis of clinical trials on saffron (*Crocus*

sativus) effectiveness and safety on erectile dysfunction and semen parameters. *Avicenna Journal of Phytomedicine*. 2018;8(3):198–209.

58. Wilborn C, Taylor L, Poole C, Foster C, Willoughby D, Kreider R. Effects of a purported aromatase and 5α-reductase inhibitor on hormone profiles in college-age men. *International Journal of Sport Nutrition and Exercise Metabolism*. 2010;20(6):457–65.
59. Maheshwari A, Verma N, Swaroop A, et al. Efficacy of Furosap™, a novel *Trigonella foenum-graecum* seed extract, in enhancing testosterone level and improving sperm profile in male volunteers. *International Journal of Medical Sciences*. 2017;14(1):58–66. doi:10.7150/ijms.17256; Steels E, Rao A, Vitetta L. Physiological aspects of male libido enhanced by standardized *Trigonella foenum-graecum* extract and mineral formulation. *Phytotherapy Research*. 2011 Sep;25(9):1294–300. doi:10.1002/ptr.3360.
60. Steels E, Rao A, Vitetta L. Physiological aspects of male libido enhanced by standardized *Trigonella foenum-graecum* extract and mineral formulation. *Phytotherapy Research*. 2011 Sep;25(9):1294–300. doi:10.1002/ptr.3360.
61. Cai T, Gacci M, Mattivi F, et al. Apple consumption is related to better sexual quality of life in young women. *Archives of Gynecology and Obstetrics*. 2014;290(1):93–98. doi:10.1007/s00404-014-3168-x.
62. Türk G, Sönmez M, Aydin M, et al. Effects of pomegranate juice consumption on sperm quality, spermatogenic cell density, antioxidant activity and testosterone level in male rats. *Clinical Nutrition*. 2008;27(2):289–96. doi:10.1016/j.clnu.2007.12.006.
63. Al-Olayan EM, El-Khadragy MF, Metwally DM, Abdel Moneim AE. Protective effects of pomegranate (*Punica granatum*) juice on testes against carbon tetrachloride intoxication in rats. *BMC Complementary and Alternative Medicine*. 2014;14(1). doi:10.1186/1472-6882-14-164; Smail NF, Al-Dujaili E. Pomegranate juice intake enhances salivary testosterone levels and improves mood and well-being in healthy men and women. *Endocrine Abstracts*. 2012;28:P313.
64. Sathyanarayana Rao T, Asha M, Hithamani G, Rashmi R, Basavaraj K, Jagannath Rao K. History, mystery and chemistry of eroticism: emphasis on sexual health and dysfunction. *Indian Journal of Psychiatry*. 2009;51(2):141. doi:10.4103/0019-5545.49457.
65. Bègue L, Bricout V, Boudesseul J, Shankland R, Duke AA. Some like it hot: testosterone predicts laboratory eating behavior of spicy food. *Physiology and Behavior*. 2015 Feb;139:375–77. doi:10.1016/j.physbeh.2014.11.061.
66. Banihani SA. Testosterone in males as enhanced by onion (*Allium Cepa* L.). *Biomolecules*. 2019;9(2):75. doi:10.3390/biom9020075.

67. Nakayama Y, Tanaka K, Hiramoto S, et al. Alleviation of the aging males' symptoms by the intake of onion-extracts containing concentrated cysteine sulfoxides for 4 weeks—randomized, double-blind, placebo-controlled, parallel-group comparative study. *Japanese Pharmacology and Therapeutics*. 2017;45(4):595–608.
68. Sathyanarayana Rao T, Asha M, Hithamani G, Rashmi R, Basavaraj K, Jagannath Rao K. History, mystery and chemistry of eroticism: emphasis on sexual health and dysfunction. *Indian Journal of Psychiatry*. 2009;51(2):141. doi:10.4103/0019-5545.49457.
69. Pizzorno L. Nothing boring about boron. *Integrative Medicine* (Encinitas). 2015;14(4):35–48.
70. How Much Boron Is Present in Avocado? Organic Facts website. https://www.organicfacts.net/forum/how-much-boron-is-present-in-avocado. Accessed February 5, 2020.
71. Patwardhan B. Bridging Ayurveda with evidence-based scientific approaches in medicine. *EPMA Journal*. 2014;5(1). doi:10.1186/1878-5085-5-19.
72. Chauhan NS, Sharma V, Dixit VK, Thakur M. A review on plants used for improvement of sexual performance and virility. *BioMed Research International*. 2014;2014:1–19. doi:10.1155/2014/868062.
73. What Is Ayurveda? The Science of Life. National Ayurvedic Medical Association website. https://www.ayurvedanama.org/. Accessed February 5, 2020.

Index

About the Author

Uma Naidoo, MD, is a board-certified psychiatrist (Harvard Medical School), professional chef (Cambridge School of Culinary Arts), and nutrition specialist (Cornell University). She is currently the director of nutritional and lifestyle psychiatry at Massachusetts General Hospital (MGH), where she consults on nutritional interventions for the psychiatrically and medically ill; is director of nutritional psychiatry at the Massachusetts General Hospital Academy; and has a private practice in Newton, Massachusetts. She also teaches at the Cambridge School of Culinary Arts. Dr. Naidoo speaks frequently at conferences at Harvard, for Goop audiences, at the New York City Jewish Community Center, and at Ivy Boston. She blogs for *Harvard Health* and *Psychology Today* and has just completed a unique video cooking series for the MGH Academy that teaches nutritional psychiatry using culinary techniques in the kitchen. She has been asked by the American Psychiatric Association to author the first text in the area of nutritional psychiatry. Baking is one of her true passions, in addition to savory cooking.

To M[illegible]

Ben

Christmas 1955

BUDDENBROOKS

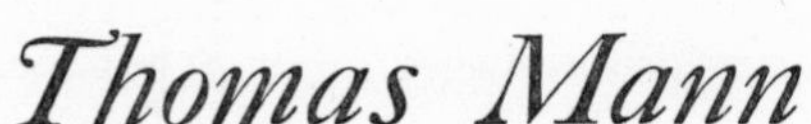

BUDDENBROOKS

Translated from the German by

H. T. LOWE-PORTER

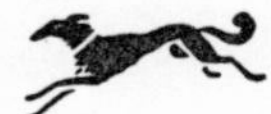

ALFRED A. KNOPF *NEW YORK*

1955

First published February 20, 1924 in two volumes
Reset and printed from new plates, October 1938
Reprinted four times
Sixth printing of reset edition, October 1955

ORIGINALLY ISSUED AS
Buddenbrooks
COPYRIGHT 1901 BY S. FISCHER VERLAG
BERLIN

This is a Borzoi Book,
published by Alfred A. Knopf, Inc.

MANUFACTURED IN THE UNITED STATES OF AMERICA

TRANSLATOR'S NOTE

Buddenbrooks was written before the turn of the century; it was first published in 1902, and became a German classic. It is one of those novels – we possess many of them in English – which are at once a work of art and the unique record of a period and a district. *Buddenbrooks* is great in its psychology, great as the monument of a vanished cultural tradition, and ultimately great by the perfection of its art: the classic purity and beautiful austerity of its style.

The translation of a book which is a triumph of style in its own language, is always a piece of effrontery. *Buddenbrooks* is so leisurely, so chiselled: the great gulf of the war divides its literary method from that of our time. Besides, the author has recorded much dialect. This difficulty is insuperable. Dialect cannot be transferred.

So the present translation is offered with humility. It was necessary to recognize that the difficulties were great. Yet it was necessary to set oneself the bold task of transferring the spirit first and the letter so far as might be; and above all, to make certain that the work of art, coming as it does to the ear, in German, like music out of the past, should, in English, at least *not* come like a translation – which is, " God bless us, a thing of naught."

H. T. Lowe-Porter

PART ONE

[3]

CHAPTER I

" AND – and – what comes next? "

" Oh, yes, yes, what the dickens does come next? *C'est la question, ma très chère demoiselle!* "

Frau Consul Buddenbrook shot a glance at her husband and came to the rescue of her little daughter. She sat with her mother-in-law on a straight white-enamelled sofa with yellow cushions and a gilded lion's head at the top. The Consul was in his easy-chair beside her, and the child perched on her grandfather's knee in the window.

" Tony," prompted the Frau Consul, " ' I believe that God ' – "

Dainty little eight-year-old Antonie, in her light shot-silk frock, turned her head away from her grandfather and stared aimlessly about the room with her blue-grey eyes, trying hard to remember. Once more she repeated " What comes next? " and went on slowly: " ' I believe that God ' – " and then, her face brightening, briskly finished the sentence: " ' created me, together with all living creatures.' " She was in smooth waters now, and rattled away, beaming with joy, through the whole Article, reproducing it word for word from the Catechism just promulgated, with the approval of an omniscient Senate, in that very year of grace 1835. When you were once fairly started, she thought, it was very like going down " Mount Jerusalem " with your brothers on the little sled: you had no time to think, and you couldn't stop even if you wanted to.

" ' And clothes and shoes,' " she said, " ' meat and drink, hearth and home, wife and child, acre and cow . . .' " But old Johann Buddenbrook could hold in no longer. He burst out laughing, in a high, half-smothered titter, in his glee at being able to make fun of the Catechism. He had probably put the child through this little examination with no other end in view. He inquired after Tony's acre and cow, asked how much she wanted for a sack of wheat, and tried to drive a bargain with her.

His round, rosy, benevolent face, which never would look cross no matter how hard he tried, was set in a frame of snow-white powdered hair, and the suggestion of a pigtail fell over the broad collar of his mouse-coloured coat. His double chin rested comfortably on a white lace frill. He still, in his seventies, adhered to the fashions of his youth: only the lace frogs and the big pockets were missing. And never in all his life had be worn a pair of trousers.

They had all joined in his laughter, but largely as a mark of respect for the head of the family. Madame Antoinette Buddenbrook, born Duchamps, tittered in precisely the same way as her husband. She was a stout lady, with thick white curls over her ears, dressed in a plain gown of striped black and grey stuff which betrayed the native quiet simplicity of her character. Her hands were still white and lovely, and she held a little velvet work-bag on her lap. It was strange to see how she had grown, in time, to look like her husband. Only her dark eyes, by their shape and their liveliness, suggested her half-Latin origin. On her grandfather's side Madame Buddenbrook was of French-Swiss stock, though born in Hamburg.

Her daughter-in-law, Frau Consul Elizabeth Buddenbrook, born Kröger, laughed the sputtering Kröger laugh and tucked in her chin as the Krögers did. She could not be called a beauty, but, like all the Krögers, she looked distinguished; she moved with graceful deliberation and had a clear, well-modulated voice. People liked her and felt confidence in her. Her reddish hair curled over her ears and was piled in a crown on top of her head; and she had the brilliant white complexion that goes with such hair, set off with a tiny freckle here and there. Her nose was rather too long, her mouth somewhat small; her most striking facial peculiarity was the shape of her lower lip, which ran straight into the chin without a curve. She had on a short bodice with high puffed sleeves, that left exposed a flawlessly modelled neck adorned with a spray of diamonds on a satin ribbon.

The Consul was leaning forward in his easy-chair, rather fidgety. He wore a cinnamon-coloured coat with wide lapels and leg-of-mutton sleeves close-fitting at the wrists, and white linen trousers with black stripes up the outside seams. His chin nestled in a stiff choker collar, around which was folded a silk cravat that flowed down amply over his flowered waistcoat.

He had his father's deep-set blue observant eyes, though their expression was perhaps more dreamy; but his features were clearer-cut and more serious, his nose was prominent and aquiline, and his cheeks, half-covered with a fair curling beard, were not so plump as the old man's.

Madame Buddenbrook put her hand on her daughter-in-law's

arm and looked down at her lap with a giggle. " Oh, *mon vieux* – he's always the same, isn't he, Betsy? "

The Consul's wife only made a motion with her delicate hand, so that her gold bangles tinkled slightly. Then, with a gesture habitual to her, she drew her finger across her face from the corner of her mouth to her forehead, as if she were smoothing back a stray hair.

But the Consul said, half-smiling, yet with mild reproach: " There you go again, Father, making fun of sacred things."

They were sitting in the " landscape-room " on the first floor of the rambling old house in Meng Street, which the firm of Johann Buddenbrook had acquired some time since, though the family had not lived in it long. The room was hung with heavy resilient tapestries put up in such a way that they stood well out from the walls. They were woven in soft tones to harmonize with the carpet, and they depicted idyllic landscapes in the style of the eighteenth century, with merry vine-dressers, busy husbandmen, and gaily beribboned shepherdesses who sat beside crystal streams with spotless lambs in their laps or exchanged kisses with amorous shepherds. These scenes were usually lighted by a pale yellow sunset to match the yellow coverings on the white enamelled furniture and the yellow silk curtains at the two windows.

For the size of the room, the furniture was rather scant. A round table, its slender legs decorated with fine lines of gilding, stood, not in front of the sofa, but by the wall opposite the little harmonium, on which lay a flute-case; some stiff arm-chairs were ranged in a row round the walls; there was a sewing-table by the window, and a flimsy ornamental writing-desk laden with knick-knacks.

On the other side of the room from the windows was a glass door, through which one looked into the semi-darkness of a pillared hall; and on the left were the lofty white folding doors that led to the dining-room. A semi-circular niche in the remaining wall was occupied by the stove, which crackled away behind a polished wrought-iron screen.

For cold weather had set in early. The leaves of the little lime-trees around the churchyard of St. Mary's, across the way, had turned yellow, though it was but mid-October. The wind whistled around the corners of the massive Gothic pile, and a cold, thin rain was falling. On Madame Buddenbrook's account, the double windows had already been put in.

It was Thursday, the day on which all the members of the family living in town assembled every second week, by established custom. To-day, however, a few intimate friends as well had been bidden to a family dinner; and now, towards four o'clock in the afternoon, the Buddenbrooks sat in the gathering twilight and awaited their guests.

Little Antonie had not let her grandfather interfere with her toboggan-ride. She merely pouted, sticking out her already prominent upper lip still further over the lower one. She was at the bottom of her Mount Jerusalem, but not knowing how to stop herself, she shot over the mark. "Amen," she said. "I know something, Grandfather."

"*Tiens!*" cried the old gentleman. "She knows something!" He made as if he were itching all over with curiosity. "Did you hear, Mamma? She knows something. Can any one tell me – ?"

"If the lightning," uttered Tony, nodding her head with every word, "sets something on fire, then it's the lightning that strikes. If it doesn't, why, then it's the thunder!" She folded her arms and looked around her like one sure of applause. But old Buddenbrook was annoyed by this display of wisdom. He demanded to know who had taught her such nonsense. It turned out that the culprit was the nursery governess, Ida Jungmann, who had lately been engaged from Marienwerder. The Consul had to come to her defence.

"You are too strict, Papa. Why shouldn't the child have her own little ideas about such things, at her age?"

"*Excusez, mon cher! . . . Mais c'est une folie!* You know I don't like the children's heads muddled with such things. 'The thunder strikes,' does it? Oh, very well, let it strike, and get along with your Prussian woman!"

The truth was, the old gentleman hadn't a good word to say for Ida Jungmann. Not that he was narrow-minded. He had seen something of the world, having travelled by coach to Southern Germany in 1813 to buy up wheat for the Prussian army; he had been to Amsterdam and Paris, and was too enlightened to condemn everything that lay beyond the gabled roofs of his native town. But in social intercourse he was more apt than his son to draw the line rigidly and give the cold shoulder to strangers. So when this young girl – she was then only twenty – had come back with his children from a visit to Western Prussia, as a sort of charity-child, the old man had made his son a scene for the act of piety, in which he spoke hardly anything but French and low German. Ida was the daughter of an inn-keeper who had died just before the Buddenbrooks' arrival in Marienwerder. She had proved to be capable in the household and with the children, and her rigid honesty and Prussian notions of caste made her perfectly suited to her position in the family. She was a person of aristocratic principles, drawing hair-line distinctions between class and class, and very proud of her position as servant of the higher orders. She objected to Tony's making friends with any schoolmate whom she reckoned as belonging only to the respectable middle class.

And now the Prussian woman herself came from the pillared hall through the glass door – a fairly tall, big-boned girl in a black frock, with smooth hair and an honest face. She held by the hand an extraordinarily thin small child, dressed in a flowered print frock, with lustreless ash-coloured hair and the manner of a little old maid. This was Clothilde, the daughter of a nephew of old Buddenbrook who belonged to a penniless branch of the family and was in business at Rostock as an estates agent. Clothilde was being brought up with Antonie, being about the same age and a docile little creature.

"Everything is ready," Mamsell Jungmann said. She had had a hard time learning to pronounce her *r's*, so now she rolled them tremendously in her throat. "Clothilde helped very well in the kitchen, so there was not much for cook to do."

Monsieur Buddenbrook sneered behind his lace frill at Ida's accent. The Consul patted his little niece's cheek and said: "That's right, Tilda. Work and pray. Tony ought to take a pattern from you; she's far too likely to be saucy and idle."

Tony dropped her head and looked at her grandfather from under her eyebrows. She knew he would defend her – he always did.

"No, no," he said, "hold your head up, Tony. Don't let them frighten you. We can't all be alike. Each according to his lights. Tilda is a good girl – but we're not so bad, either. Hey, Betsy? "

He turned to his daughter-in-law, who generally deferred to his views. Madame Antoinette, probably more from shrewdness than conviction, sided with the Consul; and thus the older and the younger generation crossed hands in the dance of life.

"You are very kind, Papa," the Consul's wife said. "Tony will try her best to grow up a clever and industrious woman. . . . Have the boys come home from school? " she asked Ida.

Tony, who from her perch on her grandfather's knee was looking out the window, called out in the same breath: "Tom and Christian are coming up Johannes Street . . . and Herr Hoffstede . . . and Uncle Doctor. . . ."

The bells of St. Mary's began to chime, ding-dong, ding-dong –

rather out of time, so that one could hardly tell what they were playing; still, it was very impressive. The big and the little bell announced, the one in lively, the other in dignified tones, that it was four o'clock; and at the same time a shrill peal from the bell over the vestibule door went ringing through the entry, and Tom and Christian entered, together with the first guests, Jean Jacques Hoffstede, the poet, and Doctor Grabow, the family physician.

CHAPTER II

Herr Jean Jacques Hoffstede was the town poet. He undoubtedly had a few verses in his pocket for the present occasion. He was nearly as old as Johann Buddenbrook, and dressed in much the same style except that his coat was green instead of mouse-coloured. But he was thinner and more active than his old friend, with bright little greenish eyes and a long pointed nose.

" Many thanks," he said, shaking hands with the gentlemen and bowing before the ladies – especially the Frau Consul, for whom he entertained a deep regard. Such bows as his it was not given to the younger generation to perform; and he accompanied them with his pleasant quiet smile. " Many thanks for your kind invitation, my dear good people. We met these two young ones, the Doctor and I " – he pointed to Tom and Christian, in their blue tunics and leather belts – " in King Street, coming home from school. Fine lads, eh, Frau Consul? Tom is a very solid chap. He'll have to go into the business, no doubt of that. But Christian is a devil of a fellow – a young *incroyable*, hey? I will not conceal my *engouement*. He must study, I think – he is witty and brilliant."

Old Buddenbrook used his gold snuff-box. " He's a young monkey, that's what he is. Why not say at once that he is to be a poet, Hoffstede? "

Mamsell Jungmann drew the curtains, and soon the room was bathed in mellow flickering light from the candles in the crystal chandelier and the sconces on the writing-desk. It lighted up golden gleams in the Frau Consul's hair.

" Well, Christian," she said, " what did you learn to-day? " It appeared that Christian had had writing, arithmetic, and singing lessons. He was a boy of seven, who already resembled his father to an almost comic extent. He had the same rather small round deep-set eyes and the same prominent aquiline nose; the lines of his face below the cheek-bones showed that it would not always retain its present child-like fulness.

" We've been laughing dreadfully," he began to prattle, his eyes darting from one to another of the circle. " What do you think Herr Stengel said to Siegmund Kostermann? " He bent his back, shook his head, and declaimed impressively: " ' Outwardly, outwardly, my dear child, you are sleek and smooth; but inwardly, my dear child, you are black and foul.' . . ." He mimicked with indiscribably funny effect not only the master's odd pronunciation but the look of disgust on his face at the " outward sleekness " he described. The whole company burst out laughing.

" Young monkey! " repeated old Buddenbrook. But Herr Hoffstede was in ecstasies. " *Charmant!* " he cried. " If you know Marcellus Stengel – that's he, to the life. Oh, that's too good! "

Thomas, to whom the gift of mimicry had been denied, stood near his younger brother and laughed heartily, without a trace of envy. His teeth were not very good, being small and yellowish. His nose was finely chiselled, and he strikingly resembled his grandfather in the eyes and the shape of the face.

The company had for the most part seated themselves on the chairs and the sofa. They talked with the children or discussed the unseasonable cold and the new house. Herr Hoffstede admired a beautiful Sèvres inkstand, in the shape of a black and white hunting dog, that stood on the escritoire. Doctor Grabow, a man of about the Consul's age, with a long mild face between thin whiskers, was looking at the table, set out with cakes and currant bread and salt-cellars in different shapes. This was the " bread and salt " that had been sent by friends for the house warming; but the " bread " consisted of rich, heavy pastries, and the salt came in dishes of massive gold, that the senders might not seem to be mean in their gifts.

" There will be work for me here," said the Doctor, pointing to the sweetmeats and threatening the children with his glance. Shaking his head, he picked up a heavy salt and pepper stand from the table.

" From Lebrecht Kröger," said old Buddenbrook, with a grimace. " Our dear kinsman is always open-handed. I did not spend as much on him when he built his summer house outside the Castle Gate. But he has always been like that – very lordly, very free with his money, a real cavalier à-la-mode. . . ."

The bell had rung several times. Pastor Wunderlich was announced; a stout old gentleman in a long black coat and powdered hair. He had twinkling grey eyes set in a face that was jovial if rather pale. He had been a widower for many years, and considered himself a bachelor of the old school, like Herr Gratjens, the broker, who entered with him. Herr Gratjens was a tall man who went around with one of his thin hands up to his eye like a telescope, as if he were examining a painting. He was a well-known art connoisseur.

Among the other guests were Senator Doctor Langhals and his wife, both friends of many years' standing; and Köppen the wine-merchant, with his great crimson face between enormous padded sleeves. His wife, who came with him, was nearly as stout as he.

It was after half past four when the Krögers put in an appearance – the elders together with their children; the Consul Krögers with their sons Jacob and Jürgen, who were about the age of Tom and Christian. On their heels came the parents of Frau Consul Kröger, the lumber-dealer Överdieck and his wife, a fond old pair who still addressed each other in public with nicknames from the days of their early love.

"Fine people come late," said Consul Buddenbrook, and kissed his mother-in-law's hand.

"But look at them when they do come!" and Johann Buddenbrook included the whole Kröger connection with a sweeping gesture, and shook the elder Kröger by the hand. Lebrecht Kröger, the cavalier à-la-mode, was a tall, distinguished figure. He wore his hair slightly powdered, but dressed in the height of fashion, with a double row of jewelled buttons on his velvet waistcoat. His son Justus, with his turned-up moustache and small beard, was very like the father in figure and manner, even to the graceful easy motions of the hands.

The guests did not sit down, but stood about awaiting the principal event of the evening and passing the time in casual talk. At length, Johann Buddenbrook the elder offered his arm to Madame Köppen and said in an elevated voice, "Well, *mesdames et messieurs*, if you are hungry . . ."

Mamsell Jungmann and the servant had opened the folding-doors into the dining-room; and the company made its way with studied ease to table. One could be sure of a good square meal at the Buddenbrooks'.

CHAPTER III

As the party began to move toward the dining-room, Consul Buddenbrook's hand went to his left breast-pocket and fingered a paper that was inside. The polite smile had left his face, giving place to a strained and care-worn look, and the muscles stood out on his temples as he clenched his teeth. For appearance's sake he made a few steps toward the dining-room, but stopped and sought his mother's eye as she was leaving the room on Pastor Wunderlich's arm, among the last of her guests.

"Pardon me, dear Herr Pastor . . . just a word with you, Mamma." The Pastor nodded gaily, and the Consul drew his Mother over to the window of the landscape-room.

"Here is a letter from Gotthold," he said in low, rapid tones. He took out the sealed and folded paper and looked into her dark eyes. "That is his writing. It is the third one, and Papa answered only the first. What shall I do? It came at two o'clock, and I ought to have given it to him already, but I do not like to upset him today. What do you think? I could call him out here. . . ."

"No, you are right, Jean; it is better to wait," said Madame Buddenbrook. She grasped her son's arm with a quick, habitual movement. "What do you suppose is in it?" she added uneasily. "The boy won't give in. He's taken it into his head he must be compensated for his share in the house. . . . No, no, Jean. Not now. To-night, perhaps, before we go to bed."

"What am I to do?" repeated the Consul, shaking his bent head. "I have often wanted to ask Papa to give in. I don't like it to look as if I had schemed against Gotthold and worked myself into a snug place. I don't want Father to look at it like that, either. But, to be honest . . . I am a partner, after all. And Betsy and I pay a fair rent for the second storey. It is all arranged with my sister in Frankfort: her husband gets compensation already, in Papa's lifetime – a quarter of the purchase price of the house. That is good business: Papa arranged it very cleverly, and it is very satisfactory from the point of view of the firm. And if Papa acts so unfriendly to Gotthold – "

"Nonsense, Jean. Your position in the matter is quite clear. But it is painful for me to have Gotthold think that his step-mother looks out after her own children and deliberately makes bad blood between him and his father!"

"But it is his own fault," the Consul almost shouted, and then, with a glance at the dining-room door, lowered his voice. "It is his fault, the whole wretched thing. You can judge for yourself. Why couldn't he be reasonable? Why did he have to go and marry that Stüwing girl and . . . the shop. . . ." The Consul gave an angry, embarrassed laugh at the last word. "It's a weakness of Father's, that prejudice against the shop; but Gotthold ought to have respected it. . . ."

"Oh, Jean, it would be best if Papa would give in."

"But ought I to advise him to?" whispered the Consul excitedly, clapping his hand to his forehead. "I am an interested party, so I ought to say, Pay it. But I am also a partner. And if Papa thinks he is under no obligation to a disobedient and rebellious son to draw the money out of the working capital of the firm . . . It is a matter of eleven thousand thaler, a good bit of money. No, no, I cannot advise him either for or against. I'd rather wash my hands of the whole affair. But the scene with Papa is so *désagréable* –"

"Late this evening, Jean. Come now; they are waiting."

The Consul put the paper back into his breast-pocket, offered his arm to his mother, and led her over the threshold into the brightly lighted dining-room, where the company had already taken their places at the long table.

The tapestries in this room had a sky-blue background, against which, between slender columns, white figures of gods and goddesses stood out with plastic effect. The heavy red damask window-curtains were drawn; stiff, massive sofas in red damask stood ranged against the walls; and in each corner stood a tall gilt candelabrum with eight flaming candles, besides those in silver sconces on the table. Above the heavy sideboard, on the wall opposite the landscape room, hung a large painting of an Italian bay, the misty blue atmosphere of which was most effective in the candle-light.

Every trace of care or disquiet had vanished from Madame Buddenbrook's face. She sat down between Pastor Wunderlich and the elder Kröger, who presided on the window side.

"*Bon appétit!*" she said, with her short, quick, hearty nod, flashing a glance down the whole length of the table till it reached the children at the bottom.

[14]

CHAPTER IV

"OUR best respects to you, Buddenbrook – I repeat, our best respects!" Herr Köppen's powerful voice drowned the general conversation as the maid-servant, in her heavy striped petticoat, her fat arms bare and a little white cap on the back of her head, passed the *potage aux fines herbes* and toast, assisted by Mamsell Jungmann and the Frau Consul's maid from upstairs. The guests began to use their soup-spoons.

"Such plenty, such elegance! I must say, you know how to do things! – I must say –" Herr Köppen had never visited the house in its former owner's time. He did not come of a patrician family, and had only lately become a man of means. He could never quite get rid of certain vulgar tricks of speech – like the repetition of "I must say"; and he said "respecks" for "respects."

"It didn't cost anything, either," remarked Herr Gratjens drily – he certainly ought to have known – and studied the wall-painting through the hollow of his hand.

As far as possible, ladies and gentlemen had been paired off, and members of the family placed between friends of the house. But the arrangement could not be carried out in every case; the two Överdiecks were sitting, as usual, nearly on each other's laps, nodding affectionately at one another. The elder Kröger was bolt upright, enthroned between Madame Antoinette and Frau Senator Langhals, dividing his pet jokes and his flourishes between the two ladies.

"When was the house built?" asked Herr Hoffstede diagonally across the table of old Buddenbrook, who was talking in a gay chaffing tone with Madame Köppen.

"Anno . . . let me see . . . about 1680, if I am not mistaken. My son is better at dates than I am."

"Eighty-two," said the Consul, leaning forward. He was sitting at the foot of the table, without a partner, next to Senator Langhals. "It was finished in the winter of 1682. Ratenkamp and Company were just getting to the top of their form. . . . Sad, how the firm broke down in the last twenty years!"

A general pause in the conversation ensued, lasting for half a minute, while the company looked down at their plates and pondered on the fortunes of the brilliant family who had built and lived in the house and then, broken and impoverished, had left it.

"Yes," said Broker Gratjens, "it's sad, when you think of the madness that led to their ruin. If Dietrich Ratenkamp had not taken that fellow Geelmaack for a partner! I flung up my hands, I know, when he came into the management. I have it on the best authority, gentlemen, that he speculated disgracefully behind Ratenkamp's back, and gave notes and acceptances right and left in the firm's name. . . . Finally the game was up. The banks got suspicious, the firm couldn't give security. . . . You haven't the least idea . . . who looked after the warehouse, even? Geelmaack, perhaps? It was a perfect rats' nest there, year in, year out. But Ratenkamp never troubled himself about it."

"He was like a man paralysed," the Consul said. A gloomy, taciturn look came on his face. He leaned over and stirred his soup, now and then giving a quick glance, with his little round deep-set eyes, at the upper end of the table.

"He went about like a man with a load on his mind; I think one can understand his burden. What made him take Geelmaack into the business – a man who brought painfully little capital, and had not the best of reputations? He must have felt the need of sharing his heavy responsibility with some one, not much matter who, because he realized that the end was inevitable. The firm was ruined, the old family *passée*. Geelmaack only gave it the last push over the edge."

Pastor Wunderlich filled his own and his neighbour's wineglass. "So you think my dear Consul," he said with a discreet smile, "that even without Geelmaack, things would have turned out just as they did?"

"Oh, probably not," the Consul said thoughtfully, addressing nobody in particular. "But I do think that Dietrich Ratenkamp was driven by fate when he took Geelmaack into partnership. That was the way his destiny was to be fulfilled. . . . He acted under the pressure of inexorable necessity. I think he knew more or less what his partner was doing, and what the state of affairs was at the warehouse. But he was paralysed."

"*Assez*, Jean," interposed old Buddenbrook, laying down his spoon. "That's one of your *idées*. . . ."

The Consul rather absently lifted his glass to his father. Lebrecht Kröger broke in: "Let's stick by the jolly present!" He took up a bottle of white wine that had a little silver stag on the stopper; and with one of his fastidious, elegant motions he held it on its side and examined the label. " C. F. Köppen," he read, and nodded to the wine-merchant. " Ah, yes, where should we be without you? "

Madame Antoinette kept a sharp eye on the servants while they changed the gilt-edged Meissen plates; Mamsell Jungmann called orders through the speaking-tube into the kitchen, and the fish was brought in. Pastor Wunderlich remarked, as he helped himself:

" This ' jolly present ' isn't such a matter of course as it seems, either. The young folk here can hardly realize, I suppose, that things could ever have been different from what they are now. But I think I may fairly claim to have had a personal share, more than once, in the fortunes of the Buddenbrook family. Whenever I see one of these, for instance – " he picked up one of the heavy silver spoons and turned to Madame Antoinette – " I can't help wondering whether they belong to the set that our friend the philosopher Lenoir, Sergeant under his Majesty the Emperor Napoleon, had in his hands in the year 1806 – and I think of our meeting in Alf Street, Madame."

Madame Buddenbrook looked down at her plate with a smile half of memory, half of embarrassment. Tom and Tony, at the bottom of the table, cried out almost with one voice, " Oh, yes, tell about it, Grandmama! " They did not want the fish, and they had been listening attentively to the conversation of their elders. But the Pastor knew that she would not care to speak herself of an incident that had been rather painful to her. He came to her rescue and launched out once more upon the old story. It was new, perhaps, to one or two of the present company. As for the children, they could have listened to it a hundred times.

" Well, imagine a November afternoon, cold and rainy, a wretched day; and me coming back down Alf Street from some parochial duty. I was thinking of the hard times we were having. Prince Blücher had gone, and the French were in the town. There was little outward sign of the excitement that reigned everywhere: the streets were quiet, and people stopped close in their houses. Prahl the master-butcher had been shot through the head, just for standing at the door of his shop with his hands in his pockets and making a menacing remark about its being hard to bear. Well, thought I to myself, I'll just have a look in at the Buddenbrooks'. Herr Buddenbrook is down with erysipelas, and Madame has a great deal to do, on account of the billeting.

" At that very moment, whom should I see coming towards me but our honoured Madame Buddenbrook herself? What a state she was in! Hurrying through the rain hatless, stumbling rather than walking, with a shawl flung over her shoulders, and her hair falling down – yes, Madame, it is quite true, it *was* falling down!

" 'This is a pleasant surprise,' I said. She never saw me, and I made bold to lay my hand on her sleeve, for my mind misgave me about the state of things. 'Where are you off to in such a hurry, my dear?' She realized who I was, looked at me, and burst out: 'Farewell, farewell! All is over – I'm going into the river!'

" 'God forbid,' cried I – I could feel that I went white. 'That is no place for you, my dear.' And I held her as tightly as decorum permitted. 'What has happened?' 'What has happened!' she cried, all trembling. 'They've got at the silver, Wunderlich! That's what has happened! And Jean lies there with erysipelas and can't do anything – he couldn't even if he were up. They are stealing my spoons, Wunderlich, and I am going into the river!'

"Well, I kept holding her, and I said what one would in such cases: 'Courage, dear lady. It will be all right. Control yourself, I beg of you. We will go and speak with them. Let us go.' And I got her to go back up the street to her house. The soldiery were up in the dining-room, where Madame had left them, some twenty of them, at the great silver-chest.

" 'Gentlemen,' I say politely, 'with which one of you may I have the pleasure of a little conversation?' They begin to laugh, and they say: 'With all of us, Papa.' But one of them steps out and presents himself, a fellow as tall as a tree, with a black waxed moustache and big red hands sticking out of his braided cuffs. 'Lenoir,' he said, and saluted with his left hand, for he had five or six spoons in his right. 'Sergeant Lenoir. What can I do for you?'

" 'Herr Officer,' I say, appealing to his sense of honour, 'after your magnificent charge, how can you stoop to this sort of thing? The town has not closed its gates to the Emperor.'

" 'What do you expect?' he answered. 'War is war. The people need these things. . . .'

" 'But you ought to be careful,' I interrupted him, for an idea had come into my head. 'This lady,' I said – one will say anything at a time like that – 'the lady of the house, she isn't a German. She is almost a compatriot of yours – she is a Frenchwoman. . . .' 'Oh, a Frenchwoman,' he repeated. And then what do you suppose he said, this big swashbuckler? 'Oh, an *émigrée?* Then she is an enemy of philosophy!'

"I was quite taken aback, but I managed not to laugh. 'You are a man of intellect, I see,' said I. 'I repeat that I consider your conduct unworthy.' He was silent for a moment. Then he got red, tossed his half-dozen spoons back into the chest, and exclaimed, ' Who told you I was going to do anything with these things but look at them? It's fine silver. If one or two of my men take a piece as a souvenir . . .'

" Well, in the end, they took plenty of souvenirs, of course. No use appealing to justice, either human or divine. I suppose they knew no other god than that terrible little Corsican. . . ."

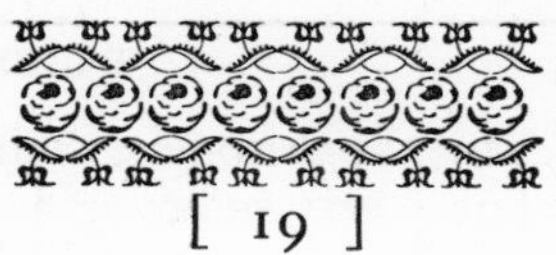

CHAPTER V

"DID you ever see him, Herr Pastor? "

The plates were being changed again. An enormous brick-red boiled ham appeared, strewn with crumbs and served with a sour brown onion sauce, and so many vegetables that the company could have satisfied their appetites from that one vegetable-dish. Lebrecht Kröger undertook the carving, and skilfully cut the succulent slices, with his elbows slightly elevated and his two long forefingers laid out along the back of the knife and fork. With the ham went the Frau Consul's celebrated "Russian jam," a pungent fruit conserve flavoured with spirits.

No, Pastor Wunderlich regretted to say that he had never set eyes on Bonaparte. Old Buddenbrook and Jean Jacques Hoffstede had both seen him face to face, one in Paris just before the Russian campaign, reviewing the troops at the Tuileries; the other in Dantzig.

"I must say, he wasn't a very cheerful person to look at," said the poet, raising his brows, as he disposed of a forkful of ham, potato, and sprouts. "But they say he was in a lively mood, at Dantzig. There was a story they used to tell, about how he would gamble all day with the Germans, and make them pay up too, and then spend the evening playing with his generals. Once he swept a handful of gold off the table, and said: '*Les Allemands aiment beaucoup ces petits Napoléons, n'est-ce pas,* Rapp? ' '*Oui, Sire, plus que le Grand!* ' Rapp answered."

There was general laughter – Hoffstede had told the story very prettily, even mimicking the Emperor's manner. Old Buddenbrook said: "Well, joking aside, one can't help having respect for his personal greatness. . . . What a nature! "

The Consul shook his head gravely.

"No, no – we of the younger generation do not see why we should revere the man who murdered the Duc d'Enghien, and butchered eight hundred prisoners in Egypt. . . ."

"All that is probably exaggerated and overdrawn," said Pastor Wunderlich. "The Duke was very likely a feather-brained and seditious person, and as for the prisoners, their execution was probably the deliberate and necessary policy of a council of war." And he went on to speak of a book at which he had been looking, by one of the Emperor's secretaries, which had appeared some years before and was well worth reading.

"All the same," persisted the Consul, snuffing a flickering candle in the sconce in front of him, "I cannot understand it – I cannot understand the admiration people have for this monster. As a Christian, as a religious man, I can find no room in my heart for such a feeling."

He had, as he spoke, the slightly inclined head and the rapt look of a man in a vision. His father and Pastor Wunderlich could be seen to exchange the smallest of smiles.

"Well, anyhow," grinned the old man, "the little napoleons aren't so bad, eh? My son has more enthusiasm for Louis Philippe," he said to the company in general.

"Enthusiasm?" repeated Jean Jacques Hoffstede, rather sarcastically. . . . That is a curious juxtaposition, Philippe Égalité and enthusiasm. . . ."

"God knows, I feel we have much to learn from the July Monarchy," the Consul said, with serious zeal. "The friendly and helpful attitude of French constitutionalism toward the new, practical ideals and interests of our time . . . is something we should be deeply thankful for. . . ."

"Practical ideals – well, ye-s –" The elder Buddenbrook gave his jaws a moment's rest and played with his gold snuff-box. "Practical ideals – well – h'm – they don't appeal to me in the least." He dropped into dialect, out of sheer vexation. "We have trade schools and technical schools and commercial schools springing up on every corner; the high schools and the classical education suddenly turn out to be all foolishness, and the whole world thinks of nothing but mines and factories and making money. . . . That's all very fine, of course. But in the long run, pretty stupid, isn't it? . . . I don't know why, but it irritates me like the deuce. . . . I don't mean, Jean, that the July Monarchy is not an admirable régime. . . ."

Senator Langhals, as well as Gratjens and Köppen, stood by the Consul. . . . They felt that high praise was due to the French government, and to similar efforts that were being made in Germany. It was worthy of all respect – Herr Köppen called it "respeck." He had grown more and more crimson from eating, and puffed audibly as he spoke. Pastor Wunderlich had not changed

colour; he looked as pale, refined, and alert as ever, while drinking down glass after glass of wine.

The candles burned down slowly in their sockets. Now and then they flickered in a draught and dispersed a faint smell of wax over the table.

There they all sat, on heavy, high-backed chairs, consuming good heavy food from good heavy silver plate, drinking full-bodied wines and expressing their views freely on all subjects. When they began to talk shop, they slipped unconsciously more and more into dialect, and used the clumsy but comfortable idioms that seemed to embody to them the business efficiency and the easy well-being of their community. Sometimes they even used an over-drawn pronunciation by way of making fun of themselves and each other, and relished their clipped phrases and exaggerated vowels with the same heartiness as they did their food.

The ladies had not long followed the discussion. Madame Kröger gave them the cue by setting forth a tempting method of boiling carp in red wine. "You cut it into nice pieces, my dear, and put it in the saucepan, add some cloves, and onions, and a few rusks, a little sugar, and a spoonful of butter, and set it on the fire. . . . But don't wash it, on any account. All the blood must remain in it."

The elder Kröger was telling the most delightful stories; and his son Justus, who sat with Dr. Grabow down at the bottom of the table, near the children, was chaffing Mamsell Jungmann. She screwed up her brown eyes and stood her knife and fork upright on the table and moved them back and forth. Even the Överdiecks were very lively. Old Frau Överdieck had a new pet name for her husband: "You good old bell-wether," she said, and laughed so hard that her cap bobbed up and down.

But all the various conversations around the table flowed together in one stream when Jean Jacques Hoffstede embarked upon his favourite theme, and began to describe the Italian journey which he had taken fifteen years before with a rich Hamburg relative. He told of Venice, Rome, and Vesuvius, of the Villa Borghese, where Goethe had written part of his Faust; he waxed enthusiastic over the beautiful Renaissance fountains that wafted coolness upon the warm Italian air, and the formal gardens through the avenues of which it was so enchanting to stroll. Some one mentioned the big wilderness of a garden outside the Castle Gate, that belonged to the Buddenbrooks.

"Upon my word," the old man said, "I still feel angry with

myself that I have never put it into some kind of order. I was out there the other day – and it is really a disgrace, a perfect primeval forest. It would be a pretty bit of property, if the grass were cut and the trees trimmed into formal shapes."

The Consul protested strenuously. "Oh, no, Papa! I love to go out there in the summer and walk in the undergrowth; it would quite spoil the place to trim and prune its free natural beauty."

"But, deuce take it, the free natural beauty belongs to me – haven't I the right to put it in order if I like?"

"Ah, Father, when I go out there and lie in the long grass among the undergrowth, I have a feeling that I belong to nature and not she to me. . . ."

"Krishan, don't eat too much," the old man suddenly called out, in dialect. "Never mind about Tilda – it doesn't hurt her. She can put it away like a dozen harvest hands, that child!"

And truly it was amazing, the prowess of this scraggy child with the long, old-maidish face. Asked if she wanted more soup, she answered in a meek drawling voice: "Ye-es, ple-ase." She had two large helpings both of fish and ham, with piles of vegetables; and she bent short-sightedly over her plate, completely absorbed in the food, which she chewed ruminantly, in large mouthfuls. "Oh, Un-cle," she replied, with amiable simplicity, to the old man's gibe, which did not in the least disconcert her. She ate: whether it tasted good or not, whether they teased her or not, she smiled and kept on, heaping her plate with good things, with the instinctive, insensitive voracity of a poor relation – patient, persevering, hungry, and lean.

CHAPTER VI

AND now came, in two great cut-glass dishes, the "Plettenpudding." It was made of layers of macaroons, raspberries, ladyfingers, and custard. At the same time, at the other end of the table, appeared the blazing plum-pudding which was the children's favourite sweet.

"Thomas, my son, come here a minute," said Johann Buddenbrook, taking his great bunch of keys from his trousers pocket. "In the second cellar to the right, the second bin, behind the red Bordeaux, two bottles – you understand?" Thomas, to whom such orders were familiar, ran off and soon came back with the two bottles, covered with dust and cobwebs; and the little dessert-glasses were filled with sweet, golden-yellow malmsey from these unsightly receptacles. Now the moment came when Pastor Wunderlich rose, glass in hand, to propose a toast; and the company fell silent to listen. He spoke in the pleasant, conversational tone which he liked to use in the pulpit; his head a little on one side, a subtle, humorous smile on his pale face, gesturing easily with his free hand. "Come, my honest friends, let us honour ourselves by drinking a glass of this excellent liquor to the health of our host and hostess in their beautiful new home. Come, then – to the health of the Buddenbrook family, present and absent! May they live long and prosper!"

"Absent?" thought the Consul to himself, bowing as the company lifted their glasses. "Is he referring to the Frankfort Buddenbrooks, or perhaps the Duchamps in Hamburg – or did old Wunderlich really mean something by that?" He stood up and clinked glasses with his father, looking him affectionately in the eye.

Broker Gratjens got up next, and his speech was rather long-winded; he ended by proposing in his high-pitched voice a health to the firm of Johann Buddenbrook, that it might continue to grow and prosper and do honour to the town.

Johann Buddenbrook thanked them all for their kindness, first as head of the family and then as senior partner of the firm – and sent Thomas for another bottle of Malmsey. It had been a mistake to suppose that two would be enough.

Lebrecht Kröger spoke too. He took the liberty of remaining seated, because it looked less formal, and gestured with his head and hands most charmingly as he proposed a toast to the two ladies of the family, Madame Antoinette and the Frau Consul. As he finished, the Plettenpudding was nearly consumed, and the Malmsey nearing its end; and then, to a universal, long-drawn " Ah-h! " Jean Jacques Hoffstede rose up slowly, clearing his throat. The children clapped their hands with delight.

" *Excusez!* I really couldn't help it," he began. He put his finger to his long sharp nose and drew a paper from his coat pocket. . . . A profound silence reigned throughout the room.

His paper was gaily parti-coloured. On the outside of it was written, in an oval border surrounded by red flowers and a profusion of gilt flourishes:

" *On the occasion of my friendly participation in a delightful house-warming party given by the Buddenbrook family. October 1835.*"

He read this aloud first; then turning the paper over, he began, in a voice that was already somewhat tremulous:

Honoured friends, my modest lay
Hastes to greet you in these walls:
May kind Heaven grant to-day
Blessing on their spacious halls.

Thee, my friend with silver hair,
And thy faithful, loving spouse,
And your children young and fair —
I salute you, and your house.

Industry and beauty chaste
See we linked in marriage band:
Venus Anadyomene
And cunning Vulcan's busy hand.

May no future storms dismay
With unkind blast the joyful hour;
May each new returning day
Blessings on your pathway shower.

Ceaselessly shall I rejoice
O'er the fortune that is yours:
As to-day I lift my voice,
May I still, while life endures.

In your splendid walls live well,
And cherish with affection true
Him who in his humble cell
Penned to-day these lines for you.

He bowed to a unanimous outburst of applause.

"Charming, Hoffstede," cried old Buddenbrook. "It was too charming for words. I drink your health."

But when the Frau Consul touched glasses with the poet, a delicate blush mantled her cheek; for she had seen the courtly bow he made in her direction when he came to the part about the Venus Anadyomene.

CHAPTER VII

THE GENERAL merriment had now reached its height. Herr Köppen felt a great need to unfasten a few buttons of his waistcoat; but it obviously wouldn't do, for not even the elderly gentlemen were permitting themselves the liberty. Lebrecht Kröger sat up as straight as he did at the beginning; Pastor Wunderlich's face was as pale as ever, his manner as correct. The elder Buddenbrook had indeed sat back a little in his chair, but he maintained perfect decorum. There was only Justus Kröger – he was plainly a little overtaken.

But where was Dr. Grabow? The butter, cheese and fruit had just been handed round; and the Frau Consul rose from her chair and unobtrusively followed the waitress from the room; for the Doctor, Mamsell Jungmann, and Christian were no longer in their places, and a smothered wail was proceeding from the hall. There in the dim light, little Christian was half lying, half crouching on the round settee that encircled the central pillar. He was uttering heart-breaking groans. Ida and the Doctor stood beside him.

"Oh dear, oh dear," said she, "the poor child is very bad!"

"I'm ill, Mamma, damned ill," whimpered Christian, his little deep-set eyes darting back and forth, and his big nose looking bigger than ever. The "damned" came out in a tone of utter despair; but the Frau Consul said: "If we use such words, God will punish us by making us suffer still more!"

Doctor Grabow felt the lad's pulse. His kindly face grew longer and gentler.

"It's nothing much, Frau Consul," he reassured her. "A touch of indigestion." He prescribed in his best bed-side manner: "Better put him to bed and give him a Dover powder – perhaps a cup of camomile tea, to bring out the perspiration. . . . And a rigorous diet, you know, Frau Consul. A little pigeon, a little French bread . . ."

"I don't want any pigeon," bellowed Christian angrily. "I don't want to eat anything, ever any more. I'm ill, I tell you, damned ill!" The fervour with which he uttered the bad word seemed to bring him relief.

Doctor Grabow smiled to himself – a thoughtful, almost a melancholy smile. He would soon eat again, this young man. He would do as the rest of the world did – his father, and all their relatives and friends: he would lead a sedentary life and eat four good, rich, satisfying meals a day. Well, God bless us all! He, Friedrich Grabow, was not the man to upset the habits of these prosperous, comfortable tradesmen and their families. He would come when he was sent for, prescribe a few days' diet – a little pigeon, a slice of French bread – yes, yes, and assure the family that it was nothing serious this time. Young as he was, he had held the head of many an honest burgher who had eaten his last joint of smoked meat, his last stuffed turkey, and, whether overtaken unaware in his counting-house or after a brief illness in his solid old four-poster, had commended his soul to God. Then it was called paralysis, a "stroke," a sudden death. And he, Friedrich Grabow, could have predicted it, on all of these occasions when it was "nothing serious this time" – or perhaps at the times when he had not even been summoned, when there had only been a slight giddiness after luncheon. Well, God bless us all! He, Friedrich Grabow, was not the man to despise a roast turkey himself. That ham with onion sauce had been delicious, hang it! And the Plettenpudding, when they were already stuffed full – macaroons, raspberries, custard . . . "A rigorous diet, Frau Consul, as I say. A little pigeon, a little French bread . . ."

CHAPTER VIII

THEY were rising from table.

"Well, ladies and gentlemen, *gesegnete Mahlzeit!* Cigars and coffee in the next room, and a liqueur if Madame feels generous. . . . Billiards for whoever chooses. Jean, you will show them the way back to the billiard-room? Madame Köppen, may I have the honour?"

Full of well-being, laughing and chattering, the company trooped back through the folding doors into the landscape-room. The Consul remained behind, and collected about him the gentlemen who wanted to play billiards.

"You won't try a game, Father?"

No, Lebrecht Kröger would stop with the ladies, but Justus might go if he liked. . . . Senator Langhals, Köppen, Gratjens, and Doctor Grabow went with the Consul, and Jean Jacques Hoffstede said he would join them later. "Johann Buddenbrook is going to play the flute," he said. "I must stop for that. *Au revoir, messieurs.*"

As the gentlemen passed through the hall, they could hear from the landscape-room the first notes of the flute, accompanied by the Frau Consul on the harmonium: an airy, charming little melody that floated sweetly through the lofty rooms. The Consul listened as long as he could. He would have liked to stop behind in an easy-chair in the landscape-room and indulge the reveries that the music conjured up; but his duties as host . . .

"Bring some coffee and cigars into the billiard-room," he said to the maid whom he met in the entry.

"Yes, Line, coffee!" Herr Köppen echoed, in a rich, well-fed voice, trying to pinch the girl's red arm. The *c* came from far back in his throat, as if he were already swallowing the coffee.

"I'm sure Madame Köppen saw you through the glass," Consul Kröger remarked.

"So you live up there, Buddenbrook?" asked Senator Langhals. To the right a broad white staircase with a carved baluster led up to the sleeping-chambers of the Consul's family in the second storey; to the left came another row of rooms. The party descended the stairs, smoking, and the Consul halted at the landing.

"The entresol has three rooms," he explained, "the breakfast-room, my parents' sleeping-chamber, and a third room which is seldom used. A corridor runs along all three. . . . This way, please. The wagons drive through the entry; they can go all the way out to Bakers' Alley at the back."

The broad echoing passageway below was paved with great square flagstones. At either end of it were several offices. The odour of the onion sauce still floated out from the kitchen, which, with the entrance to the cellars, lay on the left of the steps. On the right, at the height of a storey above the passageway, a scaffolding of ungainly but neatly varnished rafters thrust out from the wall, supporting the servants' quarters above. A sort of ladder which led up to them from the passage was their only means of ingress or egress. Below the scaffolding were some enormous old cupboards and a carved chest.

Two low, worn steps led through a glass door out to the courtyard and the small wash-house. From here you could look into the pretty little garden, which was well laid out, though just now brown and sodden with the autumn rains, its beds protected with straw mats against the cold. At the other end of the garden rose the "portal," the rococo façade of the summer house. From the courtyard, however, the party took the path to the left, leading between two walls through another courtyard to the annexe.

They entered by slippery steps into a cellar-like vault with an earthen floor, which was used as a granary and provided with a rope for hauling up the sacks. A pair of stairs led up to the first storey, where the Consul opened a white door and admitted his guests to the billiard-room.

It was a bare, severe-looking room, with stiff chairs ranged round the sides. Herr Köppen flung himself exhausted into one of them. "I'll look on for a while," said he, brushing the wet from his coat. "It's the devil of a Sabbath day's journey through your house, Buddenbrook!"

Here too the stove was burning merrily, behind a brass lattice. Through the three high, narrow windows one looked out over red roofs gleaming with the wet, grey gables and courtyards.

The Consul took the cues out of the rack. "Shall we play a *carambolage*, Senator?" he asked. He went around and closed the pockets on both tables. "Who is playing with us? Gratjens? The Doctor? All right. Then will you take the other table, Gratjens and Justus? Köppen, you'll have to play."

The wine-merchant stood up and listened, with his mouth full of smoke. A violent gust of wind whistled between the houses, lashed the window-panes with rain, and howled down the chimney.

"Good Lord!" he said, blowing out the smoke. "Do you think the *Wullenwewer* will get into port, Buddenbrook? What abominable weather!"

Yes, and the news from Travemünde was not of the best, Consul Kröger agreed, chalking his cue. Storms everywhere on the coast. Nearly as bad as in 1824, the year of the great flood in St. Petersburg. Well, here was the coffee.

They poured it out and drank a little and began their game. The talk turned upon the Customs Union, and Consul Buddenbrook waxed enthusiastic.

"An inspiration, gentlemen," he said. He finished a shot and turned to the other table, where the topic had begun. "We ought to join at the earliest opportunity."

Herr Köppen disagreed. He fairly snorted in opposition. "How about our independence?" he asked incensed, supporting himself belligerently on his cue. "How about our self-determination? Would Hamburg consent to be a party to this Prussian scheme? We might as well be annexed at once! Heaven save us, what do we want of a customs union? Aren't we well enough as we are?"

"Yes, you and your red wine, Köppen. And the Russian products are all right. But there is little or nothing else imported. As for exports, well, we send a little corn to Holland and England, it is true. But I think we are far from being well enough as we are. In days gone by a very different business went on. Now, with the Customs Union, the Mecklenburgs and Schleswig-Holstein would be opened up – and private business would increase beyond all reckoning. . . ."

"But look here, Buddenbrook," Gratjens broke in, leaning far over the table and shifting his cue in his bony hand as he took careful aim, "I don't get the idea. Certainly our own system is perfectly simple and practical. Clearing on the security of a civic oath –"

"A fine old institution," the Consul admitted.

"Do you call it fine, Herr Consul?" Senator Langhals spoke with some heat. "I am not a merchant; but to speak frankly – well, I think this civic oath business has become little short of a farce: everybody makes light of it, and the State pockets the loss. One hears things that are simply scandalous. I am convinced that our entry into the Customs Union, so far as the Senate is concerned – "

Herr Köppen flung down his cue. "Then there will be a conflick," he said heatedly, forgetting to be careful with his pronunciation. "I know what I'm sayin' – God help you, but you don't know what you're talkin' about, beggin' your pardon."

Well, thank goodness! thought the rest of the company, as Jean Jacques entered at this point. He and Pastor Wunderlich came together, arm in arm, two cheerful, unaffected old men from another and less troubled age.

"Here, my friends," he began. "I have something for you: a little rhymed epigram from the French."

He sat down comfortably opposite the billiard-players, who leaned upon their cues across the tables. Drawing a paper from his pocket and laying his long finger with the signet ring to the side of his pointed nose, he read aloud, with a mock-heroic intonation:

> "When the Maréchal Saxe and the proud Pompadour
> Were driving out gaily in gilt coach and four,
> Frelon spied the pair: 'Oh, see them,' he cried:
> 'The sword of our king – and his sheath, side by side.'"

Herr Köppen looked disconcerted for a minute. Then he dropped the "conflick" where it was and joined in the hearty laughter that echoed to the ceiling of the billiard-room. Pastor Wunderlich withdrew to the window, but the movement of his shoulders betrayed that he was chuckling to himself.

Herr Hoffstede had more ammunition of the same sort in his pocket, and the gentlemen remained for some time in the billiard-room. Herr Köppen unbuttoned his waistcoat all the way down, and felt much more at ease here than in the dining-room. He gave vent to droll low-German expressions at every turn, and at frequent intervals began reciting to himself with enormous relish:

> "When the Maréchal Saxe . . ."

It sounded quite different in his harsh bass.

[32]

CHAPTER IX

It was rather late, nearly eleven, when the party began to break up. They had reassembled in the landscape-room, and they all made their adieux at the same time. The Frau Consul, as soon as her hand had been kissed in farewell, went upstairs to see how Christian was doing. To Mamsell Jungmann was left the supervision of the maids as they set things to rights and put away the silver. Madame Antoinette retired to the entresol. But the Consul accompanied his guests downstairs, across the entry, and outside the house.

A high wind was driving the rain slantwise through the streets as the old Krögers, wrapped in heavy fur mantles, slipped as fast as they could into their carriage. It had been waiting for hours before the door. The street was lighted by the flickering yellow rays from oil lamps hanging on posts before the houses or suspended on heavy chains across the streets. The projecting fronts of some of the houses jutted out into the roadway; others had porticos or raised benches added on. The street ran steeply down to the River Trave; it was badly paved, and sodden grass sprang up between the cracks. The church of St. Mary's was entirely shrouded in rain and darkness.

"*Merci*," said Lebrecht Kröger, shaking the Consul's hand as he stood by the carriage door. "*Merci*, Jean; it was too charming!" The door slammed, and the carriage drove off. Pastor Wunderlich and Broker Gratjens expressed their thanks and went their way. Herr Köppen, in a mantle with a five-fold cape and a broad grey hat, took his plump wife on his arm and said in his gruff bass: "G'night, Buddenbrook. Go in, go in; don't catch cold. Best thanks for everything – don't know when I've fed so well! So you like my red wine at four marks? Well, g'night, again."

The Köppens went in the same direction as the Krögers, down toward the river; Senator Langhals, Doctor Grabow, and Jean Jacques Hoffstede turned the other way. Consul Buddenbrook stood with his hands in his trousers pockets and listened to their footsteps as they died away down the empty, damp, dimly-lighted street. He shivered a little in his light clothes as he stood there a few paces from his own house, and turned to look up at its grey gabled façade. His eyes lingered upon the motto carved in the stone over the entrance, in antique lettering: *Dominus providebit* – " The Lord will provide." He bowed his head a little and went in, bolting the door carefully behind him. Then he locked the vestibule door and walked slowly across the echoing floor of the great entry. The cook was coming down the stairs with a tray of glasses in her hands, and he asked her, " Where's the master, Trina? "

" In the dining-room, Herr Consul," said she, and her face went as red as her arms, for she came from the country and was very bashful.

As he passed through the dark hall, he felt in his pocket for the letter. Then he went quickly into the dining-room, where a few small candle-ends in one of the candelabra cast a dim light over the empty table. The sour smell of the onion sauce still hung on the air.

Over by the windows Johann Buddenbrook was pacing comfortably up and down, with his hands behind his back.

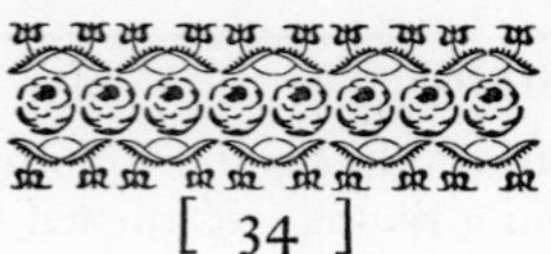

[34]

CHAPTER X

"WELL, Johann, my son, where are you going?" He stood still and put his hand out to his son – his white Buddenbrook hand, a little too short, though finely modelled. His active figure showed indistinctly against the dark red curtains, the only gleams of white being from his powdered hair and the lace frill at his throat.

"Aren't you sleepy? I've been here listening to the wind; the weather is something fearful. Captain Kloht is on his way from Riga. . . ."

"Oh, Father, with God's help all will be well."

"Well, do you think I can depend on that? I know you are on intimate terms with the Almighty – "

The Consul felt his courage rise at this display of good humour.

"Well, to get to the point," he began, "I came in here not to bid you good night, but to – you won't be angry, will you, Papa? . . . I didn't want to disturb you with this letter on such a festive occasion . . . it came this afternoon. . . ."

"*Monsieur Gotthold, voilà!*" The old man affected to be quite unmoved as he took the sealed blue paper. "Herr Johann Buddenbrook, Senior. Personal. A careful man, your step-brother, Jean! Have I answered his second letter, that came the other day? And so now he writes me a third." The old man's rosy face grew sterner as he opened the seal with one finger, unfolded the thin paper, and gave it a smart rap with the back of his hand as he turned about to catch the light from the candles. The very handwriting of this letter seemed to express revolt and disloyalty. All the Buddenbrooks wrote a fine, flowing hand; but these tall straight letters were full of heavy strokes, and many of the words were hastily underlined.

The Consul had drawn back a little to where the row of chairs stood against the wall; he did not sit down, as his father did not; but he grasped one of the high chair-backs nervously and watched the old man while he read, his lips moving rapidly, his brows drawn together, and his head on one side.

FATHER,

I am probably mistaken in entertaining any further hope of your sense of justice or any appreciation of my feelings at receiving no reply from my second pressing letter concerning the matter in question. I do not comment again on the character of the reply I received to my first one. I feel compelled to say, however, that the way in which you, by your lamentable obstinacy, are widening the rift between us, is a sin for which you will one day have to answer grievously before the judgment seat of God. It is sad enough that when I followed the dictates of my heart and married against your wishes, and further wounded your insensate pride by taking over a shop, you should have repulsed me so cruelly and remorselessly; but the way in which you now treat me cries out to Heaven, and you are utterly mistaken if you imagine that I intend to accept your silence without a struggle. The purchase price of your newly acquired house in the Mengstrasse was a hundred thousand marks; and I am aware that Johann, your business partner and your son by your second marriage, is living with you as your tenant, and after your death will become the sole proprietor of both house and business. With my step-sister in Frankfort, you have entered into agreements which are no concern of mine. But what does concern me, your eldest son, is that you carry your un-Christian spirit so far as to refuse me a penny of compensation for my share in the house. When you gave me a hundred thousand marks on my marriage and to set me up in business, and told me that a similar sum and no more should be bequeathed me by will, I said nothing, for I was not at the time sufficiently informed as to the amount of your fortune. Now I know more: and not regarding myself as disinherited in principle, I claim as my right the sum of thirty-three thousand and three hundred and thirty-three marks current, or a third of the purchase price. I make no comment on the damnable influences which are responsible for the treatment I have received. But I protest against them with my whole sense of justice as a Christian and a business man. Let me tell you for the last time that, if you cannot bring yourself to recognize the justice of my claims, I shall no longer be able to respect you as a Christian, a parent, or a man of business.

GOTTHOLD BUDDENBROOK.

"You will excuse me for saying that I don't get much pleasure out of reading that rigmarole all over again. – *Voilà!*" And Johann Buddenbrook tossed the letter to his son, with a contemptuous gesture. The Consul picked it up as it fluttered to his feet, and looked at his father with troubled eyes, while the old man took the long candle-snuffers from their place by the window and with angry strides crossed the room to the candelabrum in the corner.

"*Assez,* I say. *N'en parlons plus!* To bed with you – *en avant!*" He quenched one flame after another under the little metal cap. There were only two candles left when the elder turned again to his son, whom he could hardlly see at the far end of the room.

"*Eh bien* – what are you standing there for? Why don't you say something?"

"What shall I say, Father? I am thoroughly taken aback."

"You are pretty easily taken aback, then," Johann Buddenbrook rapped out irritably, though he knew that the reproach was far from being a just one. His son was in fact often his superior when it came to a quick decision upon the advantageous course.

"'Damnable influences,'" the Consul quoted. "That is the first line I can make out. Do you know how it makes me feel, Father? And he reproaches us with 'unchristian behaviour!'"

"You'll let yourself be bluffed by this miserable scribble, will you?" Johann Buddenbrook strode across to his son, dragging the extinguisher on its long stick behind him. "'Unchristian behaviour!' Ha! He shows good taste, doesn't he, this canting money-grabber? I don't know what to make of you young people! Your heads are full of fantastic religious humbug – practical idealism, the July Monarchy, and what not: and we old folk are supposed to be wretched cynics. And then you abuse your poor old Father in the coarsest way rather than give up a few thousand thaler. . . . So he deigns to look down upon me as a business man, does he? Well, as a business man, I know what *faux-frais* are! – *Faux-frais,*" he repeated, rolling the *r* in his throat. "I shan't make this high-falutin scamp of a son any fonder of me by giving him what he asks for, it seems to me."

"What can I say, Father? I don't care to feel that he has any justification when he talks of 'influences.' As an interested party I don't like to tell you to stick out, but – It seems to me I'm as good a Christian as Gotthold . . . but still . . ."

"'Still' – that is exactly it, Jean, you are right to say 'still.' What is the real state of the case? He got infatuated with his Mademoiselle Stüwing and wouldn't listen to reason; he made scene after scene, and finally he married her, after I had absolutely refused to give my consent. Then I wrote to him: '*Mon très cher fils:* you are marrying your shop – very well, that's an end of it. We cease to be on friendly terms from now on. I won't cut you off, or do anything melodramatic. I am sending you a hundred thousand marks as a wedding present, and I'll leave you another hundred thousand in my will. But that is absolutely all you'll get, not another shilling! ' That shut his mouth. – What have our arrangements got to do with him? Suppose you and your sister do get a bit more, and the house has been bought out of your share? "

" Father, surely you can understand how painful my position is! I ought to advise you in the interest of family harmony – but . . ." The Consul sighed. Johann Buddenbrook peered at him, in the dim light, to see what his expression was. One of the two candles had gone out of itself; the other was flickering. Every now and then a tall, smiling white figure seemed to step momentarily out of the tapestry and then back again.

" Father," said the Consul softly. " This affair with Gotthold depresses me."

" What's all this sentimentality, Jean? How does it depress you? "

" We were all so happy here to-day, Father; we had a glorious celebration, and we felt proud and glad of what we have accomplished, and of having raised the family and firm to a position of honour and respect. . . . But this bitter feud with my own brother, with your eldest son, is like a hidden crack in the building we have erected. A family should be united, Father. It must keep together. ' A house divided against itself will fall.' "

" There you are with your milk-and-water stuff, Jean! All I say is, he's an insolent young puppy."

A pause ensued. The last candle burned lower and lower.

" What are you doing, Jean? " asked Johann Buddenbrook. " I can't see you."

The Consul said shortly, " I'm calculating." He was standing erect, and the expression in his eyes had changed. They had looked dreamy all the evening; but now they stared into the candle-flame with a cold sharp gaze. " Either you give thirty-three thousand, three hundred and thirty-three marks to Gotthold, and fifteen thousand to the family in Frankfort – that makes forty-eight thousand, three hundred and thirty-five in all – or, you give nothing to Gotthold, and twenty-five thousand to the family in Frankfort. That means a gain of twenty-three thousand, three hundred and thirty-five for the firm. But there is more to it than that. If you give Gotthold a compensation for the house, you've started the ball rolling. He is likely to demand equal shares with my sister and me after your death, which would mean a loss of hundreds of thousands to the firm. The firm could not face it, and I, as sole head, could not face it either." He made a vigorous gesture and drew himself more erect than before. "No, Papa," he said, and his tone bespoke finality, "I must advise you not to give in."

"Bravo!" cried the old man. "There 's an end of it! *N'en parlons plus! En avant!* Let's get to bed."

And he extinguished the last candle. They groped through the pitch-dark hall, and at the foot of the stairs they stopped and shook hands.

"Good night, Jean. And cheer up. These little worries aren't anything. See you at breakfast!"

The Consul went up to his rooms, and the old man felt his way along the baluster and down to the entresol. Soon the rambling old house lay wrapped in darkness and silence. Hopes, fears, and ambitions all slumbered, while the rain fell and the autumn wind whistled around gables and street corners.

PART TWO

CHAPTER I

It was mid-April, two and a half years later. The spring was more advanced than usual, and with the spring had come to the Buddenbrook family a joy that made old Johann sing about the house and moved his son to the depths of his heart.

The Consul sat at the big roll-top writing-desk in the window of the breakfast-room, at nine o'clock one Sunday morning. He had before him a stout leather portfolio stuffed with papers, from among which he had drawn a gilt-edged notebook with an embossed cover, and was busily writing in it in his small, thin, flowing script. His hand hurried over the paper, never pausing except to dip his quill in the ink.

Both the windows were open, and the spring breeze wafted delicate odours into the room, lifting the curtains gently. The garden was full of young buds and bathed in tender sunshine; a pair of birds called and answered each other pertly. The sunshine was strong, too, on the white linen of the breakfast-table and the gilt borders of the old china.

The folding doors into the bed-room were open, and the voice of old Johann could be heard inside, singly softly to a quaint and ancient tune:

> A kind papa, a worthy man,
> He rocks the baby in the cradle,
> He feeds the children sugar-plums
> And stirs the porridge with a ladle.

He sat beside the little green-curtained cradle, close to the Frau Consul's lofty bed, and rocked it softly with one hand. Madame Antoinette, in a white lace cap and an apron over her striped frock, was busy with flannel and linen at the table. The old couple had given up their bedroom to the Frau Consul for the time being, to make things easier for the servants, and were sleeping in the unused room in the entresol.

Consul Buddenbrook gave scarcely a glance at the adjoining room, so absorbed was he in his work. His face wore an expression of earnest, almost suffering piety, his mouth slightly open, the chin a little dropped; his eyes filled from time to time. He wrote:

"Today, April 14, 1838, at six o'clock in the morning, my dear wife, Elizabeth Buddenbrook, born Kröger, was, by God's gracious help, happily delivered of a daughter, who will receive the name of Clara in Holy Baptism. Yea, the Lord hath holpen mightily; for according to Doctor Grabow, the birth was somewhat premature, and her condition not of the best. She suffered great pain. Oh, Lord God of Sabaoth, where is there any other God save Thee? who helpest us in all our times of need and danger, and teachest us to know Thy will aright, that we may fear Thee and obey Thy commandments! O Lord, lead us and guide us all, so long as we live upon this earth. . . ." The pen hurried glibly over the paper, with here and there a commercial flourish, talking with God in every line. Two pages further on: "I have taken out," it said, "an insurance policy for my youngest daughter, of one hundred and fifty thaler current. Lead her, O Lord, in Thy ways, give her a pure heart, O God, that she may one day enter into the mansions of eternal peace. For inasmuch as our weak human hearts are prone to forget Thy priceless gift of the sweet, blessed Jesus . . ." And so on for three pages. Then he wrote "Amen." But still the faint scratching sound of the pen went on, over several more pages. It wrote of the precious spring that refreshes the tired wanderer, of the Saviour's holy wounds gushing blood, of the broad way and the narrow way, and the glory of the Eternal God. It is true that after a while the Consul began to feel that he had written enough; that he might let well enough alone, and go in to see his wife, or out to the counting-house. Oh, fie, fie! Did one so soon weary of communion with his Lord and Saviour? Was it not robbing his God to scant Him of this service? No, he would go on, as a chastisement for these unholy impulses. He cited whole pages of Scripture, he prayed for his parents, his wife, his children, and himself, he prayed even for his brother Gotthold. And then, with a last quotation and three final "Amens," he strewed sand on the paper and leaned back with a sigh of relief.

He crossed one leg over the other and slowly turned the pages of the notebook, reading dates and entries here and there, written in his own hand, and thanking the Lord afresh as he saw how in every time of need and danger He had stretched out His hand to aid. Once he had lain so ill of small-pox that his life had been despaired of – yet it had been saved. And once, when he was a boy, a beer-vat had fallen on him. A large quantity of beer was being brewed for a wedding, in the old days when the brewing was done at home; and a vat had fallen over, pinning the boy beneath it. It had taken six people to lift it up again, and his head had been crushed so that the blood ran down in streams. He was carried into a shop, and, as he still breathed, the doctor and the surgeon were sent for. They told the father to prepare for the worst and to bow to the will of God. But the Almighty had blessed the work of healing, and the boy was saved and restored to health. The Consul dwelt a while upon this account, re-living the accident in his mind. Then he took his pen again and wrote after his last "Amen": "Yea, O God, I will eternally praise Thee!"

Another time, his life had been saved from danger by water, when he had gone to Bergen, as a young man. The account read:

"At high water, when the freight boats of the Northern Line are in, we have great difficulty getting through the press to our landing. I was standing on the edge of the scow, with my feet on the thole-pins, leaning my back against the sailboat, trying to get the scow nearer in, when, as luck would have it, the oak thole-pins broke, and I went head over heels into the water. The first time I came up, nobody was near enough to get hold of me; the second time, the scow went over my head. There were plenty of people there anxious to save me, but they had to keep the sailboat and the scow off, so that I should not come up under them; and all their shoving would probably have been in vain if a rope had not suddenly broken on one of the sailboats belonging to the Line, so that she swung further out; and this, by the grace of God, gave me room enough to come up in free water. It was only the top of my head, with the hair, that they saw; but it was enough, for they were all lying on their stomachs with their heads sticking out over the scow, and the man at the bow grabbed me by the hair, and I got hold of his arm. He was in an unsafe position himself and could not hold me, but he gave a yell, and they all took hold of him around the waist and pulled. I hung on, though he bit me to make me let go. So they got me in at last." There followed a long prayer of thanksgiving, which the Consul re-read with tear-wet eyes.

On another page he had said: "I could write much more, were I minded to reveal the passions of my youth. . . ." The Consul passed over this, and began to read here and there from the period of his marriage and the birth of his first child. The union, to be frank, could hardly be called a love-match. His father had tapped him on the shoulder and pointed out to him the daughter of the wealthy Kröger, who could bring the firm a splendid marriage portion. He had accepted the situation with alacrity; and from the first moment had honoured his wife as the mate entrusted to him by God.

After all, his father's second marriage had been of much the same kind.

" 'A kind Papa, a worthy man.' "

He could still hear old Johann softly humming in the bedroom. What a pity he had so little taste for those old records! He stood with both feet firmly planted in the present, and concerned himself seldom with the past of his family. Yet in times gone by he too had made a few entries in the gilt-edged book. The Consul turned to those pages, written in a florid hand on rather coarse paper that was already yellowing with age. They were chiefly about his first marriage. Ah, Johann Buddenbrook must have adored his first wife, the daughter of a Bremen merchant! The one brief year it had been granted him to live with her was the happiest of his life – "*l'année la plus heureuse de ma vie*," he had written there. The words were underlined with a wavy line, for all the world, even Madame Antoinette, to see.

Then Gotthold had come, and Josephine had died. And here some strange things had been written on the rough paper. Johann Buddenbrook must have openly and bitterly hated his child, even when, while still in the womb, it had caused its mother to faint and agonize under the lusty burden. It was born strong and active, while Josephine buried her bloodless face deeper in the pillows and passed away. Johann never forgave the ruthless intruder. He grew up vigorous and pushing, and Johann thought of him as his mother's murderer. This was, to the Consul's mind, incomprehensible. She had died, he thought, fulfilling the holy duty of a woman: "the love I bore to her would have passed over in all its tenderness to her child," he said to himself. It had not been so. Later the father married again, his bride being Antoinette Duchamps, the daughter of a rich and much-esteemed Hamburg family, and the two had dwelt together with mutual respect and deference.

The Consul went on turning over the pages. There at the end were written the small histories of his own children: how Tom had had the measles, and Antonie jaundice, and Christian chickenpox. There were accounts of various journeys he had taken with his wife, to Paris, Switzerland, Marienbad. Then the Consul turned back to the front of the book, to some pages written in bluish ink, in a hand full of flourishes, on paper that was like parchment, but tattered and spotted with age. Here his grandfather

Johann had set down the genealogy of the main branch of the Buddenbrooks. At the end of the sixteenth century, the first Buddenbrook of whom they had knowledge lived in Parchim, and his son had been a Senator of Grabau. Another Buddenbrook, a tailor by trade, and " very well-to-do " (this was underlined) had married in Rostock and begotten an extraordinary number of children, who lived or died, as the case might be. And again, another, this time a Johann, had lived in Rostock as a merchant, from whom the Consul's grandfather had descended, who had left Rostock to settle himself in this very town, and was the founder of the present grain business. There was much about him set down in detail: when he had had the purples, and when genuine small-pox; when he had fallen out of the malt-kiln and been miraculously saved, when he might have fallen against the beams and been crushed; how he had had fever and been delirious – all these events were meticulously described. He had also written down wise admonitions for the benefit of his descendants, like the following, which was carefully painted and framed, in a tall Gothic script set off with a border: " My son, attend with zeal to thy business by day; but do none that hinders thee from thy sleep by night." He had also stated that his old Wittenberg Bible was to descend to his eldest son, and thence from first-born to first-born in each generation.

Consul Buddenbrook reached for the old leather portfolio and took out the remaining documents. There were letters, on torn and yellow paper, written by anxious mothers to their sons abroad – which the sons had docketed: " Received and contents duly noted." There were citizens' papers, with the seal and crest of the free Hansa town; insurance policies; letters inviting this or that Buddenbrook to become god-father for a colleague's child; congratulatory epistles and occasional poems. Sons travelling for the firm to Stockholm or Amsterdam had written back, to the parent or partner at home, letters in which business was touchingly mingled with inquiries after wife and child. There was a separate diary of the Consul's journey through England and Brabant; the cover had an engraving of Edinburgh Castle and the Grass-market. Lastly, there were Gotthold's late angry letters to his father – painful documents, to offset which was the poem written by Jean Jacques Hoffstede to celebrate the house-warming.

A faint, rapid chime came from above the secretary, where there hung a dull-looking painting of an old market-square, with a church-tower that possessed a real clock of its own. It was now striking the hour, in authentic if tiny tones. The Consul closed the portfolio and stowed it away carefully in a drawer at the back of the desk. Then he went into the bed-chamber.

Here the walls and the high old bed were hung with dark flowered chintz, and there was in the air a feeling of repose, of convalescence – of calm after an anxious and painful ordeal. A mingled odour of cologne and drugs hung in the mild, dim-lighted atmosphere. The old pair bent over the cradle side by side and watched the slumbering child; and the Consul's wife lay pale and happy, in an exquisite lace jacket, her hair carefully dressed. As she put out her hand to her husband, her gold bracelets tinkled slightly. She had a characteristic way of stretching out her hand with the palm upward, in a sweeping gesture that gave it added graciousness.

" Well, Betsy, how are you? "

" Splendid, splendid, my dear Jean."

He still held her hand as he bent over and looked at the child, whose rapid little breaths were distinctly audible. For a moment he inhaled the tender warmth and the indescribable odour of well-being and cherishing care that came up from the cradle. Then he kissed the little creature on the brow and said softly: " God bless you! " He noticed how like to a bird's claws were the tiny yellow, crumpled fingers.

" She eats splendidly," Madame Antoinette said. " See how she has gained."

" I believe, on my soul, she looks like Netta," old Johann said, beaming with pride and pleasure. " See what coal-black eyes she has! "

The old lady waved him away. " How can anybody tell who she looks like yet? " she said. " Are you going to church, Jean? "

" Yes, it is ten o'clock now, and high time. I am only waiting for the children."

The children were already making an unseemly noise on the stairs, and Clothilde could be heard telling them to hush. They came in in their fur tippets – for it would still be wintry in St. Mary's – trying to be soft and gentle in the sick-room. They wanted to see the little sister, and then go to church. Their faces were rosy with excitement. This was a wonderful red-letter day, for the stork had brought not only the baby sister, but all sorts of presents as well. How tremendously strong the stork must be, to carry all that! There was a new seal-skin school-bag for Tom, a big doll for Antonie, that had real hair – imagine that! – for Christian a complete toy theatre, with the Sultan, Death, and the Devil; and a book with pictures for demure Clothilde, who accepted it with thanks, but was more interested in the bag of sweeties that fell to her lot as well.

They kissed their mother, and were allowed a peep under the green curtains of the baby's bed. Then off they went with their father, who had put on his fur coat and taken the hymn book. They were followed by the piercing cry of the new member of the family, who had just waked up.

CHAPTER II

EARLY in the summer, sometimes as early as May or June, Tony Buddenbrook always went on a visit to her grandparents, who lived outside the Castle Gate. This was a great pleasure.

For life was delightful out there in the country, in the luxurious villa with its many outbuildings, servants' quarters and stables, and its great parterres, orchards, and kitchen-gardens, which ran steeply down to the river Trave. The Krögers lived in the grand style; there was a difference between their brilliant establishment and the solid, somewhat heavy comfort of the paternal home, which was obvious at a glance, and which impressed very much the young Demoiselle Buddenbrook.

Here there was no thought of duties in house or kitchen. In the Mengstrasse, though her Mother and Grandfather did not seem to think it important, her Father and her Grandmother were always telling her to remember her dusting, and holding up Clothilde as an example. The old feudal feeling of her Mother's side of the family came out strongly in the little maid: one could see how she issued her orders to the footman or the abigail – and to her Grandmother's servants and her Grandfather's coachman as well.

Say what you will, it is pleasant to awake every morning in a large, gaily tapestried bed-chamber, and with one's first movements to feel the soft satin of the coverlet under one's hand; to take early breakfast in the balcony room, with the sweet fresh air coming up from the garden through the open glass door; to drink, instead of coffee, a cup of chocolate handed one on a tray – yes, proper birthday chocolate, with a thick slice of fresh cup-cake! True, she had to eat her breakfast alone, except on Sundays, for her grandparents never came down until long after she had gone to school. When she had munched her cake and drunk her chocolate, she would snatch up her satchel and trip down the terrace and through the well-kept front garden.

She was very dainty, this little Tony Buddenbrook. Under her straw hat curled a wealth of blond hair, slowly darkening with the years. Lively grey-blue eyes and a pouting upper lip gave her fresh face a roguish look, borne out by the poise of her graceful little figure; even the slender legs, in their immaculate white stockings, trotted along over the ground with an unmistakable air of ease and assurance. People knew and greeted the young daughter of Consul Buddenbrook as she came out of the garden gate and up the chestnut-bordered avenue. Perhaps an old market-woman, driving her little cart in from the village, would nod her head in its big flat straw hat with its light green ribbons, and call out "Mornin', little missy!" Or Matthiesen the porter, in his wide knee-breeches, white hose, and buckled shoes, would respectfully take off his hat as she passed.

Tony always waited for her neighbour, little Julie Hagenström; the two children went to school together. Julie was a high-shouldered child, with large, staring black eyes, who lived close by in a vine-covered house. Her people had not been long in the neighbourhood. The father, Herr Hagenström, had married a wife from Hamburg, with thick, heavy black hair and larger diamonds in her ears than any one had ever seen before. Her name was Semlinger. Hagenström was partner in the export firm of Strunck and Hagenström. He showed great zeal and ambition in municipal affairs, and was always acting on boards and committees and administrative bodies. But he was not very popular. His marriage had rather affronted the rigid traditions of the older families, like the Möllendorpfs, Langhals, and Buddenbrooks; and, for another thing, he seemed to enjoy thwarting their ideas at every turn – he would go to work in an underhand way to oppose their interests, in order to show his own superior foresight and energy. "Hinrich Hagenström makes trouble the whole time," the Consul would say. "He seems to take a personal pleasure in thwarting me. To-day he made a scene at the sitting of the Central Paupers' Deputation; and a few days ago in the Finance Department. . . ." "The old skunk!" Johann Buddenbrook interjected. Another time, father and son sat down to table angry and depressed. What was the matter? Oh, nothing. They had lost a big consignment of rye for Holland: Strunck and Hagenström had snapped it up under their noses. He was a fox, Hinrich Hagenström.

Tony had often heard such remarks, and she was not too well disposed toward Julie Hagenström; the two children walked together because they were neighbours, but usually they quarrelled.

"My Father owns a thousand thalers," said Julchen. She thought she was uttering the most terrible falsehood. "How much does yours?"

Tony was speechless with envy and humiliation. Then she said, with a quiet, off-hand manner: " My chocolate tasted delicious this morning. What do you have for breakfast, Julie? "

" Before I forget it," Julie would rejoin, " would you like one of my apples? Well, I won't give you any! " She pursed up her lips, and her black eyes watered with satisfaction.

Sometimes Julie's brother Hermann went to school at the same time with the two girls. There was another brother too, named Moritz, but he was sickly and did his lessons at home. Hermann was fair-haired and snub-nosed. He breathed through his mouth and was always smacking his lips.

" Stuff and nonsense! " he would say. " Papa has a lot more than a thousand thaler." He interested Tony because of the luncheon he took to school: not bread, but a soft sort of lemon bun with currants in it, and sausage or smoked goose between. It seemed to be his favourite luncheon. Tony had never seen anything like it before. Lemon bun, with smoked goose – it must be wonderful! He let her look into his box, and she asked if she might have some. Hermann said: " Not to-day, Tony, because I can't spare any. But to-morrow I'll bring another piece for you, if you'll give me something."

Next morning, Tony came out into the avenue, but there was no Julie. She waited five minutes, but there was no sign. Another minute – there came Hermann alone, swinging his lunch-box by the strap and smacking his lips.

" Now," he said, " here's a bun, with some goose between – all lean; there's not a bit of fat to it. What will you give me for it? "

" A shilling? " suggested Tony. They were standing in the middle of the avenue.

" A shilling? " repeated Hermann. Then he gave a gulp and said, " No, I want something else."

" What? " demanded Tony; for she was prepared to pay a good price for the dainty.

" A kiss! " shouted Hermann Hagenström. He flung his arms around Tony, and began kissing at random, never once touching her face, for she flung her head back with surprising agility, pushed him back with her left hand – it was holding her satchel – against his breast, while with her right hand she dealt him three or four blows in the face with all her strength. He stumbled backward; but at that moment sister Julie appeared from behind a tree, like a little black demon, and, falling upon Tony, tore off her hat and scratched her cheeks unmercifully. After this affair, naturally, the friendship was about at an end.

It was hardly out of shyness that Tony had refused the kiss. She was on the whole a forward damsel, and had given the Consul no little disquiet with her tomboy ways. She had a good little head, and did as well in the school as one could desire; but her conduct in other ways was far from satisfactory. Things even went so far that one day the schoolmistress, a certain Fräulein Agathe Vermehren, felt obliged to call upon the Frau Consul, and, flushed with embarrassment, to suggest with all due politeness that the child should receive a paternal admonition. It seemed that Tony, despite frequent correction, had been guilty, not for the first time, of creating a disturbance in the street!

There was, of course, no harm in the fact that the child knew everybody in town. The Consul quite approved of this, and argued that it displayed love of one's neighbour, a sense of human fellowship, and a lack of snobbishness. So Tony, on her way through the streets, chattered with all and sundry. She and Tom would clamber about in the granaries on the water-side, among the piles of oats and wheat, prattling to the labourers and the clerks in the dark little ground-floor offices; they would even help haul up the sacks of grain. She knew the butchers with their trays and aprons, when she met them in Broad Street; she accosted the dairy women when they came in from the country, and made them take her a little way in their carts. She knew the grey-bearded craftsmen who sat in the narrow goldsmiths' shops built into the arcades in the market square; and she knew the fish-wives, the fruit- and vegetable-women, and the porters that stood on the street corners chewing their tobacco.

So far, this was very well. But it was not all.

There was a pale, beardless man, of no particular age, who was often seen wandering up and down Broad Street with a wistful smile on his face. This man was so nervous that he jumped every time he heard a sudden noise behind him; and Tony delighted in making him jump every time she set eyes on him. Then there was an odd, tiny little woman with a large head, who put up a huge tattered umbrella at every sign of a storm. Tony would harass this poor soul with cries of "Mushroom!" whenever she had the chance. Moreover, she and two or three more of her ilk would go to the door of a tiny house in an alley off John Street, where there lived an old woman who did a tiny trade in worsted dolls; they would ring the bell and, when the old dame appeared, inquire with deceptive courtesy, if Herr and Frau Spittoon were at home — and then run away screaming with laughter. All these ragamuffinly tricks Tony Buddenbrook was guilty of — indeed, she seemed to perform them with the best conscience in the world. If one of her victims threatened her, she would step back a pace or two, toss her pretty head, pout with her pretty lip, and say "Pooh!" in a half mocking, half angry tone which meant: "Try it if you like. I am Consul Buddenbrook's daughter, if you don't know!"

Thus she went about in the town like a little queen; and like a queen, she was kind or cruel to her subjects, as the whim seized her.

CHAPTER III

JEAN JACQUES HOFFSTEDE's verdict on the two sons of Consul Buddenbrook undoubtedly hit the mark.

Thomas had been marked from the cradle as a merchant and future member of the firm. He was on the modern side of the old school which the boys attended; an able, quick-witted, intelligent lad, always ready to laugh when his brother Christian mimicked the masters, which he did with uncanny facility. Christian, on the classical side, was not less gifted than Tom, but he was less serious. His special and particular joy in life was the imitation, in speech and manner, of a certain worthy Marcellus Stengel, who taught drawing, singing, and some other of the lighter branches.

This Herr Marcellus Stengel always had a round half-dozen beautifully sharpened pencils sticking out of his pocket. He wore a red wig and a light brown coat that reached nearly down to his ankles; also a choker collar that came up almost to his temples. He was quite a wit, and loved to play with verbal distinctions, as: "You were to make a line, my child, and what have you made? You have made a dash!" In singing-class, his favourite lesson was "The Forest Green." When they sang this, some of the pupils would go outside in the corridor; and then, when the chorus rose inside: "We ramble so gaily through field and wood," those outside would repeat the last word very softly, as an echo. Once Christian Buddenbrook, his cousin Jürgen Kröger, and his chum Andreas Gieseke, the son of the Fire Commissioner, were deputed as echo; but when the moment came, they threw the coal-scuttle downstairs instead, and were kept in after school by Herr Stengel in consequence. But alas, by that time Herr Stengel had forgotten their crime. He bade his housekeeper give them each a cup of coffee, and then dismissed them.

In truth, they were all admirable scholars, the masters who taught in the cloisters of the old school – once a monastic foundation – under the guidance of a kindly, snuff-taking old head. They were, to a man, well-meaning and sweet-humoured; and they were one in the belief that knowledge and good cheer are not mutually exclusive. The Latin classes in the middle forms were heard by a former preacher, one Pastor Shepherd, a tall man with brown whiskers and a twinkling eye, who joyed extremely in the happy coincidence of his name and calling, and missed no chance of having the boys translate the word *pastor*. His favourite expression was "boundlessly limited"; but it was never quite clear whether this was actually meant for a joke or not! When he wanted to dumbfound his pupils altogether, he would draw in his lips and blow them quickly out again, with a noise like the popping of a champagne cork. He would go up and down with long strides in his class-room, prophesying to one boy or another, with great vividness, the course which his life would take. He did this avowedly with the purpose of stimulating their imaginations; and then he would set to work seriously on the business in hand, which was to repeat certain verses on the rules of gender and difficult constructions. He had composed these verses himself, with no little skill, and took much pride in declaiming them, with great attention to rhyme and rhythm.

Thus passed Tom's and Christian's boyhood, with no great events to mark its course. There was sunshine in the Buddenbrook family, and in the office everything went famously. Only now and again there would be a sudden storm, a trifling mishap, like the following:

Herr Stuht the tailor had made a new suit for each of the Buddenbrook lads. Herr Stuht lived in Bell-Founders' Street. He was a master tailor, and his wife bought and sold old clothes, and thus moved in the best circles of society. Herr Stuht himself had an enormous belly, which hung down over his legs, wrapped in a flannel shirt. The suits he made for the young Masters Buddenbrook were at the combined cost of seventy marks; but at the boys' request he had consented to put them down in the bill at eighty marks and to hand them the difference. It was just a little arrangement among themselves – not very honourable, indeed, but then, not very uncommon either. However, fate was unkind, and the bargain came to light. Herr Stuht was sent for to the Consul's office, whither he came, with a black coat over his woollen shirt, and stood there while the Consul subjected Tom and Christian to a severe cross-examination. His head was bowed and his legs far apart, his manner vastly respectful. He tried to smooth things over as much as he could for the young gentlemen, and said that what was done was done, and he would be satisfied with the seventy marks. But the Consul was greatly incensed by the trick. He gave it long and serious consideration; yet finally ended by increasing the lads' pocket-money – for was it not written: " Lead us not into temptation? "

It seemed probable that more might be expected from Thomas Buddenbrook than from his brother Christian. He was even-tempered, and his high spirits never crossed the bounds of discretion. Christian, on the other hand, was inclined to be moody: guilty at times of the most extravagant silliness, at others he would be seized by a whim which could terrify the rest of them in the most astonishing way.

The family are at table eating dessert and conversing pleasantly the while. Suddenly Christian turns pale and puts back on his plate the peach into which he has just bitten. His round, deep-set eyes, above the too-large nose, have opened wider.

" I will never eat another peach," he says.

" Why not, Christian? What nonsense! What's the matter? "

" Suppose I accidentally – suppose I swallowed the stone, and it stuck in my throat, so I couldn't breathe, and I jumped up, strangling horribly – and all of you jump up – Ugh . . . ! " and he suddenly gives a short groan, full of horror and affright, starts up in his chair, and acts as if he were trying to escape.

The Frau Consul and Ida Jungmann actually do jump up.

" Heavens, Christian! – you haven't swallowed it, have you? " For his whole appearance suggests that he has.

" No," says Christian slowly. " No " – he is gradually quieting down – " I only mean, suppose I actually *had* swallowed it! "

The Consul has been pale with fright, but he recovers and begins to scold. Old Johann bangs his fist on the table and forbids any more of these idiotic practical jokes. But Christian, for a long, long time, eats no more peaches.

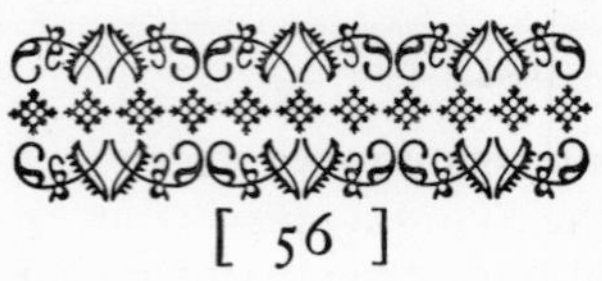

CHAPTER IV

It was not simply the weakness of age that made Madame Antoinette Buddenbrook take to her lofty bed in the bed-chamber of the entresol, one cold January day after they had dwelt some six years in Meng Street. The old lady had remained hale and active, and carried her head, with its clustering white side-curls, proudly erect to the very last. She had gone with her husband and children to most of the large dinners given in the town, and presided no whit less elegantly than her daughter-in-law when the Buddenbrooks themselves entertained. But one day an indefinable malady had suddenly made itself felt — at first in the form of a slight intestinal catarrh, for which Dr. Grabow prescribed a mild diet of pigeon and French bread. This had been followed by colic and vomiting, which reduced her strength so rapidly as to bring about an alarming decline.

Dr. Grabow held hurried speech with the Consul, outside on the landing, and another doctor was called in consultation — a stout, black-bearded, gloomy-looking man who began going in and out with Dr. Grabow. And now the whole atmosphere of the house changed. They went about on their tip-toes and spoke in whispers. The wagons were no longer allowed to roll through the great entry-way below. The family looked in each other's eyes and saw there something strange. It was the idea of death that had entered, and was holding silent sway in the spacious rooms.

But there was no idle watching, for visitors came: old Senator Duchamps, the dying woman's brother, from Hamburg, with his daughter; and a few days later, the Consul's sister from Frankfort and her husband, who was a banker. The illness lasted fourteen or fifteen days, during which the guests lived in the house, and Ida Jungmann had her hands full attending to the bedrooms and providing heavy breakfasts, with shrimps and port wine. Much roasting and baking went on in the kitchen.

Upstairs, Johann Buddenbrook sat by the sick-bed, his old Netta's limp hand in his, and stared into space with his brows knitted and his lower lip hanging. A clock hung on the wall and ticked dully, with long pauses between; not so long, however, as the pauses between the dying woman's fluttering breaths. A black-robed sister of mercy busied herself about the beef-tea which they still sought to make the patient take. Now and then some member of the family would appear at the door and disappear again.

Perhaps the old man was thinking how he had sat at the deathbed of his first wife, forty-six years before. Perhaps he recalled his frenzy of despair and contrasted it with the gentle melancholy which he felt now, as an old man, gazing into the face of his old wife – a face so changed, so listless, so void of expression. She had never given him either a great joy or a great sorrow; but she had decorously played her part beside him for many a long year – and now her life was ebbing away.

He was not thinking a great deal. He was only looking with fixed gaze back into his own past life and at life in general. It all seemed to him now quite strange and far away, and he shook his head a little. That empty noise and bustle, in the midst of which he had once stood, had flowed away imperceptibly and left him standing there, listening in wonder to sounds that died upon his ear. " Strange, strange," he murmured.

Madame Buddenbrook breathed her last brief, effortless sigh; and they prayed by her side in the dining-room, where the service was held; and the bearers lifted the flower-covered coffin to carry it away. But old Johann did not weep. He only gave the same gentle, bewildered head-shake, and said, with the same half-smiling look: " Strange, strange! " It became his most frequent expression. Plainly, the time for old Johann too was near at hand.

He would sit silent and absent in the family circle; sometimes with little Clara on his knee, to whom he would sing one of his droll catches, like

" The omnibus drives through the town "

or perhaps

" Look at the blue-fly a-buzzin' on the wall."

But he might suddenly stop in the middle, like one aroused out of a train of thought, put the child down on the floor, and move away, with his little head-shake and murmur: " Strange, strange! " One day he said: " Jean – it's about time, eh? "

It was soon afterward that neatly printed notices signed by father and son were sent about through the town, in which Johann Buddenbrook senior respectfully begged leave to announce that his increasing years obliged him to give up his former business activities, and that in consequence the firm of Johann Buddenbrook, founded by his late father anno 1768, would as from that day be transferred, with its assets and liabilities, to his son and former partner Johann Buddenbrook as sole proprietor; for whom he solicited a continuance of the confidence so widely bestowed upon him. Signed, with deep respect, Johann Buddenbrook – who would from now on cease to append his signature to business papers.

These announcements were no sooner sent out than the old man refused to set foot in the office; and his apathy so increased that it took only the most trifling cold to send him to bed, one March day two months after the death of his wife. One night more – then came the hour when the family gathered round his bed and he spoke to them: first to the Consul: " Good luck, Jean, and keep your courage up! " And then to Thomas: " Be a help to your Father, Tom! " And to Christian: " Be something worth while! " Then he was silent, gazing at them all; and finally, with a last murmured " Strange! " he turned his face to the wall. . . .

To the very end, he did not speak of Gotthold, and the latter encountered with silence the Consul's written summons to his father's death-bed. But early the next morning, before the announcements were sent out, as the Consul was about to go into the office to attend to some necessary business, Gotthold Buddenbrook, proprietor of the linen firm of Siegmund Stüwing and Company, came with rapid steps through the entry. He was forty-six years old, broad and stocky, and had thick ash-blond whiskers streaked with grey. His short legs were cased in baggy trousers of rough checked material. On the steps he met the Consul, and his eyebrows went up under the brim of his grey hat.

He did not put out his hand. " Johann," he said, in a high-pitched, rather agreeable voice, " how is he? "

" He passed away last night," the Consul said, with deep emotion, grasping his brother's hand, which held an umbrella. " The best of fathers! "

Gotthold drew down his brows now, so low that the lids nearly closed. After a silence, he said pointedly: " Nothing was changed up to the end? "

The Consul let his hand drop and stepped back. His round, deep-set blue eyes flashed as he answered, " Nothing."

Gotthold's eyebrows went up again under his hat, and his eyes fixed themselves on his brother with an expression of suspense.

" And what have I to expect from your sense of justice? " he asked in a lower voice.

It was the Consul's turn to look away. Then, without lifting his eyes, he made that downward gesture with his hand that always betokened decision; and in a quiet voice, but firmly, he answered:

"In this sad and solemn moment I have offered you my brotherly hand. But if it is your intention to speak of business matters, then I can only reply in my capacity as head of the honourable firm whose sole proprietor I have to-day become. You can expect from me nothing that runs counter to the duties I have to-day assumed; all other feelings must be silent."

Gotthold went away. But he came to the funeral, among the host of relatives, friends, business associates, deputies, clerks, porters, and labourers that filled the house, the stairs, and the corridors to overflowing and assembled all the hired coaches in town in a long row all the way down the Mengstrasse. Gotthold came, to the sincere joy of the Consul. He even brought his wife, born Stüwing, and his three grown daughters: Friederike and Henriette, who were too tall and thin, and Pfiffi, who was eighteen, and too short and fat.

Pastor Kölling of St. Mary's, a heavy man with a bullet head and a rough manner of speaking, held the service at the grave, in the Buddenbrook family burying-ground, outside the Castle Gate, at the edge of the cemetery grove. He extolled the godly, temperate life of the deceased and compared it with that of "gluttons, drunkards, and profligates" – over which strong language some of the congregation shook their heads, thinking of the tact and moderation of their old Pastor Wunderlich, who had lately died. When the service and the burial were over, and the seventy or eighty hired coaches began to roll back to town, Gotthold Buddenbrook asked the Consul's permission to go with him, that they might speak together in private. He sat with his brother on the back seat of the high, ungainly old coach, one short leg crossed over the other – and, wonderful to relate, he was gentle and conciliatory. He realized more and more, he said, that the Consul was bound to act as he was doing; and he was determined to cherish no bitter memories of his father. He renounced the claims he had put forward, the more readily that he had decided to retire from business and live upon his inheritance and what capital he had left; for he had no joy of the linen business, and it was going so indifferently that he could not bring himself to put any more money into it. . . . "His spite against our Father brought him no blessing," the Consul thought piously. Probably Gotthold thought so too.

When they got back, he went with his brother up to the breakfast-room; and as both gentlemen felt rather chilly, after standing so long in their dress-coats in the early spring air, they drank a glass of old cognac together. Then Gotthold exchanged a few courteous words with his sister-in-law, stroked the children's heads, and went away. But he appeared at the next " children's day," which took place at the Krögers', outside the Castle Gate. And he began to wind up his business at once.

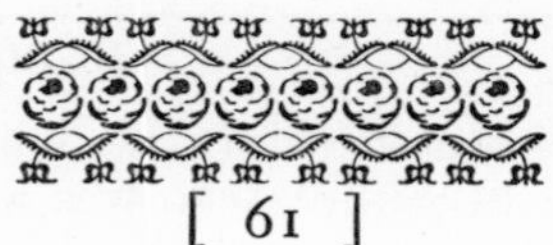

[61]

CHAPTER V

It grieved the Consul sorely that the grandfather had not lived to see the entry of his grandson into the business – an event which took place at Easter-time of the same year.

Thomas had left school at sixteen. He was grown strong and sturdy, and his manly clothes made him look still older. He had been confirmed, and Pastor Kölling, in stentorian tones, had enjoined upon him to practise the virtues of moderation. A gold chain, bequeathed him by his grandfather, now hung about his neck, with the family arms on a medallion at the end – a rather dismal design, showing on an irregularly hatched surface a flat stretch of marshy country with one solitary, leafless willow tree. The old seal ring with the green stone, once worn, in all probability, by the well-to-do tailor in Rostock, had descended to the Consul, together with the great Bible.

Thomas's likeness to his grandfather was as strong as Christian's to his father. The firm round chin was the old man's, and the straight, well-chiselled nose. Thomas wore his hair parted on one side, and it receded in two bays from his narrow veined temples. His eyelashes were colourless by contrast, and so were the eyebrows, one of which he had a habit of lifting expressively. His speech, his movements, even his laugh, which showed his rather defective teeth, were all quiet and adequate. He already looked forward seriously and eagerly to his career.

It was indeed a solemn moment when, after early breakfast, the Consul led him down into the office and introduced him to Herr Marcus the confidential clerk, Herr Havermann the cashier, and the rest of the staff, with all of whom, naturally, he had long been on the best of terms. For the first time he sat at his desk, in his own revolving chair, absorbed in copying, stamping, and arranging papers. In the afternoon his father took him through the magazines on the Trave, each one of which had a special name, like the "Linden," the "Oak," the "Lion," the "Whale." Tom was thoroughly at home in every one of them, of course, but now for the first time he entered them to be formally introduced as a fellow worker.

He entered upon his tasks with devotion, imitating the quiet, tenacious industry of his father, who was working with his jaws set, and writing down many a prayer for help in his private diary. For the Consul had set himself the task of making good the sums paid out by the firm on the occasion of his father's death. It was a conception . . . an ideal. . . . He explained the position quite fully to his wife late one evening in the landscape-room.

It was half-past eleven, and Mamsell Jungmann and the children were already asleep in the corridor rooms. No one slept in the second story now – it was empty save for an occasional guest. The Frau Consul sat on the yellow sofa beside her husband, and he, cigar in mouth, was reading the financial columns of the local paper. She bent over her embroidery, moving her lips as she counted a row of stitches with her needle. Six candles burned in a candelabrum on the slender sewing-table beside her, and the chandelier was unlighted.

Johann Buddenbrook was nearing the middle forties, and had visibly altered in the last years. His little round eyes seemed to have sunk deeper in his head, his cheek-bones and his large aquiline nose stood out more prominently than ever, and the ash-blond hair seemed to have been just touched with a powder-puff where it parted on the temples. The Frau Consul was at the end of her thirties, but, while never beautiful, was as brilliant as ever; her dead-white skin, with a single freckle here and there, had lost none of its splendour, and the candle-light shone on the rich red-blond hair that was as wonderfully dressed as ever. Giving her husband a sidelong glance with her clear blue eyes, she said:

" Jean, I wanted to ask you to consider something: if it would not perhaps be advisable to engage a man-servant. I have just been coming to that conclusion. When I think of my parents – "

The Consul let his paper drop on his knee and took his cigar out of his mouth. A shrewd look came into his eyes: here was a question of money to be paid out.

" My dear Betsy," he said – and he spoke as deliberately as possible, to gain time to muster his excuses – " do you think we need a man-servant? Since my parents' death we have kept on all three maids, not counting Mamsell Jungmann. It seems to me – "

" Oh, but the house is so big, Jean. We can hardly get along as it is. I say to Line, ' Line it's a fearfully long time since the rooms in the annexe were dusted '; but I don't like to drive the girls too hard; they have their work cut out to keep everything clean and tidy here in the front. And a man-servant would be so useful for errands and so on. We could find some honest man from the country, who wouldn't expect much. . . . Oh, before I forget it – Louise Möllendorpf is letting her Anton go. I've seen him serve nicely at table."

"To tell you the truth," said the Consul, and shuffled about a little uneasily, "it is a new idea to me. We aren't either entertaining or going out just now – "

"No, but we have visitors very often – for which I am not responsible, Jean, as you know, though of course I am always glad to see them. You have a business friend from somewhere, and you invite him to dinner. Then he has not taken a room at a hotel, so we ask him to stop the night. A missionary comes, and stops the week with us. Week after next, Pastor Mathias is coming from Kannstadt. And the wages amount to so little – "

"But they mount up, Betsy! We have four people here in the house – and think of the pay-roll the firm has! "

"So we really can't afford a man-servant? " the Frau Consul asked. She smiled as she spoke, and looked at her husband with her head on one side. "When I think of all the servants my Father and Mother had – "

"My dear Betsy! Your parents – I really must ask you if you understand our financial position? "

"No, Jean, I must admit I do not. I'm afraid I have only a vague idea – "

"Well, I can tell you in a few words," the Consul said. He sat up straight on the sofa, with one knee crossed over the other, puffed at his cigar, knit his brows a little, and marshalled his figures with wonderful fluency.

"To put it briefly, my Father had, before my sister's marriage, a round sum of nine hundred thousand marks net, not counting, of course, real estate, and the stock and good will of the firm. Eighty thousand went to Frankfort as dowry, and a hundred thousand to set Gotthold up in business. That leaves seven hundred and twenty thousand. The price of this house, reckoning off what we got for the little one in Alf Street, and counting all the improvements and new furnishings, came to a good hundred thousand. That brings it down to six hundred and twenty thousand. Twenty-five thousand to Frankfort, as compensation on the house, leaves five hundred and ninety-five thousand – which is what we should have had at Father's death if we hadn't partly made up for all these expenses through years, by a profit of some two hundred thousand marks current. The entire capital amounted to seven hundred and ninety-five thousand marks, of which another hundred thousand went to Gotthold, and a few thousand marks for the minor legacies that Father left to the Holy Ghost Hospital, the Fund for Tradesmen's Widows, and so on. That brings us down to around four hundred and twenty thousand, or another hundred thousand with your own dowry. There is the position, in round figures, aside from small fluctuations in the capital. You see, my dear Betsy, we are not rich. And while the capital has grown smaller, the running expenses have not; for the whole business is established on a certain scale, which it costs about so much to maintain. Have you followed me? "

The Consul's wife, her needle-work in her lap, nodded with some hesitation. "Quite so, my dear Jean," she said, though she was far from having understood everything, least of all what these big figures had to do with her engaging a man-servant.

The Consul puffed at his cigar till it glowed, threw back his head and blew out the smoke, and then went on:

"You are thinking, of course, that when God calls your dear parents unto Himself, we shall have a considerable sum to look forward to – and so we shall. But we must not reckon too blindly on it. Your Father has had some heavy losses, due, we all know, to your brother Justus. Justus is certainly a charming personality, but business is not his strong point, and he has had bad luck too. According to all accounts he has had to pay up pretty heavily, and transactions with bankers make dear money. Your Father has come to the rescue several times, to prevent a smash. That sort of thing may happen again – to speak frankly, I am afraid it will. You will forgive me, Betsy, for my plain speaking, but you know that the style of living which is so proper and pleasing in your Father is not at all suitable for a business man. Your Father has nothing to do with business any more; but Justus – you know what I mean – he isn't very careful, is he? His ideas are too large, he is too impulsive. And your parents aren't saving anything. They live a lordly life – as their circumstances permit them to."

The Frau Consul smiled forbearingly. She well knew her husband's opinion of the luxurious Kröger tastes.

"That's all," he said, and put his cigar into the ash-receiver. "As far as I'm concerned, I live in the hope that God will preserve my powers unimpaired, and that by His gracious help I may succeed in reëstablishing the firm on its old basis. . . . I hope you see the thing more clearly now, Betsy? "

"Quite, quite, my dear Jean," the Frau Consul hastened to reply; for she had given up the man-servant, for the evening. " Shall we go to bed? It is very late — "

A few days later, when the Consul came in to dinner in an unusually good mood, they decided at the table to engage the Möllendorpfs' Anton.

CHAPTER VI

"We shall put Tony into Fräulein Weichbrodt's boarding-school," said the Consul. He said it with such decision that so it was.

Thomas was applying himself with talent to the business; Clara was a thriving, lively child; and the appetite of the good Clothilde must have pleased any heart alive. But Tony and Christian were hardly so satisfactory. It was not only that Christian had to stop nearly every afternoon for coffee with Herr Stengel – though even this became at length too much for the Frau Consul, and she sent a dainty missive to the master, summoning him to conference in Meng Street. Herr Stengel appeared in his Sunday wig and his tallest choker, bristling with lead-pencils like lance-heads, and they sat on the sofa in the landscape-room, while Christian hid in the dining-room and listened. The excellent man set out his views, with eloquence if some embarrassment: spoke of the difference between " line " and " dash," told the tale of " The Forest Green " and the scuttle of coals, and made use in every other sentence of the phrase " in consequence." It probably seemed to him a circumlocution suitable to the elegant surroundings in which he found himself. After a while the Consul came and drove Christian away. He expressed to Herr Stengel his lively regret that a son of his should give cause for dissatisfaction. " Oh, Herr Consul, God forbid! Buddenbrook minor has a wide-awake mind, he is a lively chap, and in consequence – Just a little *too* lively, if I might say so; and in consequence – " The Consul politely went with him through the hall to the entry, and Herr Stengel took his leave. . . . Ah, no, this was far from being the worst!

The worst, when it became known, was as follows: Young Christian Buddenbrook had leave one evening to go to the theatre in company with a friend. The performance was Schiller's Wilhelm Tell; and the rôle of Tell's son Walter was played by a young lady, a certain Mademoiselle Meyer-de-la-Grange. Christian's worst, then, had to do with this young person. She wore when on the stage, whether it suited her part or not, a diamond brooch, which was notoriously genuine; for, as everybody knew, it was the gift of young Consul Döhlmann – Peter Döhlmann, son of the deceased wholesale dealer in Wall Street outside Holsten Gate. Consul Peter, like Justus Kröger, belonged to the group of young men whom the town called " fast." His way of life, that is to say, was rather loose! He had married, and had one child, a little daughter; but he had long ago quarrelled with his wife, and he led the life of a bachelor. His father had left him a considerable inheritance, and he carried on the business, after a fashion; but people said he was already living on his capital. He lived mostly at the Club or the Rathskeller, was often to be met somewhere in the street at four o'clock in the morning; and made frequent business trips to Hamburg. Above all, he was a zealous patron of the drama, and took a strong personal interest in the caste. Mademoiselle Meyer-de-la-Grange was the latest of a line of young ladies whom he had, in the past, distinguished by a gift of diamonds.

Well, to arrive at the point, this young lady looked so charming as Walter Tell, wore her brooch and spoke her lines with such effect, that Christian felt his heart swell with enthusiasm, and tears rose to his eyes. He was moved by his transports to a course that only the very violence of emotion could pursue. He ran during the entr'acte to a flower-shop opposite, where, for the sum of one mark eight and a half shillings, he got at a bargain a bunch of flowers; and then this fourteen-year-old sprat, with his big nose and his deep-lying eyes, took his way to the green-room, since nobody stopped him, and came upon Fräulein Meyer-de-la-Grange, talking with Consul Peter Döhlmann at her dressing-room door. Peter Döhlmann nearly fell over with laughing when he saw Christian with the bouquet. But the new wooer, with a solemn face, bowed in his best manner before Walter Tell, handed her the bouquet, and, nodding his head, said in a voice of well-nigh tearful conviction: " Ah, Fräulein, how *beautifully* you act! "

" Well, hang me if it ain't Krishan Buddenbrook! " Consul Döhlmann cried out, in his broadest accent. Fräulein Meyer-de-la-Grange lifted her pretty brows and asked: " The son of Consul Buddenbrook? " And she stroked the cheek of her young admirer with all the favour in the world.

Such was the story that Consul Peter Döhlmann told at the Club that night; it flew about the town like lightning, and reached the ears of the head master, who asked for an audience with Consul Buddenbrook. And how did the Father take this affair? He was, in truth, less angry than overwhelmed. He sat almost like a broken man, after telling the Frau Consul the story in the landscape-room.

"And this is our son," he said. "So is he growing up – "

"But Jean! Good heavens, your Father would have laughed at it. Tell it to my Father and Mother on Thursday – you will see how Papa will enjoy it – "

But here the Consul rose up in anger. "Ah, yes, yes! I am sure he will enjoy it, Betsy. He will be glad to know that his light blood and impious desires live on, not only in a rake like Justus, his own son, but also in a grandson of his as well! Good God, you drive me to say these things! – He goes to this – person; he spends his pocket-money on flowers for this – *lorette!* I don't say he knows what he is doing – yet. But the inclination shows itself – it shows itself, Betsy! "

Ah, yes, this was all very painful indeed. The Consul was perhaps the more beside himself for the added reason that Tony's behaviour, too, had not been of the best. She had given up, it is true, shouting at the nervous stranger to make him dance; and she no longer rang the doorbell of the tiny old woman who sold worsted dolls. But she threw back her head more pertly than ever, and showed, especially after the summer visits with her grandparents, a very strong tendency to vanity and arrogance of spirit.

One day the Consul surprised her and Mamsell Jungmann reading together. The book was Clauren's "Mimili"; the Consul turned over some of the leaves, and then silently closed it – and it was opened no more. Soon afterward it came to light that Tony – Antonie Buddenbrook, no less a person – had been seen walking outside the City wall with a young student, a friend of her brother. Frau Stuht, she who moved in the best circles, had seen the pair, and had remarked at the Möllendorpfs', whither she had gone to buy some cast-off clothing, that really Mademoiselle Buddenbrook was getting to the age where – And Frau Senator Möllendorpf had lightly repeated the story to the Consul. The pleasant strolls came to an end. Later it came out that Fräulein Antonie had made a post-office of the old hollow tree that stood near the Castle Gate, and not only posted therein letters addressed to the same student, but received letters from him as well by that means. When these facts came to light, they seemed to indicate the need of a more watchful oversight over the young lady, now fifteen years old; and she was accordingly, as we have already said, sent to boarding-school at Fräulein Weichbrodt's, Number seven, Millbank.

CHAPTER VII

THERESE WEICHBRODT was humpbacked. So humpbacked that she was not much higher than a table. She was forty-one years old. But as she had never put her faith in outward seeming, she dressed like an old lady of sixty or seventy. Upon her padded grey locks rested a cap the green ribbons of which fell down over shoulders narrow as a child's. Nothing like an ornament ever graced her shabby black frock – only the large oval brooch with her mother's miniature in it.

Little Miss Weichbrodt had shrewd, sharp brown eyes, a slightly hooked nose, and thin lips which she could compress with extraordinary firmness. In her whole insignificant figure, in her every movement, there indwelt a force which was, to be sure, somewhat comic, yet exacted respect. And her mode of speech helped to heighten the effect. She spoke with brisk, jerky motions of the lower jaw and quick, emphatic nods. She used no dialect, but enunciated clearly and with precision, stressing the consonants. Vowel-sounds, however, she exaggerated so much that she said, for instance, " botter " instead of " butter " – or even " batter! " Her little dog that was forever yelping she called Babby instead of Bobby. She would say to a pupil: " Don-n't be so stu-upid, child," and give two quick knocks on the table with her knuckle. It was very impressive – no doubt whatever about that! And when Mlle. Popinet, the Frenchwoman, took too much sugar to her coffee, Miss Weichbrodt had a way of gazing at the ceiling and drumming on the cloth with one hand while she said: " Why not take the who-ole sugar-basin? I would! " It always made Mlle. Popinet redden furiously.

As a child – heavens, what a tiny child she must have been! – Therese Weichbrodt had given herself the nickname of Sesemi, and she still kept it, even letting the best and most favoured of the day- as well as of the boarding-pupils use it. " Call me Sesemi, child," she said on the first day to Tony Buddenbrook, kissing her briefly, with a sound as of a small explosion, on the forehead. " I like it." Her elder sister, however, Madame Kethelsen, was called Nelly.

Madame Kethelsen was about forty-eight years old. She had been left penniless when her husband died, and now lived in a little upstairs bedroom in her sister's house. She dressed like Sesemi, but by contrast was very tall. She wore woollen wristlets on her thin wrists. She was not a mistress, and knew nothing of discipline. A sort of inoffensive and placid cheerfulness was all her being. When one of the pupils played a prank, she would laugh so heartily that she nearly cried, and then Sesemi would rap on the table and call out "Nelly!" very sharply – it sounded like "Nally" – and Madame Kethelsen would shrink into herself and be mute.

Madame Kethelsen obeyed her younger sister, who scolded her as if she were a child. Sesemi, in fact, despised her warmly. Therese Weichbrodt was a well-read, almost a literary woman. She struggled endlessly to keep her childhood faith, her religious assurance that somewhere in the beyond she was to be recompensed for the hard, dull present. But Madame Kethelsen, innocent, uninstructed, was all simplicity of nature. "Dear, good Nelly, what a child she is! She never doubts or struggles, she is always happy." In such remarks there was always as much contempt as envy. Contempt was a weakness of Sesemi's – perhaps a pardonable one.

The small red-brick suburban house was surrounded by a neatly kept garden. Its lofty ground floor was entirely taken up by schoolrooms and dining-room; the bedrooms were in the upper story and the attic. Miss Weichbrodt did not have a large number of pupils. As boarders she received only older girls, while the day-school consisted of but three classes, the lowest ones. Sesemi took care to have only the daughters of irreproachably refined families in her house. Tony Buddenbrook, as we have seen, she welcomed most tenderly. She even made "bishop" for supper – a sort of sweet red punch to be taken cold, in the making of which she was a past mistress. "A little more beeshop," she urged with a hearty nod. It sounded so tempting; nobody could resist!

Fräulein Weichbrodt sat on two sofa-cushions at the top of the table and presided over the meal with tact and discretion. She held her stunted figure stiffly erect, tapped vigilantly on the table, cried "Nally" or "Babby," and subdued Mlle. Popinet with a glance whenever the latter seemed about to take unto herself all the cold veal jelly. Tony had been allotted a place between two other boarders, Armgard von Schilling, the strapping blond daughter of a Mecklenburg landowner, and Gerda Arnoldsen, whose home was in Amsterdam – an unusual, elegant figure, with dark red hair, brown eyes close together, and a lovely, pale, haughty face. Opposite her sat a chattering French girl who looked like a negress, with huge gold earrings. The lean English Miss Brown, with her sourish smile, sat at the bottom of the table. She was a boarder too.

It was not hard, with the help of Sesemi's bishop, to get acquainted. Mlle. Popinet had had nightmares again last night — *ah, quel horreur!* She usually screamed " Help, thieves; help, thieves! " until everybody jumped out of bed. Next, it appeared that Gerda Arnoldsen did not take piano like the rest of them, but the violin, and that Papa — her Mother was dead — had promised her a real Stradivarius. Tony was not musical — hardly any of the Buddenbrooks and none of the Krögers were. She could not even recognize the chorals they played at St. Mary's. — Oh, the organ in the new Church at Amsterdam had a *vox humana* — a human voice — that was just wonderful. Armgard von Schilling talked about the cows at home.

It was Armgard who from the earliest moment had made a great impression on Tony. She was the first person from a noble family whom Tony had ever known. What luck, to be called *von* Schilling! Her own parents had the most beautiful old house in the town, and her grandparents belonged to the best families; still, they were called plain Buddenbrook and Kröger — which was a pity, to be sure. The granddaughter of the proud Lebrecht Kröger glowed with reverence for Armgard's noble birth. Privately, she sometimes thought that the splendid " von " went with her better than it did with Armgard; for Armgard did not appreciate her good luck, dear, no! She had a thick pigtail, good-natured blue eyes, and a broad Mecklenburg accent, and went about thinking just nothing at all on the subject. She made absolutely no pretensions to being aristocratic; in fact, she did not know what it was. But the word " aristocratic " stuck in Tony's small head; and she emphatically applied it to Gerda Arnoldsen.

Gerda was rather exclusive, and had something foreign and queer about her. She liked to do up her splendid red hair in striking ways, despite Sesemi's protests. Some of the girls thought it was " silly " of her to play the violin instead of the piano — and, be it known, " silly " was a term of very severe condemnation. Still, the girls mostly agreed with Tony that Gerda was artistocratic — in her figure, well-developed for her years; in her ways, her small possessions, everything. There was the ivory toilet set from Paris, for instance; that Tony could appreciate, for her own parents and grandparents also had treasures which had been brought from Paris.

The three girls soon made friends. They were in the same class and slept together in the same large room at the top of the house. What delightful, cosy times they had going to bed! They gossiped while they undressed – in undertones, however, for it was ten o'clock and next door Mlle. Popinet had gone to bed to dream of burglars. Eva Ewers slept with her. Eva was a little Hamburger, whose father, an amateur painter and collector, had settled in Munich.

The striped brown blinds were down, the low, red-shaded lamp burned on the table, there was a faint smell of violets and fresh wash, and a delicious atmosphere of laziness and dreams.

"Heavens," said Armgard, half undressed, sitting on her bed, "how Dr. Newmann can talk! He comes into the class and stands by the table and tells about Racine – "

"He has a lovely high forehead," remarked Gerda, standing before the mirror between the windows and combing her hair by the light of two candles.

"Oh, yes, hasn't he? " Armgard said eagerly.

"And you are taking the course just on his account, Armgard; you gaze at him all the time with your blue eyes, as if – "

"Are you in love with him? " asked Tony. "I can't undo my shoe-lace; please, Gerda. Thanks. Why don't you marry him? He is a good match – he will get to be a High School Professor."

"I think you are both horrid. I'm not in love with him, and I would not marry a teacher, anyhow. I shall marry a country gentleman."

"A nobleman? " Tony dropped her stocking and looked thoughtfully into Armgard's face.

"I don't know, yet. But he must have a large estate. Oh, girls, I just love that sort of thing! I shall get up at five o'clock every morning, and attend to everything. . . ." She pulled up the bed-covers and stared dreamily at the ceiling.

"Five hundred cows are before your mind's eye," said Gerda, looking at her in the mirror.

Tony was not ready yet; but she let her head fall on the pillow, tucked her hands behind her neck, and gazed dreamily at the ceiling in her turn.

"Of course," she said, "I shall marry a business man. He must have a lot of money, so we can furnish elegantly. I owe that to my family and the firm," she added earnestly. "Yes, you'll see, that's what I shall do."

Gerda had finished her hair for the night and was brushing her big white teeth, using the ivory-backed hand-mirror to see them better.

"I shall *probably* not marry at all," she said, speaking with some difficulty on account of the tooth-powder. "I don't see why I should. I am not anxious. I'll go back to Amsterdam and play duets with Daddy and afterwards live with my married sister."

"What a pity," Tony said briskly. "What a pity! You ought to marry here and stay here for always. Listen: you could marry one of my brothers – "

"The one with the big nose?" asked Gerda, and gave a dainty little yawn, holding the hand-mirror before her face.

"Or the other; it doesn't matter. You could furnish beautifully. Jacobs could do it – the upholsterer in Fish Street. He has lovely taste. I'd come to see you every day – "

But then there came the voice of Mlle. Popinet. It said: "Oh, mesdemoiselles! Please go to bed. It is too late to get married any more this evening!"

Sundays and holidays Tony spent in Meng Street or outside the town with her grandparents. How lovely, when it was fine on Easter Sunday, hunting for eggs and marzipan hares in the enormous Kröger garden! Then there were the summer holidays at the seashore; they lived in the Kurhaus, ate at the table-d'hôte, bathed, and went donkey-riding. Some seasons when the Consul had business, there were long journeys. But Christmases were best of all. There were three present-givings: at home, at the grandparents', and at Sesemi's, where bishop flowed in streams. The one at home was the grandest, for the Consul believed in keeping the holy feast with pomp and ceremony. They gathered in the landscape-room with due solemnity. The servants and the crowd of poor people thronged into the pillared hall, where the Consul went about shaking their purple hands. Then outside rose the voices of the choir-boys from St. Mary's in a quartette, and one's heart beat loudly with awe and expectation. The smell of the Christmas tree was already coming through the crack in the great white folding doors; and the Frau Consul took the old family Bible with the funny big letters, and slowly read aloud the Christmas chapter; and after the choir-boys had sung another carol, everybody joined in "O Tannenbaum" and went in solemn procession through the hall into the great salon, hung with tapestries that had statuary woven into them. There the tree rose to the ceiling, decorated with white lilies, twinkling and sparkling and pouring out light and fragrance; and the table with the presents on it stretched from the windows to the door. Outside, the Italians with the barrel-organ were making music in the frozen, snowy streets, and a great hubbub came over from the Christmas market in Market

Square. All the children except little Clara stopped up to late supper in the salon, and there were mountains of carp and stuffed turkey.

In these years Tony Buddenbrook visited two Mecklenburg estates. She stopped for two weeks one summer with her friend Armgard, on Herr von Schilling's property, which lay on the coast across the bay from Travemünde. And another time she went with Cousin Tilda to a place where Bernard Buddenbrook was inspector. This estate was called " Thankless," because it did not bring in a penny's income; but for a summer holiday it was not to be despised.

Thus the years went on. It was, take it all in all, a happy youth for Tony.

PART THREE

CHAPTER I

On a June afternoon, not long after five o'clock, the family were sitting before the " portal " in the garden, where they had drunk coffee. They had pulled the rustic furniture outside, for it was too close in the white-washed garden house, with its tall mirror decorated with painted birds and its varnished folding doors, which were really not folding doors at all and had only painted latches.

The Consul, his wife, Tony, Tom, and Clothilde sat in a half-circle around the table, which was laid with its usual shining service. Christian, sitting a little to one side, conned the second oration of Cicero against Catiline. He looked unhappy. The Consul smoked his cigar and read the *Advertiser*. His wife had let her embroidery fall into her lap and sat smiling at little Clara; the child, with Ida Jungmann, was looking for violets in the grass-plot. Tony, her head propped on both hands, was deep in Hoffman's " Serapion Brethren," while Tom tickled her in the back of the neck with a grass-blade, an attention which she very wisely ignored. And Clothilde, looking thin and old-maidish in her flowered cotton frock, was reading a story called " Blind, Deaf, Dumb, and Still Happy." As she read, she scraped up the biscuit-crumbs carefully with all five fingers from the cloth and ate them.

A few white clouds stood motionless in the slowly paling sky. The small town garden, with its carefully laid-out paths and beds, looked gay and tidy in the afternoon sun. The scent of the mignonette borders floated up now and then.

" Well, Tom," said the Consul expansively, and took the cigar out of his mouth, " we are arranging that rye sale I told you about, with van Henkdom and Company."

" What is he giving? " Tom asked with interest, ceasing to tickle Tony.

" Sixty thaler for a thousand kilo – not bad, eh? "

" That's very good." Tom knew this was excellent business.

" Tony, your position is not *comme il faut*," remarked the Frau Consul. Whereat Tony, without raising her eyes from her book, took one elbow off the table.

" Never mind," Tom said. " She can sit how she likes, she will always be Tony Buddenbrook. Tilda and she are certainly the beauties of the family."

Clothilde was astonished almost to death. "Good gracious, Tom," she said. It was inconceivable how she could drawl out the syllables. Tony bore the jeer in silence. It was never any use, Tom was more than a match for her. He could always get the last word and have the laugh on his side. Her nostrils dilated a little, and she shrugged her shoulders. But when the Consul's wife began to talk of the coming dance at the house of Consul Huneus, and let fall something about new patent leather shoes, Tony took the other elbow off the table and displayed a lively interest.

"You keep talking and talking," complained Christian fretfully, "and I'm having such a hard time. I wish I were a business man."

"Yes, you're always wanting something different," said Tom. Anton came across the garden with a card on his tray. They all looked at him expectantly.

"Grünlich, Agent," read the Consul. "He is from Hamburg – an agreeable man, and well recommended, the son of a clergyman. I have business dealings with him. There is a piece of business now. – Is it all right, Betsy, if I ask him to come out here?"

A middle-sized man, his head thrust a little forward of his body, carrying his hat and stick in one hand, came across the garden. He was some two-and-thirty years old; he wore a fuzzy greenish-yellow suit with a long-skirted coat, and grey worsted gloves. His face, beneath the sparse light hair, was rosy and smiling; but there was an undeniable wart on one side of his nose. His chin and upper lip were smooth-shaven; he wore long, drooping side-whiskers, in the English fashion, and these adornments were conspicuously golden-yellow in colour. Even at a distance, he began making obsequious gestures with his broad-brimmed grey hat, and as he drew near he took one last very long step, and arrived describing a half-circle with the upper part of his body, by this means bowing to them all at once.

"I am afraid I am disturbing the family circle," he said in a soft voice, with the utmost delicacy of manner. "You are conversing, you are indulging in literary pursuits – I must really beg your pardon for my intrusion."

"By no means, my dear Herr Grünlich," said the Consul. He and his sons got up and shook hands with the stranger. "You are very welcome. I am delighted to see you outside the office and in my family circle. Herr Grünlich, Betsy – a friend of mine and a keen man of business. This is my daughter Antonie, and my niece

Clothilde. Thomas you know already, and this is my second son, Christian, in High School." Herr Grünlich responded to each name with an inclination of the body.

"I must repeat," he said, "that I have no desire to intrude. I came on business. If the Herr Consul would be so good as to take a walk with me round the gardens – " The Consul's wife answered: "It will give us pleasure to have you sit down with us for a little before you begin to talk business with my husband. Do sit down."

"A thousand thanks," said Herr Grünlich, apparently quite flattered. He sat down on the edge of the chair which Tom brought, laid his hat and stick on his knees, and settled himself, running his hand over his long beard with a little hemming and hawing, as if to say, "Well, now we've got past the introduction – what next? "

The Frau Consul began the conversation. "You live in Hamburg? " she asked, inclining her head and letting her work fall into her lap.

"Yes, Frau Consul," responded Herr Grünlich with a fresh bow. "At least, my house is in Hamburg, but I am on the road a good deal. My business is very flourishing – ahem – if I may be permitted to say so."

The Frau Consul lifted her eyebrows and made respectful motions with her mouth, as if she were saying "Ah – indeed? "

"Ceaseless activity is a condition of my being," added he, half turning to the Consul. He coughed again as he noticed that Fräulein Antonie's glance rested upon him. She gave him, in fact, the cold, calculating stare with which a maiden measures a strange young man – a stare which seems always on the point of passing over into actual contempt.

"We have relatives in Hamburg," said she, in order to be saying something.

"The Duchamps," explained the Consul. "The family of my late Mother."

"Oh, yes," Herr Grünlich hastened to say. "I have the honour of a slight acquaintance with the family. They are very fine people, in mind and heart. Ahem! This would be a better world if there were more families like them in it. They have religion, benevolence, and genuine piety; in short, they are my ideal of the true Christlike spirit. And in them it is united to a rare degree with a brilliant cosmopolitanism, an elegance, an aristocratic bearing, which I find most attractive, Frau Consul."

Tony thought: "How can he know my Father and Mother so

well? He is saying exactly what they like best to hear." The Consul responded approvingly, "The combination is one that is becoming in everybody." And the Frau Consul could not resist stretching out her hand to their guest with her sweeping gesture, palm upward, while the bracelets gave a little jingle. "You speak as though you read my inmost thoughts, dear Herr Grünlich," she said.

Upon which, Herr Grünlich made another deep bow, settled himself again, stroked his beard, and coughed as if to say: "Well, let us get on."

The Frau Consul mentioned the disastrous fire which had swept Hamburg in May of the year 1842. "Yes, indeed," said Herr Grünlich, "truly a fearful misfortune. A distressing visitation. The loss amounted to one hundred and thirty-five millions, at a rough estimate. I am grateful to Providence that I came off without any loss whatever. The fire raged chiefly in the parishes of St. Peter and St. Nicholas. – What a charming garden!" he interrupted himself, taking the cigar which the Consul offered. "It is so large for a town garden, and the beds of colour are magnificent. I confess my weakness for flowers, and for nature in general. Those climbing roses over there trim up the garden uncommonly well." He went on, praising the refinement of the location, praising the town itself, praising the Consul's cigar. He had a pleasant word for each member of the circle.

"May I venture to inquire what you are reading, Fräulein Antonie?" he said smiling.

Tony drew her brows together sharply at this, for some reason, and answered without looking at him, "Hoffmann's 'Serapion Brethren.'"

"Really! He is a wonderful writer, is he not? Ah, pardon me – I forgot the name of your younger son, Frau Consul?"

"Christian."

"A beautiful name. If I may so express myself" – here he turned again to the Consul – "I like best the names which show that the bearer is a Christian. The name of Johann, I know, is hereditary in your family – a name which always recalls the beloved disciple. My own name – if I may be permitted to mention it," he continued, waxing eloquent, "is that of most of my forefathers – Bendix. It can only be regarded as a shortened form of Benedict. And you, Herr Buddenbrook, are reading – ? ah, Cicero. The works of this great Roman orator make pretty difficult reading, eh? '*Quousque tandem – Catilina*' . . . ahem. Oh, I have not forgotten quite all my Latin."

"I disagree with my late Father on this point," the Consul said. "I have always objected to the perpetual occupation of young heads with Greek and Latin. When there are so many other important subjects, necessary as a preparation for the practical affairs of life – "

"You take the words out of my mouth," Herr Grünlich hastened to say. "It is hard reading, and not by any means always unexceptionable – I forgot to mention that point. Everything else aside, I can recall passages that were positively offensive – "

There came a pause, and Tony thought "Now it's my turn." Herr Grünlich had turned his gaze upon her. And, sure enough: he suddenly started in his chair, made a spasmodic but always highly elegant gesture toward the Frau Consul and whispered ardently, "Pray look, Frau Consul, I beg of you. – Fräulein, I implore you," he interrupted himself aloud, just as if Tony could not hear the rest of what he said, "to keep in that same position for just a moment. Do you see," he began whispering again, "how the sunshine is playing in your daughter's hair? Never," he said solemnly, as if transported, speaking to nobody in particular, "have I seen more beautiful hair." It was as if he were addressing his remarks to God or to his own soul.

The Consul's wife smiled, well pleased. The Consul said, "Don't be putting notions into the girl's head." And again Tony drew her brows together without speaking. After a short pause, Herr Grünlich got up.

"But I won't disturb you any longer now – no, Frau Consul, I refuse to disturb you any longer," he repeated. "I only came on business, but I could not resist – indeed, who could resist you? Now duty calls. May I ask the Consul – "

"I hope I do not need to assure you that it would give us pleasure if you would let us put you up while you are here," said the Frau Consul. Herr Grünlich appeared for the moment struck dumb with gratitude. "From my soul I am grateful, Frau Consul," he said, and his look was indeed eloquent with emotion. "But I must not abuse your kindness. I have a couple of rooms at the City of Hamburg – "

"A *couple* of rooms," thought the Frau Consul – which was just what Herr Grünlich meant her to think.

"And, in any case," he said, as she offered her hand cordially, "I hope we have not seen each other for the last time." He kissed her hand, waited a moment for Antonie to extend hers – which she did not do – described another half-circle with his upper torso, made a long step backward and another bow, threw back his head and put his hat on with a flourish, then walked away in company with the Consul.

"A pleasant man," the Father said later, when he came back and took his place again.

"I think he's silly," Tony permitted herself to remark with some emphasis.

"Tony! Heavens and earth, what an idea!" said the Consul's wife, displeased. "Such a Christian young man!"

"So well brought up, and so cosmopolitan," went on the Consul. "You don't know what you are talking about." He and his wife had a way of taking each other's side like this, out of sheer politeness. It made them the more likely to agree.

Christian wrinkled up his long nose and said, "He was so important. 'You are conversing' – when we weren't at all. And the roses over there 'trim things up uncommonly.' He acted some of the time as if he were talking to himself. 'I am disturbing you' – 'I beg pardon' – 'I have never seen more beautiful hair.'" Christian mocked Herr Grünlich so cleverly that they all had to laugh, even the Consul.

"Yes, he gave himself too many airs," Tony went on. "He talked the whole time about himself – *his* business is good, and *he* is fond of nature, and *he* likes such-and-such names, and *his* name is Bendix – what is all that to us, I'd like to know? Everything he said was just to spread himself." Her voice was growing louder all the time with vexation. "He said all the very things you like to hear, Mamma and Papa, and he said them just to make a fine impression on you both."

"That is no reproach, Tony," the Consul said sternly. "Everybody puts his best foot foremost before strangers. We all take care to say what will be pleasant to hear. That is a commonplace."

"I think he is a good man," Clothilde pronounced with drawling serenity – she was the only person in the circle about whom Herr Grünlich had not troubled himself at all. Thomas refrained from giving an opinion.

"Enough," concluded the Consul. "He is a capable, cultured, and energetic Christian man, and you, Tony, should try to bridle your tongue – a great girl of eighteen or nineteen years old, like you! And after he was so polite and gallant to you, too. We are all weak creatures; and you, let me say, are one of the last to have a right to throw stones. Tom, we'll get to work."

Pert little Tony muttered to herself "A golden goat's beard!" and scowled as before.

CHAPTER II

Tony, coming back from a walk some days later, met Herr Grünlich at the corner of Meng Street. "I was most grieved to have missed you, Fräulein," he said. "I took the liberty of paying my respects to your Mother the other day, and I regretted your absence more than I can say. How delightful that I should meet you like this!"

Fräulein Buddenbrook had paused as he began to speak; but her half-shut eyes looked no further up than the height of Herr Grünlich's chest. On her lips rested the mocking, merciless smile with which a young girl measures and rejects a man. Her lips moved – what should she say? It must be something that would demolish this Herr Bendix Grünlich once and for all – simply annihilate him. It must be clever, witty, and effective, must at one and the same time wound him to the quick and impress him tremendously.

"The pleasure is not mutual, Herr Grünlich," said she, keeping her gaze meanwhile levelled at his chest. And after she had shot this poisoned arrow, she left him standing there and went home, her head in the air, her face red with pride in her own powers of repartee – to learn that Herr Grünlich had been invited to dinner next Sunday.

And he came. He came in a not quite new-fashioned, rather wrinkled, but still handsome bell-shaped frock coat which gave him a solid, respectable look. He was rosy and smiling, his scant hair carefully parted, his whiskers curled and scented. He ate a ragout of shell-fish, julienne soup, fried soles, roast veal with creamed potatoes and cauliflower, maraschino pudding, and pumpernickel with roquefort; and he found a fresh and delicate compliment for each fresh course. Over the sweet he lifted his dessert-spoon, gazed at one of the tapestry statues, and spoke aloud to himself, thus: "God forgive me, I have eaten far too well already. But this pudding – ! It is *too* wonderful! I must beg my good hostess for another slice." And he looked roguishly at the Consul's wife. With the Consul he talked business and politics, and spoke soundly and weightily. He discussed the theatre and the fashions with the Frau Consul, and he had a good word for Tom and Christian and Clothilde, and even for little Clara and Ida Jungmann. Tony sat in silence, and he did not undertake to engage her; only gazing at her now and then, with his head a little tilted, his face looking dejected and encouraged by turns.

When Herr Grünlich took his leave that evening, he had only strengthened the impressions left by his first visit. " A thoroughly well-bred man," said the Frau Consul. " An estimable Christian gentleman," was the Consul's opinion. Christian imitated his speech and actions even better than before; and Tony said her good nights to them all with a frowning brow, for something told her that she had not yet seen the last of this gentleman who had won the hearts of her parents with such astonishing ease and rapidity.

And, sure enough, coming back one afternoon from a visit with some girl friends, she found Herr Grünlich cosily established in the landscape-room, reading aloud to the Frau Consul out of Sir Walter Scott's "Waverley." His pronunciation was perfect, for, as he explained, his business trips had taken him to England. Tony sat down apart with another book, and Herr Grünlich softly questioned: " Our book is not to your taste, Fräulein? " To which she replied, with her head in the air, something in a sarcastic vein, like " Not in the very least."

But he was not taken aback. He began to talk about his long-dead parents and communicated the fact that his father had been a clergyman, a Christian, and at the same time a highly cosmopolitan gentleman. – After this visit, he departed for Hamburg. Tony was not there when he called to take leave. " Ida," she said to Mamsell Jungmann, " Ida, the man has gone." But Mamsell Jungmann only replied, " You'll see, child."

And eight days later, in fact, came that scene in the breakfast room. Tony came down at nine o'clock and found her father and mother still at table. She let her forehead be kissed and sat down, fresh and hungry, her eyes still red with sleep, and helped herself to sugar, butter, and herb cheese.

" How nice to find you still here, for once, Papa," she said as she held her egg in her napkin and opened it with her spoon.

" But to-day I have been waiting for our slug-a-bed," said the Consul. He was smoking and tapping on the table with his folded newspaper. His wife finished her breakfast with her slow, graceful motions, and leaned back in the sofa.

" Tilda is already busy in the kitchen," went on the Consul, " and I should have been long since at work myself, if your Mother and I had not been speaking seriously about a matter that concerns our little daughter."

Tony, her mouth full of bread and butter, looked first at her father and then her mother, with a mixture of fear and curiosity.

"Eat your breakfast, my child," said the Frau Consul. But Tony laid down her knife and cried, "Out with it quickly, Papa – please." Her father only answered: "Eat your breakfast first."

So Tony drank her coffee and ate her egg and bread and cheese silently, her appetite quite gone. She began to guess. The fresh morning bloom disappeared from her cheek, and she even grew a little pale. She said "Thank you" for the honey, and soon after announced in a subdued voice that she had finished.

"My dear child," said the Consul, "the matter we desire to talk over with you is contained in this letter." He was tapping the table now with a big blue envelope instead of the newspaper. "To be brief: Bendix Grünlich, whom we have learned, during his short stay here, to regard as a good and a charming man, writes to me that he has conceived a strong inclination for our daughter, and he here makes a request in form for her hand. What does my child say?"

Tony was leaning back in her seat, her head bent, her right hand slowly twirling the silver napkin-ring round and round. But suddenly she looked up, and her eyes had grown quite dark with tears. She said, her voice full of distress: "What does this man want of me? What have I done to him?" And she burst into weeping.

The Consul shot a glance at his wife and then regarded his empty cup, embarrassed.

"Tony dear," said the Frau Consul gently, "why this – *échauffement?* You know quite well your parents can only desire your good. And they cannot counsel you to reject forthwith the position offered you. I know you feel so far no particular inclination for Herr Grünlich, but that will come; I assure you it comes, with time. Such a young thing as you is never sure what she wants. The mind is as confused as the heart. One must just give the heart time – and keep the mind open to the advice of experienced people who think and plan only for our good."

"I don't know him the least little bit," Tony said in a dejected tone, wiping her eyes on the little white batiste serviette, stained with egg. "All I know is, he has a yellow beard, like a goat's, and a flourishing business –" Her upper lip, trembling on the verge of tears, had an expression that was indescribably touching.

With a movement of sudden tenderness the Consul jerked his chair nearer hers and stroked her hair, smiling.

"My little Tony, what should you like to know of him? You are still a very young girl, you know. You would know him no better if he had been here for fifty-two weeks instead of four. You are a child, with no eyes yet for the world, and you must trust other people who mean well by you."

"I don't understand – I don't understand," Tony sobbed helplessly, and put down her head as a kitten does beneath the hand that strokes it. "He comes here and says something pleasant to everybody, and then goes away again; and then he writes to you that he – that I – I don't understand. What made him? What have I done to him?"

The Consul smiled again. "You said that once before, Tony; and it illustrates so well your childish way of reasoning. My little daughter must not feel that people mean to urge or torment her. We can consider it all very quietly; in fact, we must consider it all very quietly and calmly, for it is a very serious matter. Meanwhile I will write an answer to Herr Grünlich's letter, without either consenting or refusing. There is much to be thought of. – Well, is that agreed? What do you say? – And now Papa can go back to his work, can't he? – Adieu, Betsy."

"Au revoir, dear Jean."

"Do take a little more honey, Tony," said the Frau Consul to her daughter, who sat in her place motionless, with her head bent. "One must eat."

Tony's tears gradually dried. Her head felt hot and heavy with her thoughts. Good gracious, what a business! She had always known, of course, that she should one day marry, and be the wife of a business man, and embark upon a solid and advantageous married life, commensurate with the position of the family and the firm. But suddenly, for the first time in her life, somebody, some actual person, in serious earnest, wanted to marry her. How did people act? To her, her, Tony Buddenbrook, were now applicable all those tremendous words and phrases which she had hitherto met with only in books: her "hand," her "consent," "as long as life shall last!" Goodness gracious, what a step to take, all at once!

"And you, Mamma? Do you too advise me to – to – to yield my consent?" She hesitated a little before the "yield my consent." It sounded high-flown and awkward. But then, this was the first occasion in her life that was worthy of fine language. She began to blush for her earlier lack of self-control. It seemed to her now not less unreasonable than it had ten minutes ago that she should marry Herr Grünlich; but the dignity of her situation began to fill her with a sense of importance which was satisfying indeed.

"*I* advise you to accept, my child? Has Papa advised you to do so? He has only not advised you not to, that is all. It would be very irresponsible of either of us to do that. The connection offered you is a very good one, my dear Tony. You would go to Hamburg on an excellent footing and live there in great style."

Tony sat motionless. She was having a sort of vision of silk portières, like those in grandfather's salon. And, as Madame Grünlich, should she drink morning chocolate? She thought it would not be seemly to ask.

"As your Father says, you have time to consider," the Frau Consul continued. "But we are obliged to tell you that such an offer does not come every day, that it would make your fortune, and that it is exactly the marriage which duty and vocation prescribe. This, my child, it is my business to tell you. You know yourself that the path which opens before you to-day is the prescribed one which your life ought to follow."

"Yes," Tony said thoughtfully. She was well aware of her responsibilities toward the family and the firm, and she was proud of them. She was saturated with her family history – she, Tony Buddenbrook, who, as the daughter of Consul Buddenbrook, went about the town like a little queen, before whom Matthiesen the porter took off his hat and made a low bow! The Rostock tailor had been very well off, to begin with; but since his time, the family fortunes had advanced by leaps and bounds. It was her vocation to enhance the brilliance of family and firm in her allotted way, by making a rich and aristocratic marriage. To the same end, Tom worked in the office. Yes, the marriage was undoubtedly precisely the right one. But – but – She saw him before her, saw his gold-yellow whiskers, his rosy, smiling face, the wart on his nose, his mincing walk. She could feel his woolly suit, hear his soft voice. . . .

"I felt sure," the Consul's wife said, "that we were accessible to quiet reason. Have we perhaps already made up our mind?"

"Oh, goodness, *no!*" cried Tony, suddenly. She uttered the "Oh" with an outburst of irritation. "What nonsense! Why should I marry him? I have always made fun of him. I never did anything else. I can't understand how he can possibly endure me. The man must have some sort of pride in his bones!" She began to drip honey upon a slice of bread.

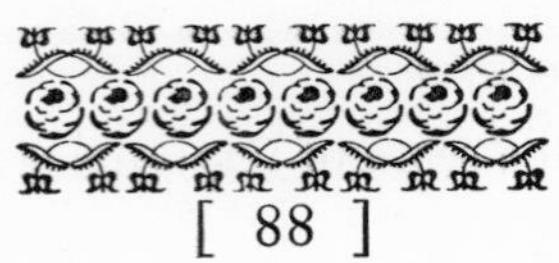

CHAPTER III

This year the Buddenbrooks took no holiday during Christian's and Clara's vacation. The Consul said he was too busy; but it was Tony's unsettled affair as well, that kept them lingering in Mengstrasse. A very diplomatic letter, written by the Consul himself, had been dispatched to Herr Grünlich; but the progress of the wooing was hindered by Tony's obstinacy. She expressed herself in the most childish way. " Heaven forbid, Mamma," she would say. " I simply can't en*dure* him! " with tremendous emphasis on the second syllable. Or she would explain solemnly, " Father " (Tony never otherwise said anything but " Papa "), " I can never yield him my consent."

And at this point the matter would assuredly have stuck, had it not been for events that occurred some ten days after the talk in the breakfast-room – in other words, about the middle of July.

It was afternoon – a hot blue afternoon. The Frau Consul was out, and Tony sat with a book alone at the window of the landscape room, when Anton brought her a card. Before she had time to read the name, a young man in a bell-skirted coat and pea-green pantaloons entered the room. It was, of course, Herr Grünlich, with an expression of imploring tenderness upon his face.

Tony started up indignantly and made a movement to flee into the next room. How could one possibly talk to a man who had proposed for one's hand? Her heart was in her throat and she had gone very pale. While he had been at a safe distance she had hugely enjoyed the solemn conferences with her Father and Mother and the suddenly enhanced importance of her own person and destiny. But now, here he was – he stood before her. What was going to happen? And again she felt that she was going to weep.

At a rapid stride, his head tipped on one side, his arms outstretched, with the air of a man who says: " Here I am, kill me if you will! " he approached. " What a providence! " he cried. " I find you here, Antonie – " (He said " Antonie "!)

Tony stood erect, her novel in her right hand. She stuck out her lips and gave her head a series of little jerks upward, relieving her irritation by stressing, in that manner, each word as she spoke it. She got out: "What is the matter with you?" – But the tears were already rising. And Herr Grünlich's own excitement was too great for him to realize the check.

"How could I wait longer? Was I not driven to return?" he said in impassioned tones. "A week ago I had your Father's letter, which filled me with hope. I could bear it no longer. Could I thus linger on in half-certainty? I threw myself into a carriage, I hastened hither, I have taken a couple of rooms at the City of Hamburg – and here I am, Antonie, to hear from your lips the final word which will make me happier than I can express."

Tony was stunned. Her tears retreated abashed. This, then, was the effect of her Father's careful letter, which had indefinitely postponed the decision. Two or three times she stammered: "You are mistaken – you are mistaken."

Herr Grünlich had drawn an arm-chair close to her seat in the window. He sat down, he obliged her to sit as well, and, bowing over her hand, which, limp with indecision, she resigned to him, he went on in a trembling voice: "Fräulein Antonie, since first I saw you, that afternoon, – do you remember that afternoon, when I saw you, a vision of loveliness, in your own family circle? – Since then, your name has been indelibly written on my heart." He went back, corrected himself, and said "graven": "Since that day, Fräulein Antonie, it has been my only, my most ardent wish, to win your beautiful hand. What your Father's letter permitted me only to hope, that I implore you to confirm to me now in all certainty. I may feel sure of your consent – I may be assured of it?" He took her other hand in his and looked deep into her wide-open, frightened eyes. He had left off his worsted gloves to-day, and his hands were long and white, marked with blue veins. Tony stared at his pink face, at his wart, at his eyes, which were as blue as a goose's.

"Oh, no, no," she broke out, rapidly, in terror. And then she added, "No, I will never yield my consent." She took great pains to speak firmly, but she was already in tears.

"How have I deserved this doubt and hesitation?" he asked in a lower, well-nigh reproachful tone. "I know you are a maiden cherished and sheltered by the most loving care. But I swear to you, I pledge you my word of honour as a man, that I would carry you in my arms, that as my wife you would lack nothing, that you would live in Hamburg a life altogether worthy of you –"

Tony sprang up. She freed her hand and, with the tears rolling down her cheeks, cried out in desperation, " No, no! I said *no!* I am refusing you – for heaven's sake, can't you understand? " Then Herr Grünlich rose up too. He took one backward step and stretched out his arms toward her, palms up. Seriously, like a man of honour and resolution, he spoke.

" Mademoiselle Buddenbrook, you understand that I cannot permit myself to be insulted? "

" But I am not insulting you, Herr Grünlich," said Tony, repenting her brusqueness. Oh, dear, oh dear, *why* did all this have to happen to her? Such a wooing as this she had never imagined. She had supposed that one only had to say: " Your offer does me great honour, but I cannot accept it," and that would be an end of the matter. " Your offer does me great honour," she said, as calmly as she could, " but I cannot accept it. And now I must go; please excuse me – I am busy – " But Herr Grünlich stood in front of her.

" You reject me? " he said gloomily.

" Yes," Tony said; adding with tact, " unfortunately."

Herr Grünlich gave a gusty sigh. He took two big steps backward, bent his torso to one side, pointed with his forefinger to the carpet and said in an awful voice: " Antonie! " Thus for the space of a moment they stood, he in a posture of commanding rage, Tony pale, weepy, and trembling, her damp handkerchief to her mouth. Then he turned from her and, with his hands on his back, measured the room twice through, as if he were at home. He paused at the window and looked out into the early dusk. Tony moved cautiously toward the glass doors, but she got only as far as the middle of the room when he stood beside her again.

" Tony! " he murmured, and gently took her hand. Then he sank, yes, he sank slowly upon his knees beside her! His two gold whiskers lay across her hand!

" Tony! " he repeated. " You behold me here – you see to what you have brought me. Have you a heart to feel what I endure? Listen. You behold a man condemned to death, devoted to destruction, a man who – who will certainly die of grief," he interrupted himself, " if you scorn his love. Here I lie. Can you find it in your heart to say: ' I despise you '? "

" No, no," Tony said quickly in a consoling tone. Her tears were conquered, pity stirred. Heavens, how he must adore her, to go on like that, while she herself felt completely indifferent! Was it to her, Tony Buddenbrook, that all this was happening? One read of it in the novels. But here in real life was a man in a frock-coat, on his knees in front of her, weeping, imploring. The idea of marrying him was simply idiotic, because she had found him silly; but just at this moment he did not seem silly; heavens, no! Honourable, upright, desperate entreaty were in his voice and face.

" No, no," she repeated, bending over him quite touched. " I don't despise you, Herr Grünlich. How can you say such a thing? Do get up – please do! "

" Then you will not kill me? " he asked again; and she answered, in a consoling, almost motherly tone, " No, no."

" That is a promise! " he cried, springing to his feet. But when he saw Tony's frightened face he got down again and went on in a wheedling tone: " Good, good, say no more, Antonie. Enough, for this time. We shall speak of this again. No more now – farewell. I will return – farewell! " He had got quickly to his feet. He took his broad grey hat from the table, kissed her hand, and was out through the glass doors in a twinkling.

Tony saw him take his stick from the hall and disappear down the corridor. She stood, bewildered and worn out, in the middle of the room, with the damp handkerchief in one of her limp hands.

CHAPTER IV

Consul Buddenbrook said to his wife: "If I thought Tony had a motive in refusing this match – But she is a child, Betsy. She enjoys going to balls and being courted by the young fellows; she is quite aware that she is pretty and from a good family. Of course, it is possible that she is consciously or unconsciously seeking a mate herself – but I know the child, and I feel sure she has never yet found her heart, as the saying goes. If you asked her, she would turn this way and that way, and consider – but she would find nobody. She is a child, a little bird, a hoyden. Directly she once says yes, she will find her place. She will have *carte blanche* to set herself up, and she will love her husband, after a few days. He is no beau, God knows. But he is perfectly presentable. One mustn't ask for five legs on a sheep, as we say in business. If she waits for somebody to come along who is an Adonis and a good match to boot – well, God bless us, Tony Buddenbrook could always find a husband, but it's a risk, after all. Every day is fishing-day, but not every day catching-day, to use another homely phrase – . Yesterday I had a long talk with Grünlich. He is a most constant wooer. He showed me all his books. They are good enough to frame. I told him I was completely satisfied. The business is young, but in fine condition – assets must be somewhere about a hundred and twenty thousand thaler, and that is obviously only the situation at the moment, for he makes a good slice every year. I asked the Duchamps. What they said doesn't sound at all bad. They don't know his connections, but he lives like a gentleman, mingles in society, and his business is known to be expanding. And some other people in Hamburg have told me things – a banker named Kesselmeyer, for instance – that I feel pleased with. In short, as you know, Betsy, I can only wish for the consummation of this match, which would be highly advantageous for the family and the firm. I am heartily sorry the child feels so pressed. She hardly speaks at all, and acts as if she were in a state of siege. But I can't bring myself to refuse him out and out. You know, Betsy, there is another thing I can't emphasize often enough: in these last years we haven't been doing any too brilliantly. Not that there's anything to complain of. Oh, no. Faithful work always finds its reward. Business goes quietly on – but a bit *too* quietly for me. And it only does that because I am eternally vigilant. We haven't perceptibly advanced since Father was taken away. The times aren't good for merchants. No, our prospects are not too bright. Our daughter is in a position to make a marriage that would undoubtedly be honourable and advantageous; she is of an age to marry, and she ought to do it. Delay isn't advisable – it isn't advisable, Betsy. Speak to her again. I said all I could, this afternoon."

Tony was besieged, as the Consul said. She no longer said no – but she could not bring herself to say yes. She could not wring a "yes" out of herself – God knew why; she did not.

Meanwhile, first her Father would draw her aside and speak seriously, and then her Mother would take up the tale, both pressing for a decision. Uncle Gotthold and family were not brought into the affair; their attitude toward the Mengstrasse was not exactly sympathetic. But Sesemi Weichbrodt got wind of it and came to give good advice, with correct enunciation. Even Mademoiselle Jungmann said, "Tony, my little one, why should you worry? You will always be in the best society." And Tony could not pay a visit to the admired silken salon outside the Castle Gate without getting a dose from old Madame Kröger: "A propos, little one, I hear there is an affair! I hope you are going to listen to reason, child."

One Sunday, as she sat in St. Mary's with her parents and brothers, Pastor Kölling began preaching from the text about the wife leaving father and mother and cleaving only to her husband. His language was so violent that she began listening with a jump, staring up to see if he were looking at her. No, thank goodness, his head was turned in the other direction, and he seemed to be preaching in general to all the faithful. Still, it was plain that this was a new attack upon her, – every word struck home. A young, a still childish girl, he said, could have as yet no will and no wisdom; and if she set herself up against the loving advice of her parents she was as deserving of punishment as the guilty are; she was one of those whom the Lord spews out of his mouth. With this phrase, which was the kind Pastor Kölling adored, she encountered a piercing glance from his eyes, as he made a threatening gesture with his right arm. Tony saw how her Father, sitting next to her, raised his hand, as though he would say, "Not so hard." But it was perfectly plain that either he or her Mother had let the

Pastor into the secret. Tony crouched in her place with her face like fire, and felt the eyes of all the world upon her. Next Sunday she flatly refused to go to church.

She moved dumbly about the house, she laughed no more, she lost her appetite. Sometimes she gave such heart-breaking sighs as would move a stone to pity. She was growing thinner too, and would soon lose her freshness. It would not do. At length the Consul said:

"This cannot go on, Betsy. We must not ill-use the child. She must get away a bit, to rest and be able to think quietly. You'll see she will listen to reason then. I can't leave, and the holidays are almost over. But there is no need for us to go. Yesterday old Schwarzkopf from Travemünde was here, and I spoke to him. He said he would be glad to take the child for a while. I'd give them something for it. She would have a good home, where she could bathe and be in the fresh air and get clear in her mind. Tom can take her – so it's all arranged. Better to-morrow than day after."

Tony was much pleased with this idea. True, she hardly ever saw Herr Grünlich, but she knew he was in town, in touch with her parents. Any day he might appear before her and begin shrieking and importuning. She would feel safer at Travemünde, in a strange house. So she packed her trunk with alacrity, and on one of the last days in July she mounted with Tom into the majestic Kröger equipage. She said good-bye in the best of spirits; and breathed more freely as they drove out of the Castle Gate.

CHAPTER V

THE ROAD to Travemünde first crosses the ferry and then goes straight ahead. The grey high-road glided away under the hoofs of Lebrecht Kröger's fat brown Mecklenburgs. The sound of their trotting was hollow and rhythmical, the sun burned hot, and dust concealed the meagre view. The family had eaten at one o'clock, an hour earlier than usual, and the brother and sister set out punctually at two. They would arrive shortly after four; for what a hired carriage could do in three hours, the Kröger pair were mettlesome enough to make in two.

Tony sat half asleep, nodding under her broad straw hat and her lace-trimmed parasol, which she held tipped back against the hood of the chaise. The parasol was twine-grey with cream-coloured lace, and matched her neat, simply cut frock. She reclined in the luxurious ease proper to the equipage, with her feet, in their white stockings and strap shoes, daintily crossed before her.

Tom was already twenty years old. He wore an extremely well cut blue suit, and sat smoking Russian cigarettes, with his hat on the back of his head. He was not very tall; but already he boasted a considerable moustache, darker in tone than his brows and eyelashes. He had one eyebrow lifted a trifle – a habit with him – and sat looking at the dust and the trees that fled away behind them as the carriage rolled on.

Tony said: "I was never so glad to come to Travemünde before – for various reasons. You needn't laugh, Tom. I wish I could leave a certain pair of yellow mutton-chops even further behind! And then, it will be an entirely different Travemünde at the Schwarzkopfs', on the sea front. I shan't be bothered with the Kurhaus society, I can tell you that much. I am not in the mood for it. Besides, that – that man could come there too as well as not. He has nerve enough – it wouldn't trouble him at all. Some day he'd be bobbing up in front of me and putting on all his airs and graces."

Tom threw away the stub of his cigarette and took a fresh one out of the box, a pretty little affair with an inlaid picture inside the lid, of an overturned troika being set upon by wolves. It was a present from a Russian customer of the Consul. The cigarettes, those biting little trifles with the yellow mouthpiece, were Tom's passion. He smoked quantities of them, and had the bad habit of inhaling the smoke, breathing it slowly out again as he talked.

"Yes," he said. "As far as that goes, the garden of the Kurhouse is alive with Hamburgers. Consul Fritsche, who has bought it, is a Hamburger himself. He must be doing a wonderful business now, Papa says. But you'll miss something if you don't take part in it a bit. Peter Döhlmann is there – he never stops in town this time of year. His business goes on at a jog-trot, all by itself, I suppose. Funny! Well – and Uncle Justus comes out for a little on a Sunday, of course, to visit the roulette table. Then there are the Möllendorpfs and the Kistenmakers, I suppose, in full strength, and the Hagenströms – "

"H'm. Yes, of course. They couldn't get on without Sarah Semlinger!"

"Her name is Laura, my child. Let us be accurate."

"And Julchen with her, of course. Julchen ought to get engaged to August Möllendorpf this summer – and she will do it, too. After all, they belong together. Disgusting, isn't it, Tom? This adventurer's family – "

"Yes, but good heavens, they are the firm of Strunck and Hagenström. That is the point."

"Naturally, they make the firm. Of course. And everybody knows *how* they do it. With their *elbows*. Pushing and shoving – entirely without courtesy or elegance. Grandfather said that Hinrich Hagenström could coin money out of paving-stones. Those were his very words."

"Yes, yes, that is exactly it. It is money talks. And this match is perfectly good business. Julchen will be a Möllendorpf, and August will get a snug position – "

"Oh, you just want to make me angry, Tom, that's all. You know how I despise that lot."

Tom began to laugh. "Goodness, one has to get along with them," he replied. "As Papa said the other day, they are the coming people; while the Möllendorpfs, for example – And one can't deny that the Hagenströms are clever. Hermann is already useful in the business, and Moritz is very able. He finished school brilliantly, in spite of his weak chest; and he is going to study law."

"That's all very well, Tom, but all the same I am glad there are families that don't have to knuckle down to them. For instance, we Buddenbrooks – "

"Oh," Tom said, "don't let's begin to boast. Every family has its own skeleton," he went on in a lower voice, with a glance at Jock's broad back. "For instance, God knows what state Uncle Julius' affairs are in. Papa shakes his head when he speaks of him, and Grandfather Kröger has had to come forward once or twice with large sums, I hear. The cousins aren't just the thing, either. Jürgen wants to study, but he still hasn't come up for his finals; and they are not very well satisfied with Jacob, at Dalbeck and Company. He is always in debt, even with a good allowance, and when Uncle Justus refuses to send any more, Aunt Rosalie does – No, I find it doesn't do to throw stones. If you want to balance the scale with the Hagenströms, you'd better marry Grünlich."

"Did we get into this wagon to discuss that subject? – Oh, yes, I suppose you're right. I ought to marry him – but I won't think about it now! I want to forget it. We are going to the Schwarzkopfs'. I've never seen them to know them: are they nice people?"

"Oh, old Diederich Schwarzkopf – he's not such a bad old chap. Doesn't speak such atrocious dialect, unless he's had more than five glasses of grog. Once he was at the office, and we went together to the Ships' Company. He drank like a tank. His father was born on a Norwegian freighter and grew up to be captain on the very same line. Diederich has had a good education; the pilot command is a responsible office, and pretty well paid. Diederich is an old bear – but very gallant with the ladies. Look out: he'll flirt with you."

"Ah – well, and his wife?"

"I don't know her, myself. She must be nice, I should think. There is a son, too. He was in first or second, in my time at school, and is a student now, I expect. Look, there's the sea. We shall be there inside a quarter of an hour."

They drove for a while along the shore on an avenue bordered with young beech-trees. There was the water, blue and peaceful in the sunshine; the round yellow light-house tower came into view, then the bay and the breakwater, the red roofs of the little town, the harbour with its sails, tackle, and shipping. They drove between the first houses, passed the church, and rolled along the front close to the water and up to a pretty little house, the verandah of which was overhung with vines.

Pilot-Captain Schwarzkopf stood before his door and took off his seaman's cap as the calèche drove up. He was a broad, stocky man with a red face, sea-blue eyes, and a bristling grizzled beard that ran fan-shaped from one ear to the other. His mouth turned down at the corners, in one of which he held a wooden pipe. His smooth-shaven, red upper lip was hard and prominent; he looked thoroughly solid and respectable, with big bones and well-rounded paunch; and he wore a coat decorated with gold braid, underneath which a white piqué waistcoat was visible.

"Servant, Mademoiselle," he said, as he carefully lifted Tony from the calèche. "We know it's an honour you do us, coming to stop with us like this. Servant, Herr Buddenbrook. Papa well? And the honoured Frau Consul? Come in, come in! My wife has some sort of a bite ready, I suppose. Drive over to Peddersen's Inn," he said in his broadest dialect to the coachman, who was carrying in the trunk. "You'll find they take good care of the horses there." Then, turning to Thomas, "you'll stop the night with us, Herr Buddenbrook? Oh, yes, you must. The horses want a bait and a rest, and you wouldn't get home until after dark."

"Upon my word, one lives at least as well here as at the Kurhouse," Tony said a quarter of an hour later, as they sat around the coffee-table in the verandah. "What wonderful air! You can smell the sea-weed from here. How frightfully glad I am to be in Travemünde again!"

Between the vine-clad columns of the verandah one could look out on the broad river-mouths, glittering in the sun; there were the piers and the boats, and the ferry-house on the "Prival" opposite, the projecting peninsula of Mecklenburg. – The clumsy, blue-bordered cups on the table were almost like basins. How different from the delicate old porcelain at home! But there was a bunch of flowers at Tony's place, the food looked inviting, and the drive had whetted her appetite.

"Yes, Mademoiselle will see, she will pick up here fast enough," the housewife said. "She looks a little poorly, if I might say so. That is the town air, and the parties."

Frau Schwarzkopf was the daughter of a Schlutup pastor. She was a head shorter than Tony, rather thin, and looked to be about fifty. Her hair was still black, and neatly dressed in a large-meshed net. She wore a dark brown dress with white crocheted collar and cuffs. She was spotless, gentle, and hospitable, urging upon her guests the currant bread that lay in a boat-shaped basket surrounded by cream, butter, sugar, and honeycomb. This basket had a border of bead-work embroidery, done by little Meta, the eight-year-old daughter, who now sat next her mother, dressed in a plaid frock, her flaxen hair in a thick pigtail.

Frau Schwarzkopf made excuses for Tony's room, whither she had already been to make herself tidy after the journey. It was so very simple –

"Oh, all the better," Tony said. It had a view of the ocean, which was the main thing. And she dipped her fourth piece of currant bread into her coffee. Tom walked with the pilot-captain about the *Wullenwewer*, now undergoing repairs in the town.

There came suddenly into the verandah a young man of some twenty years. He took off his grey felt hat, blushed, and bowed rather awkwardly.

"Well, my son," said Herr Schwarzkopf, "you are late." He presented him to the guests: "This is my son, studying to be a doctor. He is spending his vacation with us." He had mentioned the young man's name, but Tony failed to understand it.

"Pleased to meet you," said Tony, primly. Tom rose and and shook hands. Young Schwarzkopf bowed again, put down his book, and took his place at the table, blushing afresh. He was of medium height, very slender, and as fair as he could possibly be. His youthful moustaches, colourless as the hair which covered his long head, were scarcely visible; and he had a complexion to match, a tint like translucent porcelain, which grew pink on the slightest provocation. His eyes, slightly darker than his father's, had the same not very animated but good-natured quizzical expression; and his features were regular and rather pleasing. When he began to eat he displayed unusually regular teeth, glistening in close ranks of polished ivory. For the rest, he wore a grey jacket buttoned up, with flaps on the pockets, and an elastic belt at the back.

"Yes, I am sorry I am late," he said. His speech was somewhat slow and grating. "I was reading on the beach, and did not look soon enough at my watch." Then he ate silently, looking up now and then to glance at Tom and Tony.

Later on, Tony being again urged by the housewife to take something, he said, "You can rely on the honey, Fräulein Buddenbrook; it is a pure nature product – one knows what one is eating. You must eat, you know. The air here consumes one – it accelerates the process of metabolism. If you do not eat well, you will get thin." He had a pleasant, naïve, way of now and then bending forward as he spoke and looking at some other person than the one whom he addressed.

His mother listened to him tenderly and watched Tony's face to see the impression he made. But old Schwarzkopf said, "Now, now, Herr Doctor. Don't be blowing off about your metabolism – *we* don't know anything about that sort of talk." Whereupon the young man laughed, blushed again, and looked at Tony's plate.

The pilot-captain mentioned more than once his son's Christian name, but Tony could never quite catch what it was. It sounded like Moor – or Mort; but the Father's broad, flat pronunciation was impossible to understand.

They finished their meal. Herr Diederich sat blinking in the sun, his coat flung wide open over his white waistcoat, and he and his son took out their short pipes. Tom smoked his cigarettes, and the young people began a lively conversation, the subject of which was their old school and all the old school recollections. Tony took part gaily. They quoted Herr Stengel: " What! You were to make a line, and what are you making? A dash! " What a pity Christian was not here! he could imitate him so much better.

Once Tom pointed to the flowers at Tony's place and said to his sister: " That trims things up uncommonly well, as Herr Grünlich would say! " Whereat Tony, red with anger, gave him a push and darted an embarrassed glance at young Schwarzkopf.

The coffee-hour had been unusually late, and they had prolonged it. It was already half-past six, and twilight was beginning to descend over the Prival, when the captain got up.

" The company will excuse me," he said; " I've some work down at the pilot-house. We'll have supper at eight o'clock, if that suits the young folk. Or even a little later to-night, eh, Meta? And you " (here he used his son's name again), " don't be lolling about here. Just go and dig up your bones again. Fräulein Buddenbrook will want to unpack. Or perhaps the guests would like to go down on the beach. Only don't get in the way."

" Diederich, for pity's sake, why shouldn't he sit still a bit? " Frau Schwarzkopf said, with mild reproach. " And if our guests like to go down on the beach, why shouldn't he go along? Is he to see nothing at all of our visitors? "

CHAPTER VI

In her neat little room with the flower-covered furniture, Tony woke next morning with the fresh, happy feeling which one has at the beginning of a new chapter. She sat up in bed and, with her hands clasped round her knees and her tousled head flung back, blinked at the stream of light that poured through the closed shutters into the room. She began to sort out the experiences of the previous day.

Her thoughts scarcely touched upon the Grünlich affair. The town, his hateful apparition in the landscape room, the exhortations of her family and Pastor Kölling – all that lay far behind her. Here, every morning, there would be a care-free waking. These Schwarzkopfs were splendid people. Last night there had been pineapple punch, and they had made part of a happy family circle. It had been very jolly. Herr Schwarzkopf had told his best sea tales, and young Schwarzkopf stories about student life at Göttingen. How odd it was, that she still did not know his first name! And she had strained her ear to hear too, but even at dinner she did not succeed, and somehow it did not seem proper to ask. She tried feverishly to think how it sounded – was it Moor – Mord –? Anyhow, she had liked him pretty well, this young Moor or Mord. He had such a sly, good-natured laugh when he asked for the water and called it by letters and numbers, so that his father got quite furious. But it was only the scientific formula for water – that is, for ordinary water, for the Travemünde product was a much more complicated affair, of course. Why, one could find a jelly-fish in it, any time! The authorities, of course, might have what notions they chose about fresh water. For this he only got another scolding from his father, for speaking slightingly of the authorities. But Frau Schwarzkopf watched Tony all the time, to see how much she admired the young man – and really, it was most interesting, he was so learned and so jolly, all at the same time. He had given her considerable attention. She had complained that her head felt hot, while eating, and that she must have too much blood. What had he replied? He had given her a careful scrutiny, and then said, Yes, the arteries in the temples might be full; but that did not prove that she had too much blood. Perhaps, instead, it meant she had too little – or rather, that there were too few red corpuscles in it. In fact, she was perhaps a little anæmic.

The cuckoo sprang out of his carven house on the wall and cuckooed several times, clear and loud. "Seven, eight, nine," counted Tony. "Up with you!" She jumped out of bed and opened the blinds. The sky was partly overcast, but the sun was visible. She looked out over the Leuchtenfeld with its tower, to the ruffled sea beyond. On the right it was bounded by the curve of the Mecklenburg coast; but before her it stretched on and on till its blue and green streaks mingled with the misty horizon. "I'll bathe afterwards," she thought, "but first I'll eat a big breakfast, so as not to be consumed by my metabolism." She washed and dressed with quick, eager movements.

It was shortly after half-past nine when she left her room. The door of the chamber in which Tom had slept stood open; he had risen early and driven back to town. Even up here in the upper story, it smelled of coffee – that seemed to be the characteristic odour of the little house, for it grew stronger as she descended the simple staircase with its plain board baluster and went down the corridor, where lay the living-room, which was also the dining-room and the office of the pilot-captain. She went out into the verandah, looking, in her white piqué frock, perfectly fresh, and in the gayest of tempers. Frau Schwarzkopf sat with her son at the table. It was already partly cleared away, and the housewife wore a blue checked kitchen apron over her brown frock. A key-basket stood beside her.

"A thousand pardons for not waiting," she said, as she stood up. "We simple folk rise early. There is so much to be done! Schwarzkopf is in his office. I hope you don't take it ill?"

Tony excused herself in her turn. "You must not think I always sleep so late as this," she said. "I feel very guilty. But the punch last night –"

The young man began to laugh. He stood behind the table with his short pipe in his hand and a newspaper before him.

"Good morning," Tony said. "Yes, it is your fault. You kept urging me. Now I deserve only cold coffee. I ought to have had breakfast and a bathe as well, by this time."

"Oh, no, that would be rather too early, for a young lady. At seven o'clock the water was rather cold – eleven degrees. That's pretty sharp, after a warm bed."

"How do you know I wanted a warm bath, monsieur?" and

Tony sat down beside Frau Schwarzkopf. "Oh, you have kept the coffee hot for me, Frau Schwarzkopf! But I will pour it out myself, thank you so much."

The housewife looked on as her guest began to eat. "Fräulein slept well, the first night? The mattress, dear knows, is only stuffed with sea-weed – we are simple folk! And now, good appetite, and a good morning. You will surely find many friends on the beach. If you like, my son shall bear you company. Pardon me for not sitting longer, but I must look after the dinner. The joint is in the oven. We will feed you as well as we can."

"I shall stick to the honeycomb," Tony said when the two were alone. "You know what you are getting."

Young Schwarzkopf laid his pipe on the verandah rail.

"But please smoke. I don't mind it at all. At home, when I come down to breakfast, Papa's cigar-smoke is already in the room. Tell me," she said suddenly. "Is it true that an egg is as good as a quarter of a pound of meat?"

He grew red all over. "Are you making fun of me?" he asked, partly laughing but partly vexed. "I got another wigging from my Father last night for what he calls my silly professional airs."

"No, really, I was asking because I wanted to know." Tony stopped eating in consternation. "How could anybody call them airs? I should be so glad to learn something. I'm such a goose, you see. At Sesemi Weichbrodt's I was always one of the very laziest. I'm sure you know a great deal." Inwardly her thoughts ran: "Everybody puts his best foot foremost, before strangers. We all take care to say what will be pleasant to hear – that is a commonplace. . . ."

"Well, you see they are the same thing, in a way. The chemical constituents of food-stuffs –" And so on, while Tony breakfasted. Next they talked about Tony's boarding-school days, and Sesemi Weichbrodt, and Gerda Arnoldsen, who had gone back to Amsterdam, and Armgard von Schilling, whose home, a large white house, could be seen from the beach here, at least in clear weather. Tony finished eating, wiped her mouth, and asked, pointing to the paper, "Is there any news?" Young Schwarzkopf shook his head and laughed cynically.

"Oh, no. What would there be? You know these little provincial news-sheets are wretched affairs."

"Oh, are they? Papa and Mamma always take it in."

He reddened again. "Oh, well, you see I always read it, too. Because I can't get anything else. But it is not very thrilling to hear that So-and-So, the merchant prince, is about to celebrate his silver wedding. Yes, you laugh. But you ought to read other papers – the *Königsberg Gazette*, for instance, or the *Rhenish Gazette*. You'd find a different story there, entirely. There it's what the King of Prussia says."

"What does he say?"

"Well – er – I really couldn't repeat it to a lady." He got red again. "He expressed himself rather strongly on the subject of this same press," he went on with another cynical laugh, which, for a moment, made a painful impression on Tony. "The press, you know, doesn't feel any too friendly toward the government or the nobility or the parsons and junkers. It knows pretty well how to lead the censor by the nose."

"Well, and you? Aren't you any too friendly with the nobility, either?"

"I?" he asked, and looked very embarrassed. Tony rose.

"Shall we talk about this again another time?" she suggested. "Suppose I go down to the beach now. Look, the sky is blue nearly all over. It won't rain any more. I am simply longing to jump into the water. Will you go down with me?"

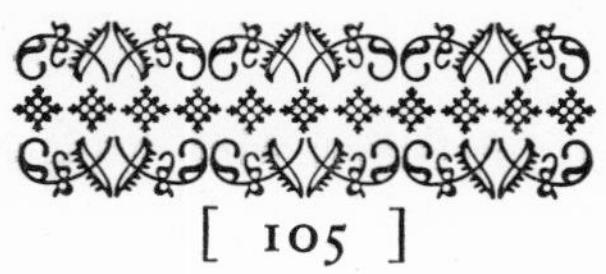

CHAPTER VII

She had put on her big straw hat, and she raised her sunshade; for it was very hot, though there was a little sea-breeze. Young Schwarzkopf, in his grey felt, book in hand, walked beside her and sometimes gave her a shy side-glance. They went along the front and walked through the garden of the Kurhouse, which lay there in the sun shadeless and still, with its rose-bushes and pebbly paths. The music pavilion, hidden among pine trees, stood opposite the Kurhouse, the pastry-cook's, and the two Swiss cottages, which were connected by a long gallery. It was about half-past eleven, and the hotel guests were probably down on the beach.

They crossed the playground, where there were many benches and a large swing, passed close to the building where one took the hot baths, and strolled slowly across the Leuchtenfeld. The sun brooded over the grass, and there rose up a spicy smell from the warm weeds and clover; blue-bottle flies buzzed and droned about. A dull, booming roar came up from the ocean, whose waters now and then lifted a crested head of spray in the distance.

"What is that you are reading?" Tony asked. The young man took the book in both hands and ran it quickly through, from cover to cover.

"Oh, that is nothing for you, Fräulein Buddenbrook. Nothing but blood and entrails and such awful things. This part treats of nodes in the lungs. What we call pulmonary catarrh. The lungs get filled up with a watery fluid. It is a very dangerous condition, and occurs in inflammation of the lungs. In bad cases, the patient simply chokes to death. And that is all described with perfect coolness, from a scientific point of view."

"Oh, horrors! But if one wants to be a doctor – I will see that you become our family physician, when old Grabow retires. You'll see!"

"Ha, ha! And what are you reading, if I may ask, Fräulein Buddenbrook?"

"Do you know Hoffmann?" Tony asked.

"About the choir-master, and the gold pot? Yes, that's very

pretty. But it is more for ladies. Men want something different, you know."

"I must ask you one thing," Tony said, taking a sudden resolution, after they had gone a few steps. "And that is, do, I beg of you, tell me your first name. I haven't been able to understand it a single time I've heard it, and it is making me dreadfully nervous. I've simply been racking my brains – I have, quite."

"You have been racking your brains?"

"Now don't make it worse – I'm sure it couldn't have been proper for me to ask, only I'm naturally curious. There's really no reason whatever why I should know."

"Why, my name is Morten," said he, and became redder than ever.

"Morten? That is a nice name."

"Oh – *nice!*"

"Yes, indeed. At least, it's prettier than to be called something like Hinz, or Kunz. It is unusual; it sounds foreign."

"You are romantic, Fräulein Buddenbrook. You have read too much Hoffmann. My grandfather was half Norwegian, and I was named after him. That is all there is to it."

Tony picked her way through the rushes on the edge of the beach. In front of them was a row of round-topped wooden pavilions, and beyond they could see the basket-chairs at the water's edge and people camped by families on the warm sand – ladies with blue sun-spectacles and books out of the loan-library; gentlemen in light suits idly drawing pictures in the sand with their walking-sticks; sun-burnt children in enormous straw hats, tumbling about, shovelling sand, digging for water, baking with wooden moulds, paddling bare-legged in the shallow pools, floating little ships. To the right, the wooden bathing-pavilion ran out into the water.

"We are going straight across to Möllendorpf's pier," said Tony. "Let's turn off."

"Certainly; but don't you want to meet your friends? I can sit down yonder on those boulders."

"Well, I suppose I ought to just greet them. But I don't want to, you know. I came here to be in peace and quiet."

"Peace? From what?"

"Why – from – from –"

"Listen, Fräulein Buddenbrook. I must ask you something. No, I'll wait till another day – till we have more time. Now I will say au revoir and go and sit down there on the rocks."

"Don't you want me to introduce you, then?" Tony asked, importantly.

"Oh, no," Morten said, hastily. "Thanks, but I don't fit very well with those people, you see. I'll just sit down over there on the rocks."

It was a rather large company which Tony was approaching while Morten Schwarzkopf betook himself to the great heap of boulders on the right, near to the bathing-house and washed by the waves. The party was encamped before the Möllendorpfs' pier, and was composed of the Möllendorpf, Hagenström, Kistenmaker, and Fritsche families. Except for Herr Fritsche, the owner, from Hamburg, and Peter Döhlmann, the idler, the group consisted of women, for it was a week-day, and most of the men were in their offices. Consul Fritsche, an elderly, smooth-shaven gentleman with a distinguished face, was up on the open pier, busy with a telescope, which he trained upon a sailboat visible in the distance. Peter Döhlmann, with a broad-brimmed straw hat and a beard with a nautical cut, stood chatting with the ladies perched on camp-stools or stretched out on rugs on the sand. There were Frau Senator Möllendorpf, born Langhals, with her long-handled lorgnon and untidy grey hair; Frau Hagenström, with Julchen, who had not grown much, but already wore diamonds in her ears, like her mother; Frau Consul Kistenmaker and her daughters; and Frau Consul Fritsche, a wrinkled little lady in a cap, who performed the duties of hospitality at the bath and went about perpetually hot and tired, thinking only about balls and routs and raffles, children's parties and sailboat excursions. At a little distance sat her paid companion.

Kistenmaker and Son was the new firm of wine-merchants which had, in the last few years, managed to put C. F. Köppen rather in the shade. The two sons, Edouard and Stephan, worked in their father's office. Consul Döhlmann possessed none of those graces of manner upon which Justus Kröger laid such stress. He was an idler pure and simple, whose special characteristic was a sort of rough good humour. He could and did take a good many liberties in society, being quite aware that his loud, brusque voice and bluff ways caused the ladies to set him down as an original. Once at a dinner at the Buddenbrooks', when a course failed to come in promptly and the guests grew dull and the hostess flustered, he came to the rescue and put them into a good humour by bellowing in his big voice the whole length of the table: "Please don't wait for me, Frau Consul!" Just now, in this same reverberating voice, he was relating questionable anecdotes seasoned with low-German idioms. Frau Senator Möllendorpf, in paroxysms of laughter, was crying out over and over again: " Stop, Herr Döhlmann, stop! for heaven's sake, don't tell any more."

They greeted Tony – the Hagenströms coldly, the others with great cordiality. Consul Fritsche even came down the steps of the pier, for he hoped that the Buddenbrooks would return next year to swell the population of the baths.

" Yours to command, Fräulein Buddenbrook," said Consul Döhlmann, with his very best pronunciation; for he was aware that Mademoiselle did not especially care for his manners.

" Mademoiselle Buddenbrook! "

" You here? "

" How lovely! "

" When did you come? "

" What a sweet frock! "

" Where are you stopping? "

" At the Schwarzkopfs'? "

" With the pilot-captain? How original! "

" How *frightfully* original."

" You are stopping in the town? " asked Consul Fritsche, the owner of the baths. He did not betray that he felt the blow.

" Will you come to our next assembly? " his wife asked.

" Oh, you are only here for a short time? " – this from another lady.

" Don't you think, darling, the Buddenbrooks rather give themselves airs? " Frau Hagenström whispered to Frau Senator Möllendorpf.

" Have you been in yet? " somebody asked. " Which of the rest of you hasn't bathed yet, young ladies? Marie? Julie, Louise? Your friends will go bathing with you, of course, Fräulein Antonie." Some of the young girls rose, and Peter Döhlmann insisted on accompanying them up the beach.

" Do you remember how we used to go back and forth to school together? " Tony asked Julie Hagenström.

" Yes, and you were always the one that got into mischief," Julie said, joining in her laugh. They went across the beach on a foot-bridge made of a few boards, and reached the bathhouse. As they passed the boulders where Morten Schwarzkopf sat, Tony nodded to him from a distance, and somebody asked, " who is that you are bowing to, Tony? "

" That was young Schwarzkopf," Tony answered. " He walked down here with me."

"The son of the pilot-captain?" Julchen asked, and peered across at Morten with her staring black eyes. He on his side watched the gay troop with rather a melancholy air. Tony said in a loud voice: "What a pity August is not here. It must be stupid on the beach."

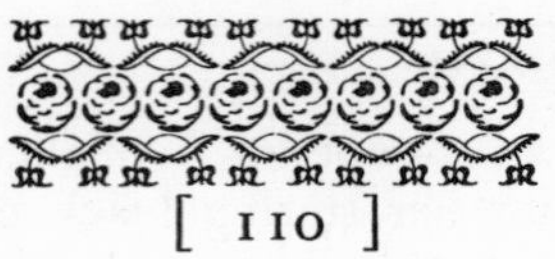

CHAPTER VIII

AND now began for Tony Buddenbrook a stretch of beautiful summer weeks, briefer, lovelier, than any she had ever spent in Travemünde. She bloomed as she felt her burden no longer upon her; her gay, pert, careless manner had come back. The Consul looked at her with satisfaction when he came on Sundays with Tom and Christian. On those days they ate at the table-d'hôte, sat under the awnings at the pastry-cook's, drinking coffee and listening to the band, and peeped into the roulette-room at the gay folk there, like Justus Kröger and Peter Döhlmann. The Consul himself never played. Tony sunned herself, took baths, ate sausages with ginger-nut sauce, and took long walks with Morten. They went out on the high-road to the next village, or along the beach to the " ocean temple " on its height, whence a wide view was to be had over land and sea; or to the woods behind the Kurhouse, where was a great bell used to call the guests to the table-d'hôte. Sometimes they rowed across the Trave to the Prival, to look for amber.

Morten made an entertaining companion, though his opinions were often dogmatic, not to say heated. He had a severe and righteous judgment for everything, and he expressed it with finality, blushing all the time. It saddened Tony to hear him call the nobility idiots and wretches and to see the contemptuous if awkward gesture that accompanied the words. She scolded him, but she was proud to have him express so freely in her presence the views and opinions which she knew he concealed from his parents. Once he confided in her: " I'll tell you something: I've a skeleton in my room at Göttingen – a whole set of bones, you know, held together by wire. I've put an old policeman's uniform on it. Ha, ha! Isn't that great? But don't say anything to my Father about it."

Tony was naturally often in the society of her town friends, or drawn into some assembly or boating party. Then Morten " sat on the rocks." And after their first day this phrase became a convenient one. To " sit on the rocks " meant to feel bored and lonely.

When a rainy day came and a grey mist covered the sea far and wide till it was one with the deep sky; when the beach was drenched and the roads streaming with wet, Tony would say: "To-day we shall both have to sit on the rocks – that is, in the verandah or sitting-room. There is nothing left to do but for you to play me some of your student songs, Morten – even if they do bore me horribly."

"Yes," Morten said, "come and sit down. But you know that when you are here, there are no rocks!" He never said such things when his father was present. His mother he did not mind.

"Well, what now?" asked the pilot-captain, as Tony and Morten both rose from table and were about to take their leave. "Where are the young folk off to?"

"I was going to take a little walk with Fräulein Antonie, as far as the temple."

"Oh, is that it? Well, my son Filius, what do you say to going up to your room and conning over your nerves? You'll lose everything out of your head before you get back to Göttingen."

But Frau Schwarzkopf would intervene: "Now, Diederich, aren't these his holidays? Why shouldn't he take a walk? Is he to have nothing of our visitor?" So Morten went.

They paced along the beach close to the water, on the smooth, hard sand that made walking easy. It was strewn with common tiny white mussel-shells, and others too, pale opalescent and longish in shape; yellow-green wet seaweed with hollow round fruit that snapped when you squeezed it; and pale, translucent, reddish-yellow jelly-fish, which were poisonous and burned your leg when you touched one bathing.

"I used to be frightfully stupid, you know," Tony said. "I wanted the bright star out of the jelly-fish, so I brought a lot home in my pocket-handkerchief and put them on the balcony, to dry in the sunshine. When I looked at them again, of course there was just a big wet spot that smelled of sea-weed."

The waves whispered rhythmically beside them as they walked, and the salt wind blew full in their faces, streaming over and about them, closing their ears to other sounds and causing a pleasant slight giddiness. They walked in this hushed, whispering peacefulness by the sea, whose every faint murmur, near or far, seemed to have a deep significance.

To their left was a precipitous cliff of lime and boulders, with jutting corners that came into view as they rounded the bay. When the beach was too stony to go on, they began to climb, and continued upward through the wood until they reached the temple. It was a round pavilion, built of rough timbers and boards, the inside of which was covered with scribbled inscriptions and poetry, carved hearts and initials. Tony and Morten seated themselves in one of the little rooms facing the sea; it smelled of wood, like the cabins at the bathhouse. It was very quiet, even solemn, up here at this hour of the afternoon. A pair of birds chattered, and the faint rustling of the leaves mingled with the sound of the sea spread out below them. In the distance they could see the rigging of a ship. Sheltered now from the wind that had been thrumming at their ears, they suddenly experienced a quiet, almost pensive mood.

Tony said, "Is it coming or going?"

"What?" asked Morten, his subdued voice sounding as if he were coming back from a far distance. "Oh – going – That is the *Bürgermeister Steenbock*, for Russia." He added after a pause: "I shouldn't like to be going with it. It must be worse there than here."

"Now," Tony said, "you are going to begin again on the nobility. I see it in your face. And it's not at all nice of you. Tell me, did you ever know a single one of them?"

"No!" Morten shouted, quite insulted. "Thank God, no."

"Well, there, then, I have – Armgard von Schilling over there, that I told you about. She was much better-natured than either of us; she hardly knew she was a *von* – she ate sausage-meat and talked about her cows."

"Oh, of course. There are naturally exceptions. Listen, Fräulein Tony. You are a woman, you see, so you take everything personally. You happen to know a single member of the nobility, and you say she is a good creature – certainly! But one does not need to know any of them to be able to judge them all. It is a question of the principle, you understand – of – the organization of the state. You can't answer that, can you? They need only to be born to be the pick of everything, and look down on all the rest of us. While we, however hard we strive, cannot climb to their level." Morten spoke with a naïve, honest irritation. He tried to fit his speech with gestures, then perceived that they were awkward, and gave it up. But he was in the vein to talk, and he went on, sitting bent forward, with his thumb between the buttons of his jacket, a defiant expression in his usually good-natured eyes. "We, the bourgeoisie – the Third Estate, as we have been called – we recognize only that nobility which consists of merit; we refuse to admit any longer the rights of the indolent aristocracy, we repudiate the class distinctions of the present day, we desire that all men should be free and equal, that no person shall be subject to another, but all subject to the law. There shall be no more privilege and arbitrary rule. All shall be sovereign children of the state; and as no middlemen exist any longer between the people and almighty God, so shall the citizen stand in direct relation to the State. We will have freedom of the press, of trade and industry, so that all men, without distinction, shall be able to strive together and receive their reward according to their merit. We are enslaved, muzzled! – What was it I wanted to say? Oh, yes! Four years ago they renewed the laws of the Confederation touching the universities and the press. Fine laws they are! No truth may be written or taught which might not agree with the established order of things. Do you understand? The truth is suppressed – forbidden to be spoken. Why? For the sake of an obsolete, idiotic, decadent class which everybody knows will be destroyed some day, anyhow. I do not think you can comprehend such meanness. It is the stupid, brutal application of force, the immediate physical strength of the police, without the slightest understanding of new, spiritual forces. And apart from all that, there is the final fact of the great wrong the King of Prussia has done us. In 1813, when the French were in the country, he called us together and promised us a Constitution. We came to the rescue, we freed Germany from the invader – "

Tony, chin in hand, stole a look at him and wondered for a moment if he could have actually helped to drive out Napoleon.

" – but do you think he kept his promise? Oh, no! The present king is a fine orator, a dreamer; a romantic, like you, Fräulein Tony. But I'll tell you something: take any general principle or conception of life. It always happens that, directly it has been found wanting and discarded by the poets and philosophers, there comes along a King to whom it is a perfectly new idea, and who makes it a guiding principle. That is what kings are like. It is not only that kings are men – they are even very distinctly average men; they are always a good way in the rear. Oh, yes, Germany is just like a students' society; it had its brave and spirited youth at the time of the great revolution, but now it is just a lot of fretful Philistines."

"Ye – es," Tony said. "But let me ask you this: Why are you so interested in Prussia? You aren't a Prussian."

"Oh, it is all the same thing, Fräulein Buddenbrook. Yes, I said Fräulein Buddenbrook on purpose, I ought even to have said Demoiselle Buddenbrook, and given you your entire title. Are the men here freer, more brotherly, more equal than in Prussia? Conventions, classes, aristocracy, here as there. You have sympathy for the nobility. Shall I tell you why? Because you belong to it yourself. Yes, yes, didn't you know it? Your father is a great gentleman, and you are a princess. There is a gulf between you and us, because we do not belong to your circle of ruling families. You can walk on the beach with one of us for the sake of your health, but when you get back into your own class, then the rest of us can go and sit on the rocks." His voice had grown quite strangely excited.

"Morten," said Tony, sadly. "You have been angry all the time, then, when you were sitting on the rocks! And I always begged you to come and be introduced."

"Now you are taking the affair personally again, like a young lady, Fräulein Tony, I'm only speaking of the principle. I say that there is no more fellowship of humanity with us than in Prussia. – And even if I were speaking personally," he went on, after a little pause, with a softer tone, out of which, however, the strange excitement had not disappeared, "I shouldn't be speaking of the present, but rather, perhaps, of the future. When you as Madame So-and-So finally vanish into your proper sphere, one is left to sit on the rocks all the rest of one's life."

He was silent, and Tony too. She did not look at him, but in the other direction, at the wooden partition. There was an uneasy stillness for some time.

"Do you remember," Morten began again, "I once said to you that there was a question I wanted to ask you? Yes, I have wanted to know, since the first afternoon you came. Don't guess. You couldn't guess what I mean. I am going to ask you another time; there is no hurry; it has really nothing to do with me; it is only curiosity. No, to-day I will only show you one thing. Look." He drew out of the pocket of his jacket the end of a narrow gaily-striped ribbon, and looked with a mixture of expectation and triumph into Tony's eyes.

"How pretty," she said uncomprehendingly. "What is it?"

Morten spoke solemnly: "That means that I belong to a students' fraternity in Göttingen. – Now you know. I have a cap in the same colours, but my skeleton in the policeman's uniform is wearing it for the holidays. I couldn't be seen with it here, you understand. I can count on your saying nothing, can't I? Because it would be very unfortunate if my father were to hear of it."

"Not a word, Morten. You can rely on me. But I don't understand – have you all taken a vow against the nobility? What is it you want?"

"We want freedom," Morten said.

"Freedom?" she asked.

"Yes, freedom, you know – *Freedom!*" he repeated; and he made a vague, awkward, fervent gesture outward and downward, not toward the side where the coast of Mecklenburg narrowed the bay, but in the direction of the open sea, whose rippling blue, green, yellow, and grey stripes rolled as far as eye could see out to the misty horizon.

Tony followed his gesture with her eye; they sat, their hands lying close together on the bench, and looked into the distance. Thus they remained in silence a long time, while the sea sent up to them its soft enchanting whispers. . . . Tony suddenly felt herself one with Morten in a great, vague yearning comprehension of this portentous something which he called "Freedom."

CHAPTER IX

"It is wonderful how one doesn't get bored, here at the seashore, Morten. Imagine lying anywhere else for hours at a time, flat on your back, doing nothing, not even thinking – "

"Yes. But I must confess that I used to be bored sometimes – only not in the last few weeks."

Autumn was at hand. The first strong wind had risen. Thin, tattered grey clouds raced across the sky. The dreary, tossing sea was covered far and wide with foam. Great, powerful waves rolled silently in, relentless, awesome; towered majestically, in a metallic dark-green curve, then crashed thundering on the sand.

The season was quite at an end. On that part of the beach usually occupied by the throng of bathers, the pavilions were already partly dismantled, and it lay as quiet as the grave, with only a very few basket-chairs. But Tony and Morten spent the afternoon in a distant spot, at the edge of the yellow loam, where the waves hurled their spray as far up as Sea-gull Rock. Morten had made her a solid sand fortress, and she leaned against it with her back, her feet in their strap shoes and white stockings crossed in front of her. Morten lay turned toward her, his chin in his hands. Now and then a sea-gull flew past them, shrieking. They looked at the green wall of wave, streaked with sea-weed, that came threateningly on and on and then broke against the opposing boulders, with the eternal, confused tumult that deafens and silences and destroys all sense of time.

Finally Morten made a movement as though rousing himself from deep thought, and said, "Well, you will soon be leaving us, Fräulein Tony."

"No; why? " Tony said absently.

"Well, it is the tenth of September. My holidays are nearly at an end, anyhow. How much longer can it last? Shall you be glad to get back to the society of your own kind? Tell me – I suppose the gentlemen you dance with are very agreeable? – No, no, that was not what I wanted to say. Now you must answer me," he said, with a sudden resolution, shifting his chin in his hands and looking at her. "Here is the question I have been waiting so long to ask. Now: who is Herr Grünlich?"

Tony sat up, looking at him quickly, her eyes shifting back and forth like those of a person recollecting himself on coming out of a dream. She was feeling again the sense of increased personal importance first experienced when Herr Grünlich proposed for her hand.

"Oh, is that what you want to know, Morten?" she said weightily. "Well, I will tell you. It was really very painful for me to have Thomas mention his name like that, the first afternoon; but since you have already heard of him – well, Herr Grünlich, Bendix Grünlich, is a business friend of my father, a well-to-do Hamburg merchant, who has asked for my hand. No, no," she replied quickly to a movement of Morten's, "I have refused him; I have never been able to make up my mind to yield him my consent for life."

"And why not? – if I may ask," said Morten awkwardly.

"Why? Oh, good heavens, because I couldn't endure him," she cried out in a passion. "You ought to have seen him, how he looked and how he acted. Among other things, he had yellow whiskers – dreadfully unnatural. I'm sure he curled them and put on gold powder, like the stuff we use for the Christmas nuts. And he was underhanded. He fawned on my Father and Mother and chimed in with them in the most shameful way –"

Morten interrupted her. "But what does this mean: 'That trims it up uncommonly'?"

Tony broke into a nervous giggle.

"Well, he talked like that, Morten. He wouldn't say 'That looks very well' or 'It goes very well with the room.' He was frightfully silly, I tell you. And very persistent; he simply wouldn't be put off, although I never gave him anything but sarcasm. Once he made such a scene – he nearly wept – imagine a man weeping!"

"He must have worshipped you," Morten said softly.

"Well, what affair was that of mine?" she cried out, astonished, turning around on her sand-heap.

"You are cruel, Fräulein Tony. Are you always cruel? Tell me: You didn't like this Herr Grünlich. But is there any one to whom you have been more gracious? Sometimes I think: Has she a cold heart? Let me tell you something: a man is not idiotic simply because he weeps when you won't look at him. I swear it. I am not sure, not at all, that I wouldn't do the same thing. You see, you are such a dainty, spoilt thing. Do you always make fun of people that lie at your feet? Have you really a cold heart? "

After the first giggle, Tony's lip began to quiver. She turned on him a pair of great distressed eyes, which slowly filled with tears as she said softly: " No, Morten, you should not think that of me – you must not think that of me."

" I don't; indeed I don't," he cried, with a laugh of mingled emotion and hardly suppressed exultation. He turned fully about, so that he lay supporting himself on his elbows, took her hands in both his, and looked straight into hers with his kind steel-blue eyes, which were excited and dreamy and exalted all at once.

" Then you – you won't mock at me if I tell you – ? "

" I know, Morten," she answered gently, looking away from him at the fine white sand sifting through the fingers of her free hand.

" You know – and you – oh, Fräulein Tony! "

" Yes, Morten. I care a great deal for you. More than for any one else I know."

He started up, making awkward gestures with his arms, like a man bewildered. Then he got to his feet, only to throw himself down again by her side and cry in a voice that stammered, wavered, died away and rose again, out of sheer joy: " Oh, thank you, thank you! I am so happy! more than I ever was in all my life! " And he fell to kissing her hands. After a moment he said more quietly: " You will be going back to town soon, Tony, and my holidays will be over in two weeks; then I must return to Göttingen. But will you promise me that you will never forget this afternoon here on the beach – till I come back again with my degree, and can ask your Father – however hard that's going to be? And you won't listen to any Herr Grünlich meantime? Oh, it won't be so long – I will work like a – like anything! it will be so easy! "

" Yes, Morten," she said dreamily, looking at his eyes, his mouth, his hands holding hers.

He drew her hand close to his breast and asked very softly and imploringly: " And won't you – may I – seal the promise? "

She did not answer, she did not look at him, but moved nearer to him on the sand-heap, and Morten kissed her slowly and solemnly on the mouth. Then they stared in different directions across the sand, and both felt furiously embarrassed.

CHAPTER X

Dearest Mademoiselle Buddenbrook,

For how long must the undersigned exist without a glimpse of his enchantress? These few lines will tell you that the vision has never ceased to hover before his spiritual eye; that never has he during these interminably anxious months ceased to think of the precious afternoon in your parental salon, when you let fall a blushing promise which filled me with bliss unspeakable! Since then long weeks have flown, during which you have retired from the world for the sake of calm and self-examination. May I now hope that the period of probation is past? The undersigned permits himself, dearest Mademoiselle, to send the enclosed ring as an earnest of his undying tenderness. With the most tender compliments, and devotedly kissing your hand, I remain,

Your obedient servant,

Grünlich.

Dear Papa,

How angry I've been! I had the enclosed letter and ring just now from Grünlich, and my head aches fearfully from excitement. I don't know what else to do but send them both to you. He simply will not understand me, and what he so poetically writes about the promise isn't in the least true, and I beg you emphatically to make it immediately perfectly clear to him that I am a thousand times less able to say yes to him than I was before, and that he must leave me in peace. He makes himself ridiculous. To you, my dearest Father, I can say that I have bound myself elsewhere, to one who adores me and whom I love more than I can say. Oh, Papa! I could write pages to you! I mean Herr Morten Schwarzkopf, who is studying to be a physician, and who as soon as that happens will ask for my hand. I know that it is the rule of the family to marry a business man, but Morten belongs to the other section of respectable men, the scholars. He is not rich, which I know is important to you and Mamma: but I must tell you that, young as I am, I have learned that riches do not make every one happy. With a thousand kisses,

Your obedient daughter,
ANTONIE.

P.S. I find the ring very poor gold, and too narrow.

MY DEAR TONY,

Your letter duly received. As regards its contents, I must tell you that I did not fail to communicate them to Herr Grünlich: the result was of such a nature as to shock me very much. You are a grown girl, and at a serious time of life, so I need not scruple to tell you the consequences that a frivolous step of yours may draw after it. Herr Grünlich, then, burst into despair at my announcement, declaring that he loved you so dearly, and could so little console himself for your loss, that he would be in a state to take his own life if you remain firm in your resolve. As I cannot take seriously what you write me of another attachment, I must beg you to master your excitement over the ring, and consider everything again very carefully. It is my Christian conviction, my dear daughter, that one must have regard for the feelings of others. We do not know that you may not be made responsible by the most high Judge if a man whose feelings you have coldly and obstinately scorned should trespass against his own life. But the thing I have so often told you by word of mouth, I must recall again to your remembrance, and I am glad to have the occasion to repeat it in writing; for though speech is more vivid and has the more immediate effect, the written word has the advantage that it can be chosen with pains and fixed in a form well-weighed and calculated by the writer, to be read over and over again, with proportionate effect. — My child, we are not born for that which, with our short-sighted vision, we reckon to be our own small personal happiness. We are not free, separate, and independent entities, but like links in a chain, and we could not by any means be what we are without those who went before us and showed us the way, by following the straight and narrow path, not looking to right or left. Your path, it seems to me, has lain all these weeks sharply marked out for you, and you would not be my daughter, nor the granddaughter of your Grandfather who rests in God, nor a worthy member of our own family, if you really have it in your heart, alone, wilfully, and light-headedly to choose your own unregulated path. Your Mother, Thomas, Christian, and I beg you, my dear Antonie, to weigh all this in your heart. Mlle. Jungmann and Clara greet you affectionately, likewise Clothilde, who has been the last several weeks with her father at Thankless. We all rejoice at the thought of embracing you once more.

With unfailing affection,

YOUR LOVING FATHER.

CHAPTER XI

It rained in streams. Heaven, earth, and sea were in flood, while the driving wind took the rain and flung it against the panes as though not drops but brooks were flowing down and making them impossible to see through. Complaining and despairing voices sounded in the chimney.

When Morten Schwarzkopf went out into the verandah with his pipe shortly after dinner to look at the sky, he found there a gentleman with a long, narrow yellow-checked ulster and a grey hat. A closed carriage, its top glistening with wet, its wheels clogged with mud, was before the door. Morten stared irresolutely into the rosy face of the gentleman. He had mutton-chop whiskers that looked as though they had been dressed with gold paint.

The gentleman in the ulster looked at Morten as one looks at a servant, blinking gently without seeing him, and said in a soft voice: " Is Herr Pilot-Captain Schwarzkopf at home? "

" Yes," stammered Morten, " I think my Father – "

Hereupon the gentleman fixed his eyes upon him; they were as blue as a goose's.

" Are you Herr Morten Schwarzkopf? " he asked.

" Yes, sir," answered Morten, trying to keep his face straight.

" Ah – indeed! " remarked the gentleman in the ulster, and went on, " Have the goodness to announce me to your Father, young man. My name is Grünlich."

Morten led the gentleman through the verandah, opened for him the right-hand door that led into the office, and went back into the sitting-room to tell his Father. Then the youth sat down at the round table, resting his elbow on it, and seemed, without noticing his Mother, who was sitting at the dark window mending stockings, to busy himself with the " wretched news-sheet " which had nothing in it except the announcements of the silver wedding of Consul So-and-So. Tony was resting in her room.

The pilot-captain entered his office with the air of a man satisfied with his meal. His uniform-coat stood open over the usual white waistcoat. His face was red, and his ice-grey beard coldly set off against it; his tongue travelled about agreeably among his teeth, making his good mouth take the most extraordinary shapes. He bowed shortly, jerkily, with the air of one conforming to the conventions as he understood them.

" Good afternoon," he said. " At your service."

Herr Grünlich, on his side, bowed with deliberation, although one corner of his mouth seemed to go down. He said softly: " Ahem! "

The office was rather a small room, the walls of which had wainscoting for a few feet and then simple plaster. Curtains, yellow with smoke, hung before the window, on whose panes the rain beat unceasingly. On the right of the door was a rough table covered with papers, above it a large map of Europe, and a smaller one of the Baltic Sea fastened to the wall. From the middle of the ceiling hung the well-cut model of a ship under full sail.

The Captain made his guest take the sloping sofa, covered with cracked oil-cloth, that stood opposite the door, and made himself comfortable in a wooden arm-chair, folding his hands across his stomach; while Herr Grünlich, his ulster tightly buttoned up, his hat on his knees, sat bolt upright on the edge of the sofa.

" My name is, I repeat, Grünlich," he said; " from Hamburg. I may say by way of introduction that I am a close business friend of Herr Buddenbrook."

" Servant, Herr Grünlich; pleased to make your acquaintance. Won't you make yourself comfortable? Have a glass of grog after your journey? I'll send right into the kitchen."

" I must permit myself to remark that my time is limited, my carriage is waiting, and I am really obliged to ask for the favour of a few words with you."

" At your service," repeated Herr Schwarzkopf, taken aback. There was a pause.

" Herr Captain," began Herr Grünlich, wagging his head with determination and throwing himself back on his seat. After this he was silent again; and by way of enhancing the effect of his address he shut his mouth tight, like a purse drawn together with strings.

" Herr Captain," he repeated, and went on without further pause, " The matter about which I have come to you directly concerns the young lady who has been for some weeks stopping in your house."

" Mademoiselle Buddenbrook? " asked the Consul.

" Precisely," assented Herr Grünlich. He looked down at the

floor, and spoke in a voice devoid of expression. Hard lines came out at the corners of his mouth.

"I am obliged to inform you," he went on in a sing-song tone, his sharp eyes jumping from one point in the room to another and then to the window, "that some time ago I proposed for the hand of Mademoiselle Buddenbrook. I am in possession of the fullest confidence of both parents, and the young lady herself has unmistakably given me a claim to her hand, though no betrothal has taken place in form."

"You don't say – God keep us!" said Herr Schwarzkopf, in a sprightly tone. "I never heard that before! Congratulations, Herr – er – Grünlich. She's a good girl – genuine good stuff."

"Thank you for the compliment," said Herr Grünlich, coldly. He went on in his high sing-song: "What brings me to you on this occasion, my good Herr Captain, is the circumstance that certain difficulties have just arisen – and these difficulties – appear to have their source in your house – ?" He spoke the last words in a questioning tone, as if to say, "Can this disgraceful state of things be true, or have my ears deceived me?"

Herr Schwarzkopf answered only by lifting his eyebrows as high as they would go, and clutching the arms of his chair with his brown, blond-felled fisherman's hands.

"Yes. This is the fact. So I am informed," Herr Grünlich said, with dreary certitude. "I hear that your son – *studiosus medicinae*, I am led to understand – has allowed himself – of course unconsciously – to encroach upon my rights. I hear that he has taken advantage of the present visit of the young lady to extract certain promises from her."

"What?" shouted the pilot-captain, gripping the arms of his chair and springing up. "That we shall soon – we can soon see – !" With two steps he was at the door, tore it open, and shouted down the corridor in a voice that would have outroared the wildest seas: "Meta, Morten! Come in here, both of you."

"I shall regret it exceedingly if the assertion of my prior rights runs counter to your fatherly hopes, Herr Captain."

Diederich Schwarzkopf turned and stared, with his sharp blue eyes in their wrinkled setting, straight into the stranger's face, as though he strove in vain to comprehend his words.

"Sir!" he said. Then, with a voice that sounded as though he had just burnt his throat with hot grog, "I'm a simple sort of a man, and don't know much about landlubber's tricks and skin games; but if you mean, maybe, that – well, sir, you can just set it down right away that you've got on the wrong tack, and are making a pretty bad miscalculation about my fatherly hopes. I know who my son is, and I know who Mademoiselle Buddenbrook is, and there's too much respect and too much pride in my carcase to be making any plans of the sort you've mentioned. – And now," he roared, jerking his head toward the door, " it's your turn to talk, boy. You tell me what this affair is; what is this I hear – hey? "

Frau Schwarzkopf and her son stood in the doorway, she innocently arranging her apron, he with the air of a hardened sinner. Herr Grünlich did not rise at their entrance. He waited, erect and composed, on the edge of the sofa, buttoned up tight in his ulster.

" So you've been behaving like a silly fool? " bellowed the captain to Morten.

The young man had his thumb stuck between the buttons of his jacket. He scowled and puffed out his cheeks defiantly.

" Yes, Father," he said, " Fräulein Buddenbrook and I – "

" Well, then, I'll just tell you you're a perfect Tom-fool, a young ninny, and you'll be packed off to-morrow for Göttingen – to-morrow, understand? It's all damned childish nonsense, and rascality into the bargain."

" Good heavens, Diederich," said Frau Schwarzkopf, folding her hands, " you can't just say that, you know. Who knows – ? " She stopped, she said no more; but it was plain from her face that a mother's beautiful dream had been shattered in that moment.

" Would the gentleman like to see the young lady? " Schwarzkopf turned to Herr Grünlich and spoke in a harsh voice.

" She is upstairs in her room asleep," Frau Schwarzkopf said with feeling.

" I regret," said Herr Grünlich, and he got up, obviously relieved. " But I repeat that my time is limited, and the carriage waits. I permit myself," he went on, describing with his hat a motion in the direction of Herr Schwarzkopf, " to acknowledge to you, Herr Captain, my entire recognition of your manly and high-principled bearing. I salute you. Good-bye."

Diederich Schwarzkopf did not offer to shake hands with him. He merely gave a jerky bow with the upper part of his heavy figure, that had an air of saying: " This is the proper thing, I suppose."

Herr Grünlich, with measured tread, passed between Morten and his mother and went out the door.

CHAPTER XII

THOMAS appeared with the Kröger calèche. The day was at hand.

The young man arrived at ten o'clock in the forenoon and took a bite with the family in the living-room. They sat together as on the first day, except that now summer was over; it was too cold and windy to sit in the verandah; and – Morten was not there. He was in Göttingen. Tony and he had not even been able to say good-bye. The Captain had stood there and said, " Well, so that's the end of that, eh! "

At eleven the brother and sister mounted into the wagon, where Tony's trunk was already fastened at the back. She was pale and shivered in her soft autumn coat – from cold, weariness, excitement, and a grief that now and then rose up suddenly and filled her breast with a painful oppression. She kissed little Meta, pressed the house-wife's hand, and nodded to Herr Schwarzkopf when he said, " Well, you won't forget us, little Miss, will you? And no bad feeling, eh? And a safe journey and best greetings to your honoured Father and the Frau Consul." Then the coach door slammed, the fat brown horses pulled at their traces, and the three Schwarzkopfs waved their handkerchiefs.

Tony crooked her neck in the corner of the coach, in order to peer out of the window. The sky was covered with white cloud-flakes; the Trave broke into little waves that hurried before the wind. Now and then drops of rain pattered against the glass. At the end of the front people sat in the doors of their cottages and mended nets; barefoot children came running to look curiously at the carriage. *They* did not have to go away!

As they left the last houses behind, Tony bent forward to look at the lighthouse; then she leaned back and closed her tired and burning eyes. She had hardly slept for excitement. She had risen early to finish her packing, and discovered no desire for breakfast. There was a dull taste in her mouth, and she felt so weak that she made no effort to dry the slow, hot tears that kept rising every minute.

But directly her eyes were shut, she found herself again in Travemünde, on the verandah. She saw Morten in the flesh before her; he seemed to speak and to lean toward her as he always did, and then look good-naturedly and searchingly at the next person, unconsciously showing his beautiful teeth as he smiled. Slowly her mind grew calm and peaceful again. She recalled everything that she had heard and learned from him in many a talk, and it solaced her to promise herself that she would preserve all this as a secret holy and inviolate and cherish it in her heart. That the King of Prussia had committed a great wrong against his people; that the local newspaper was a lamentable sheet; yes, that the laws of the League concerning universities had been renewed four years ago – all these were from now on consoling and edifying truths, a hidden treasure which she might store up within herself and contemplate whenever she chose. On the street, in the family circle, at the table she would think of them. Who knew? Perhaps she might even go on in the path prescribed for her and marry Herr Grünlich – that was a detail, after all – but when he spoke to her she could always say to herself, "I know something you don't: the nobility is in principle despicable."

She smiled to herself and was assuaged. But suddenly, in the noise of the wheels, she heard Morten's voice with miraculous clearness. She distinguished every nuance of his kindly, dragging speech as he said: "To-day we must both 'sit on the rocks,' Fräulein Tony," and this little memory overpowered her. Her breast contracted with her grief, and she let the tears flow down unopposed. Bowed in her corner, she held her handkerchief before her face and wept bitterly.

Thomas, his cigarette in his mouth, looked somewhat blankly at the high-road. "Poor Tony," he said at last, stroking her jacket. "I feel so sorry – I understand so well, you know. But what can you do? One has to bear these things. Believe me, I do understand what you feel."

"Oh, you don't understand at all, Tom," sobbed Tony.

"Don't say that. Did you know it is decided that I am to go to Amsterdam at the beginning of next year? Papa has obtained a place for me with van der Kellen and Company. That means I must say good-bye for a long, long time."

"Oh, Tom! Saying good-bye to your father and mother and sisters and brothers – that isn't anything."

"Ye-es," he said, slowly. He sighed, as if he did not wish to say more, and was silent. He let the cigarette rove from one corner of his mouth to the other, lifted one eyebrow, and turned his head away.

"Well, it doesn't last for ever," he began again after a while. "Naturally one forgets."

"But I don't want to forget," Tony cried out in desperation. "Forgetting – is that any consolation?"

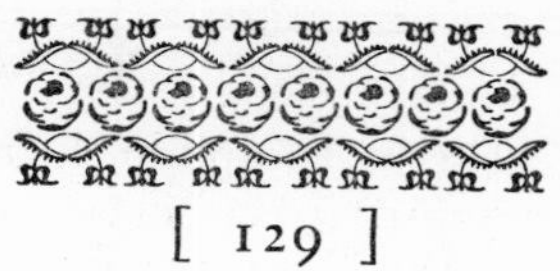

CHAPTER XIII

THEN came the ferry, and Israelsdorf Avenue, Jerusalem Hill, the Castle Field. The wagon passed the Castle Gate, with the walls of the prison rising on the right, and rolled along Castle Street and over the Koberg. Tony looked at the grey gables, the oil lamps hung across the streets, Holy Ghost Hospital with the already almost bare lindens in front of it. Oh, how everything was exactly as it had been! It had been standing here, in immovable dignity, while she had thought of it as a dream worthy only to be forgotten. These grey gables were the old, the accustomed, the traditional, to which she was returning, in the midst of which she must live. She wept no more. She looked about curiously. The pain of parting was almost dulled at the sight of these well-known streets and faces. At that moment – the wagon was rolling through Broad Street – the porter Matthiesen passed and took off his stove-pipe hat so obsequiously that it seemed he must be thinking, " Bow, you dog of a porter – you can't bow low enough."

The equipage turned into the Mengstrasse, and the fat brown horses stood snorting and stamping before the Buddenbrook door. Tom was very attentive in helping his sister out, while Anton and Line hastened up to unfasten the trunk. But they had to wait before they could enter the house. Three great lorries were being driven through, one close behind another, piled high with full corn sacks, with the firm name written on them in big black letters. They jolted along over the great boards and down the shallow steps to the cart-yard with a heavy rumbling noise. Part of the corn was evidently to be unloaded at the back of the house and the rest taken to the " Walrus," the " Lion," or the " Oak."

The Consul came out of the office with his pen behind his ear as the brother and sister reached the entry, and stretched out his arms to his daughter.

" Welcome home, my dear Tony! "

She kissed him, looking a little shame-faced, her eyes still red with weeping. But he was very tactful; he made no allusions; he only said: " It is late, but we waited with the second breakfast."

The Frau Consul, Christian, Clothilde, Clara, and Ida Jungmann stood above on the landing to greet her.

Tony slept soundly and well the first night in Mengstrasse. She rose the next morning, the twenty-second of September, refreshed and calmed, and went down into the breakfast-room. It was still quite early, hardly seven o'clock. Only Mamsell Jungmann was there, making the morning coffee.

"Well, well, Tony, my little child," she said, looking round with her small, blinking brown eyes. "Up so early?"

Tony sat down at the open desk, clasped her hands behind her head, and looked for a while at the pavement of the court, gleaming black with wet, and at the damp, yellow garden. Then she began to rummage curiously among the visiting-cards and letters on the desk. Close by the inkstand lay the well-known large copy-book with the stamped cover, gilt edges, and leaves of various qualities and colours. It must have been used the evening before, and it was strange that Papa had not put it back in its leather portfolio and laid it in its special drawer.

She took it and turned over the pages, began to read, and became absorbed. What she read were mostly simple facts well known to her; but each successive writer had followed his predecessor in a stately but simple chronicle style which was no bad mirror of the family attitude, its modest but honourable self-respect, and its reverence for tradition and history. The book was not new to Tony; she had sometimes been allowed to read in it. But its contents had never made the impression upon her that they made this morning. She was thrilled by the reverent particularity with which the simplest facts pertinent to the family were here treated. She propped herself on her elbows and read with growing absorption, seriousness and pride.

No point in her own tiny past was lacking. Her birth, her childish illnesses, her first school, her boarding-school days at Mademoiselle Weichbrodt's, her confirmation – everything was carefully entered, with an almost reverent observation of facts, in the Consul's small, flowing business hand; for was not the least of them the will and work of God, who wonderfully guided the destinies of the family? What, she mused, would there be entered here in the future after her name, which she had received from her grandmother Antoinette? All that was yet to be written there would be conned by later members of the family with a piety equal to her own.

She leaned back sighing; her heart beat solemnly. She was filled with reverence for herself: the familiar feeling of personal importance possessed her, heightened by all she had been reading. She felt thrilled and shuddery. "Like a link in a chain," Papa had written. Yes, yes. She was important precisely as a link in this chain. Such was her significance and her responsibility, such her task: to share by deed and word in the history of her family.

She turned back to the end of the great volume, where on a rough folio page was entered the genealogy of the whole Buddenbrook family, with parentheses and rubrics, indicated in the Consul's hand, and all the dates set down: from the marriage of the earliest scion of the family with Brigitta Schuren, the pastor's daughter, down to the wedding of Consul Johann Buddenbrook with Elizabeth Kröger in 1825. From this marriage, it said, four children had resulted: whereupon these were all entered, with the days and years of their birth, and their baptismal names, one after another. Under that of the eldest son it was recorded that he had entered as apprentice in his father's business in the Easter of 1842.

Tony looked a long time at her name and at the blank space next it. Then, suddenly, with a jerk, with a nervous, feverish accompaniment of sobbing breaths and quick-moving lips – she clutched the pen, plunged it rather than dipped it into the ink, and wrote, with her forefinger crooked, her hot head bent far over on her shoulder, in her awkward handwriting that climbed up the page from left to right: "Betrothed, on Sept. 22, 1845, to Herr Bendix Grünlich, Merchant, of Hamburg."

CHAPTER XIV

"I ENTIRELY agree with you, my good friend. This important matter must be settled. In short, then: the usual dowry of a young girl of our family is seventy thousand marks."

Herr Grünlich cast at his future father-in-law a shrewd, calculating glance – the glance of the genuine man of business.

"As a matter of fact," he said – and this "matter of fact" was of precisely the same length as his left-hand whisker, which he was drawing reflectively through his fingers; he let go of the end just as "of fact" was finished.

"You know, my honoured father," he began again, "the deep respect I have for traditions and principles. Only – in the present case is not this consideration for the tradition a little exaggerated? A business increases – a family prospers – in short, conditions change and improve."

"My good friend," said the Consul, "you see in me a fair-dealing merchant. You have not let me finish, or you would have heard that I am ready and willing to meet you in the circumstances, and add ten thousand marks to the seventy thousand without more ado."

"Eighty thousand, then," said Herr Grünlich, making motions with his mouth, as though to say: "Not *too* much; but it will do."

Thus they came to an affectionate settlement; the Consul jingled his keys like a man satisfied as he got up. And, in fact, his satisfaction was justified; for it was only with the eighty thousand marks that they had arrived at the dowry traditional in the family.

Herr Grünlich now said good-bye and departed for Hamburg. Tony as yet realized but little of her new estate. She still went to dances at the Möllendorpfs', Kistenmakers', and Langhals', and in her own home; she skated on the Burgfield and the meadows of the Trave, and permitted the attentions of the young gentlemen of the town. In the middle of October she went to the betrothal feast at the Möllendorpfs' for the oldest son of the house and Juliet Hagenström. "Tom," she said, "I won't go. It is disgusting." But she went, and enjoyed herself hugely. And, as for the rest, by the entry with the pen in the family history-book, she had won the privilege of going, with the Frau Consul or alone, into all the shops in town and making purchases in a grand style for her trousseau. It was to be a brilliant trousseau. Two seamstresses sat all day in the breakfast-room window, sewing, embroidering monograms, and eating quantities of house-bread and green cheese.

" Is the linen come from Lentföhr, Mamma? "

" No, but here are two dozen tea-serviettes."

" That is nice. But he promised it by this afternoon. My goodness, the sheets still have to be hemmed."

" Mamsell Bitterlich wants to know about the lace for the pillow-cases, Ida."

" It is in the right-hand cupboard in the entry, Tony, my child."

" Line – ! "

" You could go yourself, my dear."

" Oh, if I'm marrying for the privilege of running up and down stairs – ! "

" Have you made up your mind yet about the material for the wedding-dress, Tony? "

" Moiré antique, Mamma – I won't marry without moiré antique! "

So passed October and November. At Christmas time Herr Grünlich appeared, to spend Christmas in the Buddenbrook family circle and also to take part in the celebration at the Krögers'. His conduct toward his bride showed all the delicacy one would have expected from him. No unnecessary formality, no importunity, no tactless tenderness. A light, discreet kiss upon the forehead, in the presence of the parents, sealed the betrothal. Tony sometimes puzzled over this, the least in the world. Why, she wondered, did his present happiness seem not quite commensurate with the despair into which her refusal had thrown him? He regarded her with the air of a satisfied possessor. Now and then, indeed, if they happened to be alone, a jesting and teasing mood seemed to overcome him; once he attempted to fall on his knees and approach his whiskers to her face, while he asked in a voice apparently trembling with joy, " Have I indeed captured you? Have I won you for my own? " To which Tony answered, " You are forgetting yourself," and got away with all possible speed.

Soon after the holidays Herr Grünlich went back to Hamburg, for his flourishing business demanded his personal attention; and the Buddenbrooks agreed with him that Tony had had time enough before the betrothal to make his acquaintance.

The question of a house was quickly arranged. Tony, who

looked forward extravagantly to life in a large city, had expressed the wish to settle in Hamburg itself, and indeed in the Spitalstrasse, where Herr Grünlich's office was. But the bridegroom, by manly persistence, won her over to the purchase of a villa outside the city, near Eimsbüttel, a romantic and retired spot, an ideal nest for a newly-wedded pair – "*procul negotiis*." – Ah, he had not yet forgotten quite all his Latin!

Thus December passed, and at the beginning of the year '46 the wedding was celebrated. There was a splendid wedding feast, to which half the town was bidden. Tony's friends – among them Armgard von Schilling, who arrived in a towering coach – danced with Tom's and Christian's friends, among them Andreas Gieseke, son of the Fire Commissioner and now *studiosus juris;* also Stephan and Edouard Kistenmaker, of Kistenmaker and Son. They danced in the dining-room and the hall, which had been strewn with talc for the occasion. Among the liveliest of the lively was Consul Peter Döhlmann; he got hold of all the earthenware crocks he could find and broke them on the flags of the big passage.

Frau Stuht from Bell-Founders' Street had another opportunity to mingle in the society of the great; for it was she who helped Mamsell Jungmann and the two seamstresses to adjust Tony's toilette on the great day. She had, as God was her judge, never seen a more beautiful bride. Fat as she was, she went on her knees; and, with her eyes rolled up in admiration, fastened the myrtle twigs on the white moiré antique. This was in the breakfast-room. Herr Grünlich, in his long-skirted frock-coat and silk waistcoat, waited at the door. His rosy face had a correct and serious expression, his wart was powdered, and his gold-yellow whiskers carefully curled.

Above in the hall, where the marriage was to take place, the family gathered – a stately assemblage. There sat the old Krögers, a little ailing both of them, but distinguished figures always. There was Consul Kröger with his sons Jürgen and Jacob, the latter having come from Hamburg, like the Duchamps. There were Gotthold Buddenbrook and his wife, born Stüwing, with their three offspring, Friederike, Henriette, and Pfiffi, none of whom was, unfortunately, likely to marry. There was the Mecklenburg branch, represented by Clothilde's father, Herr Bernhard Buddenbrook, who had come in from Thankless and looked with large eyes at the seignorial house of his rich relations. The relatives from Frankfort had contented themselves with sending presents; the journey was too arduous. In their place were the only guests not members of the family. Dr. Grabow, the family physician, and Mlle. Weichbrodt, Tony's motherly friend – Sesemi Weichbrodt, with fresh ribbons on her cap over the side curls, and a little black dress. "Be happy, you *good* child," she said, when Tony appeared at Herr Grünlich's side in the hall. She reached up and kissed her with a little explosion on the forehead. The family was satisfied with the bride: Tony looked pretty, gay, and at her ease, if a little pale from excitement and tension.

The hall had been decorated with flowers and an altar arranged on the right side. Pastor Kölling of St. Mary's performed the service, and laid special stress upon moderation. Everything went according to custom and arrangement, Tony brought out a hearty yes, and Herr Grünlich gave his little ahem, beforehand, to clear his throat. Afterward, everybody ate long and well.

While the guests continued to eat in the salon, with the pastor in their midst, the Consul and his wife accompanied the young pair, who had dressed for their journey, out into the snowy, misty air, where the great travelling coach stood before the door, packed with boxes and bags.

After Tony had expressed many times her conviction that she should soon be back again on a visit, and that they too would not delay long to come to Hamburg to see her, she climbed in good spirits into the coach and let herself be carefully wrapped up by the Consul in the warm fur rug. Her husband took his place by her side.

"And, Grünlich," said the Consul, "the new laces are in the small satchel, on top. You take a little in under your overcoat, don't you? This excise – one has to get around it the best one can. Farewell, farewell! Farewell, dear Tony. God bless you."

"You will find good accommodation in Arensburg, won't you?" asked the Frau Consul. "Already reserved, my dear Mamma," answered Herr Grünlich.

Anton, Line, Trine, and Sophie took leave of Ma'am Grünlich. The coach door was about to be slammed, when Tony was overtaken by a sudden impulse. Despite all the trouble it took, she unwound herself again from her wrappings, climbed ruthlessly over Herr Grünlich, who began to grumble, and embraced her Father with passion. "Adieu, Papa, adieu, my good Papa." And then she whispered softly: "Are you satisfied with me?"

The Consul pressed her without words to his heart, then put her from him and shook her hands with deep feeling.

Now everything was ready. The coach door slammed, the coachman cracked his whip, the horses dashed away so that the coach windows rattled; the Frau Consul let fly her little white handkerchief; and the carriage, rolling down the street, disappeared in the mist.

The Consul stood thoughtfully next to his wife, who drew her cloak about her shoulders with a graceful movement.

"There she goes, Betsy."

"Yes, Jean, the first to leave us. Do you think she is happy with him?"

"Oh, Betsy, she is satisfied with herself, which is better; it is the most solid happiness we can have on this earth."

They went back to their guests.

CHAPTER XV

Thomas Buddenbrook went down Meng Street as far as the " Five Houses." He avoided Broad Street so as not to be accosted by acquaintances and obliged to greet them. With his hands deep in the big pockets of his warm dark grey overcoat, he walked, sunk in thought, over the hard, sparkling snow, which crunched under his boots. He went his own way, and whither it led no one knew but himself. The sky was pale blue and clear, the air biting and crisp – a still, severe, clear weather, with five degrees of frost; in short, a matchless February day.

Thomas walked down the " Five Houses," crossed Bakers' Alley, and went along a narrow cross-street into Fishers' Lane. He followed this street, which led down to the Trave parallel to Meng Street, for a few steps, and paused before a small house, a modest flower-shop, with a narrow door and dingy show-window, where a few pots of bulbs stood on a pane of green glass.

He went in, whereupon the bell above the door began to give tongue, like a little watch-dog. Within, before the counter, talking to the young saleswoman, was a little fat elderly lady in a Turkey shawl. She was choosing a pot of flowers, examining, smelling, criticizing, chattering, and constantly obliged to wipe her mouth with her handkerchief. Thomas Buddenbrook greeted her politely and stepped to one side. She was a poor relation of the Langhals', a good-natured garrulous old maid who bore the name of one of the best families without herself belonging to their set: that is, she was not asked to the large dinners, but to the small coffee circles. She was known to almost all the world as Aunt Lottchen. She turned toward the door, with her pot of flowers, wrapped up in tissue paper, under her arm; and Thomas, after greeting her again, said in an elevated voice to the shop girl, " Give me a couple of roses, please. Never mind the kind – well, La France."

Then, after Aunt Lottchen had shut the door behind her and gone away, he said in a lower voice, " Put them away again, Anna. How are you, little Anna? Here I am – and I've come with a heavy heart."

Anna wore a white apron over her simple black frock. She was wonderfully pretty. Delicately built as a fawn, she had an almost mongol type of face, somewhat prominent cheek-bones, narrow black eyes full of a soft gleam, and a pale yellow skin the like of which is rare anywhere. Her hands, of the same tint, were narrow, and more beautiful than a shop girl's are wont to be.

She went behind the counter at the right end, so that she could not be seen through the shop-window. Thomas followed on the outside of the counter and, bending over, kissed her on the lips and the eyes.

" You are quite frozen, poor boy," she said.

" Five degrees," said Tom. " I didn't notice it, I've felt so sad coming over."

He sat down on the table, keeping her hand in his, and went on: " Listen, Anna; we'll be sensible to-day, won't we? The time has come."

" Oh, dear," she said miserably, and lifted her apron to her eyes.

" It had to happen some time, Anna. No, don't weep. We were going to be reasonable, weren't we? What else is there to do? One has to bear such things."

" When? " asked Anna, sobbing.

" Day after to-morrow."

" Oh, God, no! Why to-morrow? A week longer – five days! Please, oh, please! "

" Impossible, dear Anna. Everything is arranged and in order. They are expecting me in Amsterdam. I couldn't make it a day longer, no matter how much I wanted."

" And that is so far away – so far away! "

" Amsterdam? Nonsense, that isn't far. We can always think of each other, can't we? And I'll write to you. You'll see, I'll write directly I've got there."

" Do you remember," she said, " a year and a half ago, at the Rifle-club fair? "

He interrupted her ardently. " Do I remember? Yes, a year and a half ago! I took you for an Italian. I bought a pink and put it in my button-hole. – I still have it – I am taking it with me to Amsterdam. – What a heat: how hot and dusty it was on the meadow! "

" Yes, you bought me a glass of lemonade from the next booth. I remember it like yesterday. Everything smelled of fatty-cakes and people."

" But it was fine! We knew right away how we felt – about each other! "

"You wanted to take me on the carrousel, but I couldn't go; I had to be in the shop. The old woman would have scolded."

"No, I know it wouldn't have done, Anna."

She said softly and clearly, "But that is the only thing I've refused you."

He kissed her again, on the lips and the eyes. "Adieu, darling little Anna. We must begin to say good-bye."

"Oh, you will come back to-morrow?"

"Yes, of course, and day after to-morrow early, if I can get away. – But there is one thing I want to say to you, Anna. I am going, after all, rather far away. Amsterdam *is* a long way off – and you are staying here. But – don't throw yourself away, I tell you."

She wept into her apron, holding it up with her free hand to her face. "And you – and you?"

"God knows, Anna, what will happen. One isn't young for ever – you are a sensible girl, you have never said anything about marriage and that sort of thing –"

"God forbid – that I should ask such a thing of you!"

"One is carried along – you see. If I live, I shall take over the business, and make a good match – you see, I am open with you at parting, Anna. I wish you every happiness, darling, darling little Anna. But don't throw yourself away, do you hear? For you haven't done that – with me – I swear it."

It was warm in the shop. A moist scent of earth and flowers was in the air. Outside, the winter sun was hurrying to its repose, and a pure delicate sunset, like one painted on porcelain, beautified the sky across the river. People hurried past the window, their chins tucked into their turned-up collars; no one gave a glance into the corner of the little flower-shop, at the two who stood there saying their last farewells.

PART FOUR

[143]

CHAPTER I

April 30, 1846

My dear Mamma,

A thousand thanks for your letter, in which you tell me of Armgard von Schilling's betrothal to Herr von Maiboom of Pöppenrade. Armgard herself sent me an invitation (very fine, with a gilt edge), and also a letter in which she expresses herself as enchanted with her bridegroom. He sounds like a very handsome and refined man. How happy she must be! Everybody is getting married. I have had a card from Munich too, from Eva Ewers. I hear she's getting a director of a brewery.

Now I must ask you something, dearest Mamma: Why do I hear nothing of a visit from the Buddenbrooks? Are you waiting for an official invitation from Grünlich? If so, it isn't necessary; and besides, when I remind him to ask you, he says, "Yes, yes, child, your Father has something else to do." Or do you think you would be disturbing me? Oh, dear me, no; quite the contrary! Perhaps you think you would make me homesick again? But don't you know I am a reasonable woman, already middle-aged and experienced?

I've just been to coffee at Madame Käselau's, a neighbour of mine. They are pleasant people, and our left-hand neighbours, the Gussmanns (but there is a good deal of space between the houses) are sociable people too. We have two friends who are at the house a good deal, both of whom live out here: Doctor Klaasen, of whom I must tell you more later, and Kesselmeyer, the banker, Grünlich's intimate friend. You don't know what a funny old man he is. He has a stubbly white beard and thin black and white hair on his head, that looks like down and waves in the breeze. He makes funny motions with his head, like a bird, and talks all the time, so I call him the magpie, but Grünlich has forbidden me to say that, because magpies steal, and Herr Kesselmeyer is an honourable man. He stoops when he walks, and rows along with his arms. His fuzz only reaches half-way down his head in the back, and from there on his neck is all red and seamy. There is something so awfully sprightly about him! Sometimes he pats me on the cheek and says, "You good little wifey! what a blessing for Grünlich that he has got you." Then he takes out his eye-glasses (he always wears three of them, on long cords, that are forever getting tangled up in his white waistcoat) and sticks them on his nose, which he wrinkles up to make them stop on, and looks at me with his mouth open, until I have to laugh, right in his face. But he takes no offence at that.

Grünlich is very busy; he drives into town in the morning in our little yellow wagon and often does not come back till late. Sometimes he sits down with me and reads the paper.

When we go into society – for example, to Kesselmeyer's, or to Consul Goudstikker on the Alster Dam, or Senator Bock's in City Hall Street – we have to take a hired coach. I have begged Grünlich again and again to get a coupé, for it is really a necessity out here. He has half promised, but, strange to say, he does not like to go into society with me and is evidently displeased when I visit people in the town. Do you suppose he is jealous?

Our villa, which I've already described to you in detail, dear Mamma, is really very pretty, and is much prettier by reason of the new furnishings. You could not find a flaw in the upstairs sitting-room – all in brown silk. The dining-room next is prettily wainscoted. The chairs cost twenty-five marks apiece. I sit in the "pensée-room," which we use as a sitting-room. There is also a little room for smoking and playing cards. The salon, which takes up the whole other half of the parterre, has new yellow blinds now and looks very well. Above are the bed, bath, and dressing-rooms and the servants' quarters. We have a little groom for the yellow wagon. I am fairly well satisfied with the two maid-servants. I am not sure they are quite honest, but thank God I don't have to look after every kreuzer. In short, everything is really worthy of the family and the firm.

And now, dear Mamma, comes the most important part of my letter, which I have kept till the last. A while ago I was feeling rather queer – not exactly ill and yet not quite well. I told Dr. Klaasen about it when I had the chance. He is a little bit of a man with a big head and a still bigger hat. He carries a cane with a flat round handle made of a piece of bone, and walks with it pressed against his whiskers, which are almost light-green from being dyed so many years. Well, you should have seen him! he did not answer my questions at all, but jerked his eye-glasses, twinkled his little eyes, wrinkled his nose at me – it looks like a potato – snickered, giggled, and stared so impertinently that I did not know what to do. Then he examined me, and said everything was going on well, only I must drink mineral water, because I am perhaps a little anaemic. Oh, Mamma, do tell Papa about it, so he can put it in the family book. I will write you again as soon as possible, you may be sure.

Give my love to Papa, Christian, Clara, Clothilde and Ida Jungmann. I wrote to Thomas just lately.

Your dutiful daughter,

ANTONIE.

August 2, 1846

MY DEAR THOMAS,

I have read with pleasure the news of your meeting with Christian in Amsterdam. It must have been a happy few days for both of you. I have no word as yet of your brother's further journey to England via Ostende, but I hope that with God's mercy it has been safely accomplished. It may not be too late, since Christian has decided to give up a professional career, for him to learn much that is valuable from his chief, Mr. Richardson; may he prosper and find blessing in the mercantile line! Mr. Richardson, Threadneedle Street, is, as you know, a close business friend of our house; I consider myself lucky to have placed both my sons with such friendly-disposed firms. You are now experiencing the good result of such a policy; and I feel profound satisfaction that Herr van der Kellen has already raised your salary in the quarter of a year you have been with him, and that he will continue to give you advancement. I am convinced that you have shown and will continue to show yourself, by your industry and good behaviour, worthy of these favours.

I regret to hear that your health is not so good as it should be. What you write me of nervousness reminds me of my own youth, when I was working in Antwerp and had to go to Ems to take a cure. If anything of the sort seems best for you, my son, I am ready to encourage you with advice and assistance, although I am avoiding such expense for the rest of us in these times of political unrest.

However, your Mother and I took a trip to Hamburg in the middle of June to visit your sister Tony. Her husband had not invited us, but he received us with the greatest cordiality and devoted himself to us so entirely during the two days of our visit, that he neglected his business and hardly left me time for a visit to Duchamps in the town. Antonie is in her fifth month, and her physician assures her that everything is going on in a normal and satisfactory way.

I have still to mention a letter from Herr van der Kellen, from which I was pleased to learn that you are a favoured guest in his family circle. You are now, my son, at an age to begin to harvest the fruits of the upbringing your parents gave you. It may be helpful to you if I tell you that at your age, both in Antwerp and Bergen, I formed a habit of making myself useful and agreeable to my principals; and this was of the greatest service to me. Aside from the honour of association with the family of the head of the firm, one acquires an advocate in the person of the principal's wife; and she may prove invaluable in the undesirable contingency of an oversight at the office or the dissatisfaction of your chief for some slight cause or other.

As regards your business plans for the future, my son, I rejoice in the lively interest they indicate, without being able entirely to agree with them. You start with the idea that the market for our native products – for instance, grain, rape-seed, hides and skins, wool, oil, oil-cake, bones, etc. – is our chief concern; and you think it would be of advantage for you to turn yourself to the commission branch of the business. I once occupied myself with these ideas, at a time when the competition was small (it has since distinctly increased), and I made some experiments in them. My journey to England had for its chief purpose to look out connections there for my undertakings. To this end I went as far as Scotland, and made many valuable acquaintances; but I soon recognized the precarious nature of an export trade hither, and decided to discourage further expansion in that direction. Thus I kept in mind the warning of our forefather, the founder of the firm, which he bequeathed to us, his descendants: "My son, attend with zeal to thy business by day, but do none that hinders thee from thy sleep at night."

This principle I intend to keep sacred, now as in the past, though one is sometimes forced to entertain a doubt, on contemplating the operations of people who seem to get on better without it. I am thinking of Strunck and Hagenström, who have made such notable progress while our own business seems almost at a stand-still. You know that the house has not enlarged its business since the set-back consequent upon the death of your grandfather; and I pray to God that I shall be able to turn over the business to you in its present state. I have an experienced and cautious adviser in our head clerk Marcus. If only your Mother's family would hang on to their groschen a little better! The inheritance is a matter of real importance for us.

I am unusually full of business and civic work. I have been made alderman of the Board of the Bergen Line; also city deputy for the Finance Department, the Chamber of Commerce, the Auditing Commission, and the Almshouse of St. Anne, one after the other.

Your Mother, Clara and Clothilde send greetings. Also several gentlemen – Senator Möllendorpf, Doctor Överdieck, Consul Kistenmaker, Gosch the broker, C. F. Köppen, and Herr Marcus in the office, have asked to be remembered. God's blessing on you, my dear son. Work, pray, and save.

With affectionate regards,
YOUR FATHER.

October 8, 1846

DEAR AND HONOURED PARENTS,

The undersigned is overjoyed to be able to advise you of the happy *accouchement*, half an hour ago, of your daughter, my beloved wife Antonie. It is, by God's will, a daughter; I can find no words to express my joyful emotion. The health of the dear patient, as well as of the infant, is unexceptionable. Dr. Klaasen is entirely satisfied with the way things have gone; and Frau Grossgeorgis, the midwife, says it was simply nothing at all. Excitement obliges me to lay down my pen. I commend myself to my worthy parents with the most respectful affection.

B. GRÜNLICH.

If it had been a boy, I had a very pretty name. As it is, I wanted to name her Meta, but Grünlich is for Erica.

CHAPTER II

"WHAT is the matter, Betsy?" said the Consul, as he came to the table and lifted up the plate with which his soup was covered. "Aren't you well? You don't look just right to me."

The round table in the great dining-room was grown very small. Around it there gathered in these days, besides the parents, only little Clara, now ten years old, Mamsell Jungmann, and Clothilde, as humble, lean, and hungry as ever. The Consul looked about him: every face was long and gloomy. What had happened? He himself was troubled and anxious; for the Bourse was unsteady, owing to this complicated Schleswig-Holstein affair. And still another source of disquiet was in the air; when Anton had gone to fetch in the meat course, the Consul heard what had happened. Trina, the cook, who had never before been anything but loyal and dutiful to her mistress, had suddenly shown clear signs of revolt. To the Frau Consul's great vexation, she had been maintaining relations – a sort of spiritual affinity, it seemed – with the butcher's apprentice; and that man of blood must have influenced her political views in a most regrettable way. The Consul's wife had addressed some reproach to her in the matter of an unsuccessful sauce, and she had put her naked arms akimbo and delivered herself as follows: "You jus' wait, Frau Consul; 'tain' goin' t' be much longer – there'll come another order inter the world. 'N' then *I'll* be sittin' on the sofa in a silk gownd, an' you'll be servin' me." Naturally, she received summary notice.

The Consul shook his head. He himself had had similar troubles. The old porters and labourers were of course respectful enough, and had no notions in their heads; but several here and there among the young ones had shown by their bearing that the new spirit of revolt had entered into them. In the spring there had been a street riot, although a constitution corresponding to the demands of the new time had already been drafted; which, a little later, despite the opposition of Lebrecht Kröger and other stubborn old gentlemen, became law by a decree of the Senate. The citizens met together and representatives of the people were elected. But there was no rest. The world was upside down. Every one wanted to revise the constitution and the franchise, and the citizens grumbled. "Voting by estates," said some – Consul Johann Buddenbrook among them. "Universal franchise," said the others; Hinrich Hagenström was one of these. Still others cried: "Universal voting by estates" – and dear knew what they meant by that! All sorts of ideas were in the air; for instance, the abolition of disabilities and the general extension of the rights of citizenship – even to non-Christians! No wonder Buddenbrook's Trina had imbibed such ideas about sofas and silk gowns! Oh, there was worse to come! Things threatened to take a fearful turn.

It was an early October day of the year 1848. The sky was blue, with a few light floating clouds in it, silvered by the rays of the sun, the strength of which was indeed not so great but that the stove was already going, behind the polished screen in the landscape-room. Little Clara, whose hair had grown darker and whose eyes had a rather severe expression, sat with some embroidery before the sewing-table, while Clothilde, busy likewise with her needlework, had the sofa-place near the Frau Consul. Although Clothilde Buddenbrook was not much older than her married cousin – that is to say, only twenty-one years – her long face already showed pronounced lines; and with her smooth hair, which had never been blond, but always a dull greyish colour, she presented an ideal portrait of a typical old maid. But she was content; she did nothing to alter her condition. Perhaps she thought it best to grow old early and thus to make a quick end of all doubts and hopes. As she did not own a single sou, she knew that she would find nobody in all the wide world to marry her, and she looked with humility into her future, which would surely consist of consuming a tiny income in some tiny room which her influential uncle would procure for her out of the funds of some charitable establishment for maidens of good family.

The Consul's wife was busy reading two letters. Tony related the good progress of the little Erica, and Christian wrote eagerly of his life and doings in London. He did not give any details of his industry with Mr. Richardson of Threadneedle Street. The Frau Consul, who was approaching the middle forties, complained bitterly of the tendency of blond women to grow old too soon. The delicate tint which corresponded to her reddish hair had grown dulled despite all cosmetics; and the hair itself began relentlessly to grey, or would have done so but for a Parisian tincture of which the Frau Consul had the receipt. She was determined never to grow white. When the dye would no longer perform its office, she would wear a blond wig. On top of her still artistic coiffure was a silk scarf bordered with white lace, the beginning, the first adumbration of a cap. Her silk frock was wide and flowing, its bell-shaped sleeves lined with the softest mull. A pair of gold circlets tinkled as usual on her wrist.

It was three o'clock in the afternoon. Suddenly there was a noise of running and shouting: a sort of insolent hooting and catcalling, the stamping of feet on the pavement, a hubbub that grew louder and came nearer.

"What is that noise, Mamma?" said Clara, looking out of the window and into the gossip's glass. "Look at the people! What is the matter with them? What are they so pleased about?"

"My God!" shouted the Frau Consul, throwing down her letters and springing to the window. "Is it – ? My God, it is the Revolution! It is the people!"

The truth was that the town had been the whole day in a state of unrest. In the morning the windows of Benthien the draper's shop in Broad Street had been broken by stones – although God knew what the owner had to do with politics!

"Anton," the Consul's wife called with a trembling voice into the dining-room, where the servants were bustling about with the silver. "Anton! Go below! Shut the outside doors. Make everything fast. It is a mob."

"Oh, Frau Consul," said Anton. "Is it safe for me to do that? I am a servant. If they see my livery – "

"What wicked people," Clothilde drawled without putting down her work. Just then the Consul crossed the entrance hall and came in through the glass door. He carried his coat over his arm and his hat in his hand.

"You are going out, Jean?" asked the Frau Consul in great excitement and trepidation.

"Yes, my dear, I must go to the meeting."

"But the mob, Jean, the Revolution – "

"Oh, dear me, Betsy, it isn't so serious as that! We are in God's hand. They have gone past the house already. I'll go down the back way."

"Jean, if you love me – do you want to expose yourself to this danger? Will you leave us here unprotected? I am afraid, I tell you – I am afraid."

"My dear, I beg of you, don't work yourself up like this. They will only make a bit of a row in front of the Town Hall or in the market. It may cost the government a few window-panes – but that's all."

" Where are you going, Jean? "

" To the Assembly. I am late already. I was detained by business. It would be a shame not to be there to-day. Do you think your Father is stopping away, old as he is? "

" Then go, in God's name, Jean. But be careful, I beg of you. And keep an eye on my Father. If anything hit him – "

" Certainly, my dear."

" When will you be back? " the Frau Consul called after him.

" Well, about half past four or five o'clock. Depends. There is a good deal of importance on the agenda, so I can't exactly tell."

" Oh, I'm frightened, I'm frightened," repeated the Frau Consul, walking restlessly up and down.

CHAPTER III

CONSUL BUDDENBROOK crossed his spacious ground floor in haste. Coming out into Bakers' Alley, he heard steps behind him and saw Gosch the broker, a picturesque figure in his long cloak and Jesuit hat, also climbing the narrow street to the meeting. He lifted his hat with one thin long hand, and with the other made a deferential gesture, as he said, "Well, Herr Consul – how are you?" His voice sounded sinister.

This broker, Siegismund Gosch, a bachelor of some forty years, was, despite his demeanour, the best and most honest soul in the world; but he was a wit and an oddity. His smooth-shaven face was distinguished by a Roman nose, a protruding pointed chin, sharp features, and a wide mouth drooping at the corners, whose narrow lips he was in the habit of pressing together in the most taciturn and forbidding manner. His grey hair fell thick and sombre over his brow, and he actually regretted not being hump-backed. It was his whim to assume the rôle of a wild, witty, and reckless intrigant – a cross between Mephistopheles and Napoleon, something very malevolent and yet fascinating too; and he was not entirely unsuccessful in his pose. He was a strange yet attractive figure among the citizens of the old city; still, he belonged among them, for he carried on a small brokerage business in the most modest, respectable sort of way. In his narrow, dark little office, however, he had a large book-case filled with poetry in every language, and there was a story that he had been engaged since his twentieth year on a translation of Lope de Vega's collected dramas. Once he had played the rôle of Domingo in an amateur performance of Schiller's "Don Carlos" – this was the culmination of his career. A common word never crossed his lips; and the most ordinary business expressions he would hiss between his clenched teeth, as if he were saying "Curses on you, villain," instead of some commonplace about stocks and commissions. He was, in many ways, the heir and successor to Jean Jacques Hoffstede of blessed memory, except that his character had certain elements of the sombre and pathetic, with none of the playful liveliness of that old 18th-century friend of Johann Buddenbrook.

One day he lost at a single blow, on the Bourse, six and a half thaler on two or three papers which he had bought as a speculation. This was enough. He sank upon a bench; he struck an attitude which looked as though he had lost the Battle of Waterloo; he struck his clenched fist against his forehead and repeated several times, with a blasphemous roll of the eyes: " Ha, accursed, accursed! " He must have been, at bottom, cruelly bored by the small, safe business he did and the petty transfer of this or that bit of property; for this loss, this tragic blow with which Heaven had stricken him down – him, the schemer Gosch – delighted his inmost soul. He fed on it for weeks. Some one would say, " So you've had a loss, Herr Gosch, I'm sorry to hear." To which he would answer: " Oh, my good friend, '*uomo non educato dal dolore riman sempre bambino*'*!* " Probably nobody understood that. Was it, possibly, Lope de Vega? Anyhow, there was no doubt that this Siegismund Gosch was a remarkable and learned man.

" What times we live in," he said, limping up the street with the Consul, supported by his stick. " Times of storm and unrest."

" You are right," replied the Consul. " The times are unquiet. This morning's sitting will be exciting. The principle of the estates – "

" Well, now," Herr Gosch went on, " I have been about all day in the streets, and I have been looking at the mob. There are some fine fellows in it, their eyes flaming with excitement and hatred – "

Johann Buddenbrook began to laugh. " You like that, don't you? But you have the right end of it after all, let me tell you. It is all childishness! What do these men want? A lot of uneducated rowdies who see a chance for a bit of a scrimmage."

" Of course. Though I can't deny – I was in the crowd when Berkemeyer, the journeyman butcher, smashed Herr Benthien's window. He was like a panther." Herr Gosch spoke the last word with his teeth particularly close together, and went on: " Oh, the thing has its fine side, that's certain. It is a change, at least, you know; something that doesn't happen every day. Storm, stress, violence – the tempest! Oh, the people are ignorant, I know – still, my heart, this heart of mine – it beats with theirs! " They were already before the simple yellow-painted house on the ground floor of which the sittings of the Assembly took place.

The room belonged to the beer-hall and dance-establishment of a widow named Suerkringel; but on certain days it was at the service of the gentlemen burgesses. The entrance was through a narrow whitewashed corridor opening into the restaurant on the right side, where it smelled of beer and cooking, and thence through a handleless, lockless green door so small and narrow that no one could have supposed such a large room lay behind it. The room was empty, cold, and barnlike, with a whitewashed roof in which the beams showed, and whitewashed walls. The three rather high windows had green-painted bars, but no curtains. Opposite them were the benches, rising in rows like an amphitheatre, with a table at the bottom for the chairman, the recording clerk, and the Committee of the Senate. It was covered with a green cloth and had a clock, documents, and writing-materials on it. On the wall opposite the door were several tall hat-racks with hats and coats.

The sound of voices met the Consul and his companion as they entered through the narrow door. They were the last to come. The room was filled with burgesses, hands in their trousers pockets, on their hips, or in the air, as they stood together in groups and discussed. Of the hundred and thirty members of the body at least a hundred were present. A number of delegates from the country districts had been obliged by circumstances to stop at home.

Near the entrance stood a group composed of two or three small business men, a high-school teacher, the orphan asylum " father," Herr Mindermann, and Herr Wenzel, the popular barber. Herr Wenzel, a powerful little man with a black moustache, an intelligent face, and red hands, had shaved the Consul that very morning; here, however, he stood on an equality with him. He shaved only in the best circles; he shaved almost exclusively the Möllendorpfs, Langhals, Buddenbrooks, and Överdiecks, and he owed his vote in the Assembly to his omniscience in city affairs, his sociability and ease, and his remarkable power of decision at a division.

" Have you heard the latest, Herr Consul? " he asked with round-eyed eagerness as his patron came up.

" What is there to hear, my dear Wenzel? "

" Nobody knew it this morning. Well, permit me to tell you, Herr Consul, the latest is that the crowd are not going to collect before the Town Hall, or in the market – they are coming here to threaten the burgesses. Editor Rübsam has stirred them up."

" Is it possible? " said the Consul. He pressed through the various groups to the middle of the room, where he saw his father-in-law with Senators Dr. Langhals and James Möllendorpf. " Is it true, gentlemen? " he asked, shaking hands with them.

But there was no need to answer. The whole assemblage was full of it: the peace-breakers were coming; they could be heard already in the distance.

" *Canaille!* " said Lebrecht Kröger with cold scorn. He had driven hither in his carriage. On an ordinary day the tall, distinguished figure of the once famous cavalier showed the burden of his eighty years; but to-day he stood quite erect with his eyes half closed, the corners of his mouth contemptuously drawn down, and the points of his white moustaches sticking straight up. Two rows of jewelled buttons sparkled on his black velvet waistcoat.

Not far from this group was Hinrich Hagenström, a square-built, fleshy man with a reddish beard sprinkled with grey, a heavy watch-chain across his blue-checked waistcoat, and his coat open over it. He was standing with his partner Herr Strunck, and did not greet the Consul.

Herr Benthien, the draper, a prosperous looking man, had a large group of gentlemen around him, to whom he was circumstantially describing what had happened to his show-window. " A brick, gentlemen, a brick, or at least half a brick – *crack!* through it went and landed on a roll of green rep. The rascally mob! Oh, the Government will have to take it up! It's their affair! "

And in every corner of the room unceasingly resounded the voice of Herr Stuht from Bell-Founders' Street. He had on a black coat over his woollen shirt; and he so deeply sympathized with the narrative of Herr Benthien that he never stopped saying, in outraged accents, " Infamous, un-heard-of! "

Johann Buddenbrook found and greeted his old friend G. F. Köppen, and then Köppen's rival, Consul Kistenmaker. He moved about in the crowd, pressed Dr. Grabow's hand, and exchanged a few words with Herr Gieseke the Fire Commissioner, Contractor Voigt, Dr. Langhals, the Chairman, brother of the Senator, and several merchants, lawyers, and teachers.

The sitting was not yet opened, but debate was already lively. Everybody was cursing that pestilential scribbler, Editor Rübsam; everybody knew he had stirred up the crowd – and what for? The business in hand was to decide whether they were to go on with the method of selecting representatives by estates, or whether there was to be universal and equal franchise. The Senate had already proposed the latter. But what did the people want? They wanted these gentlemen by the throats – no more and no less. It was the worst hole they had ever found themselves in, devil take it! The Senatorial Committee was surrounded, its members' opinion eagerly sought. They approached Consul Buddenbrook, as one who should know the attitude of Burgomaster Överdieck; for since Senator Doctor Överdieck, Consul Justus Kröger's brother-in-law, had been made President last year, the Buddenbrooks were related to the Burgomaster; which had distinctly enhanced the regard in which they were held.

All of a sudden the tumult began outside. Revolution had arrived under the windows of the Sitting. The excited exchange of opinions inside ceased simultaneously. Every man, dumb with the shock, folded his hands upon his stomach and looked at his fellows or at the windows, where fists were being shaken in the air and the crowd was giving vent to deafening and frantic yelling. But then, most astonishingly, as though the offenders themselves had suddenly grown aghast at their own behaviour, it became just as still outside as in the hall; and in that deep hush, one word from the neighbourhood of the lowest benches, where Lebrecht Kröger was sitting, was distinctly audible. It rang through the hall, cold, emphatic, and deliberate – the word "Canaille!" And, like an echo, came the word "Infamous," in a fat, outraged voice from the other corner of the hall. Then the hurried, trembling, whispering utterance of the draper Benthien: "Gentlemen, gentlemen! Listen! I know the house. There is a trap door on to the roof from the attic. I used to shoot cats through it when I was a lad. We can climb on to the next roof and get down safely."

"Cowardice," hissed Gosch the broker between his teeth. He leaned against the table with his arms folded and head bent, directing a blood-curdling glance through the window.

"Cowardice, do you say? How cowardice? In God's name, sir, aren't they throwing bricks? I've had enough of that."

The noise outside had begun again, but without reaching its former stormy height. It sounded quieter and more continuous, a prolonged, patient, almost comfortable hum, rising and falling; now and then one heard whistles, and sometimes single words like "principle" and "rights of citizens." The assembly listened respectfully.

After a while the chairman, Herr Dr. Langhals, spoke in a subdued tone: "Gentlemen, I think we could come to some agreement if we opened the meeting."

But this humble suggestion did not meet with the slightest support from anybody.

"No good in that," somebody said, with a simple decisiveness that permitted no appeal. It was a peasant sort of man, named Pfahl, from the Ritzerau district, deputy for the village of Little Schretstaken. Nobody remembered ever to have heard his voice raised before in a meeting, but its very simplicity made it weighty at the present crisis. Unafraid and with sure political insight, Herr Pfahl had voiced the feeling of the entire assemblage.

"God keep us," Herr Benthien said despondently. "If we sit

on the benches we can be seen from outside. They're throwing stones – I've had enough of that."

"And the cursed door is so narrow," burst out Köppen the wine-merchant, in despair. "If we start to go out, we'll probably get crushed."

"Infamous, un-heard-of," Herr Stuht intoned.

"Gentlemen," began the Chairman urgently once more. "I have to put before the Burgomaster in the next three days a draft of to-day's protocol, and the town expects its publication through the press. I should at least like to get a vote on that subject, if the sitting would come to order – "

But with the exception of a few citizens who supported the chairman, nobody seemed ready to come to the consideration of the agenda. A vote would have been useless anyhow – they must not irritate the people. Nobody knew what they wanted, so it was no good to offend them by a vote, in whatever direction. They must wait and control themselves. The clock of St. Mary's struck half past four.

They confirmed themselves and each other in this resolve of patient waiting. They began to get used to the noise that rose and fell outside, to feel quieter; to make themselves more comfortable, to sit down on the lower benches and chairs. The natural instinct toward industry, common to all these good burghers, began to assert itself: they ventured to bargain a little, to pick up a little business here and there. The brokers sat down by the wholesale dealers. These beleaguered gentlemen talked together like people shut in by a sudden storm, who speak of other things, and now and then pause to listen with respectful faces to the thunder. It was five o'clock – half-past five. It was getting dark. Now and then somebody sighed and said that the wife would be waiting with the coffee – and then Herr Benthien would venture to mention the trap-door. But most of them were like Herr Stuht, who said fatalistically, shaking his head, "I'm too fat."

Mindful of his wife's request Johann Buddenbrook had kept an eye on his father-in-law. He said to him: "This little adventure isn't disturbing you, is it, Father? "

Lebrecht Kröger's forehead showed two swollen blue veins under his white wig. He looked ill. One aristocratic old hand played with the opalescent buttons on his waistcoat; the other, with its great diamond ring, trembled on his knee.

"Fiddlesticks, Buddenbrook," he said; but his voice showed extreme fatigue. " I am sick of it, that's all." Then he betrayed himself by suddenly hissing out: " Parbleu, Jean, this infamous rabble ought to be taught some respect with a little powder and shot. *Canaille!* Scum! "

The Consul hummed assent. " Yes, yes, you are right; it is a pretty undignified affair. But what can we do? We must keep our tempers. It's getting late. They'll go away after a bit."

" Where is my carriage? I desire my carriage," said the old man in a tone of command, suddenly quite beside himself. His anger exploded; he trembled all over. " I ordered it for five o'clock: where is it? This sitting will never be held. Why should I stop any longer? I don't care about being made a fool of. My carriage! What are they doing to my coachman? Go see after it, Buddenbrook."

" My dear Father-in-Law, for heaven's sake be calm. You are getting excited. It will be bad for you. Of course I will go and see after the carriage. I think myself we have had enough of this. I will speak to the people and tell them to go home."

Close by the little green door he was accosted by Siegismund Gosch, who grasped his arm with a bony hand and asked in a gruesome whisper: " Whither away, Herr Consul? "

The broker's face was furrowed with a thousand lines. His pointed chin rose almost up to his nose, his face expressed the most desperate resolution; his grey hair streamed distractedly over brow and temples; his head was so drawn in between his shoulders that he really almost achieved his ambition of looking like a dwarf – and he rapped out: " You behold me resolved to speak to the people."

The Consul said: " No, let me do it, Gosch. I really know more of them than you do."

" Be it so," answered the broker tonelessly. " You are a bigger man than I." And, lifting his voice, he went on: " But I will accompany you, I will stand at your side, Consul Buddenbrook. Let the wrath of the outraged people tear me in pieces – "

" What a day, what a night! " he said as they went out. There is no doubt he had never felt so happy before in his life. " Ha, Herr Consul! Here are the people."

They had gone down the corridor and outside the outer door, where they stood at the top of three little steps that went down to the pavement. The street was indeed a strange sight. It was as still as the grave. At the open and lighted windows of the houses round, stood the curious, looking down upon the black mass of the insurgents before the Burgesses' House. The crowd was not much bigger than that inside the hall. It consisted of young labourers from the harbour and granaries, servants, school pupils, sailors from the merchant ships, and other people from the little streets, alleys, courts, and rabbit-hutches round about. There were even two or three women – who had probably promised themselves the same millennium as the Buddenbrooks' cook. A few of the insurrectionists, weary of standing, had sat down with their feet in the gutter and were eating sandwiches.

It was nearly six o'clock. Though twilight was well advanced, the oil lamps hung unlighted above the street. This fact, this open and unheard-of interruption of the regular order, was the first thing that really made Consul Buddenbrook's temper rise, and was responsible for his beginning to speak in a rather short and angry tone and the broadest of pronunciations:

"Now then, all of you, what is the meaning of this foolishness?"

The picnickers sprang up from the sidewalk. Those in the back ranks, beyond the foot-pavement, stood on their tiptoes. Some navvies, in the service of the Consul, took off their caps. They stood at attention, nudged each other, and muttered in low tones, "'Tis Consul Buddenbrook. He be goin' to talk. Hold yer jaw, there, Chrishan; he can jaw like the devil himself! Ther's Broker Gosch – look! What a monkey he is! Isn't he gettin' o'erwrought!"

"Carl Smolt!" began the Consul again, picking out and fastening his small, deep-set eyes upon a bow-legged young labourer of about two-and-twenty, with his cap in his hand and his mouth full of bread, standing in front of the steps. "Here, speak up, Carl Smolt! Now's the time! I've been here the whole afternoon –"

"Yes, Herr Consul," brought out Carl Smolt, chewing violently. "The thing is – ower – it's a soart o' – we're makin' a rivolution."

"What kind of nonsense is that, then?"

"Lord, Herr Consul, ye knaw what that is. We're not satisfied wi' things as they be. We demand another order o' things; tain't any more'n that – that's what it is."

"Now, listen, Carl Smolt and the rest of you. Whoever's got any sense will go home and not bother himself over any revolutions, disturbing the regular order of things –"

"The sacred order," interrupted Herr Gosch dramatically.

"The regular order, I say," finished the Consul. "Why, even the lamps aren't lighted. That's going too far with the revolution."

Carl Smolt had swallowed his mouthful by now, and, with the people at his back, stood his ground and made some objections.

" Well, Herr Consul, ye may say that. But we're only agin the principle of the voate – "

" God in heaven, you ninny," shouted the Consul, forgetting, in his excitement, to speak dialect. " You're talking the sheerest nonsense – "

" Lord, Herr Consul," said Carl Smolt, somewhat abashed, " thet's oall as it is. Rivolution it has to be. Ther's rivolution iverywheer, in Berlin, in Paris – "

" But, Smolt, what do you want? Just tell me that, if you can."

" Lord, Herr Consul, I say we wants a republic; that's wat I be sayin'."

" But, you fool, you've got one already."

" Well, Herr Consul, then we wants another."

Some of the bystanders, who understood the matter better, began to laugh rudely and heartily; and although few even heard Carl's answer, the laughter spread until the whole crowd of republicans stood shaking good-naturedly. Some of the gentlemen from inside the hall appeared at the window with curious faces and beer-mugs in their hands. The only person disappointed and painted by this turn of affairs was Siegismund Gosch.

" Now, people," shouted Consul Buddenbrook finally, " I think the best thing for you all to do is to go home."

Carl Smolt, quite crestfallen over the result he had brought about, answered: " That's right, Herr Consul. Then things'll be quieted down. And Herr Consul doesn't take it ill of me, do'e, now? Good-bye, Herr Consul! "

The crowd began to disperse, in the best of humours.

" Wait a minute, Smolt," shouted the Consul. " Have you seen the Kröger carriage? the calèche from outside the Castle Gate? "

" Yes, sir, Herr Consul. He's here; he be driven up in some court somewhere."

" Then run quick and say he's to come at once; his master wants to go home."

" Servant, Herr Consul," and, throwing his cap on his head and pulling the leather visor well down over his brows, Carl Smolt ran with great swinging strides down the street.

CHAPTER IV

When the Consul and Siegismund Gosch returned to the hall, the scene was a more comfortable one than it had been a quarter of an hour before. It was lighted by two large oil lamps standing on the Committee table, in whose yellow light the gentlemen sat or stood together, pouring out beer into shining tankards, touching glasses and talking loudly, in the gayest of humours. Frau Suerkringel, the widow, had consoled them. She had loyally taken on her enforced guests and given them good advice, recommending that they fortify themselves for the siege, which might endure some while yet. And thus she had profitably employed the time by selling a considerable quantity of her light yet exhilarating beer. As the others entered, the house-boy, in shirt-sleeves and good-natured grin, was just bringing in a fresh supply of bottles. While it was certainly late, too late to consider further the revision of the Constitution, nobody seemed inclined to interrupt the meeting and go home. It was too late for coffee, in any case.

After the Consul had received congratulatory handshakes on his success, he went up to his father-in-law. Lebrecht Kröger was the only man in the room whose mood had not improved. He sat in his place, cold, remote, and lofty, and answered the information that the carriage would be around at once by saying scornfully, in a voice that trembled more with bitterness than age: " Then the mob permits me to go home? "

With stiff movements that no longer had in them anything of the charm that had been his, he had his fur mantle put about his shoulders, and laid his arm, with a careless " *Merci*," on that of the Consul, who offered to accompany him home. The majestic coach, with two large lanterns on the box, stood in the street, where, to the Consul's great satisfaction, the lamps were now being lighted. They both got in. Silent and stiffly erect, with his eyes half-closed, Lebrecht Kröger sat with the rug over his knees, the Consul at his right hand, while the carriage rolled through the streets. Beneath the points of the old man's white moustaches two lines ran down perpendicularly from the corners of his mouth to his chin. He was gnawed by chagrin at the insult that had been offered him, and he stared, weary and chilled, at the cushions opposite.

There was more gaiety in the streets than on a Sunday evening. Obviously a holiday temper reigned. The people, delighted at the successful outcome of the revolution, were out in the gayest mood. There was singing. Here and there youngsters shouted " Hurrah! " as the carriage drove past, and threw their caps into the air.

" I really think, Father, you let the matter affect you too much," the Consul said. " When one thinks of it, what a tom-fool business the whole thing was – simply a farce." In order to get some reply from the old man he went on to talk about the revolution in lively tones. " When the propertyless class begin to realize how little they serve their own ends – why, good heavens, it's the same everywhere. I was talking this afternoon with Gosch the broker, a wonderful man, looking at everything with the eyes of a poet and writer. You see, Father, this revolution was made at the æsthetic tea-tables of Berlin. Then the people take their own skin to market – for, of course, they will be the ones to pay for it! "

" It would be a good thing if you would open the window on your side," said Herr Kröger.

Johann Buddenbrook gave him a quick glance and let the glass down hastily.

" Aren't you feeling well, dear Father? " he asked anxiously.

" Not at all," answered Lebrecht Kröger severely.

" You need food and rest," the Consul said; and in order to be doing something he drew up the fur rug closer about his father-in-law's knees.

Suddenly – the carriage was rolling through Castle Street – a wretched thing happened. Fifteen paces from the Castle Gate, in the half-dark, they passed a group of noisy and happy street urchins, and a stone flew through the open window. It was a harmless little stone, the size of a hen's egg, flung by the hand of some Chris Snut or Heine Voss to celebrate the revolution; certainly not with any bad intent, and probably not directed toward the carriage at all. It came noiselessly through the window and struck Lebrecht Kröger in his chest, which was covered with the thick fur rug. Then it rolled down over the cover and fell upon the floor of the coach.

" Clumsy fools! " said the Consul angrily. " Is everybody out of their senses this evening? It didn't hurt you, did it? "

Old Kröger was silent – alarmingly silent. It was too dark in the carriage to see his expression. He sat straighter, higher, stiffer than ever, without touching the cushions. Then, from deep within him, slowly, coldly, dully, came the single word: " Canaille."

For fear of angering him further, the Consul made no answer. The carriage clattered through the gate, and three minutes later was in the broad avenue before the gilt-tipped railings that bounded the Kröger domain. A drive bordered with chestnut trees went from the garden gate up to the terrace; and on either side of the gate a gilt-topped lantern was burning brightly. The Consul saw his father-in-law's face by this light – it was yellow and wrinkled; the firm, contemptuous set of the mouth had given way: it had changed to the lax, silly, distorted expression of a very old man. The carriage stopped before the terrace.

" Help me out," said Lebrecht Kröger; but the Consul was already out, had thrown back the rug, and offered his arm and shoulder as a support. He led the old man slowly for a few paces across the gravel to the white stone steps that went up to the dining-room. At the foot of these, the old man bent at the knee-joints. His head fell so heavily on his breast that the lower jaw clashed against the upper. His eyes rolled – grew dim; Lebrecht Kröger, the gallant, the cavalier à-la-mode, had joined his fathers.

CHAPTER V

A YEAR and two months later, on a misty, snowy morning in January of the year 1850, Herr and Madame Grünlich sat at breakfast with their little three-year-old daughter, in the brown wainscoted dining-room, on chairs that cost twenty-five marks apiece.

The panes of both windows were opaque with mist; behind them one had vague glimpses of bare trees and bushes. A red glow and a gentle, scented warmth came from the low, green-tiled stove standing in a corner. Through the open door next it one could see the foliage-plants in the " pensée-room." On the other wall, half-drawn green stuff portières gave a view of the brown satin salon and of a lofty glass door leading on to a little terrace beyond. The cracks in this door were carefully stopped with cotton-wool, and there was nothing to be seen through its panes but the whitish-grey mist beyond.

The snow-white cloth of woven damask on the round table had an embroidered green runner across it, laid with gold-bordered porcelain so translucent that it gleamed like mother-of-pearl. The tea-kettle was humming. There was a finely worked silver bread-basket in the shape of a curling leaf, with slices and rolls of fine bread; under one crystal bell were little balls of butter, under another different sorts of cheese, white, yellow, and green. There was even a bottle of wine standing before the master of the house; for Herr Grünlich had a full breakfast every morning.

His whiskers were freshly curled, and at this early hour his rosy face was rosier than ever. He sat with his back to the salon, already arrayed in a black coat and light trousers with a pattern of large checks, eating a grilled chop, in the English manner. His wife thought this very elegant, but also very disgusting – she had never brought herself to take it instead of her usual breakfast of bread and butter and an egg.

Tony was in her dressing-gown. She adored dressing-gowns. Nothing seemed more elegant to her than a handsome negligée, and as she had not been allowed to indulge this passion in the parental house she was the more given to it as a wife. She had three of these dainty clinging garments, to the fashioning of which can go so much more taste and fantasy than to a ball-gown. To-day she wore her dark red one. Its colour toned beautifully with the paper above the wainscoting, and its large-flowered stuff, of a beautiful soft texture, was embroidered all over with sprays of tiny glass beads of the same colour, while row after row of red velvet ribbons ran from neck to hem.

Her thick ash-blond hair, with its dark red velvet band, curled about her brows. She had now, as she was herself well aware, reached the highest point of her physical bloom; yet her pretty, pouting upper lip retained just the naïve, provocative expression of her childhood. The lids of her grey-blue eyes were reddened with cold water. Her hands, the white Buddenbrook hands, finely shaped if a little stumpy, their delicate wrists caressed by the velvet cuffs of her dressing-gown, handled her knife and fork and tea-cup with motions that were to-day, for some reason or other, rather jerky and abrupt. Her little daughter Erica sat near her in a high chair. She was a plump child with short blond hair, in a funny shapeless, knitted frock of pale blue wool. She held a large cup in both tiny hands, entirely concealing her face, and drank her milk with little sighs of satisfaction.

Frau Grünlich rang, and Tinka, the housemaid, came from the entry to take the child from her high chair and carry her upstairs into the play-room. "You may take her walking outside for a half-hour, Tinka," said Tony. "But not longer; and put on her thick jacket. It is very damp and foggy." She remained alone with her husband.

"You only make yourself seem absurd," she said then, after a silence, obviously continuing an interrupted conversation. "What are your objections? Give me some reason. I can't be always attending to the child."

"You are not fond of children, Antonie."

"Fond of children, indeed! I have no time. I am taken up with the housekeeping. I wake up with twenty things that must be done, and I go to bed with forty that have not been done."

"There are two servants. A young woman like you – "

"Two servants. Good. Tinka has to wash up, to clean, to serve. The cook is busy all the time. You have chops early in the morning. Think it over, Grünlich. Sooner or later, Erica must have a *bonne*, a governess."

"But to get a governess for her so soon is not suited to our means."

" Our means! Goodness, you *are* absurd! Are we beggars? Are we forced to live within the smallest limits we can? I think I brought you in eighty thousand marks – "

" Oh, you and your eighty thousand marks – ! "

" Yes, I know you like to make light of them. They were of no importance to you because you married me for love! Good. But do you still love me? You deliberately disregard my wishes. The child is not to have a governess. And I don't even speak any more of the coupé, which we need quite as much as we need food and drink. And why do you insist on our living out here in the country, if it isn't in accordance with our means to keep a carriage so that we can go into society respectably? Why do you never like it when I go in to town? You would always rather just have me bury myself out here, so I should never see a living soul. I think you are very ill-tempered."

Herr Grünlich poured some wine into his glass, lifted up one of the crystal bells, and began on the cheese. He made no reply.

" Don't you love me any more? " repeated Tony. " Your silence is so insulting, it drives me to remind you of a certain day when you entered our landscape-room. You made a fine figure of yourself! But from the very first day after our marriage you have sat with me only in the evening, and that only to read the paper. Just at first you showed some little regard for my wishes. But that's been over with for a long while now. You neglect me."

" And you? You are ruining me."

" I? I am ruining you? "

" Yes, you are ruining me with your indolence, your extravagance, and love of luxury."

" Oh, pray don't reproach me with my good upbringing! In my parents' house I never had to lift a finger. Now I have hard work to get accustomed to the housekeeping; but I have at least a right to demand that you do not refuse me the ordinary assistance. Father is a rich man; he would never dream that I could lack for service."

" Then wait for this third servant until we get hold of some of those riches."

" Oh, you are wishing for my Father's death. But I mean that we are well-to-do people in our own right. I did not come to you with empty hands."

Herr Grünlich smiled an embarrassed and dejected smile, although he was in the act of chewing his breakfast. He made no other reply, and his silence bewildered Tony.

"Grünlich," she said more quietly, "why do you smile and talk about our 'means'? Am I mistaken? Has business been bad? Have you — ?"

Just then somebody drummed on the corridor door, and Herr Kesselmeyer walked in.

CHAPTER VI

Herr Kesselmeyer entered unannounced, as a friend of the house, without hat or coat. He paused, however, near the door. His looks corresponded exactly to the description Tony had given to her Mother. He was slightly thick-set as to figure, but neither fat nor lean. He wore a black, already somewhat shiny coat, short tight trousers of the same material, and a white waistcoat, over which went a long thin watch-chain and two or three eye-glass cords. His clipped white beard was in sharp contrast with his red face. It covered his cheeks and left his chin and lips free. His mouth was small and mobile, with two yellowish pointed teeth in the otherwise vacant gum of his lower jaw, and he was pressing these into his upper lip, as he stood absently by the door with his hands in his trousers pockets and the black and white down on his head waving slightly, although there was not the least perceptible draught.

Finally he drew his hands out of his pockets, bowed, released his lip, and with difficulty freed one of the eye-glass cords from the confusion on his waistcoat. He lifted his pince-nez and put it with a single gesture astride his nose. Then he made the most astonishing grimaces, looked at the husband and wife, and remarked: "Ah, ha!"

He used this expression with extraordinary frequency and a surprising variety of inflections. He might say it with his head thrown back, his nose wrinkled up, mouth wide open, hands swishing about in the air, with a long-drawn-out, nasal, metallic sound, like a Chinese gong; or he might, with still funnier effect, toss it out, gently, *en passant;* or with any one of a thousand different shades of tone and meaning. His *a* was very clouded and nasal. To-day it was a hurried, lively "Ah ha!" accompanied with a jerk of the head, that seemed to arise from an unusually pleasant mood, and yet might not be trusted to be so; for the fact was, Banker Kesselmeyer never behaved more gaily than when he was dangerous. When he jumped about emitting a thousand "Ah ha's," lifting his glasses to his nose and letting them fall again, waving his arms, chattering, plainly quite beside himself with light-headedness, then you might be sure that evil was gnawing at his inwards. Herr Grünlich looked at him blinking, with unconcealed mistrust.

"Already – so early?" he asked.

"Ah, ha!" answered Herr Kesselmeyer, and waved one of his small, red, wrinkled hands in the air, as if to say: "Patience, there is a surprise coming." "I must speak with you, without any delay; I must speak with you."

The words sounded irresistibly comic as he rolled each one about before giving it out, with exaggerated movements of his little toothless, mobile mouth. He rolled his *r*'s as if his palate were greased. Herr Grünlich blinked more and more suspiciously.

"Come and sit down, Herr Kesselmeyer," said Tony. "I'm glad you've come. Listen. You can decide between us. Grünlich and I have been disagreeing. Now tell me: ought a three-year-old child to have a governess or not?"

But Herr Kesselmeyer seemed not to be attending. He had seated himself and was rubbing his stubbly beard with his forefinger, making a rasping sound, his mouth as wide open as possible, nose as wrinkled, while he stared over his glasses with an indescribably sprightly air at the elegantly appointed breakfast-table, the silver bread-basket, the label on the wine-bottle.

"Grünlich says I am ruining him," Tony continued.

Herr Kesselmeyer looked at her; then he looked at Herr Grünlich; then he burst out into an astonishing fit of laughter. "You are ruining him? – you? *You* are ruining him – that's it, is it? Oh good gracious, heavens and earth, you don't say! That *is* a joke. That is a tre-men-dous, tre-men-dous joke." He let out a stream of ha ha's all run in together.

Herr Grünlich was plainly nervous. He squirmed on his seat. He ran his long finger down between his collar and his neck and let his golden whiskers glide through his hand.

"Kesselmeyer," he said. "Control yourself, man. Are you out of your head? Stop laughing! Will you have some wine? Or a cigar? What are you laughing at?"

"What am I laughing at? Yes, yes, give me a glass of wine, give me a cigar. Why am I laughing? So you think your wife is ruining you?"

"She is very luxuriously inclined," Herr Grünlich said irritably.

Tony did not contradict him. She leaned calmly back, her hands in her lap on the velvet ribbons of her frock and her pert upper lip in evidence: "Yes, I am, I know. I have it from Mamma. All the Krögers are fond of luxury."

She would have admitted in the same calm way that she was frivolous, revengeful, or quick-tempered. Her strongly developed family sense was instinctively hostile to conceptions of free will and self-development; it inclined her rather to recognize and accept her own characteristics wholesale, with fatalistic indifference and toleration. She had, unconsciously, the feeling that any trait of hers, no matter of what kind, was a family tradition and therefore worthy of respect.

Herr Grünlich had finished breakfast, and the fragrance of the two cigars mingled with the warm air from the stove. " Will you take another, Kesselmeyer? " said the host. " I'll pour you out another glass of wine. – You want to see me? Anything pressing? Is it important? – Too warm here, is it? We'll drive into town together afterward. It is cooler in the smoking-room." To all this Herr Kesselmeyer simply shook his hand in the air, as if to say: " This won't get us anywhere, my dear friend."

At length they got up; and, while Tony remained in the dining-room to see that the servant-maid cleared away, Herr Grünlich led his colleague through the " pensée-room," with his head bent, drawing his long beard reflectively through his fingers. Herr Kesselmeyer rowed into the room with his arms and disappeared behind his host.

Ten minutes passed. Tony had gone into the salon to give the polished nut-wood escritoire and the curved table-legs her personal attention with the aid of a gay little feather duster. Then she moved slowly through the dining-room into the living-room with dignity and marked self-respect. The Demoiselle Buddenbrook had plainly not grown less important in her own eyes since becoming Madame Grünlich. She held herself very erect, chin in, and looked down at the world from above. She carried in one hand her little lacquered key-basket; the other was in the pocket of her gown, whose soft folds played about her. The naïve expression of her mouth betrayed that the whole of her dignity and importance were a part of a beautiful, childlike, innocent game which she was constantly playing with herself.

In the " pensée-room " she busied herself with a little brass sprinkler, watering the black earth around her plants. She loved her palms, they gave so much elegance to the room. She touched carefully a young shoot on one of the thick round stems, examined the majestically unfolded fans, and cut away a yellow tip here and there with the scissors. Suddenly she stopped. The conversation in the next room, which had for several minutes been assuming a livelier tone, became so loud that she could hear every word, though the door and the portières were both heavy.

" Don't shriek like that – control yourself, for God's sake! " she heard Herr Grünlich say. His weak voice could not stand the strain, and went off in a squeak. " Take another cigar," he went on, with desperate mildness.

" Yes, thanks, with the greatest pleasure," answered the banker, and there was a pause while he presumably helped himself. Then he said: " In short, will you or won't you: one or the other? "

" Kesselmeyer, give me an extension."

" Ah, ha! No, no, my friend. There is no question of an extension. That's not the point now."

" Why not? What is stirring you up to this? Be reasonable, for heaven's sake. You've waited this long."

" Not a day longer, my friend. Yes, we'll say eight days, but not an hour longer. But can't we rely any longer on – ? "

" No names, Kesselmeyer."

" No names. Good. But doesn't some one rely any longer on his estimable Herr Pa– "

" No hints, either. My God, don't be a fool."

" Very good; no hints, either. But have we no claim any longer on the well-known firm with whom our credit stands and falls, my friend? How much did it lose by the Bremen failure? Fifty thousand? Seventy thousand? A hundred thousand? More? The sparrows on the housetops know that it was involved, heavily involved. Yesterday – well, no names. Yesterday the well-known firm was good, and it was unconsciously protecting you against pressure. To-day its stock is flat – and B. Grünlich's stock is the flattest of the flat. Is that clear? Do you grasp it? You are the first man to notice a thing like that. How are people treating you? How do they look at you? Beck and Goudstikker are perfectly agreeable, give you the same terms as usual? And the bank? "

" They will extend."

" You aren't lying, are you? Oh, no! I know they gave you a jolt yesterday – a very, very stimulating jolt, eh? You see? Oh, don't be embarrassed. It is to your interest, of course, to pull the wool over my eyes, so that the others will be quiet. Hey, my dear friend? Well, you'd better write to the Consul. I'll wait a week."

" A part payment, Kesselmeyer! "

" Part payment, rubbish! One accepts part payment to convince oneself for the time of a debtor's ability to pay. Do I need to make experiments of that kind on you? I am perfectly well-informed about your ability to pay. Ah, ha, ah, ha! Part payment! That's a very good joke."

"Moderate your voice, Kesselmeyer. Don't laugh all the time in that cursed way. My position is so serious – yes, I admit, it is serious. But I have such-and-such business in hand – everything may still come out all right. Listen, wait a minute: Give me an extension and I'll sign it for twenty per cent."

"Nothing in it, nothing in it, my friend. Very funny, very amusing. Oh, yes, I'm in favour of selling at the right time. You promised me eight per cent, and I extended. You promised me twelve and sixteen per cent, and I extended, every time. Now, you might offer me forty per cent, and I wouldn't consider it – not for a moment. Since Brother Westfall in Bremen fell on his nose, everybody is for the moment freeing himself from the well-known firm and getting on a sound basis. As I say, I'm for selling at the right time. I've held your signatures as long as Johann Buddenbrook was good – in the meantime I could write up the interest on the capital and increase the per cent. But one only keeps a thing so long as it is rising or at least keeping steady. When it begins to fall, one sells – which is the same as saying I want my capital."

"Kesselmeyer, you are shameless."

"Ah, ha, a-ha! Shameless, am I? That's very charming, very funny. What do you want? You must apply to your father-in-law. The Credit Bank is raging – and you know you are not exactly spotless."

"No, Kesselmeyer. I adjure you to hear me quietly. I'll be perfectly frank. I confess that my situation is serious. You and the Credit Bank are not the only ones – there are notes of hand – everything seems to have gone to pieces at once!"

"Of course – naturally. It is certainly a clean-up – a liquidation."

"No, Kesselmeyer; hear me out. Do take another cigar."

"This one is not half finished. Leave me alone with your cigars. Pay up."

"Kesselmeyer, don't let me smash! – You are a friend of mine – you have eaten at my table."

"And maybe you haven't eaten at mine?"

"Yes, yes – but don't refuse me credit now, Kesselmeyer!"

"Credit? It's credit, now, is it? Are you in your senses? A new loan?"

"Yes, Kesselmeyer, I swear to you – A little – a trifle. I only need to make a few payments and advances here and there to get on my feet again and restore confidence. Help me and you will be doing a big business. As I said, I have a number of affairs on hand. They may still all come out right. You know how shrewd and resourceful I am."

"I know what a numbskull you are! A dolt, a nincompoop, my dear friend! Will you have the goodness to tell me what your resourcefulness can accomplish at this stage? Perhaps there is a bank somewhere in the wide world that will lend you a shilling? Or another father-in-law? Ah, no; you have already played your best card. You can't play it twice. – With all due respect, my dear fellow, and my highest regards."

"Speak lower, devil take you!"

"You are a fool. Shrewd and resourceful, are you? Yes, to the other chap's advantage. You're not scrupulous, I'll say that for you, but much good it's done you! You have played tricks, and wormed capital out of people by hook or crook, just to pay me my twelve or sixteen per cent. You threw your honour overboard without getting any return. You have a conscience like a butcher's dog, and yet you are nothing but a ninny, a scapegoat. There are always such people – they are too funny for words. Why is it you are so afraid to apply to the person we mean with the whole story? Isn't it because there was crooked work four years ago? Perhaps it wasn't all quite straight – what? Are you afraid that certain things – ?"

"Very well, Kesselmeyer; I will write. But suppose he refuses? Suppose he lets me down?"

"Oh – ah, ha! Then we will just have a bankruptcy, a highly amusing little bankruptcy. That doesn't bother me at all. So far as I am concerned, I have about covered my expenses with the interest you have scratched together, and I have the priority with the assets. Oh, you wait; I shan't come short. I know everything pretty well, my good friend; I have an inventory already in my pocket. Ah, ha! We shall see that no dressing-gown and no silver bread-basket gets away."

"Kesselmeyer, you have sat at my table – "

"Oh, be quiet with your table! In eight days I'll be back for the answer. I shall walk in to town – the fresh air will do me good. Good morning, my friend, good morning!"

And Herr Kesselmeyer seemed to depart – yes, he went. She heard his odd, shuffling walk in the corridor, and imagined him rowing along with his arms. . . .

Herr Grünlich entered the "pensée-room" and saw Tony standing there with the little watering-can in her hand. She looked him in the face.

"What are you looking at? Why are you staring like that?" he said to her. He showed his teeth, and made vague movements in the air with his hands, and wiggled his body from side to side. His rosy face could not become actually pale; but it was spotted red and white like a scarlet-fever patient's.

CHAPTER VII

CONSUL JOHANN BUDDENBROOK arrived at the villa at two o'clock in the afternoon. He entered the Grünlich salon in a grey travelling-cloak and embraced his daughter with painful intensity. He was pale and seemed older. His small eyes were deep in their sockets, his large pointed nose stuck out between the fallen cheeks, his lips seemed to have grown thinner, and the beard under his chin and jaws half covered by his stiff choker and high neck-band – he had lately ceased to wear the two locks running from the temples half-way down the cheeks – was as grey as the hair on his head.

The Consul had hard, nerve-racking days behind him. Thomas had had a haemorrhage; the Father had learned of the misfortune in a letter from Herr van der Kellen. He had left his business in the careful hands of his clerk and hurried off to Amsterdam. He found nothing immediately dangerous about his son's illness, but an open-air cure was necessary, in the South, in Southern France; and as it fortunately happened that a journey of convalescence had been prescribed for the young son of the head of the firm, the two young men had left for Pau as soon as Thomas was able to travel.

The Consul had scarcely reached home again when he was attacked by a fresh misfortune, which had for the moment shaken his firm to its foundations and by which it had lost eighty thousand marks at one blow. How? Discounted cheques drawn on Westfall Brothers had come back to the firm, liquidation having begun. He had not failed to cover them. The firm had at once showed what it could do, without hesitation or embarrassment. But that could not prevent the Consul from experiencing all the sudden coldness, the reserve, the mistrust at the banks, with "friends," and among firms abroad, which such an event, such a weakening of working capital, was sure to bring in its train.

Well, he had pulled himself together, and had reviewed the whole situation; had reassured, reinforced, made head. And then, in the midst of the struggle, among telegrams, letters, and calculations, this last blow broke upon him as well: B. Grünlich, his daughter's husband, was insolvent. In a long, whining, confused letter he had implored, begged, and prayed for an assistance of a hundred to a hundred and twenty thousand marks. The Consul replied curtly and non-committally that he would come to Hamburg to meet Herr Grünlich and Kesselmeyer the banker, made a brief, soothing explanation to his wife, and started off.

Tony received him in the salon. She was fond of receiving visits in her brown silk salon, and she made no exception now; particularly as she had a very profound impression of the importance of the present occasion, without comprehending in the least what it was about. She looked blooming and yet becomingly serious, in her pale grey frock with its laces at breast and wrists, its bell-shaped sleeves and long train, and little diamond clasp at the throat. " How are you, Papa? At last you have come to see us again. How is Mamma? Is there good news from Tom? Take off your things, Father dear. Will you dress? The guest-room is ready for you. Grünlich is dressing."

" Don't call him, my child. I will wait for him here. You know I have come for a talk with your husband – a very, very serious talk, my dear Tony. Is Herr Kesselmeyer here? "

" Yes, he is in the pensée-room looking at the album."

" Where is Erica? "

" Up in the nursery with Tinka. She is very well. She is bathing her doll – of course, not in real water; I mean – she is a wax-doll, she only – "

" Of course." The Consul drew a deep breath and went on: " Evidently you have not been informed as to – to the state of affairs with your husband."

He had sat down in an arm-chair near the large table, and Tony placed herself at his feet on a little seat made of three cushions on top of one another. The finger of her right hand toyed gently with the diamond at her throat.

" No, Papa," answered Tony. " I must confess I know nothing. Heavens, I am a goose! – I have no understanding at all. I heard Kesselmeyer talking lately to Grünlich – at the end it seemed to me he was just joking again – he always talks so drolly. I heard your name once or twice – "

" You heard my name? In what connection? "

" Oh, I know nothing of the connection, Papa. Grünlich has been insufferably sulky ever since that day, I must say. Until yesterday – yesterday he was in a good mood, and asked me a dozen times if I loved him, and if I would put in a good word for him with you if he had something to ask you."

"Oh!"

"Yes, he told me he had written you and that you were coming here. It is good you have come. Everything is so queer. Grünlich had the card-table put in here. There are a lot of paper and pencils on it – for you to sit at, and hold a council together."

"Listen, my dear child," said the Consul, stroking her hair. "I want to ask you something very serious. Tell me: you love your husband with your whole heart, don't you?"

"Of course, Papa," said Tony with a face of child-like hypocrisy – precisely the face of the child Tony when she was asked: "You won't tease the old doll-woman again, Tony?" The Consul was silent a minute.

"You love him so much," he asked again, "that you could not live without him, under any circumstances, even if by God's will your situation should alter so that he could no longer surround you with all these things?" And his hand described a quick movement over the furniture and portières, over the gilt clock on the étagère, and finally over her own frock.

"Certainly, Papa," repeated Tony, in the soothing tone she nearly always used when any one spoke seriously to her. She looked past her father out of the window, where a heavy veil of rain was silently descending. Her face had the expression children wear when some one tells them a fairy story and then tactlessly introduces a generalization about conduct and duty – a mixture of embarrassment and impatience, piety and boredom.

The Consul looked at her without speaking for a minute. Was he satisfied with her response? He had weighed everything thoroughly, at home and during the journey.

It is comprehensible that Johann Buddenbrook's first impulse was to refuse his son-in-law any considerable payment. But when he remembered how pressing – to use a mild word – he had been about this marriage; when he looked back into the past, and recalled the words: "Are you satisfied with me?" with which his child had taken leave of him after the wedding, he gave way to a burdensome sense of guilt against her and said to himself that the thing must be decided according to her feelings. He knew perfectly that she had not made the marriage out of love, but he was obliged to reckon with the possibility that these four years of life together and the birth of the child had changed matters; that Tony now felt bound body and soul to her husband and would be driven by considerations both spiritual and worldly to shrink from a separation. In such a case, the Consul argued, he must accommodate himself to the surrender of whatever sum was necessary.

Christian duty and wifely feeling did indeed demand that Tony should follow her husband into misfortune; and if she actually took this resolve, he did not feel justified in letting her be deprived of all the ease and comfort to which she had been accustomed since childhood. He would feel himself obliged to avert the catastrophe, and to support B. Grünlich at any price. Yet the final result of his considerations was the desire to take his daughter and her child home with him and let Grünlich go his own way. God forbid that the worst should happen!

In any case, the Consul invoked the pronouncement of the law that a continued inability to provide for wife and children justified a separation. But, before everything, he must find out his daughter's real feelings.

" I see," he said, " my dear child, that you are actuated by good and praiseworthy motives. But – I cannot believe that you are seeing the thing as, unhappily, it really is – namely, as actual fact. I have not asked what you would do in this or that case, but what you to-day, now, will do. I do not know how much of the situation you know or suspect. It is my painful duty to tell you that your husband is obliged to call his creditors together; that he cannot carry on his business any longer. I hope you understand me."

" Grünlich is bankrupt? " Tony asked under her breath, half rising from the cushions and seizing the Consul's hand quickly.

" Yes, my child," he said seriously. " You did not know it? "

" My suspicions were not definite," she stammered. " Then Kesselmeyer was not joking? " she went on, staring before her at the brown carpet. " Oh, my God! " she suddenly uttered, and sank back on her seat.

In that minute all that was involved in the word " bankrupt " rose clearly before her: all the vague and fearful hints which she had heard as a child. " Bankrupt " – that was more dreadful than death, that was catastrophe, ruin, shame, disgrace, misery, despair. " He is bankrupt," she repeated. She was so cast down and shaken by the fatal word that the idea of escape, of assistance from her father, never occurred to her. He looked at her with raised eyebrows, out of his small deep-set eyes, which were tired and sad and full of an unusual suspense. " I am asking you," he said gently, " my dear Tony, if you are ready to follow your husband into misery? " He realized at once that he had used the hard word instinctively to frighten her, and he added: " He can work himself up again, of course."

" Certainly, Papa," answered she. But it did not prevent her from bursting into tears. She sobbed into her batiste handkerchief, trimmed with lace and with the monogram A. G. She still wept just like a child; quite unaffectedly and without embarrassment. Her upper lip had the most touching expression.

Her father continued to probe her with his eyes. " That is your serious feeling, my child? " he asked. He was as simple as she.

" I must, mustn't I? " she sobbed. " Don't I have to – ? "

" Certainly not," he said. But with a guilty feeling he added: " I would not force you to it, my dear Tony. If it should be the case that your feelings did not bind you indissolubly to your husband – "

She looked at him with uncomprehending, tear-streaming eyes. " How, Papa? "

The Consul twisted and turned, and found a compromise. " My dear child, you can understand how painful it would be for me to have to tell you all the hardships and suffering that would come about through the misfortune of your husband, the breaking-up of the business and of your household. I desire to spare you these first unpleasantnesses by taking you and little Erica home with me. You would be glad of that, I think? "

Tony was silent a moment, drying her tears. She carefully breathed on her handkerchief and pressed it against her eyes to heal their inflammation. Then she asked in a firm tone, without lifting her voice: " Papa, is Grünlich to blame? Is it his folly and lack of uprightness that has brought him to this? "

" Very probably," said the Consul. " That is – no, I don't know, my child. The explanation with him and the banker has not taken place yet."

She seemed not to be listening. She sat crouched on her three silk cushions, her elbow on her knee, her chin in her hand, and with her head bowed looked dreamily into the room.

" Ah, Papa," she said softly, almost without moving her lips, " wouldn't it have been better – ? "

The Consul could not see her face – but it had the expression it often wore those summer evenings at Travemünde, as she leaned at the window of her little room. One arm rested on her Father's knee, the hand hanging down limply. This very hand was expressive of a sad and tender abandonment, a sweet, pensive longing, travelling back into the past.

" Better? " asked Consul Buddenbrook. " If what, my child? "

He was thoroughly prepared for the confession that it would have been better had this marriage not taken place; but Tony only answered with a sigh: " Oh, nothing."

She seemed rapt by her thoughts, which had borne her so far

away that she had almost forgotten the "bankrupt." The Consul felt himself obliged to utter what he would rather only have confirmed.

"I think I guess your thoughts, Tony," he said, "and I don't on my side hesitate to confess that in this hour I regret the step that seemed to me four years ago so wise and advisable. I believe, before God, I am not responsible. I think I did my duty in trying to give you an existence suitable to your station. Heaven has willed otherwise. You will not believe that your Father played lightly and unreflectingly with your happiness in those days! Grünlich came to us with the best recommendations, a minister's son, a Christian and a cosmopolitan man. Later I made business inquiries, and it all sounded as favourable as possible. I examined the connections. All that is still very dark; and the explanation is yet to come. But you don't blame me – ? "

"No, Papa – how can you say such a thing? Come, don't take it to heart, poor Papa! You look pale. Shall I give you a little cordial? " She put her arm around his neck and kissed his cheek.

"Thank you, no," he said. "There, there! It is all right. Yes, I have bad days behind me. I have had much to try me. These are all trials sent from God. But that does not help my feeling a little guilty toward you, my child. Everything depends on the question I have already asked you. Speak openly, Tony. Have you learned to love your husband in these years of marriage? "

Tony wept afresh; and covering her eyes with both hands, in which she held the batiste handkerchief, she sobbed out: "Oh, what are you asking me, Papa? I have never loved him – he has always been repulsive to me. You know that."

It would be hard to say what went on in Johann Buddenbrook. His eyes looked shocked and sad; but he bit his lips hard together, and great wrinkles came in his cheeks, as they did when he had brought a piece of business to a successful conclusion. He said softly: "Four years – "

Tony's tears ceased suddenly. With her damp handkerchief in her hand, she sat up straight on her seat and said angrily: "Four years! Yes! Sometimes, in those four years, he sat with me in the evening and read the paper."

"God gave you a child," said the Father, moved.

"Yes, Papa. And I love Erica very much, although Grünlich says I am not fond of children. I would not be parted from her, that is certain. But Grünlich – no! Grünlich, no. And now he is bankrupt. Ah, Papa, if you will take Erica and me home – oh, gladly."

The Consul compressed his lips again. He was extremely well satisfied. But the main point had yet to be touched upon; though, by the decision Tony showed, he did not risk much by asking.

"You seem not to have thought it might be possible to do something, to get help. I have already said to you that I do not feel myself altogether innocent of the situation, and – in case you should expect – hope – I might intervene, to prevent the failure and cover your husband's debts, the best I could, and float his business – "

He watched her keenly, and her bearing filled him with satisfaction. It expressed disappointment.

"How much is it? " she asked.

"What is that to the point, my child? A very large sum." And Consul Buddenbrook nodded several times, as though the weight of the very thought of such a sum swung his head back and forth. "I should not conceal from you," he went on, "that the firm has suffered losses already quite apart from this affair, and that the surrender of a sum like this would be a blow from which it would recover with difficulty. I do not in any way say this to – "

He did not finish. Tony had sprung up, had even taken a few steps backward, and with the wet handkerchief still in her hand she cried: "Good! Enough! Never! " She looked almost heroic. The words "the firm " had struck home. It is highly probable that they had more effect than even her dislike of Herr Grünlich. "You shall not do that, Papa," she went on, quite beside herself. "Do you want to be bankrupt too? Never, never! "

At this moment the hall door opened a little uncertainly and Herr Grünlich entered.

Johann Buddenbrook rose, with a movement that meant: "That's settled."

CHAPTER VIII

Herr Grünlich's face was all mottled with red; but he had dressed carefully in a respectable-looking black coat and pea-green trousers like those in which he had made his first visits in Meng Street. He stood still, with his head down, looking very limp, and said in a weak exhausted sort of voice: "Father?"

The Consul bowed, not too cordially, and straightened his neck-cloth with an energetic movement.

"Thank you for coming," said Herr Grünlich.

"It was my duty, my friend," replied the Consul. "But I am afraid it will be about all I can do for you."

Herr Grünlich threw him a quick look and seemed to grow still more limp.

"I hear," the Consul went on, "that your banker, Herr Kesselmeyer, is awaiting us – where shall the conference be held? I am at your service."

"If you will be so good as to follow me," Herr Grünlich murmured. Consul Buddenbrook kissed his daughter on the forehead and said, "Go up to your child, Antonie."

Then he went, with Herr Grünlich fluttering in front of and behind him to open the portières, through the dining-room into the living-room.

Herr Kesselmeyer stood at the window, the black and white down softly rising and falling upon his cranium.

"Herr Kesselmeyer, Herr Consul Buddenbrook, my father-in-law," said Herr Grünlich, meekly. The Consul's face was impassive. Herr Kesselmeyer bowed with his arms hanging down, both yellow teeth against his upper lip, and said: "Pleasure to meet you, Herr Consul."

"Please excuse us for keeping you waiting, Kesselmeyer," said Herr Grünlich. He was not more polite to one than to the other. "Pray sit down."

As they went into the smoking-room, Herr Kesselmeyer said vivaciously: "Have you had a pleasant journey? Ah, rain? Yes, it is a bad time of year, a dirty time. If we had a little frost, or snow, now – but rain, filth – very, very unpleasant."

"What a queer creature!" thought the Consul.

In the centre of the little room with its dark-flowered wall-paper stood a sizable square table covered with green baize. It rained harder and harder; it was so dark that the first thing Herr Grünlich did was to light the three candles on the table. Business letters on blue paper, stamped with the names of various firms, torn and soiled papers with dates and signatures, lay on the green cloth. There were a thick ledger and a metal inkstand and sand-holder, full of well-sharpened pencils and goose-quills.

Herr Grünlich did the honours with the subdued and tactful mien of a man greeting guests at a funeral. "Dear Father, do take the easy chair," he said. "Herr Kesselmeyer, will you be so kind as to sit here?"

At last they were settled. The banker sat opposite the host, the Consul presided on the long side of the table. The back of his chair was against the hall door.

Herr Kesselmeyer bent over, released his upper lip, disentangled a glass from his waistcoat and stuck it on his nose, which he wrinkled for the purpose, and opened his mouth wide. Then he scratched his stubbly beard with an ugly rasping noise, put his hands on his knees, and remarked in a sprightly tone, jerking his head toward the piles of papers: "Well, there we have the whole boiling."

"May I look into matters a little more closely?" asked the Consul, taking up the ledger. But Herr Grünlich suddenly stretched out his hands over the table – long, trembling hands marked with high blue veins – and cried out in a voice that trembled too: "A moment, Father. Just a moment. Let me make just a few explanations. Yes, you will get an insight into everything – nothing will escape your glance; but, believe me, you will get an insight into the situation of an unfortunate, not a guilty man. You see in me a man who fought unwearied against fate, but was finally struck down. I am innocent of all – "

"We shall see, my friend, we shall see," said the Consul, with obvious impatience; and Herr Grünlich took his hands away and resigned himself to his fate.

Then there were long dreadful minutes of silence. The three gentlemen sat close together in the flickering candlelight, shut in by the four dark walls. There was not a sound but the rustling of the Consul's papers and the falling rain outside.

Herr Kesselmeyer stuck his thumbs in the arm-holes of his

waistcoat and played piano on his shoulders with his fingers, looking with indescribable jocosity from one to the other. Herr Grünlich sat upright in his chair, hands on the table, staring gloomily before him, and now and then stealing an anxious glance at his father-in-law out of the tail of his eye. The Consul examined the ledger, followed columns of figures with his finger, compared dates, and did indecipherable little sums in lead-pencil on a scrap of paper. His worn features expressed astonishment and dismay at the conditions into which he now " gained an insight." Finally he laid his left arm on Herr Grünlich's and said with evident emotion: " You poor man! "

" Father," Herr Grünlich broke out. Two great tears rolled down his cheeks and ran into the golden whiskers. Herr Kesselmeyer followed their course with the greatest interest. He even raised himself a little, bent over, and looked his vis-à-vis in the face, with his mouth open. Consul Buddenbrook was moved. Softened by his own recent misfortunes, he felt himself carried away by sympathy; but he controlled his feelings.

" How is it possible? " he said, with a sad head-shake. " In so few years – "

" Oh, that's simple," answered Herr Kesselmeyer, good-temperedly. " One can easily ruin oneself in four years. When we remember that it took an even shorter time for Westfal Brothers in Bremen to go smash – " The Consul stared at him, but without either seeing or hearing him. He himself had not expressed his own actual thoughts, his real misgivings. Why, he asked himself with puzzled suspicion, why was this happening now? It was as clear as daylight that, just where he stood to-day, B. Grünlich had stood two years, three years before. But his credit had been inexhaustible, he had had capital from the banks, and for his undertakings continual endorsement from sound houses like Senator Bock and Consul Goudstikker. His paper had passed as current as banknotes. Why now, precisely now – and the head of the firm of Johann Buddenbrook knew well what he meant by this " now " – had there come this crash on all sides, this complete withdrawal of credit as if by common consent, this unanimous descent upon B. Grünlich, this disregard of all consideration, all ordinary business courtesy? The Consul would have been naïve indeed had he not realized that the good standing of his own firm was to the advantage of his son-in-law. But had the son-in-law's credit so entirely, so strikingly, so exclusively depended upon his own? Had Grünlich himself been nothing at all? And the information the Consul had had, the books he had examined – ? Well, however the thing stood, his resolution was firmer than ever not to lift a finger. They had reckoned without their host.

Apparently B. Grünlich had known how to make it appear that he was connected with the firm of Buddenbrook – well, this widely-circulated error should be set right once for all. And this Kesselmeyer – he was going to get a shock too. The clown! Had he no conscience whatever? It was very plain how shamelessly he had speculated on the probability that he, Johann Buddenbrook, would not let his daughter's husband be ruined; how he had continued to finance Grünlich long after he was unsound, and exacted from him an ever crueller rate of interest.

"Now," he said shortly, "let us get to the point. If I am asked as a merchant to say frankly what I think, I am obliged to say that if the situation is that of an unfortunate man, it is also in a great degree that of a guilty one."

"Father!" stammered Herr Grünlich.

"The name does not come well to my ears," said the Consul, quickly and harshly. "Your demands on Herr Grünlich amount, sir" – turning for a moment to the banker – "to sixty thousand marks, I believe?"

"With the back interest they come to sixty-eight thousand seven hundred and fifty-five marks and fifteen shillings," answered Herr Kesselmeyer pleasantly.

"Very good. And you would not be inclined under any circumstances to be patient for a longer time?"

Herr Kesselmeyer simply began to laugh. He laughed with his mouth open, in spasms, without a trace of scorn, even good-naturedly, looking at the Consul as though he were inviting him to join in the fun.

Johann Buddenbrook's little deep eyes clouded over and began to show red rims around them that ran down to the cheek-bones. He had only asked for form's sake, being aware that a postponement on the part of one creditor would not materially alter the situation. But the manner of this man's refusal was mortifying indeed. With a motion of the hand he pushed away everything from in front of him, laid the pencil down with a jerk on the table, and said, "Then I must express myself as unwilling to concern myself any further with this affair."

"Ah, ha!" cried Herr Kesselmeyer, shaking his hands in the air. "That's the way to talk. The Herr Consul will settle everything out of hand – we shan't have any long speeches. Without more ado." Johann Buddenbrook did not even look at him.

"I cannot help you, my friend." He turned calmly to Herr

Grünlich. "Things must go on as they have begun. Pull yourself together, and God will give you strength and consolation. I must consider our interview at an end."

Herr Kesselmeyer's face took on a serious expression which was vastly becoming to it. But then he nodded encouragingly to Herr Grünlich. The latter sat motionless at the table, only wringing his hands so hard that the fingers cracked.

"Father – Herr Consul," he said, with a trembling voice. "You will not – you cannot desire my ruin. Listen. It is a matter of a hundred and twenty thousand marks in all – you can save me! You are a rich man. Regard it as you like – as a final arrangement, as your daughter's inheritance, as a loan subject to interest. I will work – you know I am keen and resourceful – "

"I have spoken my last word," said the Consul.

"Permit me – may I ask whether you could if you would? " asked Herr Kesselmeyer, looking at him through his glasses, with his nose wrinkled up. "I suggest to the Consul that this would be a most advantageous time to display the strength of the firm of Buddenbrook."

"You would do well, sir, to leave the good name of my house to me. I do not need to throw my money in the nearest ditch in order to show how good my credit is."

"Dear me, no, of course not – ditch, ah, ha! – Ditch is very funny. But doesn't the gentleman think the failure of his son-in-law places his own credit in a bad light – er – ah – ? "

"I can only recommend you again to remember that my credit in the business world is entirely my own affair," said the Consul.

Herr Grünlich looked at his banker helplessly and began afresh: "Father! I implore you again: think what you are doing. Is it a question of me alone? I – oh, I myself might be allowed to perish. But your daughter, my wife, whom I love, whom I won after such a struggle – and our child – both innocent children – are they to be brought low as well? No, Father, I will not bear it; I will kill myself. Yes, I would kill myself with this hand. Believe me – and may heaven pardon you if it will."

Johann Buddenbrook leaned back in his arm-chair quite white, with a fast-beating heart. For the second time the emotions of this man played upon him, and their expression had the stamp of truth; again he heard, as when he told Herr Grünlich the contents of his daughter's letter from Travemünde, the same terrible threat, and again there shuddered through him all the fanatical reverence of his generation for human feelings, which yet had always been in conflict with his own hard practical sense. But the attack lasted no longer than a moment. "A hundred thousand marks," he repeated to himself; and then he said quietly and decisively: "Antonie is my daughter. I shall know how to protect her from unmerited suffering."

"What do you mean by that?" asked Herr Grünlich, slowly stiffening.

"That you will see," answered the Consul. "For the present I have nothing to add." And he got up, pushed back his chair, and turned toward the door.

Herr Grünlich sat silent, stiff, irresolute; his mouth opened and closed without a word coming out. But the sprightliness of Herr Kesselmeyer returned at this conclusive action of the Consul. Yes, it got the upper hand entirely, it passed all bounds, it became frightful. The glasses fell from his nose, which went skyward, while his little mouth, with the two triangular yellow teeth, looked as though it were splitting. He rowed with his little red hands in the air, the fuzz on his head waved up and down, his whole face, with its bristly white beard distorted and grotesque with uncontrolled hilarity, had grown the colour of cinnamon.

"Ah, ha, ha, ah, ha!" he yelled, his voice cracking. "I find that in the last – degree – funny! You ought to consider, Consul Buddenbrook, before you consign to the grave such a valuable – such a supreme specimen of a son-in-law. Anything so shrewd, so resourceful as he is, won't be born upon God's wide earth a second time. Aha! Four years ago – when the knife was at our throat, the rope around our neck – suddenly we made a match with Fräulein Buddenbrook, and spread the news on 'Change, even before it had actually come off! Congratulations, my dear friend; my best respects!"

"Kesselmeyer," groaned Herr Grünlich, making spasmodic motions with his hands, as though waving off an evil spirit. He rushed into one corner of the room, where he sat down and buried his face in his hands. The ends of his whiskers lay on his shanks, and he rocked his knees up and down in his emotion.

"How did we do that?" went on Herr Kesselmeyer. "How did we actually manage to catch the little daughter and the eighty thousand marks? O-ho, ah, ha! That is easy. Even if one has no more shrewdness and resourcefulness than a tallow candle, it is easy! You show the saviour Papa nice, pretty, clean books, in which everything is put in the right way – only that they don't quite correspond with the plain fact – for the plain fact is that three-quarters of the dowry is already debts."

The Consul stood at the door deathly pale, the handle in his hand. Shivers ran up and down his back. He seemed to be standing in this little room lighted by the flickering candles, between a swindler and an ape gone mad with spite.

"I despise your words, sir," he brought out with uncertain emphasis. "I despise your wild utterances the more that they concern me as well. I did not hand my daughter over light-headedly to misfortune; I informed myself as to my son-in-law's prospects. The rest was God's will."

He turned – he would not hear any more – he opened the door. But Herr Kesselmeyer shrieked after him: "Aha, inquiries? Where? Of Bock? Of Goudstikker? Of Petersen? Of Massmann and Timm? They were all in it. They were all in it up to their necks. They were all uncommonly pleased to be secured by the wedding – " The Consul slammed the door behind him.

CHAPTER IX

Dora the cook, about whose honesty Tony had had her doubts, was busy in the dining-room.

"Ask Madame Grünlich to come down," ordered the Consul. "Get yourself ready, my child," he said as Tony appeared. He went with her into the salon. "Get ready as soon as possible, and get Erica ready too. We are going to the city. We shall sleep to-night in a hotel and travel home to-morrow."

"Yes, Papa," Tony said. Her face was red; she was distracted and bewildered. She made unnecessary and hurried motions about her waist, as if not knowing where to begin and not grasping the actuality of the occasion.

"What shall I take, Papa?" she asked distractedly. "Everything? All our clothes? One trunk or two? Is Grünlich really bankrupt? Oh, my God! But can I take my jewelry, then? Papa, the servants must leave – I cannot pay them. Grünlich was to have given me housekeeping money to-day or to-morrow."

"Never mind, my child; things will all be arranged here. Just take what is necessary in a small trunk. They can send your own things after you. Hurry, do you hear?"

Just then the portières were parted and Herr Grünlich came into the salon. With quick steps, his arms outstretched, his head on one side, with the bearing of a man who says: "Here I am; kill me if you will," he hurried to his wife and sank down on his knees right in front of her. His appearance was pitiable. His golden whiskers were dishevelled, his coat crumpled, his neck-cloth askew, his collar open; little drops stood upon his forehead.

"Antonie!" he said. "Have you a heart that can feel? Hear me. You see before you a man who will be utterly ruined, if – yes, who will die of grief, if you deny him your love. Here I lie; can you find it in your heart to say to me: 'I despise you – I am leaving you'?"

Tony wept. It was just the same as that time in the landscape room. Once more she saw his anguished face, his imploring eyes directed upon her; again she saw, and was moved to see, that this pleading, this anguish, were real and unfeigned.

" Get up, Grünlich," she said, sobbing. " Please, please get up." She tried to raise his shoulders. " I do not despise you. How can you say such a thing? " Without knowing what else she should say, she turned helplessly to her father. The Consul took her hand, bowed to his son-in-law, and moved with her toward the hall door.

" You are going? " cried Herr Grünlich, springing to his feet.

" I have told you already," said the Consul, " that I cannot be responsible for leaving my innocent child in misfortune – and I might add that you cannot, either. No, sir, you have misprized the possession of my daughter. You may thank your Creator that the child's heart is so pure and unsuspicious that she parts from you without repulsion. Farewell."

But here Herr Grünlich lost his head. He could have borne to hear of a brief parting – of a return and a new life and perhaps the saving of the inheritance. But this was too much for his powers of self-command, his shrewdness and resource. He might have taken the large bronze plaque that stood on the étagère, but he seized instead a thin painted vase with flowers that stood next it, and threw it on the ground so that it smashed into a thousand bits.

" Ha, good, good! " he screamed. " Get along with you! Did you think I'd whine after you, you goose? You are very much mistaken, my darling. I only married you for your money; and it was not nearly enough, so you may as well go home. I'm through with you – through – through – through! "

Johann Buddenbrook ushered his daughter silently out. Then he turned, went up to Herr Grünlich, who was standing in the window with his hands behind his back staring out at the rain, touched him softly on the shoulder, and spoke with soft admonishment. " Pull yourself together. *Pray!* "

CHAPTER X

A CHASTENED mood reigned for some time at the old house in Meng Street after Madame Grünlich and her little daughter returned thither to take up their abode. The family went about rather subdued and did not speak much about " it," with the exception of the chief actor in the affair, who, on the contrary, talked about " it " inexhaustibly, and was entirely in her element.

Tony had moved with Erica into the rooms in the second storey which her parents had occupied in the time of the elder Buddenbrooks. She was a little disappointed to find that it did not occur to her Papa to engage a servant for her, and she had rather a pensive half-hour when he gently explained that it would be fitting for her to live a retired life and give up the society of the town: for though, he said, according to human judgments she was an innocent victim of the fate which God had sent to try her, still her position as a divorced wife made a very quiet life advisable, particularly at first. But Tony possessed the gift of adaptability. She could adjust herself with ease and cheerfulness to any situation. She soon grew charmed with her rôle of the injured wife returned to the house of her fathers; wore dark frocks, dressed her ash-blond hair primly like a young girl's, and felt richly repaid for her lack of society by the weight she had acquired in the household, the seriousness and dignity of her new position, and above all by the immense pleasure of being able to talk about Herr Grünlich and her marriage and to make general observations about life and destiny, which she did with the utmost gusto.

Not everybody gave her this opportunity, it is true. The Frau Consul was convinced that her husband had acted correctly and out of a sense of duty; but when Tony began to talk, she would put up her lovely white hand and say: " *Assez,* my child; I do not like to hear about it."

Clara, now twelve years old, understood nothing, and Cousin Clothilde was just as stupid. " Oh, Tony! " – that was all she could say, with drawling astonishment. But the young wife found an attentive listener in Mamsell Jungmann, who was now thirty-five years old and could boast of having grown grey in the service of the best society. "You don't need to worry, Tony, my child," she would say. "You are young; you will marry again." And she devoted herself to the upbringing of little Erica, telling her the same stories, the same memories of her youth, to which the Consul's children had listened fifteen years before; and, in particular, of that uncle who died of hiccoughs at Marienwerder "because his heart was broken."

But it was with her father that Tony talked most and longest. She liked to catch him after the noonday meal or in the morning at early breakfast. Their relations had grown closer and warmer; for her feeling had been heretofore one of awe and respect rather than affection, on account of his high position in the town, his piety, his solid, stern ability and industry. During that talk in her own salon he had come humanly near to her, and it had filled her with pride and emotion to be found worthy of that serious and confidential consultation. He, the infallible parent, had put the decision into her hands: he had confessed, almost humbly, to a sense of guilt. Such an idea would never have entered Tony's head of itself; but since he said it, she believed it, and her feeling for him had thereby grown warmer and tenderer. As for the Consul, he believed himself bound to make up to his daughter for her misfortune by redoubled love and care.

Johann Buddenbrook had himself taken no steps against his untrustworthy son-in-law. Tony and her Mother did hear from him, in the course of conversation, what dishonourable means Grünlich had used to get hold of the eighty thousand marks; but the Consul was careful to give the matter no publicity. He did not even consider going to the courts with it. He felt wounded in his pride as a merchant, and he wrestled silently with the disgrace of having been so thoroughly taken in.

But he pressed the divorce suit energetically as soon as the failure of Grünlich came out, which it soon did, thereby causing no inconsiderable losses to certain Hamburg firms.

It was this suit, and the thought that she herself was a principal in it, that gave Tony her most delicious and indescribable feelings of importance.

"Father," she said – for in these conversations she never called him "Papa" – "Father, how is our affair going on? Do you think it will be all right? The paragraph is perfectly clear; I have studied it. 'Incapacity of the husband to provide for his family': surely they will say that is quite plain. If there were a son, Grünlich would keep him – "

Another time she said: " I have thought a great deal about the four years of my marriage, Father. That was certainly the reason the man never wanted us to live in the town, which I was so anxious to do. That was the reason he never liked me even to be in the town or go into society. The danger was much greater there than in Eimsbüttel, of my hearing somehow or other how things stood. What a scoundrel! "

" We must not judge, my child," answered the Consul.

Or, when the divorce was finally pronounced: " Have you entered it in the family papers, Father? No? Then I'd better do it. Please give me the key to the escritoire." With bustling pride she wrote, beneath the lines she had set there four years ago under her name: " This marriage was dissolved by law in February, 1850." Then she put away the pen and reflected a minute.

" Father," she said, " I understand very well that this affair is a blot on our family history. I have thought about it a great deal. It is exactly as if there were a spot of ink in the book here. But never mind. That is my affair. I will erase it. I am still young. Don't you think I am still quite pretty? Though Frau Stuht, when she saw me again, said to me: ' Oh, Heavens, Mme. Grünlich, how old you've grown! ' Well, I certainly couldn't remain all my life the goose I was four years ago! Life takes one along with it. Anyhow, I shall marry again. You will see, everything can be put right by a good marriage."

" That is in God's hand, my child. It is most unfitting to speak of such things."

Tony began at this time to use very frequently the expression " Such is life "; and with the word " life " she would open her eyes wide with a charming serious look, indicating the deep insight she had acquired into human affairs and human destinies.

Thomas returned from Pau in August of that year. The dining-table was opened out again, and Tony had a fresh audience for her tale. She loved and looked up to her brother, who had felt for her pain in that departure from Travemünde, and she respected him as the future head of the firm and the family.

" Yes, yes," he said; " we've both of us gone through things, Tony."

The corner of his eyebrow went up, and his cigarette moved from one corner of his mouth to the other: his thoughts were probably with the little flower-girl with the Malay face, who had lately married the son of her employer and now herself carried on the shop in Fishers' Lane.

Thomas Buddenbrook, though still a little pale, was strikingly elegant. The last few years had entirely completed his education. His hair was brushed so that it stood out in two clumps above his ears, and his moustache was trimmed in the French mode, with sharp points that were stiffened with the tongs and stuck straight out. His stocky broad-shouldered figure had an almost military air.

His constitution was not of the best; the blue veins showed too plainly at the narrow temples, and he had a slight tendency to chills, which good Dr. Grabow struggled with in vain. In the details of his physical appearance – the chin, the nose, and especially the hands, which were wonderfully true to the Buddenbrook type – his likeness to his grandfather was more pronounced than ever.

He spoke French with a distinctly Spanish accent, and astonished everybody by his enthusiasm for certain modern writers of a satiric and polemic character. Broker Gosch was the only person in town who sympathized with his tastes. His father strongly reprehended them.

But the Father's pride and joy in his eldest son were plain to be seen; they shone in the Consul's eyes. He welcomed him joyfully home as his colleague in the firm, and himself began to work with increased satisfaction in his office – especially after the death of old Madame Kröger, which took place at the end of the year.

The old lady's loss was one to be borne with resignation. She had grown very old, and lived quite alone at the end. She went to God, and the firm of Buddenbrooks received a large sum of money, a round hundred thousand thaler, which strengthened the working capital of the business in a highly desirable way.

The Consul's brother-in-law Justus, weary of continual business disappointments, as soon as he had his hands on his inheritance settled his business and retired. The gay son of the cavalier à-la-mode was not a happy man. He had been too careless, too generous to attain a solid position in the mercantile world. But he had already spent a considerable part of his inheritance; and now Jacob, his eldest son, was the source of fresh cares to him.

The young man had become addicted to light, not to say disreputable, society in the great city of Hamburg. He had cost his father a huge sum in the course of years, and when Consul Kröger refused to give him more, the mother, a weak, sickly woman, sent money secretly to the son, and wretched clouds had sprung up between husband and wife.

The final blow came at the very time when B. Grünlich was making his failure: something happened at Dalbeck and Company in Hamburg, where Jacob Kröger worked. There had been some kind of dishonesty. It was not talked about; no questions were asked of Justus Kröger; but it got about that Jacob had a position as travelling man in New York and was about to sail. He was seen once in the town before his boat left, a foppishly dressed, unwholesome-looking youth. He had probably come hither to get more money out of his mother, besides the passage money his father sent him.

It finally came about that Justus spoke exclusively of " my son," as though he had none but the one heir, his second son, Jürgen, who would certainly never be guilty of a false step, but who seemed on the other hand to be mentally limited. He had had difficulty getting through the High School; after which he spent some time in Jena, studying law – evidently without either pleasure or profit.

Johann Buddenbrook felt keenly the cloud on his wife's family and looked with the more anxiety to the future of his own children. He was justified in placing the utmost confidence in the ability and earnestness of his older son. As for Christian, Mr. Richardson had written that he showed an unusual gift for acquiring English, but no genuine interest in the business. He had a great weakness for the theatre and for other distractions of the great city. Christian himself wrote that he had a longing to travel and see the world. He begged eagerly to be allowed to take a position " over there " – which meant in South America, perhaps in Chile. " That's simply love of adventure," the Consul said, and told him to remain with Mr. Richardson for another year and acquire mercantile experience. There followed an exchange of letters on the subject, with the result that in the summer of 1851 Christian Buddenbrook sailed for Valparaiso, where he had hunted up a position. He travelled direct from England, without coming home.

So much for his two sons. As for Tony, the Consul was gratified to see with what self-possession she defended her position in the town as a Buddenbrook born; for as a divorced wife she had naturally to overcome all sorts of prejudice on the part of the other families.

" Oh! " she said, coming back with flushed cheeks from a walk and throwing her hat on the sofa in the landscape-room. " This Juliet Möllendorpf, or Hagenström – or Semmlinger – whatever she is, the creature! – Imagine, Mamma! She doesn't speak. She doesn't say ' How do you do? ' She waits for me to speak first. What do you say to that? I passed her in Broad Street with my head up and looked straight at her."

"You go too far, Tony. There is a limit to everything. Why shouldn't you speak first? You are the same age, and she is a married woman, just as you were."

"Never, Mamma! Never under the shining sun! Such rag-tag and bob-tail!"

"*Assez,* my love. Such vulgar expressions –"

"Oh, it makes me feel perfectly beside myself!"

Her hatred of the upstart family was fed by the mere thought that the Hagenströms might now feel justified in looking down on her – especially considering the present good fortune of the clan. Old Hinrich had died at the beginning of 1851, and his son Hermann – he of the lemon buns and the boxes on the ear – was doing a very brilliant business with Herr Strunck as partner. He had married, less than a year later, the daughter of Consul Huneus, the richest man in town, who had made enough out of his business to leave each of his three children two million marks. Hermann's brother Moritz, despite his lung trouble, had a brilliant career as student, and had now settled down in the town to practise law. He had a reputation for being able, witty, and literary, and soon acquired a considerable business. He did not look like the Semmlingers, having a yellow face and pointed teeth with wide spaces between.

Even in the family Tony had to take care to hold her head up. Uncle Gotthold's temper toward his fortunate step-brother had grown more mild and resigned now that he had given up business and spent his time care-free in his modest house, munching lozenges out of a tin box – he loved sweets. Still, considering his three unmarried daughters, he could not have failed to feel a quiet satisfaction over Tony's unfortunate venture; and his wife, born Stüwing, and his three daughters, twenty-six, twenty-seven, and twenty-eight years old, showed an exaggerated interest in their cousin's misfortune and the divorce proceedings; more, in fact, than they had in her betrothal and wedding. When the "children's Thursdays" began again in Meng Street after old Madame Kröger's death, Tony found it no easy work to defend herself.

"Oh, heavens, you poor thing!" said Pfiffi, the youngest, who was little and plump, with a droll way of shaking herself at every word. A drop of water always came in the corner of her mouth when she spoke. "Has the decree been pronounced? Are you exactly as you were before?"

"Oh, on the contrary," said Henriette, who, like her elder sister, was extraordinarily tall and withered-looking. "You are much worse off than if you had never married at all."

"Yes," Friederike chimed in. "Then it is ever so much better never to have married at all."

"Oh, no, dear Friederike," said Tony, erecting her head, while she bethought herself of a telling and clever retort. "You make a mistake there. Marriage teaches one to know life, you see. One is no longer a silly goose. And then I have more prospect of marrying again than those who have never married at all!"

"Oh!" cried the others with one voice. They said it with a long hissing intake of breath which made it sound very sceptical indeed.

Sesemi Weichbrodt was too good and tactful even to mention the subject. Tony sometimes visited her former teacher in the little red house at Millbrink No. 7. It was still occupied by a troop of girls, though the boarding-school was slowly falling out of fashion. The lively old maid was also invited to Meng Street on occasion to partake of a haunch of venison or a stuffed goose. She always raised herself on tiptoe to kiss Tony on the forehead, with a little exploding noise. Madame Kethelsen, her simple sister, had grown rapidly deaf and had understood almost nothing of Tony's affair. She still laughed her painfully hearty laugh on the most unsuitable occasions, and Sesemi still felt it necessary to rap on the table and cry "Nally!"

The years went on. Gradually people forgot their feelings over Tony's affair. She herself would only think now and then of her married life, when she saw on Erica's healthy, hearty little face some expression that reminded her of Bendix Grünlich. She dressed again in colours, wore her hair in the old way, and made the same old visits into society.

Still, she was always glad that she had the chance to be away from the town for some time in the summer. The Consul's health made it necessary for him to visit various cures.

"Oh, what it is to grow old!" he said. "If I get a spot of coffee on my trousers and put a drop of cold water on it, I have rheumatism. When one is young, one can do anything." He suffered at times also from spells of dizziness.

They went to Obersalzbrunn, to Ems and Baden-Baden, to Kissingen, whence they made a delightful and edifying journey to Nuremberg and Munich and the Salzburg neighbourhood, to Ischl and Vienna, Prague, Dresden, Berlin, and home again. Madame Grünlich had been suffering from a nervous affection of the digestion, and was obliged to take a strenuous cure at the baths; but nevertheless she found the journey a highly desirable change, for she did not conceal her opinion that it was a little slow at home.

" Heavens, yes – you know how it is, Father," she would say, regarding the ceiling with a thoughtful air. " Of course, I have learned what life is like – but just for that reason it is rather a dull prospect for me to be always sitting here at home like a stupid goose. I hope you don't think I mean I do not like to be with you, Papa. I ought to be whipped if I did, it would be so ungrateful. But I only mean life is like that, you know."

The hardest thing she had to bear was the increasing piety of her parents' home. The Consul's religious fervour grew upon him in proportion as he himself felt the weight of years and infirmity; and his wife too, as she got older, began to find the spiritual side to her taste. Prayers had always been customary in the Buddenbrook house, but now for some time the family and the servants had assembled mornings and evenings in the breakfast-room to hear the Master read the Bible. And the visits of ministers and missionaries increased more and more from year to year. The godly patrician house in Meng Street, where, by the way, such good dinners were to be had, had been known for years as a spiritual haven to the Lutheran and reformed clergy and to both foreign and home missions. From all quarters of the Fatherland came long-haired, black-coated gentlemen, to enjoy the pious intercourse and the nourishing meals, and to be furnished with the sinews of their spiritual warfare. The ministers of the town went in and out as friends of the house.

Tom was much too discreet and prudent even to let any one see him smile; but Tony mocked quite openly. She even, sad to say, made fun of these pious worthies whenever she had a chance.

Sometimes when the Frau Consul had a headache, it was Tony's turn to play the housekeeper and order the dinner. One day, when a strange clergyman whose appetite was the subject of general hilarity, was a guest, Tony mischievously ordered " bacon broth," the famous local dish: a bouillon made with sour cabbage, in which was served the entire meal – ham, potatoes, beet-root, cauliflower, peas, beans, pears, sour plums, and goodness knows what, juice and all – a dish which nobody except those born to it could possibly eat.

" I do hope you are enjoying the soup, Herr Pastor," she said several times. " No? Oh, dear, who would have thought it? " And she made a very roguish face, and ran her tongue over her lips, a trick she had when she thought of some prank or other.

The fat man laid down his spoon resignedly and said mildly: " I will wait till the next course."

" Yes," the Frau Consul said hastily, " there is a little something afterwards." But a "next course" was unthinkable, after this mighty dish; and despite the French toast and apple jelly which finished the meal, the reverend guest had to rise hungry from table, while Tony tittered, and Tom, with fine self-control, lifted one eyebrow.

Another time Tony stood with Stina, the cook, in domestic discourse in the entry, when Pastor Mathias from Kannstadt, who was stopping a few days in the house, came back from a walk and rang at the outer door. Stina ran to open, with her peasant waddle, and the Pastor, with the view of saying an edifying word and testing her a little, asked in a friendly tone: "Do you love the Master?"

Perhaps he had the idea of giving her a tip if she professed herself on the side of the Saviour.

"Lord, Herr Pastor," said Stina, trembling and blushing, with wide eyes. "Which one do Herr Pastor mean? T' old un or t' young un?" Madame Grünlich did not fail to tell the story at the table, so that even the Frau Consul burst out into her sputtering Kröger laugh. The Consul, however, looked down in displeasure at his plate.

"A misunderstanding," said Herr Mathias, highly embarrassed.

CHAPTER XI

WHAT follows happened in the late summer of 1855, on a Sunday afternoon. The Buddenbrooks were sitting in the landscape-room waiting for the Consul, who was below dressing himself. They had arranged to take a holiday walk to a pleasure garden outside the City Gate, where, all except Clara and Clothilde, they were to drink coffee and, if the weather permitted, go for a row on the river. Clara and Clothide went always on Sunday evenings to the house of a friend, where they knitted stockings for little negro children.

"Papa is ridiculous," Tony said, using her habitual strong language. "Can he never be ready on time? He sits and sits and sits at his desk: something or other *must* be finished – good heavens, perhaps it is something really necessary, I don't know. But I don't believe we should actually become bankrupt if he put down his pen a quarter of an hour sooner. Well, when it is already ten minutes too late, he remembers his appointment and comes upstairs, always two steps at a time, although he knows he will get palpitation at the top. And it is like that at every company, before every expedition. Isn't it possible for him to leave himself time enough? And stop soon enough? It's so irresponsible of him; you ought to talk to him about it, Mamma." She sat on the sofa beside her Mother, dressed in the changeable silk that was fashionable that summer; while the Frau Consul wore a heavy grey ribbed silk trimmed with black lace, and a cap of lace and stiffened tulle, tied under her chin with a satin bow. The lappets of her cap fell down on her breast. Her smooth hair was still inexorably reddish-blond in colour, and she held a work-bag in both her white delicately veined hands. Tom was lounging in an easy-chair beside her smoking his cigarette, while Clara and Clothilde sat opposite each other at the window. It was a mystery how much good and nourishing food that poor Clothilde could absorb daily without any result whatever! She grew thinner and thinner, and her shapeless black frock did not conceal the fact. Her face was as long, straight, and expressionless as ever, her hair as smooth and ash-coloured, her nose as straight, but full of large pores and getting thick at the end.

"Don't you think it will rain?" said Clara. The young girl had the habit of not elevating her voice at the end of a question and of looking everybody straight in the face with a pronounced and rather forbidding look. Her brown frock was relieved only by a little stiff turn-over collar and cuffs. She sat straight up, her hands in her lap. The servants had more respect for her than for any one else in the family; it was she who held the services morning and evening now, for the Consul could not read aloud without getting a feeling of oppression in the head.

"Shall you take your new Baschlik?" she asked again. "The rain will spoil it. It would be a pity. I think it would be better to put off the party."

"No," said Tom. "The Kistenmakers are coming. It doesn't matter. The barometer went down so suddenly – . There will be a storm – it will pour, but not last long. Papa is not ready yet; so we can wait till it is over."

The Frau Consul raised a protesting hand. "You think there will be a severe storm, Tom? You know I am afraid of them."

"No," Tom answered. "I was down at the harbour this morning talking to Captain Kloot. He is infallible. There will be a heavy rain, but no wind."

The second week in September had brought belated hot weather with it. There was a south-west wind, and the city suffered more than in July. A strange-looking dark blue sky hung above the roof-tops, pale on the skyline as it is in the desert. After sunset a sultry breath, like a hot blast from an oven, streamed out of the small houses and up from the pavement of the narrow streets. Today the wind had gone round to the west, and at the same time the barometer had fallen sharply. A large part of the sky was still blue, but it was slowly being overcast by heavy grey-blue clouds that looked like feather pillows.

Tom added: "It would be a good thing if it did rain, I think. We should collapse if we had to walk in this atmosphere. It is an unnatural heat. Hotter than it ever was in Pau."

Ida Jungmann, with little Erica's hand in hers, came into the room. The child looked a droll little figure in her stiffly starched cotton frock; she smelled of starch and soap. She had Herr Grünlich's eyes and his rosy skin, but the upper lip was Tony's.

The good Ida was already quite grey, almost white, although not out of the forties. It was a trait of her family: the uncle that died had had white hair at thirty. But her little brown eyes looked as shrewd and faithful as ever. She had been now for twenty years with the Buddenbrooks, and she realized with pride that she was indispensable. She oversaw kitchen, larders, linen and china cupboards, she made the most important purchases, she read to little Erica, made clothes for her dolls, and fetched her from school, with a slice of French bread, to take her walking on the Mill-wall. Every lady said to Frau Consul or her daughter: " What a treasure your Mamsell is, my dear! Goodness, she is worth her weight in gold! Twenty years – and she will be useful at sixty and more; these wiry people are. What faithful eyes she has! I envy you, my love." But Ida Jungmann was very reserved. She knew her own position, and when some ordinary nurse-girl came and sat down with her charge on the same bench and tried to enter into conversation, Ida Jungmann would say: " There is a draught here, Erica," and get up and go.

Tony drew her little daughter to her and kissed the rosy cheeks, and the Frau Consul stretched out her hand with rather an absent smile; for she was looking anxiously at the sky, which grew darker and darker. Her left hand fingered the sofa pillows nervously, and her light eyes wandered restlessly to the window.

Erica was allowed to sit next her Grandmother, and Ida sat up straight on a chair and began to knit. Thus all waited silently for the Consul. The air was heavy. The last bit of blue had disappeared; the dark grey sky lowered heavy and swollen over them. The colours in the room changed, the yellow of furniture and hangings and the tones of the landscapes on the walls were all quenched, like the gay shades in Tony's frock and the brightness of their eyes. Even the west wind, which had been playing in the churchyard of St. Mary's and whirling the dust around in the darkening street, was suddenly quiet.

This breathless moment of absolute calm came without warning, like some unexpected, soundless, awful event. The sultriness grew heavier, the atmosphere seemed to increase its weight in a second; it oppressed the brain, it rested on the heart, it prevented the breathing. A swallow flew so low over the pavement that its wings touched. And this pressure that one could not lift, this tension, this growing weight on the whole organism, would have become unbearable had it lasted even the smallest part of a second longer, if at its height there had not come a relief, a release – a little break somewhere, soundless, yet perceptible; and at the same moment, without any premonitory drops, the rain fell down in sheets, filling the gutters and overflowing the pavements.

Thomas, whose illness had taught him to pay attention to his nerves, bent over in this second, made a motion toward his head, and flung away his cigarette. He looked around the circle to see if the others had felt anything. He thought his Mother had, perhaps; the others did not seem to be aware. The Frau Consul was looking out now into the thick-streaming rain, which quite hid the church from view; she sighed " Thank God."

" There," said Tony, " that will cool the air in two minutes. But the drops will be hanging on the trees outside – we can drink coffee in the verandah. Open the window, Tilda."

The noise of the rain grew louder. It almost roared. Everything pattered, streamed, rushed, foamed. The wind came up and blew the thick veils of water, tore them apart, and flung them about. It grew cooler every minute.

Lina, the maid-servant, came running through the hall and burst so suddenly into the room that Ida Jungmann called out sharply: " I say, what do you mean – ? " Lina's expressionless blue eyes were wide open, her jaws worked without making a sound –

" Oh, Frau Consul," she got out, at last. " Come, come quick! oh, what a scare – "

" Yes," Tony said, " she's probably broken something again. Very likely the good porcelain. Oh, these servants of yours, Mamma! "

But the girl burst out: " Oh, no, Ma'am Grünlich – if that's all it was! – It's the Master – I were bringing him his boots, and there he sits and can't speak, on his chair, and I says to myself, there's something wrong there; the Herr Consul – "

" Get Grabow," cried Thomas and ran out of the room.

" My God – oh, my God! " cried the Frau Consul, putting her hands to her face and hurrying out.

" Quick, get a wagon and fetch Grabow," Tony repeated breathlessly.

Everybody flew downstairs and through the breakfast-room into the bedroom.

But Johann Buddenbrook was already dead.

PART FIVE

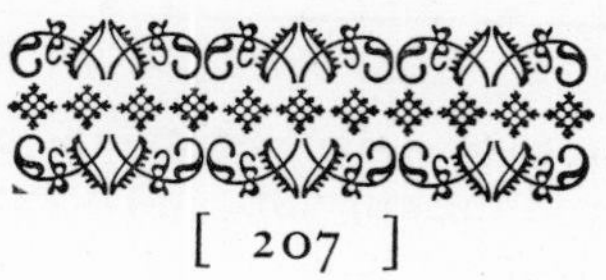

[207]

CHAPTER I

"Good evening, Justus," said the Frau Consul. "How are you? Sit down."

Consul Kröger embraced her tenderly and shook hands with his elder niece, who was also present in the dining-room. He was now about fifty-five years old, and wore a heavy round whisker as well as his moustache, leaving his chin free. It was quite grey. His scanty hair was carefully combed over the broad pink expanse of his skull. The sleeve of his elegant frock-coat had a broad mourning band.

"Do you know the latest, Betsy?" he asked. "Yes, Tony, this will particularly interest you. To put it briefly, our property outside the Castle Gate is sold – guess to whom? Not to one man, but to two: for the house is to be pulled down, and a hedge run through diagonally, and Benthien will build himself a dog-kennel on the right side, and Sorenson one on the left. God bless us!"

"Whoever heard the like?" said Frau Grünlich, folding her hands in her lap and gazing up at the ceiling. "Grandfather's property! Well, now the estate is all haggled up. Its great charm was its extent: there was really too much of it, but that was what made it elegant. The large garden, all the way down to the Trave, the house set far back with the drive, and the chestnut avenue. So it is to be divided. Benthien will stand in front of one door and Sorenson in front of the other. I say, 'God bless us,' too, Uncle Justus! I suppose there is nobody grand enough these days to occupy the whole thing. It is good that Grandpapa is not here to see it."

The sense of mourning still lay too heavily on the air for Tony to give expression to her outraged feelings in livelier or stronger terms. It was the day on which the will had been read, two weeks after the death of the Consul, at half-past five in the afternoon. Frau Consul Buddenbrook had invited her brother to Meng Street, in order that he might talk over the provisions made by the deceased with Thomas and with Herr Marcus the confidential clerk. Tony had announced her intention to be present at the settlements. This attention, she said, she owed to the firm as well as to the family, and she took pains to give the meeting the character of a family council. She had closed the curtains, and despite the two oil lamps on the green-covered dining-table, drawn out to its full extent, she had lighted all the candles in the great gilded candelabrum as well. And, though there was no particular need of them, she had put on the table a quantity of writing paper and sharpened pencils.

Tony's black frock gave her figure a maidenly slimness. She, of them all, was perhaps most deeply moved by the death of the Consul, to whom she had drawn so close in the last months that even to-day the thought of him made her burst out twice in bitter weeping; yet the prospect of this family council, this solemn little conference in which she could bear a worthy part, had power to flush her pretty cheek, brighten her glance, and give her motions dignity and even joy. The Frau Consul, on the other hand, worn with anxiety and grief and the thousand formalities of the funeral and the mourning, looked ailing. Her face, framed in the black lace of her cap-strings, seemed paler, and her light blue eyes were tired and dull. But there was not a single white hair to be seen in her smooth red-blond coiffure. Was this still the Parisian tonic, or was it the wig? Mamsell Jungmann alone knew, and she would not have betrayed the secret even to the other ladies of the family.

They sat at the end of the table and waited for Herr Marcus and Thomas to come out of the office. The painted statues seemed to stand out white and proud on their pedestals against the sky-blue background.

The Frau Consul said: "The thing is – I bade you come, my dear Justus – in short, it is about Clara, the child. My beloved husband left to me the choice of a guardian for her – she will need one for three years. I know you do not want to be overburdened with responsibilities. You have duties to your wife and sons – "

"My son, Betsy."

"Yes, yes, we must be Christlike and merciful, Justus. As we forgive our debtors, it says. Think of our gracious Father in Heaven."

Her brother looked at her, a little aggrieved. Such turns of phrase had come in the past only from the mouth of the Consul.

"Enough," she went on. "There are as good as no obligations connected with this service of love. I should like to ask you to accept it."

"Gladly, Betsy; of course, I'll do it with pleasure. May I not see my ward? A little too serious, isn't she, the good child – ? "

Clara was called. She slowly appeared, all black and pallid, her movements melancholy and full of restraint. She had spent the time since her father's death in her room praying almost without ceasing. Her dark eyes were immobile; she seemed frozen with grief and awe.

Uncle Justus the gallant stepped up to her, bowed as he pressed her hand, and murmured something appropriate. She went out, after receiving the Frau Consul's kiss on her stiff lips.

"How is Jürgen?" began the Frau Consul again. Does it agree with him in Wismar?"

"Very well," answered Justus Kröger, sitting down again with a shrug of the shoulders. "I think he has found his place now. He is a good lad, Betsy, a lad of principle, but – after he had failed twice in the examination, it seemed best – He did not like the law himself, and the position in the post-office at Wismar is quite suitable. Tell me – I hear Christian is coming?"

"Yes, Justus, he is coming. May God watch over him on the seas! I wrote to him the next day after Jean's death, but he hasn't even had the letter yet, and then he will take about two months with the sailing-vessel after that. But he must come, Justus; I must see him. Tom says Jean would never have been willing for Christian to give up his position in Valparaiso; but I ask you – nearly eight years since I have seen him! And then, under the circumstances! No, I must have them all about me in this painful time – that is a natural feeling for a mother."

"Surely, surely," said Consul Kröger; for she had begun to weep.

"Thomas agrees with me now, too," she went on; "for where will Christian be better off than in his own father's business, in Tom's business? He can stay here, work here. I have been in constant fear that the climate over there might be bad for him – "

Thomas Buddenbrook, accompanied by Herr Marcus, came into the room. Friederich Wilhelm Marcus, for years the dead Consul's confidential clerk, was a tall man in a brown-skirted coat with a mourning band. He spoke softly, hesitatingly stammering a little and considering each word before he uttered it. He had a habit of slowly and cautiously stroking the red-brown moustache that grew over his mouth with the extended middle and index fingers of his left hand; or he would rub his hands together and let his round brown eyes wander so aimlessly about that he gave the impression of complete confusion and absent-mindedness, though he was always most watchfully bent on the matter in hand.

Thomas Buddenbrook, now the youthful head of the great house, displayed real dignity in manner and bearing. But he was pale. His hands in particular, on one of which shone the Consul's signet ring with the green stone, were as white as the cuffs beneath his black sleeves – a frozen whiteness which showed that they were quite dry and cold. He had extraordinarily sensitive hands, with beautifully cared-for oval bluish fingernails. Sometimes, in a difficult situation, they would take positions or make little nervous movements that were indescribably expressive of shrinking sensibility and painful reserve. This was an individual trait strange heretofore to the rather broad, though finely articulated Buddenbrook hand.

Tom's first care was to open the folding doors into the landscape-room in order to get the benfit of the warmth from the stove burning there behind the wrought-iron lattice. Then he shook hands with Consul Kröger and sat down at the table with Herr Marcus opposite him. He looked at his sister Tony, and his eyebrow went up in surprise. But she flung her head back and tucked in her chin in a way that warned him to suppress any comment on her presence.

"Well, and one may not say Herr Consul?" asked Justus Kröger. "The Netherlands hope in vain that you should represent them, Tom, my dear chap?"

"Yes, Uncle Justus, I thought it was better. You see, I could have taken over the Consulate along with so many other responsibilities, but in the first place I am a little too young – and then I spoke to Uncle Gotthold, and he was very pleased to accept it."

"Very sensible, my lad; very politic. And very gentlemanly."

"Herr Marcus," said the Frau Consul, "my dear Herr Marcus!" And with her usual sweeping gesture she reached out her hand, which he took slowly, with a respectful side-glance: "I have asked you to come up – you know what the affair is; and I know that you are agreed with us. My beloved husband expressed in his final arrangements the wish that after his death you would put your loyal and well-tried powers at the service of the firm, not as an outsider but as partner."

"Certainly, Frau Consul," said Herr Marcus, "I must protest that I know how to value the honour your offer does me, being aware, as I am, that the resources I can bring to the firm are but small. In God's name, I know nothing better to do than thankfully to accept the offer you and your son make me."

"Yes, Marcus. And I thank you in my turn, most warmly, for your willingness to share with me the great responsibilities which would perhaps be too heavy for me alone." Thomas Buddenbrook spoke quickly and whole-heartedly, reaching his hand across the table to his partner; for they were already long since agreed on the subject, and this was only the formal expression.

"Company is trumpery – you will spoil our chat, between you," said Consul Kröger. "And now, shall we run through the provisions, my children? All I have to look out for is the dowry of my ward. The rest is not my affair. Have you a copy of the will here, Betsy? And have you made a rough calculation, Tom?"

"I have it in my head," said Thomas; and he began, leaning back, looking into the landscape-room, and moving his gold pencil back and forth on the table, to explain how matters stood. The truth was that the Consul's estate was more considerable than any one had supposed. The dowry of his oldest daughter, indeed, was gone, and the losses which the firm had suffered in the Bremen failure in 1851 had been a heavy blow. And the year '48, as well as the present year '55, with their unrest and interval of war, had brought losses. But the Buddenbrook share of the Kröger estate of four hundred thousand current marks had been full three hundred thousand, for Justus had already had much of his beforehand. Johann Buddenbrook had continually complained, as a merchant will; but the losses of the firm had been made good by the accrued profits of some fifteen years, amounting to thirty thousand thaler, and thus the property, aside from real estate, amounted in round figures, to seven hundred thousand marks.

Thomas himself, with all his knowledge of the business, had been left in ignorance by his father of this total. The Frau Consul took the announcement with discreet calm; Tony put on an adorable expression of pride and ignorance, and then could not repress an anxious mental query: Is that a lot? Are we very rich now? Herr Marcus slowly rubbed his hands, apparently in absence of mind, and Consul Kröger was obviously bored. But the sum filled Tom himself, as he stated it, with such a rush of excited pride that the effort at self-control made him seem dejected. "We must have already passed the million," he said. He controlled his voice, but his hands trembled. "Grandfather could command nine hundred thousand marks in his best time; and we've made great efforts since then, and had successes, and made fine *coups* here and there. And Mamma's dowry, and Mamma's inheritance! There was the constant breaking up – well, good heavens, that lay in the nature of things! Please forgive me if I speak just now in the sense of the firm and not of the family. These dowries and payments to Uncle Gotthold and to Frankfort, these hundreds of thousands which had to be drawn out of the business – and then there were only two heirs beside the head of the firm. Good; we have our work cut out for us, Marcus." The thirst for action, for power and success, the longing to force fortune to her knees, sprang up quick and passionate in his eyes. He felt all the world looking at him expectantly, questioning if he would know how to command prestige for the firm and the family and protect its name. On exchange he had been meeting measuring side-looks out of jovial, mocking old eyes, that seemed to be saying " So you're taking it on, my son! " " I *am!* " he thought.

Friederich Wilhelm Marcus rubbed his hands circumspectly, and Justus Kröger said: " Quietly, quietly, my dear chap. Times aren't what they were when your grandfather was a Prussian army contractor."

There began now a detailed conversation upon the provisions of the will, in which they all joined, and Consul Kröger took a lighter tone, referring to Thomas as " his Highness the reigning Prince " and saying, " The warehouses will go with the crown, according to tradition." In general, of course, it was decided that as far as possible everything should be left together, that Frau Elizabeth Buddenbrook should be considered the sole heir, and that the entire property should remain in the business. Herr Marcus announced that as partner he should be able to strengthen the working capital by a hundred and twenty thousand marks current. A sum of fifty thousand marks was set aside as a private fortune for Thomas, and the same for Christian, in case he wished to establish himself separately. Justus Kröger paid close attention to the passage that ran: " The fixing of the dowry of my beloved daughter Clara I leave to the discretion of my dear wife." " Shall we say a hundred thousand? " he suggested, leaning back, one leg crossed over the other, and turning up his short grey moustache with both hands. He was affability itself. But the sum was fixed at eighty thousand. " In case of a second marriage of my dearly loved older daughter Antonie, in view of the fact that eighty thousand marks have already been applied to her first marriage, the sum of seventeen thousand thaler current must not be exceeded." Frau Antonie waved her arm with a graceful but excited gesture which tossed back her flowing sleeve; she looked at the ceiling and said loudly: " Grünlich, indeed! " It sounded like a challenge, like a little trumpet-call. " You know, Herr Marcus," she said, " about that man. We are sitting, one fine afternoon, perfectly innocent, in the garden, in front of the door – you know the portal, Herr Marcus. Well! Who appears? a person with gold-coloured whiskers – the scoundrel! "

" Yes," Thomas said. " We will talk about Herr Grünlich afterward."

" Very well; but you are a clever creature, and you will admit, Tom, that in this life things don't always happen fairly and squarely. That's been my experience, though a short time ago I was too simple to realize it."

" Yes," Tom said. They went into detail, noting the Consul's instructions about the great family Bible, about his diamond buttons, and many, many other matters.

Justus Kröger and Herr Marcus stopped for supper.

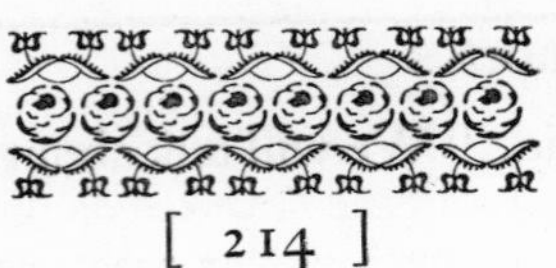

CHAPTER II

In the beginning of February, 1856, after eight years' absence, Christian Buddenbrook returned to the home of his fathers. He arrived in the post-coach from Hamburg, wearing a yellow suit with a pattern of large checks, that had a distinctly exotic look. He brought the bill of a swordfish and a great sugar-cane, and received the embraces of his mother with a half-embarrassed, half-absent air.

He wore the same air when, on the next afternoon after his arrival, the family went to the cemetery outside the Castle Gate to lay a wreath on the grave. They stood together on the snowy path in front of the large tablet on which were the names of those resting there, surrounding the family arms cut in the stone. Before them was the upright marble cross that stood at the edge of the bare little churchyard grove. They were all there except Clothilde, who was at Thankless, nursing her ailing father.

Tony laid the wreath on the tablet, where her father's name stood on the stone in fresh gold letters: then, despite the snow, she knelt down by the grave to pray. Her black veil played about her, and her full skirt lay spread out in picturesque folds. God alone knew how much grief and religious emotion – and, on the other hand, how much of a pretty woman's self-conscious pleasure – there was in the bowed attitude. Thomas was not in the mood to think about it. But Christian looked sidewise at his sister with a mixture of mockery and misgiving, as if to say: "Can you really carry that off? Shan't you feel silly when you get up? How uncomfortable!" Tony caught this look as she rose, but she was not in the least put out. She tossed her head back, arranged her veil and skirt, and turned with dignified assurance to go; whereupon Christian was obviously relieved.

The deceased Consul's fanatical love of God and of the Saviour had been an emotion foreign to his forebears, who never cherished other than the normal, every-day sentiments proper to good citizens. The two living Buddenbrooks had in their turn their own idiosyncrasies. One of these appeared to be a nervous distaste for the expression of feeling. Thomas had certainly felt the death of his father with painful acuteness, much as his grandfather had felt the loss of his. But he could not sink on his knees by his grave. He had never, like his sister Tony, flung himself across the table sobbing like a child; and he shrank from hearing the heart-broken words in which Madame Grünlich, from roast to dessert, loved to celebrate the character and person of her dead father. Such outbursts he met with composed silence or a reserved nod. And yet, when nobody had mentioned or was thinking of the dead, it would be just then that his eyes would fill with slow tears, although his facial expression remained unchanged.

It was different with Christian. He unfortunately did not succeed in preserving his composure at the naïve and childish outpourings of his sister. He bent over his plate, turned his head away, and looked as though he wanted to sink through the floor; and several times he interrupted her with a low, tormented " Good God, Tony! " his large nose screwed into countless tiny wrinkles.

In fact, he showed disquiet and embarrassment whenever the conversation turned to the dead. It seemed as though he feared and avoided not only the indelicate expression of deep and solemn feeling, but even the feeling itself.

No one had seen him shed a tear over the death of his father; and his long absence alone hardly explained this fact. A more remarkable thing, however, was that he took his sister Tony aside again and again to hear in vivid detail the events of that fatal afternoon; for Madame Grünlich had a gift of lively narration.

" He looked yellow? " he asked for the fifth time. " What was it the girl shrieked when she came running in to you? He looked quite yellow, and died without saying another word? What did the girl say? What sort of sound was it he made? " Then he would be silent – silent a long time – while his small deep-set eyes travelled round the room in thought.

" Horrible," he said suddenly, and a visible shudder ran over him as he got up. He would walk up and down with the same unquiet and brooding eyes. Madame Grünlich felt astonished to see that Christian, who for some unknown reason was so embarrassed when she bewailed her father aloud, liked to reproduce with a sort of dreadful relish the dying efforts to speak which he had inquired about in detail of Line the maid-servant.

Christian had certainly not grown better looking. He was lean and pallid. The skin was stretched over his skull very tightly; his large nose, with a distinct hump, stuck out fleshless and sharp between his cheek-bones, and his hair was already noticeably scantier.

His neck was too thin and long and his lean legs decidedly bowed. His London period seemed to have made a lasting impression upon him. In Valparaiso, too, he had mostly associated with Englishmen; and his whole appearance had something English about it which somehow seemed rather appropriate. It was partly the comfortable cut and durable wool material of his clothing, the broad, solid elegance of his boots, his crotchety expression, and the way in which his red-blond moustache drooped over his mouth. Even his hands had an English look: they were a dull porous white from the hot climate, with round, clean, short-trimmed nails.

" Tell me," he said, abruptly, " do you know that feeling – it is hard to describe – when you swallow something hard, the wrong way, and it hurts all the way down your spine? " His whole nose wrinkled as he spoke.

" Yes," said Tony; " that is quite common. You take a drink of water – "

" Oh," he said in a dissatisfied tone. " No, I don't think we mean the same thing." And a restless look floated across his face.

He was the first one in the house to shake off his mourning and re-assume a natural attitude. He had not lost the art of imitating the deceased Marcellus Stengel, and he often spoke for hours in his voice. At the table he asked about the theatre – if there were a good company and what they were giving.

" I don't know," said Tom, with a tone that was exaggeratedly indifferent, in order not to seem irritated. " I haven't noticed lately."

But Christian missed this altogether and went on to talk about the theatre. " I am too happy for words in the theatre. Even the *word* ' theatre ' makes me feel happy. I don't know whether any of you have that feeling. I could sit for hours and just look at the curtain. I feel as I used to when I was a child and we went in to the Christmas party here. Even the sound of the orchestra beforehand! I would go if only to hear that and nothing more. I like the love scenes best. Some of the heroines have such a fetching way of taking their lovers' heads between their hands. But the actors – in London and Valparaiso I have known a lot of actors. At first I was very proud to get to know them in ordinary life. In the theatre I watched their every movement. It is fascinating. One of them says his last speech and turns around quietly and goes deliberately, without the least embarrassment, to the door, although he knows that the eyes of the whole audience are on his back. How can he do that? I used to be continually thinking about going behind the scenes. But now I am pretty much at home there, I must say. Imagine: once, in an operetta – it was in London – the curtain went up one evening when I was on the stage! I was talking with Miss Waterhouse, a very pretty girl. Well, suddenly there was the whole audience! Good Lord, I don't know how I got off the stage."

Madame Grünlich was the only one who laughed, to speak of, in the circle round the table. But Christian went on, his eyes wandering back and forth. He talked about English *café-chantant* singers; about an actress who came on in powdered wig, and knocked with a long cane on the ground and sang a song called: "That's Maria." "Maria, you know – Maria is the most scandalous of the lot. When somebody does something perfectly shocking, why – 'that's Maria' – the bad lot, you know – utterly depraved!" He said this last with a frightful expression and raised his right hand with the fingers formed into a ring.

"*Assez*, Christian," said the Frau Consul. "That does not interest us in the least."

But Christian's gaze flickered absently over her head; he would probably have stopped without her suggestion, for he seemed to be sunk in a profound, disquieting dream of Maria and her depravity, while his little round deep eyes wandered back and forth.

Suddenly he said: "Strange – sometimes I can't swallow. Oh, it's no joke. I find it very serious. It enters my head that perhaps I can't swallow, and then all of a sudden I can't. The food is already swallowed, but the muscles – right here – they simply refuse. It isn't a question of will-power. Or rather, the thing is, I don't dare really will it."

Tony cried out, quite beside herself: "Christian! Good Lord, what nonsense! You don't dare to make up your mind to swallow! What are you talking about? You are absurd!"

Thomas was silent. But the Frau Consul said: "That is nerves, Christian. Yes, it was high time you came home; the climate over there would have killed you in the end."

After the meal Christian sat down at the little harmonium that stood in the dining-room and imitated a piano virtuoso. He pretended to toss back his hair, rubbed his hands, and looked around the room; then, without a sound, without touching the bellows – for he could not play in the least, and was entirely unmusical, like all the Buddenbrooks – he bent quite over and began to belabour the bass, played unbelievable passages, threw himself back, looked in ecstasy at the ceiling, and banged the key-board in a triumphant finale. Even Clara burst out laughing. The illusion was convincing; full of assurance and charlatanry and irresistible comicality of the burlesque, eccentric English-American kind; so certain of its own effect that the result was not in the least unpleasant.

"I have gone a great deal to concerts," he said. "I like to watch how the people behave with their instruments. It is really beautiful to be an artist."

Then he began to play again, but broke off suddenly and became serious, as though a mask had fallen over his features. He got up, ran his hand through his scanty hair, moved away, and stood silent, obviously fallen into a bad mood, with unquiet eyes and an expression as though he were listening to some kind of uncanny noise.

"Sometimes I find Christian a little strange," said Madame Grünlich to her brother Thomas, one evening, when they were alone. "He talks so, somehow. He goes so unnaturally into detail, seems to me – or what shall I say? He looks at things in such a strange way; don't you think so?"

"Yes," said Tom, "I understand what you mean very well, Tony. Christian is very incautious – undignified – it is difficult to express what I mean. Something is lacking in him – what people call equilibrium, mental poise. On the one hand, he does not know how to keep his countenance when other people make naïve or tactless remarks – he does not understand how to cover it up, and he just loses his self-possession altogether. But the same thing happens when he begins to be garrulous himself, in the unpleasant way he has, and tells his most intimate thoughts. It gives one such an uncanny feeling – it is just the way people speak in a fever, isn't it? Self-control and personal reserve are both lacking in the same way. Oh, the thing is quite simple: Christian busies himself too much with himself, with what goes on in his own insides. Sometimes he has a regular mania for bringing out the deepest and the pettiest of these experiences – things a reasonable man does not trouble himself about or even want to know about, for the simple reason that he would not like to tell them to any one else. There is such a lack of modesty in so much communicativeness. You see, Tony, anybody, except Christian, may say that he loves the theatre. But he would say it in a different tone, more *en passant*, more modestly, in short. Christian says it in a tone that says: 'Is not my passion for the stage something very marvellous and interesting?' He struggles, he behaves as if he were really wrestling to express something supremely delicate and difficult.

"I'll tell you," he went on after a pause, throwing his cigarette through the wrought-iron lattice into the stove: "I have thought a great deal about this curious and useless self-preoccupation, because I had once an inclination to it myself. But I observed that it made me unsteady, hare-brained, and incapable – and control, equilibrium, is, at least for me, the important thing. There will always be men who are justified in this interest in themselves, this detailed observation of their own emotions; poets who can express with clarity and beauty their privileged inner life, and thereby enrich the emotional world of other people. But the likes of us are simple merchants, my child; our self-observations are decidedly inconsiderable. We can sometimes go so far as to say that the sound of orchestra instruments gives us unspeakable pleasure, and that we sometimes do not dare try to swallow – but it would be much better, deuce take it, if we sat down and accomplished something, as our fathers did before us."

"Yes, Tom, you express my views exactly. When I think of the airs those Hagenströms put on – oh, Heavens, what truck! Mother doesn't like the words I use, but I find they are the only right ones. Do you suppose they think they are the only good family in town? I have to laugh, you know; I really do."

CHAPTER III

THE HEAD of the firm of Johann Buddenbrook had measured his brother on his arrival with a long, scrutinizing gaze. He had given him passing and unobtrusive observation during several days; and then, though he did not allow any sign of his opinion to appear upon his calm and discreet face, his curiosity was satisfied, his mind made up. He talked with him in the family circle in a casual tone on casual subjects and enjoyed himself like the others when Christian gave a performance. A week later he said to him: " Well, shall we work together, young man? So far as I know, you consent to Mamma's wish, do you not? As you know, Marcus has become my partner, in proportion to the quota he has paid in. I should think that, as my brother, you could ostensibly take the place he had – that of confidential clerk. What your work would be – I do not know how much mercantile experience you have really had. You have been loafing a bit, so far – am I right? Well, in any case, the English correspondence will suit you. But I must beg one thing of you, my dear chap. In your position as brother of the head of the house, you will actually have a superior position to the others; but I do not need to tell you that you will impress them far more by behaving like their equal and doing your duty, than you will by making use of privileges and taking liberties. Are you willing to keep office hours and observe appearances? "

And then he made a proposal in respect of salary, which Christian accepted without consideration, with an embarrassed and inattentive face that betrayed very little love of gain and a great zeal to settle the matter quickly. Next day Thomas led him into the office; and Christian's labours for the old firm began.

The business had taken its uninterrupted and solid course after the Consul's death. But soon after Thomas Buddenbrook seized the reins, a fresher and more enterprising spirit began to be noticeable in the management. Risks were taken now and then. The credit of the house, formerly a conception, a theory, a luxury, was consciously strained and utilized. The gentlemen on 'Change nodded at each other. " Buddenbrook wants to make money with both hands," they said. They thought it was a good thing that Thomas had to carry the upright Friederich Wilhelm Marcus along with him, like a ball and chain on his foot. Herr Marcus' influence was the conservative force in the business. He stroked his moustache with his two fingers, punctiliously arranged his writing materials and glass of water on his desk, looked at everything on both sides and top and bottom; and, five or six times in the day, would go out through the courtyard into the wash-kitchen and hold his head under the tap to refresh himself.

"They complement each other," said the heads of the great houses to each other; Consul Heneus said it to Consul Kistenmaker. The small families echoed them; and the dockyard and warehouse hands repeated the same opinion. The whole town was interested in the way young Buddenbrook would "take hold." Herr Stuht in Bell Founders' Street would say to his wife, who knew the best families: "They balance each other, you see."

But the personality of the business was plainly the younger partner. He knew how to handle the personnel, the ship-captains, the heads in the warehouse offices, the drivers and the yard hands. He could speak their language with ease and yet keep a distance between himself and them. But when Herr Marcus spoke in dialect to some faithful servant it sounded so outlandish that his partner would simply begin to laugh, and the whole office would dissolve in merriment.

Thomas Buddenbrook's desire to protect and increase the prestige of the old firm made him love to be present in the daily struggle for success. He well knew that his assured and elegant bearing, his tact and winning manners were responsible for a great deal of good trade.

"A business man cannot be a bureaucrat," he said to Stephen Kistenmaker, of Kistenmaker and Sons, his former school-fellow. He had remained the oracle of this old playmate, who listened to his every word in order to give it out later as his own. "It takes personality – that is my view. I don't think any great success is to be had from the office alone – at least, I shouldn't care for it. I always want to direct the course of things on the spot, with a look, a word, a gesture – to govern it with the immediate influence of my will and my talent – my luck, as you call it. But, unfortunately, personal contact is going out of fashion. The times move on, but it seems to me they leave the best behind. Relations are easier and easier; the connections better and better; the risk gets smaller – but the profits do too. Yes, the old people were better off. My grandfather, for example – he drove in a four-horse coach to

Southern Germany, as commissary to the Prussian army – an old man in pumps, with his head powdered. And there he played his charms and his talents and made an astonishing amount of money, Kistenmaker. Oh, I'm afraid the merchant's life will get duller and duller as time goes on."

It was feelings like these that made him relish most the trade he came by through his own personal efforts. Sometimes, entirely by accident, perhaps on a walk with the family, he would go into a mill for a chat with the miller, who would feel himself much honoured by the visit; and quite *en passant*, in the best of moods, he would conclude a good bargain. His partner was incapable of that sort of thing.

As for Christian, he seemed at first to devote himself to his task with real zest and enjoyment, and to feel exceptionally well and contented. For several days he ate with appetite, smoked his short pipe, and squared his shoulders in the English jacket, giving expression to his sense of ease and well-being. In the morning he went to the office at about the same time as Thomas, and sat opposite his brother and Herr Marcus in a revolving arm-chair like theirs. First he read the paper, while he comfortably smoked his morning cigarette. Then he would fetch out an old cognac from his bottom desk drawer, stretch out his arms in order to feel himself free to move, say "Well!" and go to work good-naturedly, his tongue roving about among his teeth. His English letters were extraordinarily able and effective, for he wrote English as he spoke it, simply and fluently, without effort.

He gave expression to his mood in his own way in the family circle.

"Business is really a fine, gratifying calling," he said. "Respectable, satisfying, industrious, comfortable. I was really born to it – fact! And as a member of the house! – well, I've never felt so good before. You come fresh into the office in the morning, and look through the paper, smoke, think about this and that, take some cognac, and then go to work. Comes midday; you eat with your family, take a rest, then to work again. You write, on smooth, good business paper, with a good pen, rule, paper-knife, stamp – everything first-class and all in order. You keep at it, get things done one after the other, and finish up. To-morrow is another day. When you go home to supper, you feel thoroughly satisfied – satisfied in every limb. Even your hands – "

"Heavens, Christian," cried Tony. "What rubbish! How can your hands feel satisfied? "

"Why, yes, of course – can't you understand that? I mean – "

He made a painstaking effort to express and explain. "You can shut your fist, you see. You don't make a violent effort, of course, because you are tired from your work. But it isn't flabby; it doesn't make you feel irritable. You have a sense of satisfaction in it; you feel easy and comfortable – you can sit quite still without feeling bored."

Every one was silent. Then Thomas said in a casual tone, so as not to show that he disagreed: "It seems to me that one doesn't work for the sake of – " He broke off and did not continue. "At least, I have different reasons," he added after a minute. But Christian did not hear. His eyes roamed about, sunk in thought; and he soon began to tell a story of Valparaiso, a tale of assault and murder of which he had personal knowledge. "Then the fellow ripped out his knife – " For some reason Thomas never applauded these tales. Christian was full of them, and Madame Grünlich found them vastly entertaining. The Frau Consul, Clara, and Clothilde sat aghast, and Mamsell Jungmann and Erica listened with their mouths open. Thomas used to make cool sarcastic comments and act as if he thought Christian was exaggerating or hoaxing – which was certainly not the case. He narrated with colour and vividness. Perhaps Thomas found unpleasant the reflection that his younger brother had been about and seen more of the world than he! Or were his feelings of repulsion due to the glorification of disorder, the exotic violence of these knife- and revolver-tales? Christian certainly did not trouble himself over his brother's failure to appreciate his stories. He was always too much absorbed in his narrative to notice its success or lack of success with his audience, and when he had finished he would look pensively or absently about the room.

But if in time the relations between the two brothers came to be not of the best, Christian was not the one who thought of showing or feeling any animosity against his brother. He silently took for granted the pre-eminence of his elder, his superior capacity, earnestness, and respectability. But precisely this casual, indiscriminate acknowledgment irritated Thomas, for it had the appearance of setting no value upon superior capacity, earnestness, or respectability.

Christian appeared not to notice the growing dislike of the head of the firm. Thomas's feelings were indeed quite justifiable; for unfortunately Christian's zeal for business visibly decreased, even after the first week, though more after the second. His little preparations for work, which, in the beginning, wore the air of a prolonged and refined anticipation: the reading of the paper, the after-breakfast cigarette, the cognac, began to take more and more time, and finally used up the whole morning. It gradually came about that Christian freed himself largely from the constraint of office hours. He appeared later and later with his breakfast cigarette to begin his preparations for work; he went at midday to eat at the Club, and came back late or not at all.

This Club, to which mostly unmarried business men belonged, occupied comfortable rooms in the first story of a restaurant, where one could eat and meet in unrestrained and sometimes not altogether harmless conversation – for there was a roulette table. Even some of the more light-minded fathers of families, like Justus Kröger and, of course, Peter Döhlmann, were members, and police senator Crema was here " the first man at the hose." That was the expression of Dr. Gieseke – Andreas Gieseke, the son of the Fire Commissioner and Christian's old schoolmate. He had settled as a lawyer in the town, and Christian renewed the friendship with him, though he ranked as rather a wild fellow. Christian – or, as he was called everywhere, Chris – had known them all more or less in the old days, for nearly all of them had been pupils of Marcellus Stengel. They received him into the Club with open arms; for, while neither business men nor scholars found him a genius, they recognized his amusing social gifts. It was here that he gave his best performances and told his best stories. He did the virtuoso at the club piano and imitated English and transatlantic actors and opera singers. But the best things he did were stories of his affairs with women, related in the most harmless and entertaining way imaginable – adventures that had befallen him on shipboard, on trains, in St. Paul's, in Whitechapel, in the virgin forest. There was no doubt that Christian's weakness was for women. He narrated with a fluency and power that entranced his listeners, in an exhaustless stream, with his somewhat plaintive, drawling voice, burlesque and innocent, like an English humourist. He told a story about a dog that had been sent in a satchel from Valparaiso to San Francisco and was mangy to boot. Goodness knew what was the point of the anecdote – in his mouth it was indescribably comic. And while everybody about him writhed with laughter, unable to leave off, he himself sat there cross-legged, a strange, uneasy seriousness in his face with its great hooked nose, his thin, long neck, his sparse light-red hair and little round deep-set eyes. It almost seemed as if the laugh were at his expense, as if they were laughing at him. But that never occurred to him.

At home his favourite tales were about his office in Valparaiso. He told of the extreme heat there, and about a young Londoner, named Johnny Thunderstorm, a ne'er-do-well, an extraordinary chap, whom he had " never seen do a stroke of work, God damn me," and who yet was a remarkable business man.

" Good God, the heat! " he said. " Well, the chief came into the office – there we all lay, eight of us, like flies, and smoked cigarettes to keep the mosquitoes away. Good God! Well, the chief said: ' You are not working, gentlemen? ' ' No, sir,' says Johnny Thunderstorm, ' as you see, sir! ' And we all blew our cigarette-smoke in his face. Good God! "

" Why do you keep saying ' good God '? " asked Thomas irritably. But his irritation was at bottom because he felt that Christian told this story with particular relish just because it gave him a chance to sneer at honest work.

The Mother would discreetly change the subject. There were many hateful things in the world, thought the Frau Consul, born Kröger. Brothers could despise and dislike each other, dreadful as it sounded; but one didn't mention such things. They had to be covered up and ignored.

CHAPTER IV

IN May it happened that Uncle Gotthold – Consul Gotthold Buddenbrook, now sixty years old – was seized with a heart attack one night and died in the arms of his wife, born Stüwing.

The son of poor Madame Josephine had had the worst of it in life, compared with the younger and stronger brother and sister born of Madame Antoinette. But he had long since resigned himself to his fortunes; and in his later years, especially after his nephew turned over to him the Consulate of the Netherlands, he ate his lozenges out of his tin box and harboured the friendliest feelings. It was his ladies who kept up the feud now: not so much his good-natured wife as the three elderly damsels, who could not look at Frau Consul, or Antonie, or Thomas, without a spark in their eyes.

On the traditional " children's day," at four o'clock, they all gathered in the big house in Meng Street, to eat dinner and spend the evening. Sometimes Consul Kröger or Sesemi Weichbrodt came too, with her simple sister. On these occasions the three Miss Buddenbrooks from Broad Street loved to turn the conversation to Tony's former marriage and to dart sharp glances at each other while they egged Madame Grünlich on to use strong language. Or they would make general remarks on the subject of the undignified vanity of dyeing one's hair. Or they would enquire particularly after Jacob Kröger, the Frau Consul's nephew. They made jokes at the expense of poor, innocent, Clothilde – jokes not so harmless as those which the charity girl received in good part every day from Tom and Tony. They made fun of Clara's austerity and bigotry. They were quick to find out that Tom and Christian were not on the best of terms; also, that they did not need to pay much attention to Christian anyhow, for he was a sort of Tomfool. As for Thomas himself, who had no weak point for them to ferret out, and who always met them with a good-humoured indulgence, that signified " I understand what you mean, and I am very sorry " – him they treated with respect tinctured with bitterness. Next came the turn of little Erica. Rosy and plump as she was, they found her alarmingly backward in her growth. And

Pfiffi in a series of little shakes drew attention several times to the child's shocking resemblance to the deceiver Grünlich.

But now they stood with their mother about their Father's death-bed, weeping; and a message was sent to Meng Street, though the feeling was not entirely wanting that their rich relations were somehow or other to blame for this misfortune too.

In the middle of the night the great bell downstairs rang; and as Christian had come home very late and was not feeling up to much, Tom set out alone in the spring rain.

He came just in time to see the last convulsive motions of the old gentleman. Then he stood a long time in the death-chamber and looked at the short figure under the covers, at the dead face with the mild features and white whiskers. "You haven't had a very good time, Uncle Gotthold," he thought. "You learned too late to make concessions and show consideration. But that is what one has to do. If I had been like you, I should have married a shop girl years ago. But for the sake of appearances – ! I wonder if you really wanted anything different? You were proud, and probably felt that your pride was something idealistic; but your spirit had little power to rise. To cherish the vision of an abstract good; to carry in your heart, like a hidden love, only far sweeter, the dream of preserving an ancient name, an old family, an old business, of carrying it on, and adding to it more and more honour and lustre – ah, that takes imagination, Uncle Gotthold, and imagination you didn't have. The sense of poetry escaped you, though you were brave enough to love and marry against the will of your father. And you had no ambition, Uncle Gotthold. The old name is only a burgher name, it is true, and one cherishes it by making the grain business flourish, and oneself beloved and powerful in a little corner of the earth. Did you think: 'I will marry her whom I love, and pay no attention to practical considerations, for they are petty and provincial?' Oh, we are travelled and educated enough to realize that the limits set to our ambition are small and petty enough, looked at from outside and above. But everything in this world is comparative, Uncle Gotthold. Did you know one can be a great man, even in a small place; a Cæsar even in a little commercial town on the Baltic? But that takes imagination and idealism – and you didn't have it, whatever you may have thought yourself."

Thomas Buddenbrook turned away. He went to the window and looked out at the dim grey gothic façade of the Town Hall opposite, shrouded in rain. He had his hands behind his back and a smile on his intelligent face.

The office and title of the Royal Consulate of the Netherlands, which Thomas Buddenbrook might have taken after his father's death, went back to him now, to the boundless satisfaction of Tony Grünlich; and the curving shield with the lions, the arms, and the crown was once more to be seen on the gabled front of the house in Meng Street, under the " Dominus providebit."

Soon after this was accomplished, in June of the same year, the young Consul set out to Amsterdam on a business journey the duration of which he did not know.

CHAPTER V

DEATHS in the family usually induce a religious mood. It was not surprising, after the decease of the Consul, to hear from the mouth of his widow expressions which she had not been accustomed to use.

But it was soon apparent that this was no passing phase. Even in the last years of the Consul's life, his wife had more and more sympathized with his spiritual cravings; and it now became plain that she was determined to honour the memory of her dead by adopting as her own all his pious conceptions.

She strove to fill the great house with the spirit of the deceased – that mild and Christlike spirit which yet had not excluded a certain dignified and hearty good cheer. The morning and evening prayers were continued and lengthened. The family gathered in the dining-room, and the servants in the hall, to hear the Frau Consul or Clara read a chapter out of the great family Bible with the big letters. They also sang a few verses out of the hymn-book, accompanied by the Frau Consul on the little organ. Or, often, in place of the chapter from the Bible, they had a reading from one of those edifying or devotional books with the black binding and gilt edges – those Little Treasuries, Jewel-Caskets, Holy Hours, Morning Chimes, Pilgrims' Staffs, and the like, whose common trait was a sickly and languishing tenderness for the little Jesus, and of which there were all too many in the house.

Christian did not often appear at these devotions. Thomas once chose a favourable moment to disparage the practice, half-jestingly; but his objection met with a gentle rebuff. As for Madame Grünlich, she did not, unfortunately, always conduct herself correctly at the exercises. One morning when there was a strange clergyman stopping with the Buddenbrooks, they were invited to sing to a solemn and devout melody the following words: –

I am a reprobate,
A warped and hardened sinner;
I gobble evil down
Just like the joint for dinner.

Lord, fling thy cur a bone
Of righteousness to chew
And take my carcass home
To Heaven and to you.

Whereat Frau Grünlich threw down her book and left the room, bursting with suppressed giggles.

But the Frau Consul made more demands upon herself than upon her children. She instituted a Sunday School, and on Sunday afternoon only little board-school pupils rang at the door of the house in Meng Street. Stine Voss, who lived by the city wall, and Mike Stuht from Bell-Founders' Street, and Fike Snut from the river-bank or Groping Alley, their straw-coloured locks smoothed back with a wet comb, crossed the entry into the garden-room, which for a long time now had not been used as an office, and in which rows of benches had been arranged and Frau Consul Buddenbrook, born Kröger, in a gown of heavy black satin, with her white refined face and still whiter lace cap, sat opposite to them at a little table with a glass of sugar-water and catechized them for an hour.

Also, she founded the " Jerusalem evenings," which not only Clara and Clothilde but also Tony were obliged to attend, willy-nilly. Once a week they sat at the extension table in the dining-room by the light of lamps and candles. Some twenty ladies, all of an age when it is profitable to begin to look after a good place in heaven, drank tea or bishop, ate delicate sandwiches and puddings, read hymns and sermons aloud to each other, and did embroidery, which at the end of the year was sold at a bazaar and the proceeds sent to the mission in Jerusalem.

This pious society was formed in the main from ladies of the Frau Consul's own social rank: Frau Senator Langhals, Frau Consul Möllendorpf, and old Frau Consul Kistenmaker belonged; but other, more worldly and profane old ladies, like Mme. Köppen, made fun of their friend Betsy. The wives of the clergymen of the town were all members, likewise the widowed Frau Consul Buddenbrook, born Stüwing, and Sesemi Weichbrodt and her simple sister. There is, however, no rank and no discrimination before Jesus; and so certain humble oddities were also guests at the Jerusalem evenings – for example, a little wrinkled creature, rich in the grace of God and knitting-patterns, who lived in the Holy Ghost Hospital and was named Himmelsburger. She was the last of her name – " the last Himmelsburger," she called herself humbly, and ran her knitting-needle under her cap to scratch her head.

But far more remarkable were two other extraordinary old

creatures, twins, who went about hand in hand through the town doing good deeds, in shepherdess hats out of the eighteenth century and faded clothes out of the long, long ago. They were named Gerhardt, and asserted that they descended in a direct line from Paul Gerhardt. People said they were by no means poor; but they lived wretchedly and gave away all they had. "My dears," remarked the Frau Consul, who was sometimes rather ashamed of them, "God sees the heart, I know; but your clothes are really a little – one must take some thought for oneself." But she could not prevent them kissing their elegant friend on the brow with the forbearing, yearning, pitying superiority of the poor in heart over the worldly great who seek salvation. They were not at all stupid. In their homely shrivelled heads – for all the world like ancient parrots – they had bright soft brown eyes and they looked out at the world with a wonderful expression of gentleness and understanding. Their hearts were full of amazing wisdom. They knew that in the last day all our beloved gone before us to God will come with song and salvation to fetch us home. They spoke the words "the Lord" with the fluent authority of early Christians, as if they had heard out of the Master's own mouth the words, "Yet a little while and ye shall see me." They possessed the most remarkable theories concerning inner light and intuition and the transmission of thought. One of them, named Lea, was deaf, and yet she nearly always knew what was being talked about!

It was usually the deaf Gerhardt who read aloud at the Jerusalem evenings, and the ladies found that she read beautifully and very affectingly. She took out of her bag an old book of a very disproportionate shape, much taller than it was broad, with an inhumanly chubby presentment of her ancestor in the front. She held it in both hands and read in a tremendous voice, in order to catch a little herself of what she read. It sounded as if the wind were imprisoned in the chimney:

"If Satan me would swallow."

"Goodness!" thought Tony Grünlich, "how could Satan want to swallow her?" But she said nothing and devoted herself to the pudding, wondering if she herself would ever become as ugly as the two Miss Gerhardts.

She was not happy. She felt bored and out of patience with all the pastors and missionaries, whose visits had increased ever since the death of the Consul. According to Tony they had too much to say in the house and received entirely too much money. But this last was Tom's affair, and he said nothing, while his sister now and then murmured something about people who consumed widows' homes and made long prayers.

She hated these black gentlemen bitterly. As a mature woman who knew life and was no longer a silly innocent, she found herself unable to believe in their irreproachable sanctity. " Mother," she said, " oh dear, I know I must not speak evil of my neighbours. But one thing I must say, and I should be surprised if life had not taught you that too, and that is that not all those who wear a long coat and say 'Lord, Lord' are always entirely without blemish."

History does not say what Tom thought of his sister's opinion on this point. Christian had no opinion at all. He confined himself to watching the gentlemen with his nose wrinkled up, in order to imitate them afterward at the club or in the family circle.

But it is true that Tony was the chief sufferer from the pious visitants. One day it actually happened that a missionary named Jonathan, who had been in Arabia and Syria – a man with great, reproachful eyes and baggy cheeks – was stopping in the house, and challenged her to assert that the curls she wore on her forehead were consistent with true Christian humility. He had not reckoned with Tony Grünlich's skill at repartee. She was silent a moment, while her mind worked rapidly; and then out it came. " May I ask you, Herr Pastor, to concern yourself with your own curls? " With that she rustled out, shoulders up, head back, and chin well tucked in. Pastor Jonathan had very few curls on his head – it would be nearer truth to say that he was quite bald.

And once she had an even greater triumph. There was a certain Pastor Trieschke from Berlin. His nickname was Teary Trieschke, because every Sunday he began to weep at an appropriate place in his sermon. Teary Trieschke had a pale face, red eyes, and cheek-bones like a horse's. He had been stopping for eight or ten days with the Buddenbrooks, conducting devotions and holding eating contests with poor Clothilde, turn about. He happened to fall in love with Tony – not with her immortal soul, oh no, but with her upper lip, her thick hair, her pretty eyes and charming figure. And the man of God, who had a wife and numerous children in Berlin, was not ashamed to have Anton leave a letter in Madame Grünlich's bedroom in the upper storey, wherein Bible texts and a kind of fawning sentimentality were surpassingly mingled. She found it when she went to bed, read it, and went with a firm step downstairs into the Frau Consul's bedroom, where by the candle-light she read aloud the words of the soul-saver to her Mother, quite unembarrassed and in a loud voice; so that Teary Trieschke became impossible in Meng Street.

"They are all alike," said Madame Grünlich; "ah, they are all alike. Oh, heavens, what a goose I was once! But life has destroyed my faith in men. Most of them are scoundrels – alas, it is the truth. Grünlich – " The name was, as always, like a summons to battle. She uttered it with her shoulders lifted and her eyes rolled up.

CHAPTER VI

Sievert Tiburtius was a small, narrow man with a large head and a thin, long, blond beard parted in the middle, so that he sometimes put the ends back over his shoulders. A quantity of little woolly ringlets covered his round head. His ears were large and outstanding, very much curled up at the edges and pointed at the tips like the ears of a fox. His nose sat like a tiny flat button in his face, his cheek-bones stood out, and his grey eyes, usually drawn close together and blinking about rather stupidly, could at certain moments widen quite extraordinarily, and get larger and larger, protruding more and more until they almost sprang out of their sockets.

This Pastor Tiburtius, who came from Riga, had preached for some years in central Germany, and now touched at the town on his way back home, where a living had been offered to him. Armed with the recommendation of a brother of the cloth who had eaten at least once in Meng Street of mock-turtle soup and ham with onion sauce, he waited upon the Frau Consul and was invited to be her guest for a few days. He occupied the spacious guest-chamber off the corridor in the first storey. But he stopped longer than he had expected. Eight days passed, and still there was this or that to be seen: the dance of death and the apostle-clock in St. Mary's, the Town Hall, the ancient Ships' Company, the Cathedral clock with the movable eyes. Ten days passed, and he spoke repeatedly of his departure, but at the first word of demur from anybody would postpone anew.

He was a better man than Herr Jonathan or Teary Trieschke. He thought not at all about Frau Antonie's curls and wrote her no letters. Strange to say, he paid his attentions to Clara, her younger and more serious sister. In her presence, when she spoke, entered or left the room, his eyes would grow surprisingly larger and larger and open out until they nearly jumped out of his head. He would spend almost the entire day in her company, in spiritual or worldly converse or reading aloud to her in his high voice and with the droll, jerky pronunciation of his Baltic home.

Even on the first day he said: "Permit me to say, Frau Consul, what a treasure and blessing from God you have in your daughter Clara. She is certainly a wonderful child."

"You are right," replied the Frau Consul. But he repeated his opinion so often that she began looking him over with her pale blue eyes, and led him on to speak of his home, his connections, and his prospects. She learned that he came of a mercantile family, that his mother was with God, that he had no brothers and sisters, and that his old father had retired and lived on his income in Riga – an income which would some time fall to him, Pastor Tiburtius. He also had a sufficient living from his calling.

Clara Buddenbrook was now in her nineteenth year. She had grown to be a young lady of an austere and peculiar beauty, with a tall, slender figure, dark, smooth hair, and stern yet dreamy eyes. Her nose was slightly hooked, her mouth a little too firmly closed. In the household she was most intimate with her poor and pious cousin Clothilde, whose father had lately died, and whose idea it was to "establish herself" soon – which meant to go into a pension somewhere with the money and furniture which she had inherited. Clara had nothing of Clothilde's meek and hungry submissiveness. On the contrary, with the servants and even with her brothers and sister and mother, a commanding tone was usual with her. Her low voice, which seemed only to drop with decision and never to rise with a question, had an imperious sound and could often take on a short, hard, impatient, haughty quality – on days, for example, when Clara had a headache.

Before the father's death had shrouded the family in mourning, she had taken part with irreproachable dignity in the society of her parents' house and other houses of like rank. But when the Frau Consul looked at her, she could not deny that, despite the stately dowry and Clara's domestic prowess, it would not be easy to marry her off. None of the godless, jovial, claret-drinking merchants of their circle would answer in the least; a clergyman would be the only suitable partner for this earnest and God-fearing maiden. After the Frau Consul had conceived this joyful idea, she responded with friendliness to the delicate advances of Pastor Tiburtius.

And truly the affair developed with precision. On a warm, cloudless July afternoon the family took a walk: the Frau Consul, Antonie, Christian, Clara, Clothilde, Erica Grünlich, and Mamsell Jungmann, with Pastor Tiburtius in their midst, went out far beyond the Castle Gate to eat strawberries and clotted milk or porridge at a wooden table laid out-of-doors, going after the meal into the large nut-garden which ran down to the river, in the shade of all sorts of fruit-trees, between currant and gooseberry bushes, asparagus and potato patches.

Sievert Tiburtius and Clara Buddenbrook stopped a little behind the others. He, much the smaller of the two, with his beard parted back over his shoulders, had taken off his broad-brimmed black hat from his big head; and he wiped his brow now and then with his handkerchief. His eyes were larger than usual and he carried on with her a long and gentle conversation, in the course of which they both stood still, and Clara, with a serious, calm voice said her "Yes."

After they returned, the Frau Consul, a little tired and overheated, was sitting alone in the landscape-room, when Pastor Tiburtius came and sat beside her. Outside there reigned the pensive calm of the Sabbath afternoon; and they sat inside and held, in the brightness of the summer evening, a long, low conversation, at the end of which the Frau Consul said: "Enough, my dear Herr Pastor. Your offer coincides with my motherly plans for my daughter; and you on your side have not chosen badly – that I can assure you. Who would have thought that your coming and your stay here in our house would be so wonderfully blest! I will not speak my final word to-day, for I must write first to my son, the Consul, who is at present, as you know, away. You will travel to-morrow, if you live and have your health, to Riga, to take up your work; and we expect to go for some weeks to the seashore. You will receive word from me soon, and God grant that we shall have a happy meeting."

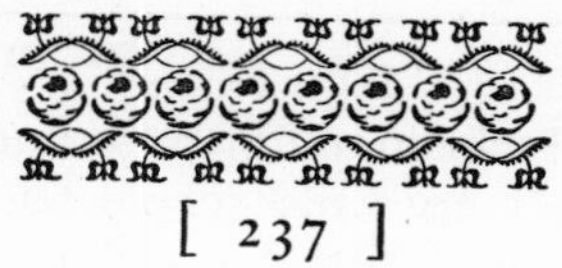

CHAPTER VII

AMSTERDAM, July 30th, 1856
HOTEL HET HASSJE

MY DEAR MOTHER,

I have just received your important letter, and hasten to thank you for the consideration you show me in asking for my consent in the affair under discussion. I send you, of course, not only my hearty agreement, but add my warmest good-wishes, being thoroughly convinced that you and Clara have made a good choice. The fine name Tiburtius is known to me, and I feel sure that Papa had business relations with the father. Clara comes into pleasant connections, in any case, and the position as pastor's wife will be very suited to her temperament.

And Tiburtius has gone back to Riga, and will visit his bride again in August? Well, it will be a gay time then with us in Meng Street – gayer than you realize, for you do not know the reason why I was so joyfully surprised by Mademoiselle Clara's betrothal, nor what a charming company it is likely to be. Yes, my dear good Mother: I am complying with the request to send my solemn consent to Clara's betrothal from the Amstel to the Baltic. But I do so on condition that you send me a similar consent by return of post! I would give three solid gulden to see your face, and even more that of our honest Tony, when you read these lines. But I will come to the point.

My clean little hotel is in the centre of the town with a pretty view of the canal. It is not far from the Bourse; and the business on which I came here – a question of a new and valuable connection, which you know I prefer to look after in person – has gone successfully from the first day. I have still considerable acquaintance here from the days of my apprenticeship; so, although many families are at the shore now, I have been invited out a good deal. I have been at small evening companies at the Van Henkdoms and the Moelens, and on the third day after my arrival I had to put on my dress clothes to go to a dinner at the house of my former chief, van der Kellen, which he had arranged out of season in my honour. Whom did I take in to dinner? Should you like to guess? Fräulein Arnoldsen, Tony's old school-fellow. Her father, the great merchant and almost greater violin artist, and his married daughter and her husband were also of the party.

I well remember that Gerda – if I may call her so – from the beginning, even when she was a young girl at school at Fräulein Weichbrodt's on the Millbrink, made a strong impression on me, never quite obliterated. But now I saw her again, taller, more developed, lovelier, more animated. Please spare me a description, which might so easily sound overdrawn – and you will soon see each other face to face.

You can imagine we had much to talk about at the table, but we had left the old memories behind by the end of the soup, and went on to more serious and fascinating matters. In music I could not hold my own with her, for we poor Buddenbrooks know all too little of that, but in the art of the Netherlands I was more at home, and in literature we were fully agreed.

Truly the time flew. After dinner I had myself presented to old Herr Arnoldsen, who received me with especial cordiality. Later, in the salon, he played several concert pieces, and Gerda also performed. She looked wonderful as she played, and although I have no notion of violin playing, I know that she knew how to sing upon her instrument (a real Stradivarius) so that the tears nearly came into my eyes. Next day I went to call on the Arnoldsens. I was received at first by an elderly companion, with whom I spoke French, but then Gerda came, and we talked as on the day before for perhaps an hour, only that this time we drew nearer together and made still more effort to understand and know each other. The talk was of you, Mamma, of Tony, of our good old town, and of my work.

And on that day I had already taken the firm resolve: this one or no one, now or never! I met her again by chance at a garden party at my friend van Svindren's, and I was invited to a musical evening at the Arnoldsens', in the course of which I sounded the young lady by a half-declaration, which was received encouragingly. Five days ago I went to Herr Arnoldsen to ask for permission to win his daughter's hand. He received me in his private office. "My dear Consul," he said, "you are very welcome, hard as it will be for an old widower to part from his daughter. But what does she say? She has already held firmly to her resolve never to marry. Have you a chance?" He was extremely surprised when I told him that Fräulein Gerda had actually given me ground for hope.

He left her some time for reflection, and I imagine that out of pure selfishness he dissuaded her. But it was useless. She had chosen me – since yesterday evening the betrothal is an accomplished fact.

No, my dear Mother, I am not asking a written answer to this letter, for I am leaving to-morrow. But I am bringing with me the Arnoldsens' promise that father, daughter, and married sister will visit us in August, and then you will be obliged to confess that she is the very wife for me. I hope you see no objection in the fact that Gerda is only three years younger than I? I am sure you never thought I would marry a chit out of the Möllendorpf-Langhals, Kistenmaker-Hagenström circle.

And now for the dowry. I am almost frightened to think how Stephan Kistenmaker and Hermann Hagenström and Peter Döhlmann and Uncle Justus and the whole town will blink at me when they hear of the dowry. For my future father-in-law is a millionaire. Heavens, what is there to say? We are such complex, contradictory creatures! I deeply love and respect Gerda Arnoldsen; and I simply will not delve deep down enough in myself to find out how much the thought of the dowry, which was whispered into my ear that first evening, contributed to my feeling. I love her: but it crowns my happiness and pride to think that when she becomes mine, our firm will at the same time gain a very considerable increase of capital.

I must close this letter, dear Mother; considering that in a few days, we shall be talking over my good fortune together, it is already too long. I wish you a pleasant and beneficial stay at the baths, and beg you to greet all the family most heartily for me. Your loving and obedient son,

T.

CHAPTER VIII

THAT year there was indeed a merry midsummer holiday in the Buddenbrook home. At the end of July Thomas returned to Meng Street and visited his family at the shore several times, like the other business men in the town. Christian had allotted full holidays unto himself, as he complained of an indefinite ache in his left leg. Dr. Grabow did not seem to treat it successfully, and Christian thought of it so much the more.

" It is not a pain – one can't call it a pain," he expatiated, rubbing his hand up and down his leg, wrinkling his big nose, and letting his eyes roam about. " It is a sort of ache, a continuous, slight, uneasy ache in the whole leg and on the left side, the side where the heart is. Strange. I find it strange – what do you think about it, Tom? "

" Well, well," said Tom, " you can have a rest and the sea-baths."

So Christian went down to the shore to tell stories to his fellow-guests, and the beach resounded with their laughter. Or he played roulette with Peter Döhlmann, Uncle Justus, Dr. Gieseke, and other Hamburg high-fliers.

Consul Buddenbrook went with Tony, as always when they were in Travemünde, to see the old Schwarzkopfs on the front. " Good-day, Ma'am Grünlich," said the pilot-captain, and spoke low German out of pure good feeling.

" Well, well, what a long time ago that was! And Morten, he's a doctor in Breslau and has all the practice in the town, the rascal." Frau Schwarzkopf ran off and made coffee, and they supped in the green verandah as they used to – only all of them were a good ten years older, and Morten and little Meta were not there, she having married the magistrate of Haffkrug. And the captain, already white-haired and rather deaf, had retired from his office – and Madame Grünlich was not a goose any more! Which did not prevent her from eating a great many slices of bread and honey, for, as she said: " Honey is a pure nature product – one knows what one is getting."

At the beginning of August the Buddenbrooks, like most of the other families, returned to town; and then came the great moment when, almost at the same time, Pastor Tiburtius from Prussia and the Arnoldsens from Holland arrived for a long visit in Meng Street.

It was a very pretty scene when the Consul led his bride for the first time into the landscape-room and took her to his mother, who received her with outstretched arms. Gerda had grown tall and splendid. She walked with a free and gracious bearing; with her heavy dark-red hair, her close-set brown eyes with the blue shadows round them, her large, gleaming teeth which showed when she smiled, her straight strong nose and nobly formed mouth, this maiden of seven-and-twenty years had a strange, aristocratic, haunting beauty. Her face was white and a little haughty, but she bowed her head as the Frau Consul with gentle feeling took it between her hands and kissed the pure, snowy forehead. " Yes, you are welcome to our house and to our family, you dear, beautiful, blessed creature," she said. " You will make him happy. Do I not see already how happy you make him? " And she drew Thomas forward with her other arm, to kiss him also.

Never, except perhaps in Grandfather's time, was there more gay society in the great house, which accommodated its guests with ease. Pastor Tiburtius had modestly chosen a bed-chamber in the back building next the billiard-room. But the rest divided the unoccupied space on the ground floor next the hall and in the first storey: Gerda; Herr Arnoldsen, a quick, clever man at the end of the fifties, with a pointed grey beard and a pleasant impetuosity in every motion; his oldest daughter, an ailing-looking woman; and his son-in-law, an elegant man of the world, who was turned over to Christian for entertainment in the town and at the club.

Antonie was overjoyed that Sievert Tiburtius was the only parson in the house. The betrothal of her adored brother rejoiced her heart. Aside from Gerda's being her friend, the parti was a brilliant one, gilding the family name and the firm with such new glory! And the three-hundred-thousand-mark dowry and the thought of what the town and particularly the Hagenströms would say to it, put her in a state of prolonged and delightful enchantment. Three times daily, at least, she passionately embraced her future sister-in-law.

" Oh, Gerda," she cried, " I love you – you know I always did love you. I know you can't stand me – you used to hate me; but – "

" Why, Tony! " said Fräulein Arnoldsen. " How could I have

hated you? Did you ever do anything to me?" For some reason, however – probably out of mere wantonness and love of talking – Tony asserted stoutly that Gerda had always hated her, while she on her side had always returned the hate with love. She took Thomas aside and told him: "You have done very well, Tom. Oh, heavens, how well you have done! If Father could only see this – it is just dreadful that he cannot! Yes, this wipes out a lot of things – not least the affair with that person whose name I do not even like to speak."

Which put it into her head to take Gerda into an empty room and tell her with awful detail the story of her married life with Bendix Grünlich. Then they talked for hours about boarding-school days and the bed-time gossip; of Armgard von Schilling in Mecklenburg and Eva Ewers in Munich. Tony paid little or no attention to Sievert Tiburtius and his bethrothed – which troubled them not at all. The lovers sat quietly together hand in hand, and spoke gently and earnestly of the beautiful future before them.

As the year of mourning was not quite over, the two betrothals were celebrated only in the family. But Gerda quickly became a celebrity in the town. Her person formed the chief subject of conversation on the Bourse, at the club, at the theatre, and in society. "Tip-top," said the gallants, and clucked their tongues, for that was the latest Hamburg slang for a superior article, whether a brand of claret, a cigar, or a "deal." But among the solid, respectable citizens there was much head-shaking. "Something queer about her," they said. "Her hair, her face, the way she dresses – a little too unusual." Sorenson expressed it: "She has a certain something about her!" He made a face as if he were on the Bourse and somebody had made him a doubtful proposition. But it was all just like Consul Buddenbrook: a little pretentious, not like his forebears. Everybody knew – not least Benthien the draper – that he ordered his clothes from Hamburg: not only the fine new-fashioned materials for his suits – and he had a great many of them, cloaks, coats, waistcoats, and trousers – but his hats and cravats and linen as well. He changed his shirt every day, sometimes twice a day, and perfumed his handkerchief and his moustache, which he wore cut like Napoleon III. All this was not for the sake of the firm, of course – the house of Johann Buddenbrook did not need that sort of thing – but to gratify his own personal taste for the superfine and aristocratic – or whatever you might call it. And then the quotations from Heine and other poets which he dropped sometimes in the most practical connections, in business or civic matters! And now, his bride – well, Consul Buddenbrook himself had "a certain something" about him! All this, of course, with the greatest respect; for the family was highly esteemed, the firm very, very "good," and the head of it an able and charming man who loved his city and would still serve her well. It was really a devilishly fine match for him; there was talk of a hundred thousand thaler down; but of course . . . Among the ladies there were some who found Gerda "silly"; which, it will be recalled, was a very severe judgment.

But the man who gazed with furious ardour at Thomas Buddenbrook's bride, the first time he saw her on the street, was Gosch the broker. "Ah!" he said in the club or the Ships' Company, lifting his glass and screwing up his face absurdly, "what a woman! Hera and Aphrodite, Brunhilda and Melusina all in one! Oh, how wonderful life is!" he would add. And not one of the citizens who sat about with their beer on the hard wooden benches of the old guild-house, under the models of sailing vessels and big stuffed fish hanging down from the ceiling, had the least idea what the advent of Gerda Arnoldsen meant in the yearning life of Gosch the broker.

The little company in Meng Street, not committed, as we have seen, to large entertainments, had the more leisure for intimacy with each other. Sievert Tiburtius, with Clara's hand in his, talked about his parents, his childhood, and his future plans. The Arnoldsens told of their people, who came from Dresden, only one branch of them having been transplanted to Holland.

Madame Grünlich asked her brother for the key of the secretary in the landscape-room, and brought out the portfolio with the family papers, in which Thomas had already entered the new events. She proudly related the Buddenbrook history, from the Rostock tailor on; and when she read out the old festival verses:

> Industry and beauty chaste
> See we linked in marriage band:
> Venus Anadyomene,
> And cunning Vulcan's busy hand

she looked at Tom and Gerda and let her tongue play over her lips. Regard for historical veracity also caused her to narrate events connected with a certain person whose name she did not like to mention!

On Thursday at four o'clock the usual guests came. Uncle Justus brought his feeble wife, with whom he lived an unhappy existence. The wretched mother continued to scrape together money out of the housekeeping to send to the degenerate and disinherited Jacob in America, while she and her husband subsisted on almost nothing but porridge. The Buddenbrook ladies from Broad Street also came; and their love of truth compelled them to say, as usual, that Erica Grünlich was not growing well and that she looked more than ever like her wretched father. Also that the Consul's bride wore a rather conspicuous coiffure. And Sesemi Weichbrodt came too, and standing on her tip-toes, kissed Gerda with her little explosive kiss on the forehead and said with emotion: " Be happy, my dear child."

At table Herr Arnoldsen gave one of his witty and fanciful toasts in honour of the two bridal pairs. While the rest drank their coffee he played the violin, like a gipsy, passionately, with abandonment – and with what dexterity! . . . Gerda fetched her Stradivarius and accompanied him in his passages with her sweet cantilena. They performed magnificent duets at the little organ in the landscape-room, where once the Consul's grandfather had played his simple melodies on the flute.

" Sublime! " said Tony, lolling back in her easy chair. " Oh, heavens, how sublime that is! " And she rolled up her eyes to the ceiling to express her emotions. " You know how it is in life," she went on, weightily. " Not everybody is given such a gift. Heaven has unfortunately denied it to me, though I used to pray for it at night. I am a goose, a silly creature. You know, Gerda – I am the elder and have learned to know life – let me tell you, you ought to thank your Creator every day on your knees, for being such a gifted creature! "

" Oh, please," said Gerda, with a laugh, showing her beautiful large white teeth.

Later they all ate wine jelly and discussed their plans for the near future. At the end of that month or the beginning of September, it was decided, Sievert Tiburtius and the Arnoldsens would go home. Then, directly after Christmas, Clara's wedding would be celebrated with due solemnity in the great hall. The Frau Consul, health permitting, would attend Tom's wedding in Amsterdam. But it must be put off until the beginning of the next year, that there might be a little pause for rest between. It was no use for Thomas to protest. " Please," said the Frau Consul, and laid her hand on his sleeve. " Sievert should have the precedence, I think."

The Pastor and his bride had decided against a wedding journey. Gerda and Thomas, however, were to take a trip to northern Italy, as far as Florence, and be gone about two months. In the meantime Tony, with the help of the upholsterer Jacobs in Fish Street.

was to make ready the charming little house in Broad Street, the property of a bachelor who had moved to Hamburg. The Consul was already arranging for its purchase. Oh, Tony would furnish it to the Queen's taste. "It will be perfect," she said. They were all sure it would.

Christian looked on while the two bridal pairs held hands, and listened to the talk about weddings and trousseaux and bridal journeys. His nose looked bigger and his legs more crooked than ever. He felt an indefinite sort of pain in the left one, and stared solemnly at them all out of his little round deep-set eyes. Finally, in the accents of Marcellus Stengel, he said to his cousin Clothilde, who sat elderly, dried-up, silent, and hungry, at table among the happy throng: "Well, Tilda, let's *us* get married too – I mean, of course each one for himself."

[246]

CHAPTER IX

Some six months later Consul Buddenbrook returned with his bride from Italy. The March snows lay in Broad Street as the carriage drove up at five o'clock before the front door of their simple painted façade. A few children and grown folk had stopped to watch the home-coming pair descend. Frau Antonie Grünlich stood proudly in the doorway, behind her the two servant-maids, with white caps, bare arms, and thick striped skirts – she had engaged them beforehand for her sister-in-law. Flushed with pleasure and industry, she ran impetuously down the steps; Gerda and Thomas climbed out of the trunk-laden carriage wrapped in their furs; and she drew them into the house in her embrace.

"Here you are! You lucky people, to have travelled so far in the world. 'Knowest thou the house? High-pillared are its walls!' Gerda, you are more beautiful than ever; here, I must kiss you – no, so, on the mouth. How are you, Tom, old fellow? – yes, I must kiss you too. Marcus says everything has gone well here. Mother is waiting for you at home, but you can first just make yourselves comfortable. Will you have some tea? Or a bath? Everything is ready – you won't complain. Jacobs did his best – and I have done all I could, too."

They went together into the vestibule, and the servants brought in the luggage with the help of the coachman. Tony said: "The rooms here in the parterre you will probably not need for the present. *For the present*," she repeated, running her tongue over her upper lip. "Look, this is pretty," and she opened a door directly next the vestibule. "Simple oak furniture, ivy at the windows. Over there, the other side of the corridor, is another room, a larger one. Here on the right are the kitchen and larder. But let's go up. I will show you everything." They went up the stairs, which were covered with a dark red runner. Above, behind a glass partition, was a narrow corridor which led to the dining-room. This had dark red damask wall-paper, a heavy round table upon which the samovar was steaming, a massive sideboard, and chairs of carved nut-wood, with rush seats. Then there was a comfortable sitting-room upholstered in grey, separated by portières from a small salon with a bay-window and furniture in green striped rep. A fourth of this whole storey was occupied by a large hall with three windows.

Then they went into the sleeping-room, on the right of the corridor. It had flowered hangings and solid mahogany beds. Tony passed on to a small door with open-work carving in the opposite wall, and displayed a winding stair leading from the bedroom to the lower floors, the bathroom, and the servants' quarters.

"It is pretty here. I shall stop here," said Gerda, and sank with a deep breath into the reclining chair beside one of the beds.

The Consul bent over and kissed her forehead. "Tired? I feel like that too. I should like to tidy up a bit."

"I'll look after the tea," said Tony Grünlich, "and wait for you in the dining-room."

The tea stood steaming in the Meissenware cups when Thomas entered. "Here I am," he said. "Gerda would like to rest a little. She has a headache. Afterward we will go to Meng Street. Well, how is everything, my dear Tony – all right? Mother, Erica, Christian? But now," he went on with his most charming manner, "our warmest thanks – Gerda's too – for all your trouble, you good soul. How pretty you have made everything! Nothing is missing. – I only need a few palms for my wife's bay-window; and I must look about for some suitable oil paintings. But tell me, now, how are you? What have you been doing all this time?"

He had drawn up a chair for his sister beside himself, and slowly drank his tea and ate a biscuit as they talked.

"Oh, Tom," she answered. "What should I be doing? My life is over."

"Nonsense, Tony – you and your life! But it *is* pretty tiresome, is it?"

"Yes, Tom, it is very tiresome. Sometimes I just have to shriek, out of sheer boredom. It has been nice to be busy with this house, and you don't know how happy I am at your return. But I am not happy here – God forgive me, if that is a sin. I am in the thirties now, but I'm still not quite old enough to make intimate friends with the last of the Himmelsburgers, or the Miss Gerhardts, or any of mother's black friends that come and consume widows' homes. I don't believe in them, Tom; they are wolves in sheep's clothing – a generation of vipers. We are all weak creatures with sinful hearts, and when they begin to look down on me for a poor worldling I laugh in their faces. I've always thought that all men are the same, and that we don't need any intercessors between us and God. You know my political beliefs. I think the citizens – "

"Then you feel lonely?" Tom asked, to bring her back to her starting-point. "But you have Erica."

"Yes, Tom, and I love the child with my whole heart – although a certain person did use to declare that I am not fond of children. But you see – I am perfectly frank; I am an honest woman and speak as I think, without making words – "

"Which is splendid of you, Tony."

"Well, in short – it is sad, but the child reminds me too much of Grünlich. The Buddenbrooks in Broad Street think she is very like him too. And then, when I see her before me I always think: 'You are an old woman with a big daughter, and your life is over. Once for a few years you were alive; but now you can grow to be seventy or eighty years old, sitting here and listening to Lea Gerhardt read aloud. That is such an awful thought, Tom, that a lump comes in my throat. Because I still feel so young, and still long to see life again. And besides, I don't feel comfortable – not only in the house, but in the town. You know I haven't been struck blind. I have my eyes in my head and see how things are; I am not a stupid goose any more, I am a divorced woman – and I am made to feel it, that's certain. Believe me, Tom, it lies like a weight on my heart, to know that I have besmirched our name, even if it was not any fault of mine. You can do whatever you will, you can earn money and be the first man in the town – but people will still say: 'Yes, but his sister is a divorced woman.' Julchen Möllendorpf, the Hagenström girl – she doesn't speak to me! Oh, well, she is a goose. It is the same with all families. And yet I can't get rid of the hope that I could make it all good again. I am still young – don't you think I am still rather pretty? Mamma cannot give me very much again, but even what she can give is an acceptable sum of money. Suppose I were to marry again? To confess the truth, Tom, it is my most fervent wish. Then everything would be put right and the stain wiped out. Oh, if I could only make a match worthy of our name, and set myself up again – do you think it is entirely out of the question?"

"Not in the least, Tony. Heaven forbid! I have always thought of it. But it seems to me that in the first place you must get out a little, have a little change, and brighten up a bit."

"Yes, that's it," she cried eagerly. "Now I must tell you a little story."

Thomas was well pleased. He leaned back in his chair and smoked his second cigarette. The twilight was coming on.

"Well, then, while you were away, I almost took a situation –

a position as companion in Liverpool! Would you have thought it was shocking? Oh, I know it would have been undignified! But I was so wildly anxious to get away. The plan came to nothing. I sent my photograph to the lady, and she wrote that she must decline my services, because I was too pretty – there was a grown son in the house. 'You are too pretty,' she wrote! I don't know when I have been so pleased."

They both laughed heartily.

"But now I have something else in mind," went on Tony. "I have had an invitation, from Eva Ewers, to go to Munich. Her name is Eva Niederpaur now; her husband is superintendent of a brewery. Well, she has asked me to visit her, and I think I will take advantage of the invitation. Of course, Erica could not go with me. I would put her in Sesemi Weichbrodt's pension. She would be well taken care of. Have you any objection?"

"Not at all. It is necessary, in any case, that you should make some new connections."

"Yes, that's it," she said gratefully. "But now, Tom. I have been talking the whole time about myself; I am a selfish thing. Now, tell me your affairs. Oh, heavens, how happy you must be!"

"Yes, Tony," he said with emphasis. There was a pause. He blew out the smoke across the table and continued: "In the first place, I am very glad to be married and set up an establishment. You know I should not make a good bachelor. It has a side to it that suggests loneliness and also laziness – and I am ambitious, as you know. I don't feel that my career is finished, either in business or – to speak half jestingly – in politics. And a man gains the confidence of the world better if he is a family man and a father. Though I came within an ace of not doing it, after all! I am a bit fastidious. For a long time I thought it would not be possible to find the right person. But the sight of Gerda decided me. I felt at once that she was the only one for me: though I know there are people in town who don't care for my taste. She is a wonderful creature; there are few like her in the world. She is nothing like you, Tony, to be sure. You are simpler, and more natural too. My lady sister is simply more temperamental," he continued, suddenly taking a lighter tone. "Oh, Gerda has temperament too – her playing shows that; but she can sometimes be a little cold. In short, she is not to be measured by the ordinary standards. She is an artist, an individual, a puzzling, fascinating creature."

"Yes, yes," Tony said. She had given her brother the closest attention. It was nearly dark, and she had not thought of lighting the lamps.

The corridor door opened, and there stood before them in the twilight, in a pleated piqué house-frock, white as snow, a slender figure. The heavy dark-red hair framed her white face, and blue shadows lay about her close-set brown eyes. It was Gerda, mother of future Buddenbrooks.

PART SIX

[253]

CHAPTER I

Thomas Buddenbrook took a solitary early breakfast in his pretty dining-room. His wife usually left her room late, as she was subject to headaches and vapours in the morning. The Consul went at once to Meng Street, where the offices still were, took his second breakfast with his mother, Christian and Ida Jungmann in the entresol, and met Gerda only at dinner, at four in the afternoon.

The ground floor of the old house still preserved the life and movement of a great business; but the upper storeys were empty and lonely. Little Erica had been received as a boarder by Mademoiselle Weichbrodt, and poor Clothilde had moved with her few sticks of furniture into a cheap pension with the widow of a high school teacher, a Frau Dr. Krauseminz. Even Anton had left the house, and gone over to the young pair, where he was more needed. When Christian was at the club, the Frau Consul and Ida Jungmann sat at four o'clock dinner alone at the round table, in which there was now not a single extra leaf. It looked quite lost in the great spaces of the dining-temple with its images of the gods.

The social life of Meng Street had been extinguished with the death of Consul Johann Buddenbrook. Except for the visits of this or that man of God, the Frau Consul saw no guests but the members of her family, who still came on Thursday afternoons. But the first great dinner had already been given by the young pair in Broad Street. Tables were laid in both dining- and living-room, and there were a hired cook and waiters and Kistenmaker wines. It began at five o'clock, and its sounds and smells were still in the air at eleven. All the business and professional men were present, married pairs and bachelors as well: all the tribe of Langhals, Hagenströms, Huneuses, Kistenmakers, Överdiecks, and Möllendorpfs. It finished off with whist and music. They talked about it in glowing terms on the Bourse for a whole week. The young Frau Consul certainly knew how to entertain! When she and the Consul were alone, in the room lighted by burned-down candles, with the furniture disarranged and the air thick with heavy odours of rich food, wine, cigars, coffee, perfume, and the scent of the flowers from the ladies' toilettes and the table decorations, he pressed her hand and said: " Very good, Gerda. We do not need to be ashamed. This sort of thing is necessary. I have no great fondness for balls, and having the young people jumping about here; and, besides, there is not room. But we must entertain the settled people. A dinner like that costs a bit more – but it is well spent."

" You are right," she had answered, and arranged the laces through which her bosom shimmered like marble. " I much prefer the dinners to the balls myself. A dinner is so soothing. I had been playing this afternoon, and felt a little queer. My brain feels quite dead now. If I were to be struck by lightning I should not change colour."

Next morning at half past eleven the Consul sat down beside his Mother at the breakfast table, and she read a letter aloud to him:

MUNICH, April 2, 1857
MARIENPLATZ 5

MY DEAR MOTHER,

I must beg your pardon – it is a shame that I have not written before in the eight days I have been here. My time has been so taken up with all the things there are to see – I'll tell you about them afterwards. Now I must ask if all the dear ones, you and Tom and Gerda and Erica and Christian and Tilda and Ida, are well – that is the most important thing.

Ah, what all I have seen in these days! – the Pinakothek and the Glyptothek and the Hofbräuhaus and the Court Theatre and the churches, and quantities of other things! I must tell you of them when I see you; otherwise I should kill myself writing. We have also had a drive in the Isar valley, and for to-morrow an excursion to the Wurmsee is arranged. So it goes on. Eva is very sweet to me, and her husband, Herr Niederpaur, the brewery superintendent, is an agreeable man. We live in a very pretty square in the town, with a fountain in the middle, like ours at home in the market place, and the house is quite near the Town Hall. I have never seen such a house. It is painted from top to bottom, in all colours – St. Georges killing dragons, and old Bavarian princes in full robes and arms. Imagine!

Yes, I like Munich extremely. The air is very strengthening to the nerves, and for the moment I am quite in order with my stomach trouble. I enjoy drinking the beer – I drink a good deal, the more so as the water is not very good. But I cannot quite get used to the food. There are too few vegetables and too much flour, for instance in the sauces, which are pathetic. They have no idea of a proper joint of veal, for the butchers cut everything very badly. And I miss the fish. It is quite mad to be eating so much cucumber and potato salad with the beer – my tummy rebels audibly.

Yes, one has to get used to a great deal. It is a real foreign country. The strange currency, the difficulty of understanding the common people – I speak too fast to them and they seem to talk gibberish to me – and then the Catholicism. I hate it, as you know; I have no respect for it –

Here the Consul began to laugh, leaning back in the sofa with a piece of bread and herb cheese in his hand.

" Yes, Tom, you are laughing," said his Mother, and tapped with her middle finger on the table. " But it pleases me very much that she holds fast to the faith of her fathers and shuns the unevangelical gim-crackery. I know that you felt a certain sympathy for the papal church, while you were in France and Italy: but that is not religion in you, Tom – it is something else, and I understand what. We must be forbearing; yet in these things a frivolous feeling of fascination is very much to be regretted. I pray God that you and your Gerda – for I well know that she does not belong to those firm in the faith – will in the course of time feel the necessary seriousness. You will forgive your mother her words, I know."

On top of the fountain (she continued reading) there is a Madonna, and sometimes she is crowned with a wreath, and the common people come with rose garlands and kneel down and pray – which looks very pretty, but it is written: " Go into your chamber." You often see monks here in the street; they look very respectable. But – imagine, Mamma! – yesterday in Theatiner Street some high dignitary of the church was driving past me in his coach; perhaps it was an archbishop; anyway, an elderly man – well, this gentleman throws me an ogling look out of the window, like a lieutenant of the Guard! You know, Mother, I've no great opinion of your friends the ministers and missionaries, but Teary Trieschke was certainly nothing compared to this rakish old prince of the Church.

" Horrors! " interjected the Frau Consul, shocked.

" That's Tony, to the life," said the Consul.

" How is that, Tom? "

" Well, perhaps she just invited him a trifle – to try him, you know. I know Tony. And I am sure the 'ogling look' delighted her hugely, which was probably what the old gentleman wanted."

The Frau Consul did not take this up, but continued to read:

Day before yesterday the Niederpaurs entertained in the evening. It was lovely, though I could not always follow the conversation, and I found the tone sometimes rather questionable. There was a singer there from the Court opera, who sang songs, and a young artist, who asked me to sit for him, which I refused, as I thought it not suitable. I enjoyed myself most with a Herr Permaneder. Would you ever think there could be such a name? He is a hop-dealer, a nice, jolly man, in middle life and a bachelor. I had him at table, and stuck to him, for he was the only Protestant in the party. He is a citizen of Munich, but his family comes from Nuremberg. He assured me that he knew our firm very well by name, and you can imagine how it pleased me, Tom, to hear the respectful tone in which he said that. He asked how many there are of us, and things like that. He asked about Erica and Grünlich too. He comes sometimes to the Niederpaurs', and is probably going to-morrow to Wurmsee with us.

Well, adieu, dear Mamma; I can write no more. If I live and prosper, as you always say, I shall stop here three or four weeks more, and when I come back I will tell you more of Munich, for in a letter it is hard to know where to begin. I like it very much; that I must say – though one would have to train a cook to make decent sauces. You see, I am an old woman, with my life behind me, and I have nothing more to look forward to on earth. But if, for example, Erica should – if she lives and prospers – marry here, I should have nothing against it; that I must say.

Again the Consul was obliged to stop eating and lean back in his chair to laugh.

" She is simply priceless, Mother. And when she tries to dissimulate, she is incomparable. She is a thousand miles away from being able to carry it off."

" Yes, Tom," said the Frau Consul, " she is a good child, and deserves good fortune." And she finished the letter.

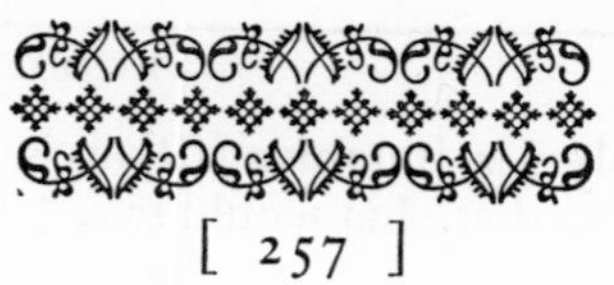

CHAPTER II

At the end of April Frau Grünlich returned home. Another epoch was behind her, and the old existence began again – attending the daily devotions and the Jerusalem evenings and hearing Lea Gerhardt read aloud. Yet she was obviously in a gay and hopeful mood.

Her brother, the Consul, fetched her from the station – she had come from Buchen – and drove her through the Holsten Gate into the town. He could not resist paying her the old compliment – how, next to Clothilde, she was the prettiest one in the family; and she answered: " Oh, Tom, I hate you! To make fun of an old lady like that – "

But he was right, nevertheless: Madame Grünlich kept her good looks remarkably. You looked at the thick ash-blond hair, rolled at the sides, drawn back above the little ears, and fastened on the top of the head with a broad tortoise-shell comb; at the soft expression of her grey-blue eyes, her pretty upper lip, the fine oval and delicate colour of her face – and you thought of three-and-twenty, perhaps; never of thirty. She wore elegant hanging gold earrings, which, in a somewhat different form, her grandmother had worn before her. A loose bodice of soft dark silk, with satin revers and flat lace epaulettes, gave her pretty bosom an enchanting look of softness and fulness.

She was in the best of tempers. On Thursday, when Consul Buddenbrook and the ladies from Broad Street, Consul Kröger, Clothilde, Sesemi Weichbrodt and Erica came to tea, she talked vividly about Munich. The beer, the noodles, the artist who wanted to paint her, and the court coaches had made the greatest impressions. She mentioned Herr Permaneder in passing; and Pfiffi Buddenbrook let fall a word or two to the effect that such a journey might be very agreeable, but did not seem to have any practical results. Frau Grünlich passed this by with dignity, though she put back her head and tucked in her chin. She fell into the habit now, whenever the vestibule bell rang through the entry, of hurrying to the landing to see who had come. What might that mean? Probably only Ida Jungmann, Tony's governess and year-long confidante, knew that. Ida would say, " Tony, my child, you will see: he'll come."

The family was grateful to the returned traveller for her cheering presence; for the atmosphere of the house sadly needed brightening. The relations between the head of the firm and his younger brother had not improved. Indeed, they had grown sadly worse. Their Mother, the Frau Consul, followed with anxious misgivings the course of events and had enough to do to mediate between the two. Her hints to visit the office more regularly were received in absent silence by Christian. He met his brother's remonstrances with a mortified air, making no defence, and for a few days would apply himself with somewhat more zeal to the English correspondence. But there developed more and more in the elder an irritated contempt for the younger brother, not decreased by the fact that Christian received his occasional rebukes without seeming offence, only looking at him with the usual absent disquiet in his eyes.

Tom's irritable activity and the condition of his nerves would not let him listen sympathetically or even patiently to Christian's detailed accounts of his increasing symptoms. To his mother or sister, he referred to them with disgust as " the silly phenomena of an obstinate introspection."

The ache, the indefinite ache in Christian's left leg, had yielded by now to treatment; but the trouble in swallowing came on often at table, and there was lately a difficulty in breathing, an asthmatic trouble, which Christian thought for several weeks was consumption. He explained its nature and activity at length to his family, his nose wrinkled up the while. Dr. Grabow was called in. He said the heart and lungs were operating soundly, but the occasional difficulty in breathing was due to muscular sluggishness, and ordered first the use of a fan and secondly that of a green powder which one burned, inhaling the smoke. Christian used the fan in the office, and to a remonstrance on the part of the chief answered that in Valparaiso every man in the office was provided with a fan on account of the heat: " Johnny Thunderstorm – good God! " But one day, after he had been wriggling about on his chair for some time, nervous and restless, he took his powder out of his pocket and made such a strong and violent-smelling reek in the room that some of the men began to cough violently, and Herr Marcus grew quite pale. There was an open explosion, a scandal, a dreadful talking-to which would have led to a break at once, but that the Frau Consul once more covered everything all up, reasoned them out of it, and set things going again.

But this was not all. The life Christian led outside the house, mainly with his old schoolmate Lawyer Gieseke, was observed by the Consul with disgust. He was no prig, no spoil-sport. He knew very well that his native town, this port and trading city, where men walked the streets proud of their irreproachable reputation as business men, was by no means of spotless morality. They made up to themselves for the tedious hours spent in their offices, by dinners with heavy wines and heavy dishes – and by other things. But the broad mantle of civic respectability concealed this side of their life. Thomas Buddenbrook's first law was to preserve "the *dehors*"; wherein he showed himself not so different from his fellow burghers. Lawyer Gieseke was a member of the professional class, whose habits of life were much like those of the merchants. That he was also a "good fellow," anybody could see who looked at him. But, like the other easy men of pleasure in the community, he knew how to avoid trouble by wearing the proper expression and saying the proper thing. And in political and professional matters, he had a reputation of irreproachable respectability. His betrothal to Fräulein Huneus had just been announced; whereby he married a considerable dowry and a place in the best society. He was active in civic affairs, and he had his eye on a seat in the Council – even, ultimately, on the seat of old Burgomaster Överdieck.

But his friend Christian Buddenbrook – the same who could go calmly up to Mlle. Meyer-de-la-Grange, present her his bouquet, and say, "Oh, Fräulein, how beautifully you act!" – Christian had been developed by character and circumstances into a free-liver of the naïve and untrammelled type. In affairs of the heart, as in all others, he was disinclined to govern his feelings or to practise discretion for the sake of preserving his dignity. The whole town had laughed over his affair with an obscure actress at the summer theatre. Frau Stuht in Bell Founders' Street – the same who moved in the best society – told everybody who would listen how Chris had been seen again walking by daylight in the open street with the person from the Tivoli.

Even that did not actually offend people. There was too much candid cynicism in the community to permit a display of serious moral disapproval. Christian Buddenbrook, like Consul Peter Döhlmann – whose declining business put him into somewhat the same artless class – was a popular entertainer and indispensable to gentlemen's companies. But neither was taken seriously. In important matters they simply did not count. It was a significant fact that the whole town, the Bourse, the docks, the club, and the street called them by their first names – Peter and Chris. And enemies, like the Hagenströms, laughed not only at Chris's stories and jokes, but at Chris himself, too.

He thought little or nothing of this. If he noticed it, it passed out of his mind again after a momentary disquiet. But his brother the Consul knew it. Thomas knew that Christian afforded a point of attack to the enemies of the family – and there were already too many such points. The connection with the Överdiecks was distant and would be quite worthless after the Burgomaster's death. The Krögers played no rôle now; they lived retired, after the misfortunes with their son. The marriage of the deceased uncle Gotthold was always unpleasant. The Consul's sister was a divorced wife, even if one did not quite give up hope of her remarrying. And his brother was a laughing-stock in the town, a man with whose clownishness industrious men amused their leisure and then laughed good-naturedly or maliciously. He contracted debts, too, and at the end of the quarter, when he had no more money, would quite openly let Dr. Gieseke pay for him – which was a direct reflection on the firm. Thomas's contemptuous ill will, which Christian bore with quiet indifference, expressed itself in all the trifling situations that come up between members of a family. If the conversation turned upon the Buddenbrook family history, Christian might be in the mood to speak with serious love and admiration of his native town and of his ancestors. It sat rather oddly on him, to be sure, and the Consul could not stand it: he would cut short the conversation with some cold remark. He despised his brother so much that he could not even permit him to love where he did. If Christian had uttered the same sentiments in the dialect of Marcellus Stengel, Tom could have borne it better. He had read a book, a historical work, which had made such a strong impression on him that he spoke about it and praised it in the family. Christian would by himself never have found out the book; but he was impressionable and accessible to every influence; so he also read it, found it wonderful, and described his reactions with all possible detail. That book was spoiled for Thomas for ever. He spoke of it with cold and critical detachment. He pretended hardly to have read it. He completely gave it over to his brother, to admire all by himself.

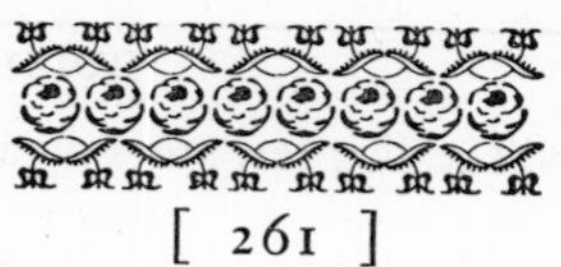

CHAPTER III

CONSUL BUDDENBROOK came from the "Harmony" – a reading-club for men, where he had spent the hour after second breakfast – back into Meng Street. He crossed the yard from behind, entered the side of the garden by the passage which ran between vine-covered walls and connected the back and front courtyards, and called into the kitchen to ask if his brother were at home. They should let him know when he came in. Then he passed through the office (where the men at the desks bent more closely over their work) into the private room; he laid aside his hat and stick, put on his working coat, and sat down in his place by the window, opposite Herr Marcus. Between his pale eyebrows were two deep wrinkles. The yellow end of a Russian cigarette roamed from one corner of his mouth to the other. The movements with which he took up paper and writing materials were so short and jerky that Herr Marcus ran his two fingers up and down his beard and gave his colleague a long, scrutinizing look. The younger men glanced at him with raised eyebrows. The Head was angry.

After half an hour, during which nothing was heard but the scratching of pens and the sound of Herr Marcus discreetly clearing his throat, the Consul looked over the green half-blind and saw Christian coming down the street. He was smoking. He came from the club, where he had eaten and also played a bit. He wore his hat a little awry on his head, and swung his yellow stick, which had come from "over there" and had the bust of a nun for a handle. He was obviously in good health and the best of tempers. He came humming into the office, said "Good morning, gentlemen," although it was a bright spring afternoon, and took his place to "do a bit of work." But the Consul got up and, passing him, said without looking at him, "Oh, may I have a few words with you?" Christian followed him. They walked rather rapidly through the entry. Thomas held his hands behind his back, and Christian involuntarily did the same, turning his big bony hooked nose toward his brother. The red-blond moustache drooped, English fashion, over his mouth. While they went across the court,

Thomas said: “ We will walk a few steps up and down the garden, my friend.”

“ Good,” answered Christian. Then there was a long silence again, while they turned to the left and walked, by the outside way, past the rococo “ portal ” right round the garden, where the buds were beginning to swell. Finally the Consul said in a loud voice, with a long breath, “ I have just been very angry, on account of your behaviour.”

“ My – ? ”

“ Yes. I heard in the ‘ Harmony ’ about a remark of yours that you dropped in the club last evening. It was so obnoxious, so incredibly tactless, that I can find no words – the stupidity called down a sharp snub on you at once. Do you care to recall what it was? ”

“ I know now what you mean. Who told you that? ”

“ What has that to do with it? Döhlmann. – In a voice loud enough so that all the people who did not already know the story could laugh at the joke.”

“ Well, Tom, I must say I was ashamed of Hagenström.”

“ You were ashamed – *you* were – ! Listen to me,” shouted the Consul, stretching out both hands in front of him and shaking them in excitement. “ In a company consisting of business as well as professional men, you make the remark, for everybody to hear, that, when one really considers it, every business man is a swindler – you, a business man yourself, belonging to a firm that strains every nerve and muscle to preserve its perfect integrity and spotless reputation! ”

“ Good heavens, Thomas, it was a joke! – although, really – ” Christian hesitated, wrinkling his nose and stooping a little. In this position he took a few steps.

“ A joke! ” shouted the Consul. “ I think I can understand a joke, but you see how your joke was understood. ‘ For my part, I have the greatest respect for my calling.’ That was what Hermann Hagenström answered you. And there you sat, a good-for-nothing, with no respect for yours – ”

“ Tom, you don’t know what you are talking about. I assure you he spoiled the whole joke. After everybody laughed, as if they agreed with me, there sat this Hagenström and brought out with ridiculous solemnity, ‘ For my part – ’ Stupid fool! I was really ashamed for him. I thought about it a long time in bed last night, and I had a quite remarkable feeling – you know how it feels – ”

“ Stop chattering, stop chattering, I beg you,” interrupted the

Consul. He trembled with disgust in his whole body. " I agree – I agree with you that his answer was not in the right key, and that it was tasteless. But that is just the kind of people you pick out to say such things to! – if it is necessary to say them at all – and so you lay yourself open to an insolent snub like that. Hagenström took the opening to – give not only you but us a slap. Do you understand what ' for my part ' meant? It meant: ' You may have such ideas going about in your brother's office, Herr Buddenbrook.' That's what it meant, you idiot."

" Idiot – ? " said Christian. He looked disturbed and embarrassed.

" And finally, you belong not to yourself alone; I'm supposed to be indifferent when you make yourself personally ridiculous – and when don't you make yourself personally ridiculous? " Thomas cried. He was pale, and the blue veins stood out on his narrow temples, from which the hair went back in two bays. One of his light eyebrows was raised; even the long, stiff pointed ends of his moustache looked angry as he threw his words down at Christian's feet on the gravel with quick sidewise gestures. " You make yourself a laughing-stock with your love affairs, your harlequinades, your diseases and your remedies."

Christian shook his head vehemently and put up a warning finger. " As far as that goes, Tom, you don't understand very well, you know. The thing is – every one must attend to his own conscience, so to speak. I don't know if you understand that. – Grabow has ordered me a salve for the throat muscles. Well – if I don't use it, if I neglect it, I am quite lost and helpless, I am restless and uncertain and worried and upset, and I can't swallow. But if I have been using it, I feel that I have done my duty, I have a good conscience, I am quiet and calm and can swallow famously. The salve does not do it, you know, but the thing is that an idea like that, you understand, can only be destroyed by another idea, an opposite one. I don't know whether you understand me – "

" Oh, yes – oh, yes! " cried the Consul, holding his head for a moment with both hands. " Do it, do it, but don't talk about it – don't gabble about it. Leave other people alone with your horrible nuances. You make yourself ridiculous with your absurd chatter from morning to night. I must tell you, and I repeat it, I am not interested in how much you make a fool of yourself personally. But I forbid your compromising the firm in the way you did yesterday evening."

Christian did not answer, except to run his hand slowly over his sparse red-brown locks, while his eyes roamed unsteadily and absently, and unrest sat upon his face. Undoubtedly he was still busy with the idea which he had just been expressing.

There was a pause. Thomas stalked along with the calmness of despair. " All business men are swindlers, you say," he began afresh. " Good. Are you tired of it? Are you sorry you are a business man? You once got permission from Father – "

" Why, Tom," said Christian reflectively, " I would really rather study. It must be nice to be in the university. One attends when one likes, at one's own free will, sits down and listens, as in the theatre – "

" As in the theatre! Yes, I think your right place is that of a comedian in a café chantant. I am not joking. I am perfectly convinced that is your secret ideal." Christian did not deny it; he merely gazed aimlessly about. " And you have the cheek to make such a remark – when you haven't the slightest notion of work, and spend your days storing up a lot of feelings and sensations and episodes you hear in the theatre and when you are loafing about, God knows where; you take these and pet them and study them and chatter about them shamelessly! "

" Yes, Tom," said Christian. He was a little depressed, and rubbed his hand again over his head. " That is true: you have expressed it quite correctly. That is the difference between us. You enjoy the theatre yourself; and you had your little affairs too, once on a time, between ourselves! And there was a time when you preferred novels and poetry and all that. But you have always known how to reconcile it with regular work and a serious life. I haven't that. I am quite used up with the other; I have nothing left over for the regular life – I don't know whether you understand – "

" Oh, so you see that? " cried Thomas, standing still and folding his arms on his breast. " You humbly admit that, and still you go on the same old way? Are you a dog, Christian? A man has some pride, by God! One doesn't live a life that one may not know how to defend oneself. But so you are. That is your character. If you can only see a thing and understand and describe it – . No, my patience is at an end, Christian." And the Consul took a quick backward step and made a gesture with his arms straight out. " It is at an end, I tell you. – You draw your pay, and stay away from the office. That isn't what irritates me. Go and trifle your life away, as you have been doing, if you choose. But you compromise us, all of us, wherever you are. You are a growth, a fester, on the body of our family. You are a disgrace to us here in this town, and if this house were mine, I'd show you the door! " he screamed, making a wild sweeping gesture over the garden, the court, and the whole property. He had no more control of himself. A long-stored-up well of hatred poured itself out.

" What is the matter with you, Thomas? " said Christian. He was seized with unaccustomed anger, standing there in a position common to bow-legged people, like a questionmark, with head, stomach, and knees all prominent. His little deep eyes were wide open and surrounded by red rims down to the cheek-bones, as his Father's used to be in anger. " How are you speaking to me? What have I done to you? I'll go, without being thrown out. Shame on you! " he added with downright reproach, accompanying the word with a short, snapping motion in front of him, as if he were catching a fly.

Strange to say, Thomas did not meet this outburst by more anger. He bent his head and slowly took his way around the garden. It seemed to quiet him, actually to do him good to have made his brother angry at last — to have pushed him finally to the energy of a protest.

" Believe me," he said quietly, putting his hands behind his back again, " this conversation is truly painful to me. But it had to take place. Such scenes in the family are frightful, but we must speak out once for all. Let us talk the thing over quietly, young one. You do not like your present position, it seems? "

" No, Tom; you are right about that. You see, at first I was very well satisfied. I know I'm better off here than in a stranger's business. But what I want is the independence, I think. I have always envied you when I saw you sit there and work, for it is really no work at all for you. You work not because you must, but as master and head, and let others work for you, and you have the control, make your calculations, and are free. It is quite different."

" Good, Christian. Why couldn't you have said that before? You can make yourself free, or freer, if you like. You know Father left you as well as me an immediate inheritance of fifty thousand marks current; and I am ready at any moment to pay out this sum for a reasonable and sound purpose. In Hamburg, or anywhere else you like, there are plenty of safe but limited firms where they could use an increase of capital, and where you could enter as a partner. Let us think the matter over quietly, each by himself, and also speak to Mother at a good opportunity. I must get to work, and you could for the present go on with the English correspondence." As they crossed the entry, he added, " What do you say, for instance, to H. C. F. Burmeester and Company in Hamburg? Import and export. I know the man. I am certain he would snap at it."

That was in the end of May of the year 1857. At the beginning of June Christian travelled via Buchen to Hamburg – a heavy loss to the club, the theatre, the Tivoli, and the liberal livers of the town. All the "good fellows," among them Dr. Gieseke and Peter Döhlmann, took leave of him at the station, and brought him flowers and cigars, and laughed to split their sides – recalling, no doubt, all the stories Christian had told them. And Lawyer Gieseke, amidst general applause, fastened to Christian's overcoat a great favour made out of gold paper. This favour came from a sort of inn in the neighbourhood of the port, a place of free and easy resort where a red lantern burned above the door at night, and it was always very lively. The favour was awarded to the departing Chris Buddenbrook for his distinguished services.

CHAPTER IV

THE OUTER bell rang, and Frau Grünlich appeared on the landing to look down into the court – a habit she had lately formed. The door was hardly opened below when she started, leaned over still more, and then sprang back with one hand pressing her handkerchief to her mouth and the other holding up her gown. She hurried upstairs.

On the steps to the second storey she met Ida Jungmann, to whom she whispered in a suffocated voice. Ida gave a joyous shriek and answered with some Polish gibberish.

The Frau Consul was sitting in the landscape room, crocheting a shawl or some such article with two large wooden needles. It was eleven o'clock in the morning.

The servant came through the hall, knocked on the glass door, and waddled in to bring the Frau Consul a visiting-card. She took the card, got out her sewing-glasses, and read it. Then she looked again at the girl's red face; then read again; then looked up again at the girl. Finally she said calmly but firmly:

"What *is* this, my dear? What does it mean?"

On the card was printed: "X. Noppe and Company." The "X. Noppe" and the "and" were crossed out with a lead-pencil, so that only the "Company" was left. "Oh, Frau Consul," said the maid, "there's a gentleman, but he doesn't speak German, and he do go on so –"

"Ask the gentleman in," said the Frau Consul; for she understood now that it was the "Company" who desired admittance. The maid went. Then the glass door was opened again to let in a stocky figure, who remained in the shadowy background of the room for a moment and said with a drawling pronunciation something that seemed as if it might have been: "I have the honour –"

"Good morning," said the Frau Consul. "Will you not come in?" And she supported herself on the sofa-cushion and rose a little; for she did not know yet whether she ought to rise all the way or not.

"I take the liberty," replied the gentleman in a pleasant sing-song; while he bowed in the politest manner, and took two steps forward. Then he stood still again and looked around as if searching for something – perhaps for a place to put his hat and stick, for he had brought both – the stick being a horn crutch with the top shaped like a claw and a good foot and a half long – into the room with him.

He was a man of forty years. Short-legged and chubby, he wore a wide-open coat of brown frieze and a light flowered waistcoat which covered the gentle protuberant curve of his stomach and supported a gold watch-chain with a whole bouquet of charms made of horn, bone, silver, and coral. His trousers were of an indefinite grey-green colour and too short. The material must have been extraordinarily stiff, for the edges stood out in a circle around the legs of his short, broad boots. He had a bullet head, untidy hair, and a stubby nose, and the light-blond curly moustache drooping over his mouth made him look like a walrus. By way of contrast, the imperial between his chin and his underlip stood out rather bristly. His cheeks were extremely fat and puffy, crowding his eyes into two narrow light-blue cracks with wrinkles at the corners. The whole face looked swollen and had a funny expression of fierceness, mingled with an almost touching good nature. Directly below his tiny chin a steep line ran into the white neck-cloth: his goiterous neck could not have endured a choker. In fact, the whole lower part of his face and his neck, the back of his head, his cheeks and nose, all ran rather formlessly in together. The whole skin of the face was stretched to an immoderate tightness and showed a roughness at the ear-joinings and the sides of the nose. In one of his short fat white hands the visitor held his stick; in the other his green Tyrolese hat, decorated with a chamois beard.

The Frau Consul had taken off her glasses and was still rising from her sofa-pillow.

" What can I do for you? " she asked politely but pointedly.

The gentleman, with a movement of decision, laid his hat and stick on the lid of the harmonium. He rubbed his free hands with satisfaction and looked at the Frau Consul out of his kindly, light-blue eyes. " I beg the gracious lady's pardon for the card," he said. " I had no other by me. My name is Permaneder – Alois Permaneder, from Munich. Perhaps you might have heard my name from your daughter." He said all this in a puzzling dialect with a rather loud, coarse voice; but there was a confidential gleam from the cracks of his eyes, which seemed to say: " I'm sure we understand each other already."

The Frau Consul had now risen entirely and went forward with her hand outstretched and her head inclined in greeting.

" Herr Permaneder! Is it you? Certainly my daughter has spoken of you. I know how much you contributed to make her visit in Munich pleasant and entertaining. And so some wind has blown you all the way up here? "

" That's it; you're just right there," said Herr Permaneder. He sat down by the Frau Consul in the armchair which she gracefully indicated to him, and began to rub his short round thighs comfortably with both hands.

" I beg your pardon? " asked the Frau Consul. She had not understood a single word of his remark.

" You've guessed it, that's the point," answered Herr Permaneder, as he stopped rubbing his knees.

" How nice! " said the Frau Consul blankly. She leaned back in her chair with feigned satisfaction and folded her hands. Actually, she was quite as much at sea as before, and inly wondering if Antonie were really able to follow the windings of the Bavarian tongue. But Herr Permaneder – though his appearance hardly led one to expect that he possessed acute sensibilities – saw through her at once. He bent forward, making – God knows why – circles in the air with his hand, and, struggling after clarity, enunciated the words: " The gracious lady is surprised? "

" Yes, Herr Permaneder, yes! " she cried, with disproportionate joy, for she had really understood him. Perhaps they could manage after all! But now there came a pause. To fill it out, Herr Permaneder gave a sort of groan, and followed it up by an exclamation in the broadest of dialect: something that shocked the Frau Consul because it sounded so like swearing, though it probably wasn't – at least, she hoped not! Should she ask him to repeat it?

" Ah – what did you say? " she ventured, turning her light eyes a little away, that he might not see the bewilderment they expressed.

Herr Permaneder obliged by repeating, with extraordinary loudness and coarseness. Surely it was something about a crucifix! Horrors!

" How nice! " she stammered again, with desperate finality; and thus this subject also was disposed of. It might be better to talk a little oneself. " May one ask," she went on, " what brings you so far, Herr Permaneder? It is a good long journey from Munich."

" A little business," said Herr Permaneder, as before, and waved his broad hand in the air. It was really touching, the efforts he made. " A little business, my dear lady, with the brewery at Walkmill."

" Oh, yes – you are hop merchants, of course, my dear Herr Permaneder: Noppe and Company, isn't it? I am sure I have heard good things of your firm from my son," said the Frau Consul cordially. Again she felt as if she were almost upon firm ground. Herr Permaneder waved away the compliment. That was nothing to mention. No, the main thing was, he wanted to pay his respects to the Frau Consul and – see Frau Grünlich again. That was enough to make the journey repay the trouble it cost.

The Frau Consul did not understand it all, but she got the general drift, and was glad. " Oh, thank you," she said, with the utmost heartiness, and again offered him her hand, with the palm outstretched.

" But we must call my daughter," she added, and stood up and went toward the embroidered bell-pull near the glass door.

" Oh, Lord, yes, I'll be glad to see her! " cried the hop merchant, and turned his chair and himself toward the door at one and the same time.

The Frau Consul said to the servant: " Ask Madame Grünlich to come down, my dear."

Then she went back to her sofa, and Herr Permaneder turned himself and his chair around again.

" Lord, yes, I'll be glad! " he repeated, while he stared at the hangings and the furniture and the great Sèvres inkstand on the escritoire. But then he sighed heavily, several times over, rubbed his knees, and gave vent to his favourite outlandish phrase. The Frau Consul thought it more discreet not to inquire again into his meaning; besides, he muttered it under his breath, with a sort of groan, though his mood, otherwise, appeared to be anything but despondent.

And now Frau Grünlich appeared. She had made a little toilette, put on a light blouse, and dressed her hair. Her face looked fresher and prettier than ever, and the tip of her tongue played in the corner of her mouth.

Scarcely had she entered when Herr Permaneder sprang up and went to meet her with tremendous enthusiasm. He vibrated all over. He seized both her hands, shook them and cried: " Well, Frau Grünlich! Well, well, *grüss Gott!* Well, and how's it been going with you? What you been doing up here? Yes, yes! *Grüss Gott!* Lord, I'm just silly glad to see you. Do you think sometimes of little old Munich and what a gay time we had? Oh, my, oh, my! And here we are again. Who would 'a' thought it? "

Tony, on her side, greeted him with great vivacity, drew up a chair, and began to chat with him about her weeks in Munich. Now the conversation went on without hitches, and the Frau Consul followed it, smiling and nodding encouragingly at Herr Permaneder. She would translate this or that expression into her own tongue, and then lean back into the sofa again, well pleased with her own intelligence.

Herr Permaneder had to explain to Frau Antonie in her turn the reason of his appearance. But he laid small stress on the "little business" with the brewery, and it was obviously not the occasion of his visit at all. He asked with interest after the second daughter and the sons of the Frau Consul, and regretted loudly the absence of Clara and Christian, as he had always wanted to get acquainted with the whole family.

He said his stay in the town was of indefinite length, but when the Frau Consul said: "I am expecting my son for second breakfast at any moment, Herr Permaneder. Will you give us the pleasure of your company?" he accepted the invitation almost before she gave it, with such alacrity that it was plain he had expected it.

The Consul came. He had found the breakfast-room empty, and appeared in his office coat, tired and preoccupied, to take a hasty bite. But when he saw the strange guest with the frieze jacket and the fantastic watch-chain, he became all charm. He had heard his name often enough from Frau Antonie, and he threw a quick glance at his sister as he greeted Herr Permaneder in his most fascinating manner. He did not sit down. They went directly down to the entresol, where Mamsell Jungmann had laid the table and set the samovar – a real samovar, a present from Pastor Tiburtius and Clara.

"You've got it good here," said Herr Permaneder, as he let himself down in his chair and looked at the variety of cold meats on the table. His grammar, now and then, was of the most artless and disarming quality.

"It isn't Munich beer, of course, Herr Permaneder, but still it is better than our domestic brew." And the Consul poured him a glass of the brown foaming porter, which he was accustomed to drink himself at midday.

"Thank you kindly, neighbour," said Herr Permaneder, quite unaware of the outraged look Mamsell Jungmann cast at him. But he drank so moderately of the porter that the Frau Consul had a bottle of red wine brought up; whereat he grew visibly gayer and began to talk with Frau Grünlich again. He sat, on account of his prominent stomach, well away from the table, with his legs far apart, and one of his arms, with the plump white hand, hanging down over the chair-back. He put his round head with its walrus moustache on one side and blinked out of the cracks of his eyes naïvely as he listened to Tony's conversation. He looked offensively comfortable. As he had had no experience with sprats, she daintily dismembered them for him, commenting the while on life in general.

"Oh, Heavens, how sad it is, Herr Permaneder, that everything good and lovely in this world is so fleeting," she said, referring to her Munich visit. She laid down her knife and fork a moment and looked earnestly up at the ceiling. She made charming if unsuccessful efforts to speak Bavarian.

During the meal there was a knock at the door, and the office boy brought in a telegram. The Consul read it, letting the long ends of his moustache run through his fingers. He was plainly preoccupied with the contents of the message; but, even as he read it, he asked in the easiest tone: "Well, how is business, Herr Permaneder? – That will do," he said immediately to the apprentice, who disappeared.

"Oh, well, neighbour," answered Herr Permaneder, turning himself about toward the Consul's side with the awkwardness of a man who has a thick, stiff neck, and letting his other arm hang over the chair-back. "There's naught to speak of – it's a fair plague. You see, Munich" – he pronounced the name of his native city in such a way that one could only guess what he meant – "Munich is no commercial town. Everybody wants his peace and quiet and his beer – nobody gets despatches while he's eating; not there. You're a different cut up here – Holy Sacrament! Yes, thank you kindly, I'll take another glass. Tough luck, that's what it is; tough luck. My partner, Noppe, wanted to go to Nuremberg, because they have a Bourse there and are keen on business, but I won't forsake my Munich. Not me! That would be a fine thing to do! You see, there's no competition, and the export trade is just silly. Even in Russia they'll be beginning soon to plant and build for themselves."

Then he suddenly threw the Consul a quick, shrewd look and said: "Oh, well, neighbour, 'tain't so bad as it sounds. Yon's a fair little business. We make money with the joint-stock brewery, that Niederpaur is director of. That was just a small affair, but we've put it on its legs and lent it credit – cash too, four per cent on security – and now we can do business at a profit, and we've collared a blame good trade already." Herr Permaneder declined cigars and cigarettes and asked leave to smoke his pipe. He drew the long horn bowl out of his pocket, enveloped himself in a reek of smoke, and entered upon a business conversation with the Consul, which glided into politics, and Bavaria's relations with Prussia, and King Max, and the Emperor Napoleon. He garnished his views with disjointed sighs and some perfectly unintelligible Munich phrases.

Mamsell Jungmann, out of sheer astonishment, continually forgot to chew, even when she had food in her mouth. She blinked speechlessly at the guest out of her bright brown eyes, standing her knife and fork perpendicularly on the table and swaying them back and forth. This room had never before beheld Herr Permaneder's like. Never had it been filled by such reeking pipesmoke; such unpleasantly easy manners were foreign to it. The Frau Consul abode in cordial miscomprehension, after she had made inquiries and received information as to the sufferings of the little protestant oasis among the Munich papists. Tony seemed to grow somewhat absent and restive in the course of the meal. But the Consul was highly entertained, asked his mother to order up another bottle of wine, and cordially invited Herr Permaneder to a visit in Broad Street – his wife would be charmed. A good three hours after his arrival the hop dealer began to show signs of leaving – emptied his glass, knocked out his pipe, called something or other " bad luck," and got up.

" I have the honour, madame. Good day, Frau Grünli' and Herr Consul – servant, servant." At this Ida Jungmann actually shivered and changed colour. " Good day, Freilein," he said to her, and he repeated " Good day " at the door.

The Frau Consul and her son exchanged a glance. Herr Permaneder had announced his intention of stopping at the modest inn on the Trave whither he had gone on arrival. The Frau Consul went toward him again. " My daughter's Munich friend," she began, " lives so far away that we shall have no opportunity to repay her hospitality. But if you, my dear sir, would give us the pleasure of your company while you are in town – you would be very welcome." She held her hand out to him; and lo! Herr Permaneder accepted this invitation as blithely as he had the one to dinner. He kissed the hands of both ladies – and a funny sight he was as he did so – fetched his hat and stick from the landscape room, and promised to have his trunk brought at once and to be on the spot at four o'clock, after transacting his business. Then he allowed the Consul to convoy him down the stairs. But even at the vestibule door he turned again and shook hands violently. " No offience, neighbour," he said – " your sister is certainly a great girl – no doubt about it. Good day," and he disappeared, still wagging his head.

The Consul felt an irresistible drawing to go up again and see the ladies. Ida Jungmann had gone to look after the linen for the guest-room. The Frau Consul still sat at the breakfast table, her light eyes fixed on a spot on the ceiling. She was lightly drumming with her white fingers on the cloth. Tony sat at the window, her arms folded, gazing straight ahead of her with a severe air. Silence reigned.

"Well?" said Thomas, standing in the door and taking a cigarette out of the box ornamented with the troika. His shoulders shook with laughter.

"A pleasant man," commented the Frau Consul innocently.

"Quite my opinion." The Consul made a quick, humorous turn toward Tony, as if he were asking her in the most respectful manner for her opinion as well. She was silent, and looked neither to the right nor to the left.

"But I think, Tom, he ought to stop swearing," went on the Frau Consul with mild disapproval. "If I understood him correctly, he kept using the words Sacrament and Cross."

"Oh, that's nothing, Mother – he doesn't mean anything by that."

"And perhaps a little too easy-mannered, Tom?"

"Oh, yes; that is south-German," said the Consul, breathing the smoke slowly out into the room. He smiled at his mother and stole glances at Tony. His mother saw the glances not at all.

"You will come to dinner to-day with Gerda. Please do me the favour, Tom."

"Certainly, Mother, with the greatest of pleasure. To tell the truth, I promise myself much pleasure from this guest, don't you? He is something different from your ministers, in any case."

"Everybody to his taste, Tom."

"Of course. I must go now. – Oh, Tony," he said, the door-handle in his hand, "you have made a great impression on him. No, no joke. Do you know what he called you down there just now? A great girl! Those were his very words."

But here Frau Grünlich turned around and said clearly: "Very good, Tom. You are repeating his words – and I don't know that he would mind; but even so I am not sure it was just the nicest thing to do. But this much I do know: and this much I am going to say: that in this life it does not depend on how things are said and expresed, but on how they are felt and meant in the heart; and if you make fun of Herr Permaneder's language and find him ridiculous – "

"Who? Why? Tony, what an idea! Why are you getting excited – ? "

"*Assez,*" said the Frau Consul, casting an imploring glance at her son. It meant "Spare her! "

"Please don't be angry, Tony," he said. "I didn't mean to provoke you. And now I will go and see that somebody from the warehouse brings Herr Permaneder's trunk. Au revoir."

CHAPTER V

Herr Permaneder moved into Meng Street; he ate dinner with Thomas Buddenbrook and his wife the following day; and on the third, a Thursday, he made the acquaintance of Justus Kröger and his wife, the three ladies from Broad Street, who found him "frightfully funny" (they said fr-*right*fully), Sesemi Weichbrodt, who was rather stern with him, and poor Clothilde and little Erica, to whom he gave a bag of bonbons.

The man was invincibly good-humoured. His sighs, in fact, meant nothing, and seemed to arise out of an excess of comfort. He smoked his pipe, talked in his curious dialect, and displayed an inexhaustible power of sitting still. He kept his place long after the meal was finished, in the most easy attitude possible, and smoked, drank, and chatted. His presence gave to the life in the old home a new and strange tone; his very being brought something unharmonious into the room. But he disturbed none of the traditional customs of the house. He was faithful to morning and evening prayers, asked permission to attend one of the Frau Consul's Sunday School classes, and even appeared on a Jerusalem evening in the drawing-room and was presented to the guests, but withdrew affrighted when Lea Gerhardt began to read aloud.

He was soon known in the town. They spoke in the great houses about the Buddenbrooks' guest from Bavaria; but neither in the family nor on the Bourse did he make connections, and as it was already the time when people were making ready to go to the shore, the Consul refrained from introducing Herr Permaneder into society. But he devoted himself with zeal to the guest, taking time from his business and civic engagements to show him about the town and point out the mediæval monuments – churches, gates, fountains, market, Town Hall, and Ship Company. He made him acquainted with his own nearest friends on Exchange and entertained him in every way. His mother took occasion one day to thank him for his self-sacrifice; but he only remarked drily: "Why, ye-es, Mother – what wouldn't one do?"

The Frau Consul left this unanswered. She did not even smile or move her eyelids, but shifted the gaze of her light eyes and changed the subject.

She preserved an even, hearty friendliness toward Herr Permaneder – which could hardly be said of her daughter. On the third or fourth day after his arrival the hop dealer let it be known that he had concluded his business with the local brewery. But a week and a half had passed since then, and he had been present for two children's afternoons. On these occasions, Frau Grünlich had sat blushing and watching his every motion, casting quick embarrassed glances at Thomas and the three Buddenbrook cousins. She talked hardly at all, sat for long minutes stiff and speechless, or even got up and left the room.

The green blinds in Frau Grünlich's sleeping-room were gently stirred by the mild air of a June night, for the windows were open. It was a large room, with simple furniture covered in grey linen. On the night table at the side of the high bed several little wicks burned in a glass with oil and water in it, filling the room with faint, even light. Frau Grünlich was in bed. Her pretty head was sunk softly in the lace-edged pillow, and her hands lay folded on the quilted coverlet. But her eyes, too thoughtful to close themselves, slowly followed the movements of a large insect with a long body, which perpetually besieged the glass with a million soundless motions of his wings. Near the bed there was a framed text hanging on the wall, between two old copper-plate views of the town in the Middle Ages. It said: "Commit your ways unto the Lord." But what good is a text like that when you are lying awake at midnight, and you have to decide for your whole life, and other people's too, whether it shall be yes or no?

It was very still. The clock ticked away on the wall, and the only other sound was Mamsell Jungmann's occasional cough. Her room was next to Tony's, divided only by curtains from it. She still had a light. The born-and-bred Prussian was sitting under the hanging lamp at her extension-table, darning stockings for little Erica. The child's deep, peaceful breathing could be heard in the room, for Sesemi's pupils were having summer holidays and Erica was at home again.

Frau Grünlich sighed and sat up a little, propping her head on her hand. "Ida," she called softly, "are you still sitting there mending?"

"Yes, yes, Tony, my child," Ida answered. "Sleep now; you will be getting up early in the morning, and you won't get enough rest."

“ All right, Ida. You will wake me at six o’clock? ”

“ Half past is early enough, child. The carriage is ordered for eight. Go on sleeping, so you will look fresh and pretty.”

“ Oh, I haven’t slept at all yet.”

“ Now, Tony, that is a bad child. Do you want to look all knocked up for the picnic? Drink seven swallows of water, and then lie down and count a thousand.”

“ Oh, Ida, do come here a minute. I can’t sleep, I tell you, and my head aches for thinking. Feel – I think I have some fever, and there is something the matter with my tummy again. Or is it because I am anæmic? The veins in my temples are all swollen and they beat so that it hurts; but still, there may be too little blood in my head.”

A chair was pushed back, and Ida Jungmann’s lean, vigorous figure, in her unfashionable brown gown, appeared between the portières.

“ Now, now, Tony – fever? Let me feel, my child – I’ll make you a compress.”

She went with her long firm masculine tread to the chest for a handkerchief, dipped it into the water-basin, and, going back to the bed, laid it on Tony’s forehead, stroking her brow a few times with both hands.

“ Thank you, Ida; that feels good. – Oh, please sit down a few minutes, good old Ida. Sit down on the edge of the bed. You see, I keep thinking the whole time about to-morrow. What shall I do? My head is going round and round.”

Ida sat down beside her, with her needle and the stocking drawn over the darner again in her hand, and bent over them the smooth grey head and the indefatigable bright brown eyes. “ Do you think he is going to propose to-morrow? ” she asked.

“ No doubt of it at all. He won’t lose this opportunity. It happened with Clara on just such an expedition. I could avoid it, of course, I could keep with the others all the time and not let him get near me. But then, that would settle it! He is leaving day after to-morrow, he said, and he cannot stay any longer if nothing comes of it to-day. It *must* be decided to-day. – But what shall I say, Ida, when he asks me? You’ve never been married, so of course you know nothing about life, *really;* but you are a truthful woman, and you have some sense – and you are forty-two years old! Do tell me what you think. – I do so need advice! ”

Ida Jungmann let the stocking fall into her lap.

“ Yes, yes, Tony child, I have thought a great deal about it. But what I think is, there is nothing to advise about. He can’t go away without speaking to you and your Mamma, and if you didn't want him, you should have sent him away before now."

"You are right there, Ida; but I could not do it – I suppose because it *is to be!* But now I keep thinking: 'It isn't too late yet; I can still draw back!' So I am lying here tormenting myself – "

"Do you like him, Tony? Tell me straight out."

"Yes, Ida. It would not be the truth if I should say no. He is not handsome – but that isn't the important thing in this life; and he is as good as gold, and couldn't do anything mean – at least, he seems so to me. When I think about Grünlich – oh, goodness! He was all the time saying how clever and resourceful he was, and all the time hiding his villainy. Permaneder is not in the least like that. You might say he is too easy-going and takes life too comfortably – and that is a fault too; because he will never be a millionaire that way, and he really is too much inclined to let things go and muddle along – as they say down there. They are all like that down there, Ida – that is what I mean. In Munich, where he was among his own kind and everybody spoke and looked as he does, I fairly loved him, he seemed so nice and faithful and comfy. And I noticed it was mutual – but part of that, I dare say, was that he takes me for a rich woman, richer probably than I am; because Mother cannot do much more for me, as you know. But I hardly think that will make much difference to him – a great lot of money would not be to his taste. – But – what was I saying, Ida? "

"That is in Munich, Tony. But here – "

"Oh, here, Ida! You know how it was already: up here he was torn right out of his own element and set against everybody here, and they are all ever so much stiffer, and – more dignified and serious. Here I really often blush for him, though it may be unworthy of me. You know – it even happened several times that he said 'me' instead of 'I.' But they say that down there; even the most cultured people do, and it doesn't hurt anything – it slips out once in a while and nobody minds. But up here – here sits Mother on one side and Tom on the other, looking at him and lifting their eyebrows, and Uncle Justus gives a start and fairly snorts, the way the Krögers do, and Pfiffi Buddenbrook gives her Mother a look, or Friederike or Henriette, and I feel so mortified I want to run out of the room, and it doesn't seem as if I *could* marry him – "

"Oh, childie – it would be Munich that you would live in with him."

"You are right, Ida. But the engagement! – and if I have to

feel the whole time mortified to death before the family and the Kistenmakers and the Möllendorpfs, because they think he is common – Oh, Grünlich was much more refined, though he was certainly black within, as Herr Stengel would have said. – Oh, Ida, my head! do wet the compress again."

"But it must be so, in the end," she went on again, drawing a long breath as the compress went on; "for the main point is and remains that I must get married again, and not stick about here any longer as a divorced woman. Ah, Ida, I think so much about the past these days: about the time when Grünlich first appeared, and the scenes he made me – scandalous, Ida! – and then about Travemünde and the Schwarzkopfs –" She spoke slowly, and her eyes rested for a while dreamily on a darn in Erica's stocking. "And then the betrothal, and Eimsbüttel, and our house. It was quite elegant, Ida. When I think of my morning-gowns – It would not be like that with Permaneder; one gets more modest as life goes on – And Dr. Klaasen and the baby, and Banker Kesselmeyer – and then the end. It was frightful; you can't imagine how frightful it was. And when you have had such dreadful experiences in life – But Permaneder would never go in for anything filthy like that. That is the last thing in the world I should expect of him, and we can rely on him too in a business way, for I really think he makes a good deal with Noppe at the Niederpaur brewery. And when I am his wife, you'll see, Ida, I will take care that he has ambition and gets ahead and makes an effort and is a credit to me and all of us. *That*, at least, he takes upon himself when he marries a Buddenbrook!"

She folded her hands under her head and looked at the ceiling. "Yes, ten years ago and more, I married Grünlich. Ten years! And here I am at the same place again, saying yes to somebody else. You know, Ida, life is very, very serious. Only the difference is that then it was a great affair, and they all pressed me and tormented me, whereas now they are all perfectly quiet and take it for granted that I am going to say yes. Of course you know, Ida, that this engagement to Alois – I say Alois, because of course it is to be – has nothing very gay or festive about it, and it isn't really a question of my happiness at all. I am making this second marriage with my eyes open, to make good the mistake of my first one, as a duty which I owe our name. Mother thinks so, and so does Tom."

"But oh, dear, Tony – if you don't like him, and if he won't make you happy –"

"Ida, I know life, and I am not a little goose any more. I have the use of my senses. I don't say that Mother would actually insist on it – when there is a dispute over anything she usually avoids it and says '*Assez!*' But Tom wants it. I know Tom. He thinks: 'Anybody! Anybody who isn't absolutely impossible.' For this time it is not a question of a brilliant match, but just one that will make good the other one. That is what he thinks. As soon as Permaneder appeared, you may be sure that Tom made all the proper inquiries about his business, and found it was all right – and then, as far as he was concerned, the matter was settled. Tom is a politician – he knows what he wants. Who was it threw Christian out? That is strong language, Ida, but that was really the truth of it. And why? Because he was compromising the firm and the family. And in his eyes I do the same thing – not with words or acts, but by my very existence as a divorced woman. He wants that put an end to, and he is right. I love him none the less for that – nor, I hope, does he me. In all these years, I have always longed to be out in the world again; it is so dull here in this house. God punish me if that is a sin: but I am not much more than thirty, and I still feel young. People differ about that. You had grey hair at thirty, like all your family and that uncle that died at Marienwerder."

More and more observations of the same kind followed as the night wore on; and every now and again she would say: "It is to be, after all." But at length she went to sleep, and slept for five hours on end, deeply and peacefully.

CHAPTER VI

A MIST lay over the town. But – or so said Herr Longuet, the livery man in John Street, as he himself drove the covered char-à-banc up to the door of the house in Meng Street: " The sun will be out before an hour is over " – which was most encouraging.

The Frau Consul, Antonie, Herr Permaneder, Erica, and Ida had breakfast together and gathered one after another, ready for the expedition, in the great entry, to wait for Gerda and Tom. Frau Grünlich, in a cream-coloured frock with a satin tie, looked her best, despite the loss of sleep the night before. Her doubts and fears seemed to be laid to rest, and her manner was assured, calm, and almost formal as she talked with their guest and fastened her glove-button. She had regained the tone of the old days. The well-known conviction of her own importance, of the weightiness of her own decisions, the consciousness that once more a day had come when she was to inscribe herself decisively in the family history – all this filled her heart and made it beat higher. She had dreamed of seeing that page in the family papers on which she would write down the fact of her betrothal – the fact that should obliterate and make void the black spot which the page contained. She looked forward to the moment when Tom would appear and she would greet him with a meaning nod.

He came with his wife, somewhat tardily, for the young Frau Consul was not used to make such an early toilette. He looked well and happy in his light-brown checked suit, the broad revers of which showed the white waistcoat beneath; and his eyes had a smile in them as he noted Tony's incomparably dignified mien. Gerda, with her slightly exotic, even morbid beauty, which was always in great contrast to her sister-in-law's healthy prettiness, was not in a holiday mood. Probably she had risen too early. The deep lilac background of her frock suited oddly with her dark-red hair and made her skin look whiter and more even-toned than ever, and the bluish shadows deeper and darker in the corners of her close-set brown eyes. She rather coldly offered her mother-in-law her brow to kiss, gave her hand to Herr Permaneder with an almost ironical expression on her face, and answered only by a deprecating smile when Tony clapped her hands and cried out in her hearty way: " Oh, Gerda, how *lovely* you always look! "

She had a real distaste for expeditions like to-day's, especially in summer and most especially on Sunday. She lived in the twilight of her curtained living-rooms, and dreaded the sun, the dust, the crowds of townsfolk in their holiday clothes, the smell of coffee, beer, and tobacco; and above everything else in the world she hated getting hot and upset. When the expedition to Swartau and the " Giant Bush " was arranged, in order to give the Munich guest a glimpse of the surroundings of the old town, Gerda said lightly to her husband: " Dearest, you know how I am made: I only like peace and quiet. I was not meant for change and excitement. You'll let me off, won't you? "

She would not have married him if she had not felt sure of his essential agreement with her in these matters.

" Oh, heavens, yes; you are right, of course, Gerda. It is mostly imagination that one enjoys oneself on such parties. Still, one goes, because one does not like to seem odd, either to oneself or to the others. Everybody has that kind of vanity; don't you think so? People get the idea that you are solitary or else unhappy, and they have less respect for you. And then, there is something else, Gerda dear. We all want to pay a little court to Herr Permaneder. Of course you see what the situation is. Something is going on; it would be a real pity if it came to nothing."

" I do not see, my dear friend, why my presence – but no matter. Let it be as you wish. Let us indulge."

They went into the street. And the sun actually began at that moment to pierce the morning mist. The bells of St. Mary's were ringing for Sunday, and the twittering of birds filled the air. The coachman took off his hat, and the Frau Consul greeted him with the patriarchal kindness which sometimes put Thomas a little on edge: " Good morning, my friend! – Well, get in now, my dears. It is just time for early service, but to-day we will praise God with full hearts in his own free out-of-doors; shall we not, Herr Permaneder? "

" That's right, Frau Consul."

They climbed one after another up the steps through the narrow back door of the wagon and made themselves comfortable on the cushioned seats, which – doubtless in honour of Herr Permaneder – were striped blue and white, the Bavarian colours. The door slammed, Herr Longuet clucked to the horses and shouted " Gee " and " Haw," the strong brown beasts tugged at the harness, and the wagon rolled down Meng Street along the Trave and out the Holsten gate and then to the right along the Swartau Road.

Fields, meadows, tree-clumps, farmyards. They stared up into the high, thin blue mist above them for the larks they heard singing there. Thomas, smoking his cigarette, looked about keenly, and when they came to the grain he called Herr Permaneder's attention to its condition. The hop dealer was in a mood of childlike anticipation. He had perched his green hat with the goat's beard on the side of his head, and was balancing his big stick with the horn handle on the palm of his broad white hand and even on his underlip – a feat which, though he never quite succeeded in accomplishing it, was always greeted with applause from little Erica. He repeated over and over remarks like: " 'Twon't be the Zugspitz, but we'll climb a bit and have a little lark – kind of a little old spree, hey, Frau Grünli'? "

Then he began to relate with much liveliness stories of mountain-climbing with knapsack and alpenstock, the Frau Consul rewarding him with many an admiring " You don't say! " He came by some train of thought or other to Christian, and expressed the most lively regret for his absence – he had heard what a jolly chap he was.

" He varies," the Consul said drily. " On a party like this he is inimitable, it is true. – We shall have crabs to eat, Herr Permaneder," he said in a livelier tone; " crabs and Baltic shrimps! You have had them a few times already at my Mother's, but friend Dieckmann, the owner of the 'Giant Bush,' serves especially fine ones. And ginger-nuts, the famous ginger-nuts of these parts. Has their fame reached even as far as the Isar? Well, you shall try them."

Two or three times Frau Grünlich stopped the wagon to pick poppies and corn-flowers by the roadside, and each time Herr Permaneder testified to his desire to get out and help her, if it were not for his slight nervousness at climbing in and out of the wagon.

Erica rejoiced at every crow she saw; and Ida Jungmann, wearing her mackintosh and carrying her umbrella, as she always did even in the most settled weather, rejoiced with her like a good governess who shares not only outwardly but inwardly in the childish emotions of her charge. She entered heartily into Erica's pleasure, with her rather loud laugh that sounded like a horse neighing. Gerda, who had not seen her growing grey in the family service, looked at her repeatedly with cold surprise.

They were in Oldenberg. The beech groves came in sight.

They drove through the village, across the market square with its well, and out again into the country, over the bridge that spanned the little river Au, and finally drew up in front of the one-story inn, " The Giant Bush." It stood at the side of a flat open space laid out with lawns and sandy paths and country flower-beds; beyond it, the forest rose gradually like an amphitheatre. Each stage was reached by rude steps formed from the natural rocks and tree roots; and on each one white-painted tables, benches, and chairs stood placed among the trees.

The Buddenbrooks were by no means the first guests. A couple of plump maids and a waiter in a greasy dress-coat were hurrying about the square carrying cold meat, lemonades, milk, and beer up to the tables, even the more remote ones, which were already occupied by several families with children.

Herr Dieckmann, the landlord, appeared personally, in shirt-sleeves and a little yellow-embroidered cap, to help the guests dismount, and Longuet drove off to unhitch. The Frau Consul said: " My good man, we will take our walk first, and after an hour or so we should like luncheon served up above – but not too high up; say perhaps at the second landing."

" You must show what you are made of, Herr Dieckmann," added the Consul. " We have a guest who is used to good living."

" Oh, no such thing," Herr Permaneder protested. " A beer and cheese – "

But Herr Dieckmann could not understand him, and began with great fluency: " Everything we have, Herr Consul: crabs, shrimps, all sorts of sausages, all sorts of cheese, smoked eel, smoked salmon, smoked sturgeon – "

" Fine, Dieckmann; give us what you have. And then – six glasses of milk and a glass of beer – if I am not mistaken, Herr Permaneder? "

" One beer, six milks – sweet milk, buttermilk, sour milk, clotted milk, Herr Consul? "

" Half and half, Herr Dieckmann: sweet milk and buttermilk. In an hour, then." They went across the square.

" First, Herr Permaneder, it is our duty to visit the spring," said Thomas. " The spring, that is to say, is the source of the Au; and the Au is the tiny little river on which Swartau lies, and on which, in the grey Middle Ages, our own town was situated – until it burned down. There was probably nothing very permanent about it at that time, and it was rebuilt again, on the Trave. But there are painful recollections connected with the Au. When we were schoolboys we used to pinch each other's arms and say:

'What is the name of the river at Swartau?' Of course, it hurt, and the involuntary answer was the right one. – Look!" he interrupted himself suddenly, ten steps from the ascent, "they've got ahead of us." It was the Möllendorpfs and the Hagenströms.

There, on the third landing of the wooded terrace, sat the principal members of those affiliated families, at two tables shoved close together, eating and talking with the greatest gusto. Old Senator Möllendorpf presided, a pallid gentleman with thin, pointed white mutton-chops; he suffered from diabetes. His wife, born Langhals, wielded her lorgnon; and, as usual, her hair stood up untidily all over her head. Her son Augustus was a blond young man with a prosperous exterior, and there was Julie his wife, born Hagenström, little and lively, with great blank black eyes and diamond earrings that were nearly as large. She sat between her brothers, Hermann and Moritz. Consul Hermann Hagenström had begun to get very stout with good living: people said he began the day with *paté de foie gras.* He wore a full, short reddish-blond beard, and he had his mother's nose, which came down quite flat on the upper lip. Dr. Moritz was narrow-chested and yellow-skinned, and he talked very gaily, showing pointed teeth with gaps between them. Both brothers had their ladies with them – for the lawyer had married, some years since, a Fräulein Puttfarken from Hamburg, a lady with butter-coloured hair and wonderful cold, regular, English features of more than common beauty; Dr. Hagenström had not been able to reconcile with his reputation as connoisseur the idea of taking a plain wife. And, finally, there were the little daughter of Hermann and the little son of Moritz, two white-frocked children, already as good as betrothed to each other, for the Huneus-Hagenström money must be kept together, of course. They all sat there eating ham and scrambled eggs.

Greetings were exchanged when the Buddenbrook party passed at a little distance the company seated at the table. The Frau Consul bowed confusedly; Thomas lifted his hat, his lips moving in a courteous and conventional greeting, and Gerda inclined her head with formal politeness. But Herr Permaneder, stimulated by the climb, swung his green hat unaffectedly and shouted in a loud, bluff voice: "Hearty good morning to all of you!" whereat Frau Senator Möllendorpf made use of her lorgnon. Tony, for her part, flung back her head and tucked in her chin as much as possible, while her shoulders went up ever so slightly, and she greeted the party as if from some remote height – which meant that she stared straight ahead directly over the broad brim of Julie Möllendorpf's elegant hat. Precisely at this moment, her decision of the night before became fixed, unalterable resolve.

"Thanks be to goodness, Tom, we are not going to eat for another hour. I'd hate to have that Julie watching us. Did you see how she spoke? Hardly at all. I only had a glimpse of her hat, but it looked frightfully bad taste."

"Well, as far as that goes, I don't know about the hat – but you were certainly not much more cordial than she was, my love. And don't get irritated – it makes for wrinkles."

"Irritated, Tom? Not at all. If these people think they are the first and foremost, why, one can only laugh at them, that's all. What difference is there between this Julie and me, if it comes to that? She only drew a fool, instead of a knave, for a husband; and if she were in my position now, we should see if she would find another one."

"How can you tell that you will find another one?"

"A fool, Thomas?"

"Very much better than a knave."

"It doesn't have to be either. But it is not a fit subject for discussion."

"Quite right. The others are ahead of us – Herr Permaneder is climbing lustily."

The shady forest road grew level, and it was not long before they reached the "spring," a pretty, romantic spot with a wooden bridge over a little ravine, steep cliffs, and overhanging trees with their roots in the air. The Frau Consul had brought a silver collapsible cup, and they scooped up the water from the little stone basin directly under the source and refreshed themselves with the iron-impregnated spring. And here Herr Permaneder had a slight attack of gallantry, and insisted on Frau Grünlich tasting his cup before presenting it to him. He ran over with friendliness and displayed great tact in chatting with the Frau Consul and Thomas, as well as with Gerda and Tony, and even with little Erica. Gerda, who had up to now been suffering from the heat and a kind of silent and rigid nervousness, began to feel like herself again. They came back to the inn by a shorter way, and sat down at a groaning table on the second of the wooded terraces; and it was Gerda who gave expression in friendly terms to the general regret over Herr Permaneder's early departure, now that they were just becoming a little acquainted and finding less and less difficulty with the language. She was ready to swear that she had heard her friend and sister-in-law, Tony, use several times the most unadulterated Munich dialect!

Herr Permaneder forbore to commit himself on the subject of his departure. Instead, he devoted himself for the time to the dainties that weighted down the table – dainties such as he seldom saw the other side of the Danube.

They sat and consumed the good things at their leisure – what little Erica liked far better than anything else were the serviettes made of tissue paper, much nicer than the big linen ones at home. With the waiter's permission she put a few in her pocket as a souvenir. When they had finished, they still sat; Herr Permaneder smoked several very black cigars with his beer, Thomas smoked cigarettes, and the whole family chatted a long time with their guest. It was noticeable that Herr Permaneder's leaving was not mentioned again; in fact, the future was left shrouded in darkness. Rather, they turned to memories of the past or talked of the political events of recent years. Herr Permaneder shook with laughter over some dozens of stories of the late Herr Consul, which his widow related, and then in his turn told about the Munich Revolution, and about Lola Montez, in whom Frau Grünlich displayed an unbounded interest. The hour after luncheon slowly wore on, and little Erica came back laden with daisies, grasses, and ladies' smocks from an expedition with Ida Jungmann, and recalled the fact that the ginger-nuts were still to be bought. They started on their walk down to the village, not before Frau Consul, who was the hostess of the occasion, had paid the bill with a good-sized gold-piece.

They gave orders at the inn that the wagon should be ready in half an hour, so that there would be time for a rest in town before dinner, and then they rambled slowly down, in the dusty sunshine, to the handful of cottages that formed the village.

After they crossed the bridge they fell naturally into little groups, in which they continued after that to walk: Mamsell Jungmann with her long stride in the van, with little Erica jumping tirelessly alongside, hunting for butterflies; then the Frau Consul, Thomas, and Gerda together; and lastly, at some distance, Frau Grünlich and Herr Permaneder. The first pair made considerable noise, for the child shouted for joy, and Ida joined in with her neighing, good-natured laugh. In the middle, all three were silent; for the dust had driven Gerda into another fit of depression, and the old Frau Consul, and her son as well, were plunged in thought. The couple behind were quiet too, but their quietness was only apparent, for in reality Tony and her Bavarian guest were conversing in subdued and intimate tones. And what was the subject of their discourse? It was Herr Grünlich. . . .

Herr Permaneder had made the pointed remark that little Erica was a dear and pretty child, but that she had not the slightest resemblance to her mother. To which Tony had answered: " She is altogether like her father in looks, and one may say that it is not at all to her disadvantage, for as far as looks go, Grünlich was a gentleman. He had golden-yellow whiskers – very uncommon; I never saw anything like them." When Tony visited the Niederpaurs in Munich, she had already told Herr Permaneder in considerable detail the story of her first marriage; but now he asked again all the particulars of it, listening with anxiously sympathetic blinks to the details of the bankruptcy.

" He was a bad man, Herr Permaneder, or Father would never have taken me away from him – of that you may be sure. Life has taught me that not everybody in the world has a good heart. I have learned that, young as I am for a person who, as you might say, has been a widow for ten years. He was a bad man, and his banker, Kesselmeyer, was a worse one – and a silly puppy into the bargain. I won't say that I consider myself an angel and perfectly free from all blame – don't misunderstand me. Grünlich neglected me, and even when he was with me he just sat and read the paper; and he deceived me, and kept me in Eimsbüttel, because he was afraid if I went to town I would find out the mess he was in. But I am a weak woman, and I have my faults too, and I've no doubt I did not always go the right way to work. I know I gave him cause to worry and complain over my extravagance and silliness and my new dressing-gowns. But it is only fair to say one thing: I was just a child when I was married, a perfect goose, a silly little thing. Just imagine: only a short time before I was engaged, I didn't even so much as know that the Confederation decrees concerning the universities and the press had been renewed four years before! And fine decrees they were, too! Ah, me, Herr Permaneder! The sad thing is that one lives but once – one can't begin life over again. And one would know so much better the second time! "

She was silent; she looked down at the road – but she was very intent on the reply Herr Permaneder would make, for she had not unskilfully left him an opening, it being only a step to the idea that, even though it was impossible to begin life anew, yet a new and better married life was not out of the question. Herr Permaneder let the chance slip and confined himself to laying the blame on Herr Grünlich, with such violence that his very chin-whiskers bristled.

"Silly ass! If I had the fool here I'd give it to him! What a swine!"

"Fie, Herr Permaneder! No, you really mustn't. We must forgive and forget—'Vengeance is mine, saith the Lord.' Ask Mother. Heaven forbid—I don't know where Grünlich is, nor what state his affairs are in, but I wish him the best of fortune, even though he doesn't deserve it."

They had reached the village and stood before the little house which was at the same time the bakery. They had stopped walking, almost without knowing it, and were hardly aware that Ida, Erica, the Frau Consul, Thomas, and Gerda had disappeared through the funny, tiny little door, so low that they had to stoop to enter. They were absorbed in their conversation, though it had not got beyond these trifling preliminaries.

They stood by a hedge with a long narrow flower-bed beneath it, in which some mignonette was growing. Frau Grünlich, rather hot, bent her head and poked industriously with her parasol in the black loam. Herr Permaneder stood close to her, now and then assisting her excavations with his walking-stick. His little green hat with the tuft of goat's beard had slid back on his forehead. He was stooping over the bed too, but his small, bulging pale-blue eyes, quite blank and even a little reddish, gazed up at her with a mixture of devotion, distress, and expectancy. It was odd to see how his very moustache, drooping down over his mouth, took the same expression.

"Likely, now," he ventured, "likely, now, ye've taken a silly fright, and are too damned scared of marriage ever to try it again—hey, Frau Grünlich?"

"How clumsy!" thought she. "Must I say yes to that?" Aloud she answered: "Well, dear Herr Permaneder, I must confess that it would be hard for me to yield to anybody my consent for life; for life has taught me, you see, what a serious step that is. One needs to be sure that the man in question is a thoroughly noble, good, kind soul—"

And now he actually ventured the question whether she could consider him such a man—to which she answered: "Yes, Herr Permaneder, I do." Upon which there followed the few short murmured words which clinched the betrothal and gave Herr Permaneder the assurance that he might speak to Thomas and the Frau Consul when they reached home.

When the other members of the party came forth, laden with bags of ginger-nuts, Thomas let his eye rove discreetly over the heads of the two standing outside, for they were embarrassed to the last degree. Herr Permaneder simply made no effort to conceal the fact, but Tony was hiding her embarrassment under a well-nigh majestic dignity.

They hurried back to the wagon, for the sky had clouded over and some drops began to fall.

Tony was right: her brother had, soon after Herr Permaneder appeared, made proper inquiries as to his situation in life. He learned that X. Noppe and Company did a thoroughly sound if somewhat restricted business, operating with the joint-stock brewery managed by Herr Niederpaur as director. It showed a nice little income, Herr Permaneder's share of which, with the help of Tony's seventeen thousand, would suffice for a comfortable if modest life. The Frau Consul heard the news, and there was a long and particular conversation among her, Herr Permaneder, Antonie, and Thomas, in the landscape-room that very evening, and everything was arranged. It was decided that little Erica should go to Munich too, this being her Mother's wish, to which her betrothed warmly agreed.

Two days later the hop-dealer left for home – "Noppe will be raising the deuce if I don't," he said. But in July Frau Grünlich was again in his native town, accompanied by Tom and Gerda. They were to spend four or five weeks at Bad Kreuth, while the Frau Consul with Erica and Ida were on the Baltic coast. While in Munich, the four had time to see the house in Kaufinger Street which Herr Permaneder was about to buy. It was in the neighborhood of the Niederpaurs' – a perfectly remarkable old house, a large part of which Herr Permaneder thought to let. It had a steep, ladderlike pair of stairs which ran without a turning from the front door straight up to the first floor, where a corridor led on each side back to the front rooms.

Tony went home the middle of August to devote herself to her trousseau. She had considerable left from her earlier equipment, but new purchases were necessary to complete it. One day several things arrived from Hamburg, among them a morning-gown – this time not trimmed with velvet but with bands of cloth instead.

Herr Permaneder returned to Meng Street well on in the autumn. They thought best to delay no longer. As for the wedding festivities, they went off just as Tony expected and desired, no great fuss being made over them. "Let us leave out the formalities," said the Consul. "You are married again, and it is simply as if you always had been." Only a few announcements were sent – Madame Grünlich saw to it that Julie Möllendorpf, born Hagenström, received one – and there was no wedding journey. Herr Permaneder objected to making "such a fuss," and Tony, just back from the summer trip, found even the journey to Munich too long. The wedding took place, not in the hall this time, but in the church of St. Mary's, in the presence of the family only. Tony wore the orange-blossom, which replaced the myrtle, with great dignity, and Doctor Kölling preached on moderation, with as strong language as ever, but in a weaker voice.

Christian came from Hamburg, very elegantly dressed, looking a little ailing but very lively. He said his business with Burmeister was "tip-top"; thought that he and Tilda would probably get married "up there" – that is to say, "Each one for himself, of course"; and came very late to the wedding from the visit he paid at the club. Uncle Justus was much moved by the occasion, and with his usual lavishness presented the newly wedded pair with a beautiful heavy silver epergne. He and his wife practically starved themselves at home, for the weak woman was still paying the disinherited and outcast Jacob's debts with the house-keeping money. Jacob was rumoured to be in Paris at present. The Buddenbrook ladies from Broad Street made the remark: "Well, let's hope it will last, this time." The unpleasant part of this lay in the doubt whether they really hoped it. Sesemi Weichbrodt stood on her tip-toes, kissed her pupil, now Frau Permaneder, explosively on the forehead, and said with her most pronounced vowels: "Be happy, you go-od che-ild!"

CHAPTER VII

In the morning at eight o'clock Consul Buddenbrook, so soon as he had left his bed, stolen through the little door and down the winding stair into the bathroom, taken a bath, and put on his night-shirt again – Consul Buddenbrook, we say, began to busy himself with public affairs. For then Herr Wenzel, barber and member of the Assembly, appeared, with his intelligent face and his red hands, his razors and other tools, and the basin of warm water which he had fetched from the kitchen; and the Consul sat in a reclining-chair and leaned his head back, and Herr Wenzel began to make a lather; and there ensued almost always a conversation that began with the weather and how you had slept the night before, went on to politics and the great world, thence to domestic affairs in the city itself, and closed in an intimate and familiar key on business and family matters. All this prolonged very much the process in hand, for every time the Consul said anything Herr Wenzel had to stop shaving.

" Hope you slept well, Herr Consul? "

" Yes, thanks, Wenzel. Is it fine to-day? "

" Frost and a bit of snow, Herr Consul. In front of St. James's the boys have made another slide, more than ten yards long – I nearly sat down, when I came from the Burgomaster's. The young wretches! "

" Seen the papers? "

" The *Advertiser* and the *Hamburg News* – yes. Nothing in them but the Orsini bombs. Horrible. It happened on the way to the opera. Oh, they must be a fine lot over there."

" Oh, it doesn't signify much, I should think. It has nothing to do with the people, and the only effect will be that the police will be doubled and there will be twice as much interference with the press. He is on his guard. Yes, it must be a perpetual strain, for he has to introduce new projects all the time, to keep himself in power. But I respect him, all the same. At all events, he can't be a fool, with his traditions, and I was very much impressed with the cheap bread affair. There is no doubt he does a great deal for the people."

" Yes, Herr Kistenmaker says so too."

" Stephan? We were talking about it yesterday."

" It looks bad for Frederick William of Prussia. Things won't last much longer as they are. They say already that the prince will be made Regent in time."

" It will be interesting to see what happens then. He has already shown that he has liberal ideas and does not feel his brother's secret disgust for the Constitution. It is just the chagrin that upsets him, poor man. What is the news from Copenhagen? "

" Nothing new, Herr Consul. They simply won't. The Confederation has declared that a united government for Holstein and Lauenburg is illegal – they won't have it at any price."

" Yes, it is unheard-of, Wenzel. They dare the Bundestag to put it into operation – and if it were a little more lively – oh, these Danes! – Careful with that chapped place, Wenzel. – There's our direct-line Hamburg railway, too. That has cost some diplomatic battles, and will cost more before they get the concession from Copenhagen."

" Yes, Herr Consul. The stupid thing is that the Altona-Kiel Railway Company is against it – and, in fact, all Holstein is. Dr. Överdieck, the Burgomaster, was saying so just now. They are dreadfully afraid of Kiel prospering much."

" Of course, Wenzel. A new connection between the North Sea and the Baltic. – You'll see, the Kiel-Altona line will keep on intriguing. They are in a position to build a rival railway: East Holstein, Neuminster, Neustadt – yes, that is quite on the cards. But we must not let ourselves be bullied, and we must have a direct route to Hamburg."

" Herr Consul must take the matter up himself."

" Certainly, so far as my powers go, and wherever I have any influence. I am interested in the development of our railways – it is a tradition with us from 1851 on. My Father was a director of the Buchen line, which is probably the reason why I was elected so young. I am only thirty-three years old, and my services so far have been very inconsiderable."

" Oh, Herr Consul! How can the Herr Consul say that after his speech in the Assembly – ? "

" Yes, that made an impression, and I've certainly shown my good will, at least. I can only be grateful that my Father, Grandfather, and great-Grandfather prepared the way for me, and that I inherited so much of the respect and confidence they received from the town; for without it I could not move as I am now able to. For instance, after '48 and the beginning of this decade, what did my Father not do towards the reform of our postal service? Think how he urged in the Assembly the union of the Hamburg diligences with the postal service; and how in 1850 he forced the Senate by continuous pressure to join the German-Austrian Postal Union! If we have cheap letter postage now, and stamps and book post, and letter-boxes, and telegraphic connection with Hamburg and Travemünde, he is not the last one to be grateful to. Why, if he and a few other people had not kept at the Senate continually, we should most likely still be behind the Danish and the Thurn-and-Taxis postal service! So when I have an opinion nowadays on these subjects, people listen to me."

"The Herr Consul is speaking God's truth. About the Hamburg line, Doctor Överdieck was saying to me only three days ago: 'When we get where we can buy a suitable site for the station in Hamburg, we will send Consul Buddenbrook to help transact the business, for in such dealings he is better than most lawyers.' Those were his very words."

"Well, that is very flattering to me, Wenzel. – Just put a little more lather on my chin, will you? It wants a bit more cleaning up. – Yes, the truth is, we mustn't let the grass grow under our feet. I am saying nothing against Överdieck, but he is getting on. If I were Burgomaster I'd make things move a little faster. I can't tell you how pleased I am that they are installing gas for the street-lighting, and the miserable old oil-lamps are disappearing – I admit I had a little something to do with that change. Oh, how much there is to do! Times are changing, Wenzel, and we have many responsibilities toward the new age. When I think back to my boyhood – you know better than I do what the town looked like then: the streets without sidewalks, grass growing a foot high between the paving-stones, and the houses with porticos and benches sticking out into the streets – and our buildings from the time of the Middle Ages spoilt with clumsy additions, and all tumbling down because, while individuals had money and nobody went hungry, the town had none at all and just muddled along, as my brother-in-law calls it, without ever thinking of repairs. That was a happy and comfortable generation, when my grandfather's crony, the good Jean Jacques Hoffstede, strolled about the town and translated improper little French poems. They had to end, those good old times; they have changed, and they will have to change still more. Then the population was thirty-seven thousand: now it is fifty, you know, and the whole character of the place is altering. There is so much building, and the suburbs are spreading out, and we are able to have good streets and restore the old monuments out of our great period. Yet even all that is merely superficial. The most important matter is still outstanding, my dear Wenzel. I mean, of course, the *ceterum censeo* of my dear Father: the customs union. We must join, Wenzel; there should be no longer any question about it, and you must all help me fight for it. As a business man, believe me, I am better informed than the diplomats, and the fear that we should lose independence and freedom of action is simply laughable in this case. The Mecklenburg and Schleswig-Holstein Inland would take us in, which is the more desirable for the reason that we do not control the northern trade quite to the extent that we once did. – That's enough. Please give me the towel, Wenzel," concluded the Consul.

Then the market price of rye, which stood at fifty-five thaler and showed disquieting signs of falling still further, was talked about, and perhaps there was a mention of some event or other in the town; and then Herr Wenzel vanished by the basement route and emptied the lather out of his shiny basin on to the pavement in the street. And the Consul mounted the winding stair into the bedroom, and found Gerda awake, and kissed her on the forehead. Then he dressed.

These little morning sessions with the lively barber formed the introduction to busy days, full to running over with thinking, talking, writing, reckoning, doing business, going about in the town. Thanks to his travel, his interests, and his knowledge of affairs, Thomas Buddenbrook's mind was the least provincial in the district; and he was certainly the first to realize the limitations of his lot. The lively interest in public affairs which the years of the Revolution had brought in, was suffering throughout the whole country from a period of prostration and arrest, and that field was too sterile to occupy a vigorous talent; but Thomas Buddenbrook possessed the spirit to take to himself that wise old saying that all human achievement is of a merely symbolic value, and thus to devote all that he had of capacity, enthusiasm, energy, and strength of will to the service of the community as well as to the service of his own name and firm. He stood in the front rank of his small society and was seriously ambitious to give his city greatness and power within her sphere – though he had the intellect, too, to smile at himself for the ambition even while he cherished it.

He ate his breakfast, served by Anton, and went to the office in Meng Street, where he remained about an hour, writing two or three pressing letters and telegrams, giving this or that instruction, imparting to the wheels of industry a small push, and then leaving them to revolve under the cautious eye of Herr Marcus.

He went to assemblies and committee meetings, visited the Bourse, which was held under the Gothic arcades in the Market Square, inspected dockyards and warehouses, talked with the captains of the ships he owned, and transacted much and various business all day long until evening, interrupted only by the hasty luncheon with his Mother and dinner with Gerda; after which he took a half-hour's rest on the sofa with his cigarette and the newspaper. Customs, rates, construction, railways, posts, almonry – all this as well as his own business occupied him; and even in matters commonly left to professionals he acquired insight and judgment, especially in finance, where he early showed himself extremely gifted.

He was careful not to neglect the social side. True, he was not always punctual, and usually appeared at the very last minute, when the carriage waited below and his wife sat in full toilette. "I'm sorry, Gerda," he would say; "I was detained"; and he would dash upstairs to don his evening clothes. But when he arrived at a dinner, a ball, or an evening company, he showed lively interest and ranked as a charming *causeur*. And in entertaining he and his wife were not behind the other rich houses. In kitchen and cellar everything was "tip-top," and he himself was considered a most courteous and tactful host, whose toasts were wittier than the common run. His quiet evenings he spent at home with Gerda alone, smoking, listening to her music, or reading with her some book of her selection.

Thus his labours enforced success, his consequence grew in the town, and the firm had excellent years, despite the sums drawn out to settle Christian and to pay Tony's second dowry. And yet there were troubles which had, at times, the power to lame his courage for hours, weaken his elasticity, and depress his mood.

There was Christian in Hamburg. His partner, Herr Burmeester, had died quite suddenly of an apoplectic stroke, in the spring of the year 1858. His heirs drew their money out of the business, and the Consul strongly advised Christian against trying to continue it with his own means, for he knew how difficult it is to carry on a business already established on definite lines if the working capital be suddenly diminished. But Christian insisted upon the continuation of his independence. He took over the assets and the liabilities of H. C. F. Burmeester and Company, and trouble was to be looked for.

Then there was the Consul's sister Clara in Riga. Her marriage with Pastor Tiburtius had remained unblest with children – but then, as Clara Buddenbrook she had never wanted children, and probably had very little talent for motherhood. Now her husband wrote that her health left much to be desired. The severe headaches from which she had suffered even as a girl were now recurring periodically, to an almost unbearable extent.

That was disquieting. And even here at home there was another source of worry – for, as yet, there was no certainty whatever that the family name would live. Gerda treated the subject with sovereign indifference which came very near to being repugnance. Thomas concealed his anxiety. But the old Frau Consul took the matter in hand and consulted Grabow.

"Doctor – just between ourselves – something is bound to happen *sometime*, isn't it? A little mountain air at Kreuth, a little seashore at Glucksberg or Travemünde – but they don't seem to work. What do you advise?" Dr. Grabow's pleasant old prescription: "a nourishing diet, a little pigeon, a slice of French bread," didn't seem strong enough, either, to fit the case. He ordered Pyrmont and Schlangenbad.

Those were three worries. And Tony? Poor Tony!

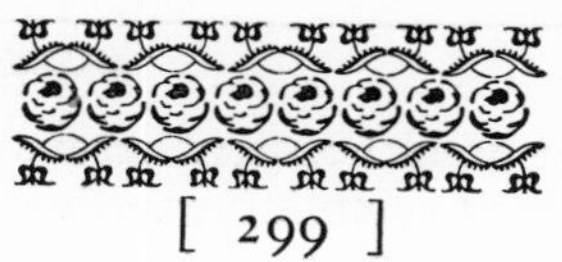

CHAPTER VIII

SHE wrote: ". . . And when I say 'croquettes,' she doesn't understand me, because here they are called 'meaties'; and when she says 'broccoli,' how could any Christian know she means cauliflower? When I say 'baked potatoes,' she screams 'How?' at me, until I remember to say 'roast potatoes,' which is what they call them here. 'How' means 'What did you say?' And she is the second one I've had – I sent away the first one, named Katy, because she was so impertinent – or at least, I thought she was. I'm getting to see now that I may have been mistaken, for I'm never quite sure whether people here mean to be rude or friendly. This one's name is Babette. She has a very pleasing exterior, with something southern, the way some of them have here; black hair and eyes, and teeth that any one might envy. She is willing, too, and I am teaching her how to make some of our home dishes. Yesterday we had sorrel and currants, but I wish I hadn't, for Permaneder objected so much to the sorrel – he picked the currants out with a fork – that he would not speak to me the whole afternoon, but just growled; and I can tell you, Mother, that life is not so easy."

Alas, it was not only the sorrel and the "meaties" that were embittering Tony's life. Before the honeymoon was over she had had a blow so unforeseen, so unexpected, so incomprehensible, that it took away all her joy in life. She could not get over it. And here it was.

Not until after the Permaneder couple had been some weeks in Munich had Consul Buddenbrook liquidated the sum fixed by his Father's will as his sister's second marriage portion. That sum, translated into gulden, had at last safely reached Herr Permaneder's hands, and Herr Permaneder had invested it securely and not unprofitably. But then, what he had said, quite unblushingly and without embarrassment, to his wife, was this: "Tonerl" – he called her "Tonerl" – "Tonerl, that's good enough for me. What do we want of more? I been working my hide off all my days; now I'd like to sit down and have a little peace and quiet, damned if I wouldn't. Let's rent the parterre and the second floor, and still we'll have a good house, where we can sit and eat our bit of pig's meat without screwing ourselves up and putting on so much lug. And in the evening I can go to the Hofbräu house. I'm no swell – I don't care about scraping money together. I want my comfort. I quit to-morrow and go into private life."

"Permaneder!" she had cried; and for the first time she had spoken his name with that peculiar throaty sound which her voice always had when she uttered the name of Grünlich.

"Oh, shut up! Don't take on!" was all he answered. There had followed, thus early in their life together, a quarrel, serious and violent enough to endanger the happiness of any marriage. He came off victorious. Her passionate resistance was shattered upon his urgent longing for "peace and quiet." It ended in Herr Permaneder's withdrawing the capital he had in the hop business, so that now Herr Noppe, in his turn, could strike the "and Company" off his card. After which Tony's husband, like most of the friends whom he met around the table in the Hofbräu House, to play cards and drink his regular three litres of beer, limited his activities to the raising of rents in his capacity of landlord, and to an undisturbed cutting of coupons.

The Frau Consul was notified quite simply of this fact. But Frau Permaneder's distress was evident in the letters which she wrote to her brother. Poor Tony! Her worst fears were more than realized. She had always known that Herr Permaneder possessed none of that "resourcefulness" of which her first husband had had so much; but that he would so entirely confound the expectations she had expressed to Mamsell Jungmann on the eve of her betrothal – that he would so completely fail to recognize the duties he had taken upon himself when he married a Buddenbrook – that she had never dreamed.

But these feelings must be overcome; and her family at home saw from her letters how she resigned herself. She lived on rather monotonously with her husband and Erica, who went to school; she attended to her housekeeping, kept up friendly relations with the people who rented the parterre and the first storey and with the Niederpaur family in Marienplatz; and she wrote now and then of going to the theatre with her friend Eva. Herr Permaneder did not care for the theatre. And it came out that he had grown to more than forty years of age in his beloved Munich without ever having seen the inside of the Pinakothek.

Time passed. But Tony could feel no longer any true happiness in her new life, since the day when Herr Permaneder received her dowry and settled himself down to enjoy his ease.

Hope was no more. She would never be able to write home to announce new ventures and new successes. Just as life was now – free from cares, it was true, but so limited, so lamentably "unrefined," – just so it would remain until the end. It weighed upon her. It was plain from her letters that this very lowness of tone was making it harder for her to adapt herself to the south-German surroundings. In small matters, of course, things grew easier. She learned to make herself understood by the servants and errand-boys, to say "meaties" instead of "croquettes," and to set no more fruit soup before her husband after the one he had called a "sickening mess." But, in general, she remained a stranger in her new home; and she never ceased to taste the bitterness of the knowledge that to be a born Buddenbrook was not to enjoy any particular prestige in her adopted home. She once related in a letter the story of how she met in the street a mason's apprentice, carrying a mug of beer in one hand and holding a large white radish by its tail in the other; who, waving his beer, said jovially: "Neighbour, can ye tell us the time?" She made a joke of it, in the telling; yet even so, a strong undercurrent of irritation betrayed itself. You might be quite certain that she threw back her head and vouchsafed to the poor man neither answer nor glance in his direction. But it was not alone this lack of formality and absence of distinctions that made her feel strange and unsympathetic. She did not live deeply, it is true, into the life or affairs of her new home; but she breathed the Munich air, the air of a great city, full of artists and citizens who habitually did nothing: an air with something about it a little demoralizing, which she sometimes found it hard to take good-humouredly.

The days passed. And then it seemed that there was after all a joy in store – in fact, the very one which was longed for in vain in Broad Street and Meng Street. For not long after the New Year of 1859 Tony felt certain that she was again to become a mother.

The joy of it trembled in her letters, which were full of the old childish gaiety and sense of importance. The Frau Consul, who, with the exception of the summer holiday, confined her journeyings more and more to the Baltic coast, lamented that she could not be with her daughter at this time. Tom and Gerda made plans to go to the christening, and Tony's head was full of giving them an elegant reception. Alas, poor Tony! The visit which took place was sad indeed, and the christening – Tony had cherished visions of a ravishing little feast, with flowers, sweetmeats, and chocolate – never took place at all. The child, a little girl, only entered into life for a tiny quarter of an hour; then, though the doctor did his best to set the pathetic little mechanism going, it faded out of being.

Consul Buddenbrook and his wife arrived in Munich to find Tony herself not out of danger. She was far more ill than before, and a nervous weakness from which she had already suffered prevented her from taking any nourishment at all for several days. Then she began to eat, and on their departure, the Buddenbrooks felt reassured as far as her health was concerned. But in other ways there was much reason for anxiety; for it had been all too plain, especially to the Consul's observant eye, that not even their common loss would suffice to bring husband and wife together again.

There was nothing against Herr Permaneder's good heart. He was truly shaken by the death of the child; big tears rolled down out of his bulging eyes upon his puffy cheeks and on into his frizzled beard. Many times he sighed deeply and gave vent to his favourite expression. But, after all, Tony felt that his "peace and quiet" had not suffered any long interruption. After a few evenings, he sought the Hofbräu House for consolation, and was soon, as he always said, "muddling along" again in his old, good-natured, comfortable, grumbling way, with the easy fatalism natural to him.

But from now on Tony's letters never lost their hopeless, even complaining tone. "Oh, Mother," she wrote, "why do I have to bear everything like this? First Grünlich and the bankruptcy, and then Permaneder going out of business—and then the baby! How have I deserved all these misfortunes?"

When the Consul read these outpourings, he could never quite forego a little smile: for, notwithstanding all the real pain they showed, he heard an undertone of almost comic pride, and he knew that Tony Buddenbrook, as Madame Grünlich or as Madame Permaneder, was and would remain a child. She bore all her mature experiences almost with a child's unbelief in their reality, yet with a child's seriousness, a child's self-importance, and, above all, with a child's power to throw them off at will.

She could not understand how she had deserved her misfortunes; for even while she mocked at her mother's piety, she herself was so full of it that she fervently believed in justice and righteousness on this earth.

Poor Tony! The death of her second child was neither the last nor the hardest blow that fell upon her. As the year 1859 drew to a close, something frightful indeed happened.

CHAPTER IX

It was a day toward the end of November — a cold autumn day with a hazy sky. It looked almost as if there would be snow, and a mist was rising, pierced through every now and then by the sun. It was one of those days, common in a seaport town, when a sharp north-east wind whistled round the massive church corners and influenzas were to be had cheap.

Consul Thomas Buddenbrook entered the breakfast-room toward midday, to find his Mother, with her spectacles on her nose, bent over a paper on the table.

"Tom," she said; and she looked at him, holding the paper with both hands, as if she hesitated to show it to him. "Don't be startled. But it is not very good news. I don't understand — It is from Berlin. Something must have happened."

"Give it to me, please," he said shortly. He lost colour, and the muscles stood out on his temples as he clenched his teeth. His gesture as he stretched out his hand was so full of decision that it was as if he said aloud: "Just tell me quickly. Don't prepare me for it!"

He read the lines still standing; one of his light eyebrows went up, and he drew the long ends of his moustache through his fingers. It was a telegram, and it said: "Don't be frightened. Am coming at once with Erica. All is over. Your unhappy Antonie."

"'At once . . . at once,'" he said, with irritation, looking at the Frau Consul and giving his head a quick shake. "What does she mean by 'at once'?"

"That is just a way of putting it, Tom; it doesn't mean anything particular. She means by the next train, or something like that."

"And from Berlin! What is she doing in Berlin? How did she get to Berlin?"

"I don't know, Tom; I don't understand it. The dispatch only came ten minutes ago. But something must have happened, and we must just wait to see what it is. God in his mercy will turn it all to good. Sit down, my son, and eat your luncheon."

He took his chair, and mechanically he poured out a glass of porter.

"'All is over,'" he repeated. And then "'Antonie.' How childish!"

He ate and drank in silence.

After a while the Frau Consul ventured to say: "It must be something about Permaneder, don't you think, Tom?"

He shrugged his shoulders without looking up.

As he went away he said, with his hand on the door-knob, "Well, we must wait and see. As she is not likely to burst into the house in the middle of the night, she will probably reach here some time to-morrow. You will let me know, won't you?"

The Frau Consul waited from hour to hour. She had slept very badly, and in the night she rang for Ida Jungmann, who now slept in the back room of the entresol. She had Ida make her some *eau sucrée;* and she sat up in bed for a long time and embroidered. And now the forenoon passed in nervous expectancy. When the Consul came to second breakfast, he said that Tony could not arrive before the three-thirty-three train from Buchen. At that hour the Frau Consul seated herself in the landscape-room and tried to read, out of a book with a black leather cover decorated with a gold palm-leaf.

It was a day like its predecessor: cold, mist, wind. The stove crackled away behind its wrought iron screen. The old lady trembled and looked out of the window whenever she heard a wagon. At four o'clock, when she had stopped watching and almost stopped thinking about her daughter, there was a stir below in the house. She hastily turned toward the window and wiped away the damp with her handkerchief. Yes, a carriage had stopped below, and some one was coming up the steps.

She grasped the arms of her chair with both hands to rise. But then she thought better of it and sank back. She only turned her head as her daughter entered, and her face wore an almost defensive expression. Tony burst impetuously into the room: Erica remained outside at the glass door, with her hand in Ida Jungmann's.

Frau Permaneder wore a fur wrap and a large felt hat with a veil. She looked very pale and ailing, and her upper lip trembled as it used to when the little Tony was about to weep. Her eyes were red. She raised her arms and let them drop, and then she fell on her knees at her Mother's side, burying her face in the folds of her gown and sobbing bitterly. It was as though she had rushed straight hither from Munich all in one breath, and now lay there, having gained the goal of her headlong flight, exhausted but safe. The Frau Consul sat a moment quite still.

"Tony!" she said then, with gentle remonstrance. She drew the long hatpins out of Frau Permaneder's hat and laid it on the window-seat; then she stroked gently and soothingly her daughter's thick ash-blond hair.

"What is it, my child? What has happened?"

But she saw that patience was her only weapon; for it was long before her question drew out any reply.

"Mother!" uttered Frau Permaneder. "Mamma!" But that was all.

The Frau Consul looked toward the glass door and, still embracing her daughter, stretched out her hand to her grandchild, who stood there shyly with her finger to her mouth.

"Come, child; come here and say how do you do. You have grown so big, and you look so strong and well, for which God be thanked. How old are you now, Erica?"

"Thirteen, Grandmamma."

"Good gracious! A young lady!" She kissed the little maiden over Tony's head and told her: "Go up with Ida now – we shall soon have dinner. Just now Mamma and I want to talk."

They were alone.

"Now, my dear Tony? Can you not stop crying? When God sends us a heavy trial, we must bear it with composure. 'Take your cross upon you,' we are told. Would you like to go up first and rest a little and refresh yourself, and then come down to me again? Our good Jungmann has your room ready. Thanks for your telegram – of course, it shocked us a good deal –"

She stopped. For Tony's voice came, all trembling and smothered, out of the folds of her gown: "He is a wicked man – a wicked man! Oh, he is –"

Frau Permaneder seemed not able to get away from this dreadful phrase. It possessed her altogether. She buried her face deeper and deeper in the Frau Consul's lap and clenched her fist beside the Frau Consul's chair.

"Do you mean your husband, my child?" asked the old lady, after a pause. "It ought not to be possible for me to have such a thought in my mind, I know; but you leave me nothing else to think, Tony. Has Herr Permaneder done you an injury? Are you making a complaint of him?"

"Babette," Frau Permaneder brought out. "Babette –"

"Babette?" repeated the Frau Consul, inquiringly. Then she

leaned back in her chair, and her pale eyes wandered toward the window. She understood now. There was a pause, broken by Tony's gradually decreasing sobs.

"Tony," said the Frau Consul after a little space, "I see now that there has been an injury done you—that you have cause to complain. But was it necessary to give the sense of injury such violent expression? Was it necessary to travel here from Munich, with Erica, and to make it appear—for other people will not be so sensible as we are—that you have left him permanently; that you will not go back to him?"

"But I won't go back to him—never!" cried Frau Permaneder, and she lifted up her head with a jerk and looked at her Mother wildly with tear-stained eyes, and then buried her face again. The Frau Consul affected not to have heard.

"But now," she went on, in a louder key, slowly nodding her head from one side to the other, "now that you are here, I am glad you are. For you can unburden your heart, and tell me everything, and then we shall see how we can put things right, by taking thought, and by mutual forbearance and affection."

"Never," Tony said again. "Never!" And then she told her story. It was not all intelligible, for she spoke into the folds of her Mother's stuff gown, and broke into her own narrative with explosions of passionate anger. But what had happened was somewhat as follows:

On the night of the twenty-fourth of the month, Madame Permaneder had gone to sleep very late, having been disturbed during the day by the nervous digestive trouble to which she was subject. She had been awakened about midnight, out of a light slumber, by a confused and continuous noise outside on the landing—a half-suppressed, mysterious noise, in which one distinguished the creaking of the stairs, a sort of giggling cough, smothered, protesting words, and, mixed with these, the most singular snarling sounds. But there was no doubt whence they proceeded. Frau Permaneder had hardly, with her sleepy senses, taken them in before she interpreted them as well, in such a way that she felt the blood leave her cheeks and rush to her heart, which contracted and then went on beating with heavy, oppressed pulsations. For a long, dreadful minute she lay among the pillows as if stunned, as if paralysed. Then, as the shameless disturbance did not stop, she had with trembling hands kindled a light, had left her bed, thrilling with horror, repulsion, and despair, had opened the door and hurried out on to the landing in her slippers, the light in her hand—to the top of the "ladder" that went straight up from the house door to the first storey. And there, on the upper steps, in all its actuality, was indeed the very scene she had pictured in her mind's eye as she listened to the compromising noises. It was an unseemly and indecent scuffle, a sort of wrestling match between Babette the cook and Herr Permaneder. The girl must have been busied late about the house, for she had her bunch of keys and her candle in her hand as she swayed back and forth in the effort to fend her master off. He, with his hat on the back of his head, held her round the body and kept making essays, now and then successfully, to press his face, with its great walrus moustache, against hers. As Antonie appeared, Babette exclaimed something that sounded like "Jesus, Mary, and Joseph!" – and "Jesus, Mary, and Joseph!" echoed Herr Permaneder likewise, as he let go. Almost in the same second the girl vanished, and there was Herr Permaneder left standing before his wife, with drooping head, drooping arms, drooping moustaches too; and all he could get out was some idiotic remark like "Holy Cross, what a mess!" When he ventured to lift his eyes, she was no longer there. She was in the bed-chamber, half-sitting, half-lying on the bed, repeating over and over again with frantic sobbing, "Shame, shame!" He leaned rather flabbily in the doorway and jerked his shoulder in her direction – had he been closer, the gesture would have been a nudge in the ribs. "Hey, Tonerl – don't be a fool, you know. Say – you know Franz, the Ramsau Franz, he had his name-day to-day, and we're all half-seas over." Strong alcoholic fumes pervaded the room as he spoke; and they brought Frau Permaneder's excitement to a climax. She sobbed no more, she was no longer weak and faint. Carried away by frenzy, incapable of measuring her words, she poured out her disgust, her abhorrence, her complete and utter contempt and loathing of him and all his ways. Herr Permaneder did not take it meekly. His head was hot; for he had treated his friend Franz not only to many beers, but to "champagne wine" as well. He answered and answered wildly – the quarrel reached a height far greater than the one that had signalized Herr Permaneder's retirement into private life, and it ended in Frau Antonie gathering her clothes together and withdrawing into the living-room for the night. And at the end he had flung at her a word – a word which she would not repeat – a word that should never pass her lips – a word . . .

This was the major content of the confession which Frau Permaneder had sobbed into the folds of her mother's gown. But the "word," the word that in that fearful night had sunk into her very depths – no, she would not repeat it; no, she would not, she asseverated, – although her mother had not in the least pressed her to do so, but only nodded her head, slowly, almost imperceptibly, as she looked down on Tony's lovely ash-blond hair.

"Yes, yes," she said; "this is very sad, Tony. And I understand it all, my dear little one, because I am not only your Mamma, but I am a woman like you as well. I see now how fully your grief is justified, and how completely your husband, in a moment of weakness, forgot what he owed to you and – "

"In a moment – ? " cried Tony. She sprang up. She made two steps backward and feverishly dried her eyes. "A moment, Mamma! He *forgot* what he owed to me and to our name? He never *knew* it, from the very beginning! A man that quietly sits down with his wife's dowry – a man without ambition or energy or will-power! A man that has some kind of thick soup made out of hops in his veins instead of blood – and I verily believe he has! And to let himself down to such common doings as this with Babette – and when I reproached him with his good-for-nothingness, to answer with a word that – a word – "

And, arrived once more at the word, the word she would not repeat, quite suddenly she took a step forward and said, in a completely altered, a quieter, milder, interested tone: "How perfectly sweet! Where did you get that, Mamma? " She motioned with her chin toward a little receptacle, a charming basket-work stand woven out of reeds and decorated with ribbon bows, in which the Frau Consul kept her fancy-work.

"I bought it, some time ago," answered the old lady. "I needed it."

"Very smart," Tony said, looking at it with her head on one side. The Frau Consul looked at it too, but without seeing it, for she was in deep thought.

"Now, my dear daughter," she said at last, putting out her hand again, "however things are, you are here, and welcome a hundred times to your old home. We can talk everything over when we are calmer. Take your things off in your room and make yourself comfortable. Ida! " she called into the dining-room, lifting her voice, "lay a place for Madame Permaneder, and one for Erica, my dear."

CHAPTER X

TONY returned to her bed-chamber after dinner. During the meal her Mother had told her that Thomas was aware of her expected arrival; and she did not seem particularly anxious to meet him.

The Consul came at six o'clock. He went into the landscape-room and had a long talk with his Mother.

"How is she?" he asked. "How does she seem?"

"Oh, Tom, I am afraid she is very determined. She is terribly wrought up. And this word – if I only knew what it was he said –"

"I will go up and see her."

"Yes, do, Tom. But knock softly, so as not to startle her, and be very calm, will you? Her nerves are upset. That is the trouble she has with her digestion – she has eaten nothing. Do talk quietly with her."

He went up quickly, skipping a step in his usual way. He was thinking, and twisting the ends of his moustache, but as he knocked, his face cleared – he was resolved to handle the situation as long as possible with humour.

A suffering voice said "Come in," and he opened the door, to find Frau Permaneder lying on the bed fully dressed. The bed curtains were flung back, the down quilt was underneath her back, and a medicine bottle stood on the night-table. She turned round a little and propped her head on her hand, looking at him with her pouting smile. He made a deep bow and spread out his hands in a solemn gesture.

"Well, dear lady! To what are we indebted for the honour of a visit from this personage from the royal city of –?"

"Oh, give me a kiss, Tom," she said, sat up to offer him her cheek, and then sank back again. "Well, how are you, my dear boy? Quite unchanged, I see, since I saw you in Munich."

"You can't tell much about it with the blinds down, my dear. And you ought not to steal my thunder like that, either. It is more suitable for me to say –" he held her hand in his, and at the same time drew up a chair beside the bed – "as I so often have, that you and Tilda –"

" Oh, for shame, Tom! – How is Tilda? "

" Well, of course. Madame Krauseminz sees she doesn't starve. Which doesn't prevent her eating for the week ahead when she comes here on Thursday."

She laughed very heartily – as she had not for a long time back, in fact. Then she broke off with a sigh, and asked: " And how is business? "

" Oh, we get on. Mustn't complain."

" Thank goodness, here everything is as it should be. Oh, Tom, I don't feel much like chatting pleasantly about trifles! "

" Pity. One should preserve one's sense of humour, *quand même*."

" All that is at an end, Tom. – You know all? "

" ' You know all '! " he repeated. He dropped her hand and pushed back his chair. " Goodness gracious, how that sounds! ' All '! What-all lies in that ' all '? ' My love and grief I gave thee,' eh? No, listen! "

She was silent. She swept him with an astonished and deeply offended glance.

" Yes, I expected that look," he said, " for without that look you would not be here. But, dear Tony, let me take the thing as much too lightly as you take it too seriously. You will see we shall complement each other very nicely – "

" Too seriously, Thomas? *I* take it too seriously? "

" Yes. – For heaven's sake, don't let's make a tragedy of it! Let us take it in a lower key, not with ' all is at an end ' and ' your unhappy Antonie.' Don't misunderstand me, Tony. You well know that no one can be gladder than I that you have come. I have long wished you would come to us on a visit by yourself, without your husband, so that we could be *en famille* together once more. But to come now, like this – my dear child, I beg your pardon, but it was – foolish. Yes – let me finish! Permaneder has certainly behaved very badly, as I will give him to understand pretty clearly – don't be afraid of that – "

" As to how he has behaved himself, Thomas," she interrupted him, raising herself up to lay a hand upon her breast, " as far as that goes, I have already given him to understand that – and not only ' given him to understand,' I can tell you! I am convinced that further discussion with that man is entirely out of place." And she let herself fall back again and looked sternly and fixedly at the ceiling.

He bowed, as if under the weight of her words, and kept on looking down at his knee and smiling.

"Well, then, I won't send him a stiff letter. It is just as you say. In the end it is after all your affair, and it is quite enough if you put him in his place – it is your duty as his wife. After all, there are some extenuating circumstances. There was a birthday celebration, and he came home a little bit exalted, so to speak, and was guilty of a false step, an unseemly blunder – "

"Thomas," said she, "I do not understand you. I do not understand your tone. You – a man with your principles! But you did not see him. You did not see how drunk he looked – "

"He looked ridiculous enough, I'm sure. But that is it, Tony. You will not see how comic it was – but probably that is the fault of your bad digestion. You caught your husband in a moment of weakness, and you have seen him make himself look ridiculous. But that ought not to outrage you to such an extent. It ought to amuse you a little, perhaps, but bring you closer together as human beings. I will say that I don't mean you could have just let it pass with a laugh and said nothing about it – not at all. You left home; that was a demonstration of a rather extreme kind, perhaps – a bit too severe – but, after all, he deserved it. I imagine he is feeling pretty down in the mouth. I only mean that you must get to take the thing differently – not so insulted – a little more politic point of view. We are just between ourselves. Let me tell you something, Tony. In any marriage, the important thing is, on which side the moral ascendency lies. Understand? Your husband has laid himself open, there is no doubt of that. He compromised himself and made a laughable spectacle – laughable, precisely because what he did was actually so harmless, so impossible to take seriously. But, after all, his dignity is impaired – and the moral advantage has passed over to you. If you know how to use it wisely, your happiness is assured. If you go back, say in a couple of weeks – certainly I must insist on keeping you for ourselves as long as that – if you go back to Munich in a couple of weeks, you will see – "

"I will not go back to Munich, Thomas."

"I beg your pardon?" he asked, putting his hand to his ear and screwing up his face as he bent forward.

She was lying on her back with her head sunk in the pillow, so that her chin stood out with an effect of severity. "Never," she said. And she gave a long, audible outward breath and cleared her throat, also at length and deliberately. It was like a dry cough, which had of late become almost a habit with her, and had probably to do with her digestive trouble. There followed a pause.

"Tony," he said suddenly, getting up and slapping his hand

on the arm of his chair, "you aren't going to make a scandal!"

She gave a side glance and saw him all pale, with the muscles standing out on his temples. Her position was no longer tenable. She bestirred herself and, to hide the fear she really felt of him, grew angry in her turn. She sat up quickly and put her feet to the floor. With glowing cheeks and a frowning brow, making hasty motions of the head and hands, she began: "Scandal, Thomas! You want to tell me not to make a scandal, when I have been insulted, and people spit in my face? Is that worthy of a brother, you will permit me to ask? Circumspection, tact – they are very well in their place. But there are limits, Tom – I know just as much of life as you do, and I tell you there is a point where the care for appearances leaves off, and cowardice begins! I am astonished that such a stupid goose as I am have to tell you this – yes, I am a stupid goose, and I should not be surprised if Permaneder never loved me at all, for I am an ugly old woman, very likely, and Babette is certainly prettier than I am! But did that give him a right to forget the respect he owed to my family, and my upbringing, and all my feelings? You did not see the way he forgot himself, Tom; and since you did not see it, you cannot understand, for I can never tell you how disgusting he was. You did not hear the word that he called after me, your sister, when I took my things and went out of the room, to sleep on the sofa in the living-room. But *I* heard it, and it was a word that – a word – Oh, it was that word, let me tell you, Thomas, that caused me to spend the whole night packing my trunk, to wake Erica early in the morning, and to leave the place, rather than to remain in the neighbourhood of a man who could utter such words. And to such a man, as I said before, I will never, never return, not so long as I have any self-respect, or care in the least what becomes of me in my life on this earth."

"And will you now have the goodness, to tell me what this cursed word was? Yes or no?"

"Never, Thomas! Never would I permit that word to cross my lips. I know too well what I owe to you and to myself within these walls."

"Then it's no use talking with you!"

"That may easily be. I am sure I do not want to discuss it any further."

"What do you expect to do? Get a divorce?"

"Yes, Tom; such is my firm determination. I feel that I owe it to myself, my child, and my family."

"That is all nonsense, of course," he said in a dispassionate tone.

He turned on his heel and moved away, as if his words had settled the matter. "It takes two to make a divorce, my child. Do you think Permaneder will just say yes and thank you kindly? The idea is absurd."

"Oh, you can leave that to me," she said, quite undismayed. "You mean he will refuse on account of the seventeen thousand marks current. But Grünlich wasn't willing, either, and they made him. There are ways and means, I'm sure. I'll go to Dr. Gieseke. He is Christian's friend, and he will help me. Oh, yes, of course, I know it was not the same thing then. It was 'incapacity of the husband to provide for his family.' You see, I know my way about in these affairs. Dear me, you act as if this were the first time in my life that I got a divorce! But even so, Tom. Perhaps there is nothing that applies to this case. Perhaps it is impossible — you may be right. But it is all the same; my resolve is fixed. Let him keep the money. There are higher things in life. He will never see me again, either way."

She coughed again. She had left the bed and seated herself in an easy-chair, resting one elbow on its arm. Her chin was so deeply buried in her hand that her four bent fingers clutched her under lip. She sat with her body turned to the right, staring with red, excited eyes out of the window.

The Consul walked up and down, sighed, shook his head, shrugged his shoulders. He paused in front of her, fairly wringing his hands.

"You are a child, Tony, a child," said he in a discouraged, almost pleading tone. "Every word you have spoken is the most utter childish nonsense. Will you make an effort, now, if I beg you, to think about the thing for just one minute like a grown woman? Don't you see that you are acting as if something very serious and dreadful had happened to you — as if your husband had cruelly betrayed you and heaped insults on you before all the world? Do try to realize that nothing of the sort has happened! Not a single soul in the world knows anything about that silly affair that happened at the top of your staircase in Kaufinger Street. Your dignity, and ours, will suffer no slightest diminution if you go calmly and composedly back to Permaneder — of course, with your nose in the air! But, on the other hand, if you don't go back, if you give this nonsense so much importance as to make a scandal out of it, then you will be wounding our dignity indeed."

She jerked her chin out of her hand and stared him in the face.

"That's enough, Thomas Buddenbrook. Be quiet now; it's my turn. Listen. So you think there is no shame and no scandal so long as people don't get to hear it? Ah, no! The shame that gnaws at us secretly and eats away our self-respect – that is far, far worse. Are we Buddenbrooks the sort of people to be satisfied if everything looks ' tip-top,' as you say here, on the outside, no matter how much mortification we have to choke down, inside our four walls? I cannot help feeling astonished at you, Tom. Think of our Father and how he would act to-day – and then judge as he would! No, no! Clean and open dealings must be the rule. Why, you can open your books any day, for all the world to see, and say, ' Here they are, look at them.' We should all of us be just the same. I know how God has made me. I am not afraid. Let Julchen Möllendorpf pass me in the street and not speak, if she wants to. Let Pfiffi Buddenbrook sit here on Thursday afternoons and shake all over with spite, and say, ' Well, that is the second time! But, *of course*, both times the men were to blame! ' I feel so far above all that now, Thomas – farther than I can tell you! I know I have done what I thought was right. But if I am to be so afraid of Julchen Möllendorpf and Pfiffi Buddenbrook as to swallow down all sorts of insults and let myself be cursed out in a drunken dialect that isn't even grammar – to stop with a man in a town where I have to get used to that kind of language and the kind of scenes I saw that night at the top of the stairs – where I have to forget my origin and my upbringing and everything that I am, and learn to disown it altogether in order to act as if I were satisfied and happy – *that* is what *I* call undignified – *that* is what *I* call scandalous, I tell you! "

She broke off, buried her chin once more in her hand, and stared out of the window. He stood before her, his weight on one leg, his hands in his trousers pockets. His eyes rested on her unseeing, for he was in deep thought, and slowly moving his head from side to side.

" Tony," he said. " You're telling the truth. I knew it all along; but you betrayed yourself just now. It is not the man at all. It is the place. It isn't this other idiotic business – it is the whole thing all together. You couldn't get used to it. Tell the truth."

" Thomas," she cried, " it is the truth! " She sprang up as she spoke, and pointed straight into his face with her outstretched hand. Her own face was red. She stood there in a warlike pose, one hand grasping the chair, gesticulating with the other, and made a long, agitated, passionate speech that welled up in a resistless tide. The Consul stared at her amazed. Scarcely would she pause to draw breath, when new words would come gushing and bubbling forth. Yes, she found words for everything; she gave full expression to all the accumulated disgust of her Munich years. Unassorted, confused, she poured it all out, one thing after another; she kept nothing back. It was like the bursting of a dam – an assertion of desperate integrity; something elemental, a force of nature, that brooked no restraint.

"It is the truth!" she cried. "Say it again, Thomas! Oh, I can tell you plainly, I am no stupid goose any longer; I know what I have to expect. I don't faint away at my time of life, to hear that dirty work goes on now and then. I've known people like Teary Trieschke, and I was married to Bendix Grünlich, and I know the dissipated creatures there are here in this town. I am no country innocent, I tell you; and the affair with Babette wouldn't have made me go off the handle like that, just by itself. No, Thomas, the thing was that it filled the cup to overflowing – and that didn't take much, for it was full already, and had been for a long time – a long time. It would have taken very little to make it run over. And then this happened! The knowledge that I could not depend on Permaneder even in that way – that put the top on everything. It knocked the bottom out of the cask. It brought to a head all at once my intention to get away from Munich, that had been slowly growing in my mind a long time before that, Tom; for I cannot live down there – I swear it before God and all His heavenly hosts! How wretched I have been, Thomas, you can never know. When you were there on a visit, I concealed everything, for I am a tactful woman and do not burden others with my complainings, nor wear my heart on my sleeve on a week-day. I have always been rather reserved. But I have suffered, Tom, suffered with my entire being – with my whole personality, so to speak. Like a plant, a flower that has been transplanted into a foreign soil – if I may make such a comparison. You will probably find it a most unsuitable one, for I am really an ugly old woman – but I could not be planted in a more foreign soil than that, and I would just as lief go and live in Turkey! Oh, we should never be transplanted, we northern folk! We should stick to the shore of our own bay; we can only really thrive upon our native soil! You all used to laugh at my taste for the nobility. Yes, in these years I have often thought of what somebody said to me once, in times gone by. A very clever man. 'Your sympathies are with the nobility,' he said. 'Shall I tell you why? Because you yourself belong to the nobility. Your father is a great gentleman, and you are a princess. A gulf lies between you and the rest of us who do not belong to the governing classes.' Yes, Tom. We feel like the nobility, and we realize the difference; we should never try to live where we are not known, where no one understands our worth, for we shall have nothing but chagrin, and be laughed at for our arrogance. Yes, they all found me ridiculously arrogant. They did not say so, but I felt it every minute, and that made me suffer, too. Do you think I feel arrogant, Tom – in a place where they eat cake with a knife, and the very princes speak bad grammar, and if a gentleman picks up a lady's fan it is supposed to be a love-affair. Get used to it? To people without dignity, morals, energy, ambition, self-respect, or good manners, lazy and frivolous, stupid and shallow at the same time? – no, never, never, as long as I am a Buddenbrook and your sister! Eva Ewers managed it – but Eva is not a Buddenbrook, and she has a husband that amounts to something. It was different with me. You think back, Tom, from the very beginning: I come from a home where people work and get things accomplished and have a purpose in life, and I go down there to Permaneder – and he sits himself down with my dowry – Oh, that was genuine enough, that was characteristic – but it was the only good thing there was about it! And then? I was going to have a baby; that would have made everything up to me. And what happens? It dies. I don't blame Permaneder for that, of course; I don't mean that. God forbid. He did everything he could – and he didn't go to the café for several days. But, after all, it belonged to the same thing. It made me no happier, as you can well believe. But I didn't give in, and I didn't grumble. I was alone, and misunderstood, and pointed at for being arrogant; but I said to myself: 'You yielded him your consent for life. He is lumpy and lazy, and he caused you a cruel disappointment. But his heart is pure, and he means well.' And then I had to bear the sight of him in that last unspeakable minute. And I said to myself: 'He understands you no better and respects you no more and no less than the others do, and he calls you names that one of our workmen up here wouldn't throw at a dog!' I knew then that nothing bound me to him any more, and that it was an indignity for me to stay. When I was driving from the station this afternoon, I passed Nielsen the porter, and he took off his hat and made me a deep bow, and I bowed back to him – not arrogantly, not a bit – I waved my hand, just the way Father used to. And here I am. You can do what you like: you can harness up all your work-horses – but you can never drag me back to Munich again. And to-morrow I go to Gieseke!"

Thus she spoke; and, finishing, sank back exhausted in her chair and stared again out of the window.

Tom was alarmed, shaken, stupefied. He stood before her and

found no words. He raised his arms up shoulder-high, drawing a long breath. Then he let them fall against his thighs.

"Well, that's an end of it," he said. His voice was calm, and he turned and went toward the door.

Her face wore now the same expression, the same half-pouting, half-injured smile, as when he entered.

"Tom?" she said, with a rising inflection. "Are you vexed with me?"

He held the oval doorknob in one hand and made a gesture of weary protest with the other. "Oh, no. Not at all."

She put out her hand and tipped her head on one side. "Come here, Tom. Your poor sister has had a hard time. Life is hard on her. She has much to bear. And at this minute she has nobody, in all the world – "

He came back; he took her hand; but wearily, indifferently, not looking at her face. Suddenly her lip began to quiver.

"You must go on alone now," she said. "There's nothing good to be looked for from Christian, and I am finished. Failed. Gone to pieces. I can do no more. I am a poor, useless woman, dependent on you all for my living. I could never have dreamed, Tom, that I should be no help to you at all. Now you stand quite alone, and upon you it depends to keep up the honour and dignity of the family. May God help you in the task."

Two large, clear, childish tears rolled down over her cheeks, which were beginning to show, very faintly, the first signs of age.

CHAPTER XI

Tony lost no time. She went resolutely about her affair. In the hope of quieting her, of bringing her slowly to a different frame of mind, the Consul said but little. He asked only one thing: that she should be very quiet and stop entirely in the house – and Erica as well. Perhaps it would blow over. The town did not need to know. The family Thursday afternoon was put off on some pretext.

But on the very next day she wrote to Dr. Gieseke and summoned him to Meng Street. She received him alone, in the middle corridor room on the first floor, where a fire was laid, and she had arranged a heavy table with ink and writing materials and a quantity of foolscap paper from the office. They sat down in two easy-chairs.

"Doctor Gieseke," said Tony. She folded her arms, flung back her head, and looked at the ceiling while she spoke. "You are a man of experience, both professionally and personally. I can speak openly with you." And thereupon she revealed to him the whole story about Babette and what had happened in her sleeping-chamber. Dr. Gieseke regretted being obliged to explain to her that neither the affair on the stairs nor the insult she had undoubtedly received, the precise nature of which she hesitated to divulge, was sufficient ground for a divorce.

"Very good," she said. "Thank you."

And then, at her request, he gave an exposition of the existing legal grounds for divorce, and an even longer discourse after it, which had for its subject-matter the law touching dowry rights. She listened with open mind and strained attention; and then, with cordial thanks, dismissed Dr. Gieseke for the time being.

She went downstairs and demanded audience of her brother in his private office.

"Thomas," she said, "please write to the man at once – I do not like to mention his name. As far as the money goes, I am perfectly informed on that subject. Let him speak. Me he shall never see again, whatever he decides. If he agrees to a divorce, we will ask him to give an accounting and restore my *dos*. If he refuses, we need not be discouraged. For, as you probably know, Permaneder's right to my *dos* is, legally speaking, a property right. We grant that. But on the other hand, thank goodness, I have certain material rights on my side – "

The Consul walked up and down with his hands behind his back, his shoulders twitching nervously. Tony's face, as she uttered the word *dos* was too unutterably self-satisfied!

He had no time. Heaven knew he had no time. Let her have patience, and wait, and bethink herself a hundred times. His nearest duty was a journey to Hamburg – indeed, he must go the very next day, for the purpose of a personal interview with Christian. Christian had written for help, for money which would have to come out of the Frau Consul's inheritance. His business was in frightful condition; he was in constant difficulties. Yet he seemed to amuse himself royally and went everywhere, to theatres, restaurants, and concert halls. To judge from the debts now coming to light, which he had been able to pile up on the credit of his family name, he had been living far, far beyond his means. And they knew in Meng Street, and at the club – yes, the whole town knew – who was responsible. It was a certain female, a certain Aline Puvogel, who lived alone with her two pretty children. Christian was not the only Hamburg business man who possessed her favours and spent money on her.

In short, Tony's intentions in the matter of her divorce were not the only dark spot in the Consul's sky; and the journey to Hamburg was pressing. Besides, it was altogether likely that they would hear from Herr Permaneder.

The Consul went to Hamburg, and came back angry and depressed. No word had come from Munich, and he felt obliged to take the first step. He wrote; wrote rather coldly, with curt condescension, to this effect: Antonie, during her life with Permaneder, had been subjected to great disappointments – that would not be denied. Without going into detail, it was evident that she could never find happiness in this marriage. Her wish that it should be dissolved must be justified, to the mind of any reasonable person; and her determination not to return to Munich was entirely unshakable. And he put the question as to what were Herr Permaneder's feelings in view of the facts which he had just stated.

There were more days of suspense. And then came Herr Permaneder's reply.

He answered as no one had expected him to answer – not Dr.

Gieseke, nor the Frau Consul, not Thomas, nor Antonie herself. He agreed, quite simply, to a divorce.

He wrote that he deeply regretted what had happened, but that he respected Antonie's wishes, as he saw that he and she had "never hit it off." If it were true that she had suffered during those years through him, he begged her to forget and forgive. As he would probably never see her and Erica again, he sent them both his hearty good wishes for all happiness on this earth. And he signed himself, Alois Permaneder. In a postscript he offered to make immediate restitution of the dowry. He had enough without it to lead a life free from care. He did not require to have notice given, for business there was none to wind up, the house belonged to him, and the money was ready any time.

Tony felt a slight twinge of shame, and was almost inclined, for the first time, to admit that Herr Permaneder's indifference to money matters might have something good about it.

Now it was Dr. Gieseke's turn again. He communicated with the husband, and a plea of "mutual incompatibility" was set up as ground for the divorce. The hearing began – Tony's second divorce case. She talked about it night and day, and the Consul lost his temper several times. Tony was in no state to share his feelings. She was entirely taken up with words like "tangibilities," "improvabilities," "accessions," "productivity," "dowry rights," and the like, which she used in season and out of season, with marvellous fluency, her shoulders slightly raised. One point in Dr. Gieseke's long disquisitions had made a great impression on her: it had to do with "treasure" found in any piece of property that has constituted part of a dowry, which was to be regarded as a component part of the dowry, to be liquidated if the marriage came to an end. About this "treasure" – which was, of course, non-existent – she talked to every soul she knew: Ida Jungmann, Uncle Justus, poor Clothilde, the Broad Street Buddenbrooks – and they, when they heard how matters stood, just folded their hands in their laps and looked at each other in speechless joy that this satisfaction, too, had been vouchsafed them. Therese Weichbrodt was told of it – Erica had gone to stay at the pension again – and Madame Kethelson too, though this last, for more than one reason, understood not a single word.

Then came the day when the divorce was pronounced; when the last formalities were gone through, and Tony asked Thomas for the family papers and set down this last event with her own hand. Yes, it was done. All that remained was to get used to it.

She did it gallantly. She bore, with unscathed dignity, the tiny dagger-thrusts of the ladies from Broad Street; she met the Hagenströms and Möllendorpfs on the street and looked with chilling indifference straight over their heads; and she quite gave up going into society – the more easily that it had for some years past forsaken her Mother's house for her brother's. She had her own immediate family, the Frau Consul, Tom, and Gerda; she had Ida Jungmann and her motherly friend Sesemi Weichbrodt; and she had Erica, upon whose future she probably built her own last secret hopes, and upon whose aristocratic upbringing she expended much care and thought.

Thus she lived, and thus time went on.

Later, in some way that was never quite clear, there came to certain members of the family knowledge of that "word," the desperate word which had escaped from Herr Permaneder on that never-to-be-forgotten night.

What was it, then, that he had said?

"Go to the devil, you filthy sprat-eating slut!"

And thus Tony Buddenbrook's second marriage came to an end.

PART SEVEN

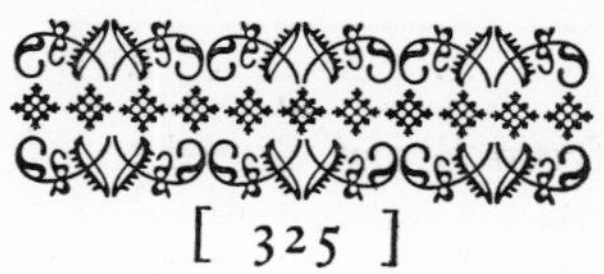

CHAPTER I

A CHRISTENING – a christening in Broad Street!

All, everything is there that was dreamed of by Madame Permaneder in the days of her expectancy. In the dining-room, the maid-servant, moving noiselessly so as not to disturb the services in the next room, is filling the cups with steaming hot chocolate and whipped cream. There are quantities of cups, crowded together on the great round tray with the gilded shell-shaped handles. And Anton the butler is cutting a towering layer-cake into slices, and Mamsell Jungmann is arranging flowers and sweets in silver dessert-dishes, with her head on one side, and both little fingers stuck out.

Soon the company will have seated themselves in the salon and sitting-room, and all these delicacies will be handed round. It is to be hoped they will hold out, since it is the whole family which has gathered here, in the broader, if not quite in the broadest sense of the word. For it is, through the Överdiecks, connected distantly with the Kistenmakers, and through them with the Möllendorpfs – and so on. One simply must draw the line somewhere! But the Överdiecks are represented, and, indeed, by no less a personage than the head of the family, the venerable Doctor Kaspar Överdieck, reigning Burgomaster, more than eighty years old.

He came in a carriage, and mounted the steps leaning on his staff and Thomas Buddenbrook's arm. His presence enhances the dignity of the occasion – and, beyond a question, this occasion is worthy of every dignity!

For within, in the salon, there is a flower-decked small table, serving as an altar, with a young priest in black vestments and a stiff snowy ruff like a millstone round his neck, reciting the service; and there is a great, strapping, particularly well-nourished person, richly arrayed in red and gold, bearing upon her billowing arms a small something, half smothered in laces and satin bows: an heir – a first-born son! A Buddenbrook! Do we really grasp the meaning of the fact?

Can we realize the thrill of that first whisper, that first little hint that travelled from Broad Street to Mengstrasse? Or Frau Permaneder's speechless ecstasy, as she embraced her mother, her brother, and – very gently – her sister-in-law? And now, with the spring – the spring of the year 1861 – he has come: he, the heir of so many hopes, whom they have expected for so many years, talked of him, longed for him, prayed to God and tormented Dr. Grabow for him; at length he has come – and looks most unimposing.

His tiny hands play among the gilt trimmings of his nurse's bodice; his head, in a lace cap trimmed with pale blue ribbons, lies sidewise on the pillow, turned heedlessly away from the preacher; he stares out into the room, at all his relatives, with an old, knowing look. Those eyes, under their long-lashed lids, blend the light blue of the Father's and the brown of the Mother's iris into a pale, indefinite, changeful golden-brown; but bluish shadows lie in the deep corners on both sides of the nose, and these give the little face, which is hardly yet a face at all, an aged look not suited to its four weeks of existence. But, please God, they mean nothing – for has not his Mother the same? And she is in perfectly good health. And anyhow, he lives – he lives, and is a son; which was the cause, four weeks ago, for great rejoicing.

He lives – and it might have been otherwise. The Consul will never forget the grip of good Dr. Grabow's hand, as he said to him, four weeks ago, when he could leave the mother and child: "Give thanks to God, my dear friend – there wasn't much to spare." The Consul has not dared to ask his meaning. He put from him in horror the thought that his son – this tiny creature, yearned for in vain so many years – had slipped into the world without breath to cry out, almost – *almost* – like Antonie's second daughter. But he knows that that hour, four weeks ago, was a desperate one for mother and child; and he bends tenderly over Gerda, who reclines in an easy-chair in front of him, next his Mother, her feet, in patent-leather shoes, crossed before her on a velvet cushion.

How pale she still is! And how strangely lovely in her pallor, with that heavy dark-red hair and those mysterious eyes that rest upon the preacher in half-veiled mockery! Herr Andreas Pringsheim, *pastor marianus*, succeeded thus young to the headship of St. Mary's after old Kölling's sudden death. He holds his chin in the air and his hands prayerfully folded beneath it. He has short, curly blond hair and a smooth-shaven, bony face, with a somewhat theatrical range of expression, from fanatical zeal to an exalted serenity. He comes from Franconia, where he has been for some years, serving a small Lutheran community among Catholics; and his effort after a clear and moving delivery has resulted in exaggerated mannerisms; an *r* rolled upon his front teeth and long, obscure, or crudely accented vowel-sounds.

He gives thanks to God, in a voice now low and soft, now loud and swelling – and the family listen: Frau Permaneder, clothed in a dignity that hides her pride and her delight; Erica Grünlich, now almost fifteen years old, a blooming young girl with a long braid and her father's rosy skin; and Christian, who has arrived that morning, and sits letting his deep-set eyes rove from side to side all over the room. Pastor Tiburtius and his wife have not shrunk from the long journey, but have come from Riga to be present at the ceremony. The ends of Sievert Tiburtius' long, thin whiskers are parted over his shoulders, and his small grey eyes now and then open wider and wider, most unexpectedly, and grow larger and more prominent till they almost jump out of his head. Clara's gaze is dark and solemn and severe, and she sometimes lifts her hand to a head that always seems to ache. But they have brought a splendid present to the Buddenbrooks: a huge brown bear stuffed in a standing position. A relative of the Pastor's shot him somewhere in the heart of Russia, and now he stands below in the vestibule with a card-tray between his paws.

The Krögers have their son Jürgen visiting them; he is a post-office official in Rostock, a quiet, simply-dressed man. Where Jacob is, nobody knows but his mother, who was an Överdieck. She, poor, weak woman, secretly sells the household silver to send money to the disinherited son. And the ladies Buddenbrook are there, deeply rejoiced over the happy family event – which does not prevent Pfiffi from remarking that the child looks rather unhealthy: a view which the Frau Consul, born Stüwing, and likewise Friederike and Henriette, feel bound to endorse. But poor Clothilde, lean, grey, resigned, and hungry, is moved by the words of Pastor Pringsheim and the prospect of layer-cake and chocolate. The guests not belonging to the family are Herr Friedrich Wilhelm Marcus and Sesemi Weichbrodt.

Now the Pastor turns to the god-parents and instructs them in their duty. Justus Kröger is one. Consul Buddenbrook refused at first to ask him. "Why invite the old man to commit a piece of folly?" he says. "He has frightful scenes with his wife every day over Jacob; their little property is slowly melting away – out of pure worry he is even beginning to be careless in his dress! But you know what will happen: if we ask him, he will send the child a heavy gold service and refuse to be thanked for it!" But when

Uncle Justus heard who was to be asked in his place – Stephan Kistenmaker had been mentioned – he was so enormously piqued that they had to ask him after all. The gold mug he presented was, to Thomas's great relief, not exaggeratedly heavy.

And the second god-father? It is this dignified old gentleman with the snow-white hair, high neck-band, and soft black broadcloth coat with the red handkerchief sticking out of the back pocket, sitting here bent over his stick, in the most comfortable arm-chair in the house. It is, of course, Burgomaster Dr. Överdieck. It is a great event – a triumph! Good heavens, how could it have come about? he is hardly even a relative! The Buddenbrooks must have dragged the old man in by the hair! In fact, it *is* rather a feat: a little intrigue planned by the Consul and Madame Permaneder. At first it was merely a joke, born of the great relief of knowing that mother and child were safe. "A boy, Tony," cried the Consul. "He ought to have the Burgomaster for godfather!" But she took it up in earnest, whereupon he considered the matter seriously and agreed to make a trial. They hid behind Uncle Justus, and got him to send his wife to her sister-in-law, the wife of Överdieck the lumber dealer. She accepted the task of preparing the old father-in-law; then Thomas Buddenbrook made a visit to the head of the state and paid his respects – and the thing was done.

Now the nurse lifts up the child's cap, and the Pastor cautiously sprinkles two or three drops out of the gilt-lined silver basin in front of him, upon the few hairs of little Buddenbrook, as he slowly and impressively names the names with which he is baptizing him: Justus, Johann, Kaspar. Follows a short prayer, and then the relatives file by to bestow a kiss upon the brow of the unconcerned little creature. Therese Weichbrodt comes last, to whom the nurse has to stoop with her burden; in return for which Sesemi gives him two kisses, that go off with small explosions, and says, between them: "You good che-ild!"

Three minutes later, the guests have disposed themselves in salon and living-room, and the sweets are passed. Even Pastor Pringsheim, the toes of his broad, shiny boots showing under his black vestments, sits and sips the cool whipped cream off his hot chocolate, chatting easily the while, and wearing his serene expression, which is most effective by way of contrast with his sermon. His manner says, as plainly as words: "See how I can lay aside the priest and become the jolly ordinary guest!" He is a versatile, an accommodating sort of man. To the Frau Consul he speaks rather unctuously, to Thomas and Gerda like a man of the world, and with Frau Permaneder he is downright jocose, making jokes and gesturing fluently. Now and then, whenever he thinks of it, he folds his hands in his lap, tips back his head, glooms his brows, and makes a long face. When he laughs he draws the air in through his teeth in little jerks.

Suddenly there is a stir in the corridor, the servants are heard laughing, and in the doorway appears a singular figure, come to offer congratulations. It is Grobleben: Grobleben, from whose thin nose, no matter what the time of year, there ever hangs a drop, which never falls. Grobleben is a workman in one of the Consul's granaries, and he has an extra job, too, at the house, as boots. Every morning early he appears in Broad Street, takes the boots from before the door, and cleans them below in the court. At family feasts he always appears in holiday attire, presents flowers, and makes a speech, in a whining, unctuous voice, with the drop pendent from his nose. For this, he always gets a piece of money – but that is *not* why he does it!

He wears a black coat – an old one of the Consul's – greased leather top-boots, and a blue woollen scarf round his neck. In his wizened red hand he holds a bunch of pale-coloured roses, which are a little past their best, and slowly shed their petals on the carpet. He blinks with his small red eyes, but apparently sees nothing. He stands still in the doorway, with his flowers held out in front of him, and begins straightway to speak. The old Frau Consul nods to him encouragingly and makes soothing little noises, the Consul regards him with one eyebrow lifted, and some of the family – Frau Permaneder, for instance – put their handkerchiefs to their mouths.

"I be a poor man, yer honour 'n' ladies 'n' gentlemen, but I've a feelin' hairt; 'n' the happiness of my master comes home to me, it do, seein's he's allus been so good t' me; 'n' so I've come, yer honour 'n' ladies 'n' gentlemen, to congratulate the Herr Consul 'n' the Frau Consul, 'n' the whole respected family, from a full hairt, 'n' that the child may prosper, for that they desarve fr'm God 'n' man, for such a master as Consul Buddenbrook there aren't so many, he's a noble gentleman, 'n' our Lord will reward him for all. . . ."

"Splendid, Grobleben! That was a beautiful speech. Thank you very much, Grobleben. What are the roses for?"

But Grobleben has not nearly done. He strains his whining voice and drowns the Consul out.

". . . 'n' I say th' Lord will reward him, him and the whole respected family; 'n' when his time has come to stan' before His throne, for stan' we all must, rich *and* poor, 'n' one'll have a fine polished hard-wood coffin 'n' 'tother 'n' old box, yet all on us must come to mother earth at th' last, yes, we must all come to her at th' last – to mother earth – to mother – "

"Oh, come, come, Grobleben! This isn't a funeral, it's a christening. Get along with your mother earth!"

". . . 'n' these be a few flowers," concludes Grobleben.

"Thank you, Grobleben, thank you. This is too much – what did you pay for them, man? But I haven't heard such a speech as that for a long time! Wait a minute – here, go out and give yourself a treat, in honour of the day!" And the Consul puts his hand on the old man's shoulder and gives him a thaler.

"Here, my good man," says the Frau Consul. "And I hope you love our blessed Lord?"

"I be lovin' him from my hairt, Frau Consul, thet's the holy truth!" And Grobleben gets another thaler from her, and a third from Frau Permaneder, and retires with a bow and a scrape, taking the roses with him by mistake, except for those already fallen on the carpet.

The Burgomaster takes his leave now, and the Consul accompanies him down to his carriage. This is the signal for the party to break up – for Gerda Buddenbrook must rest. The old Frau Consul, Tony, Erica, and Mamsell Jungmann are the last to go.

"Well, Ida," says the Consul, "I have been thinking it over: you took care of us all, and when little Johann gets a bit older – He still has the monthly nurse now, and after that he will still need a day-nurse, I suppose – but will you be willing to move over to us when the time comes?"

"Yes, indeed, Herr Consul, if your wife is satisfied."

Gerda is content to have it so, and thus it is settled.

In the act of leaving, however, and already at the door, Frau Permaneder turns. She comes back to her brother and kisses him on both cheeks, and says: "It has been a lovely day, Tom. I am happier than I have been for years. We Buddenbrooks aren't quite at the last gasp yet, thank God, and whoever thinks we are is mightily mistaken. Now that we have little Johann – it is so beautiful that he is christened Johann – it looks to me as if quite a new day will dawn for us all!"

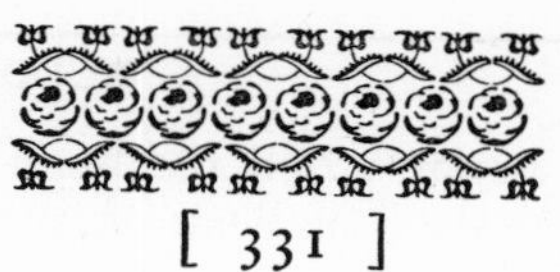

CHAPTER II

Christian Buddenbrook, proprietor of the firm of H. C. F. Burmeester and Company of Hamburg, came into his brother's living-room, holding in his hand his modish grey hat and his walking-stick with the nun's bust. Tom and Gerda sat reading together. It was half past nine on the evening of the christening day.

"Good evening," said Christian. "Oh, Thomas, I must speak with you at once. – Please excuse me, Gerda. – It is urgent, Thomas."

They went into the dark dining-room, where the Consul lighted a gas-jet on the wall, and looked at his brother. He expected nothing good. Except for the first greeting, he had had no opportunity to speak with Christian, but he had looked at him, during the service, and noted that he seemed unusually serious, and even more restless than common: in the course of Pastor Pringsheim's discourse he had left the room for several minutes. Thomas had not written him since the day in Hamburg when he had paid over into his brother's hands an advance of 10,000 marks current on his inheritance, to settle his indebtedness. "Just go on as you are going," he had said, "and you'll soon run through all your money. As far as I am concerned, I hope you will cross my path very little in future. You have put my friendship to too hard a test in these three years." Why was he here now? Something must be driving him.

"Well?" asked the Consul.

"I'm done," Christian said. He let himself down sidewise on one of the high-backed chairs around the dining-table, and held his hat and stick between his thin knees.

"May I ask what it is you are done with, and what brings you to me?" said the Consul. He remained standing.

"I'm done," repeated Christian, shaking his head from side to side with frightful earnestness and letting his little round eyes stray restlessly back and forth. He was now thirty-three years old, but he looked much older. His reddish-blond hair was grown so thin that nearly all the cranium was bare. His cheeks were sunken, the cheek-bones protruded sharply, and between them, naked, fleshless, and gaunt, stood the huge hooked nose.

" If it were only this — ! " he went on, and ran his hand down the whole of his left side, very close, but not touching it. " It isn't a pain, you know — it is a misery, a continuous, indefinite ache. Dr. Drögemuller in Hamburg tells me that my nerves on this side are all too short. Imagine, on my whole left side, my nerves aren't long enough! Sometimes I think I shall surely have a stroke here, on this side, a permanent paralysis. You have no idea. I never go to sleep properly. My heart doesn't beat, and I start up suddenly, in a perfectly terrible fright. That happens not once but ten times before I get to sleep. I don't know if you know what it is. I'll tell you about it more precisely. It is — "

" Not now," the Consul said coldly. " Am I to understand that you have come here to tell me this? I suppose not."

" No, Thomas. If it were only that — but it is not that — alone. It is the business. I can't go on with it."

" Your affairs are in confusion again? " The Consul did not start, he did not raise his voice. He asked the question quite calmly, and looked sidewise at his brother, with a cold, weary glance.

" No, Thomas. For to tell you the truth — it is all the same now — I never really was in order, even with the ten thousand, as you know yourself. They only saved me from putting up the shutters at once. The thing is — I had more losses at once, in coffee — and with the failure in Antwerp — That's the truth. So then I didn't do any more business; I just sat still. But one has to live — so now there are notes and other debts — five thousand thaler. You don't know the hole I'm in. And on top of everything else, this agony — "

" Oh, so you just sat still, did you? " cried the Consul, beside himself. His self-control was gone now. " You let the wagon stick in the mud and went off to enjoy yourself! You think I don't know the kind of life you've been living — theatres and circus and clubs — and women — "

" You mean Aline. Yes, Thomas, you have very little understanding for that sort of thing, and it's my misfortune, perhaps, that I have so much. You are right when you say it has cost me too much; and it will cost me a goodish bit more, for — I'll tell you something, just here between two brothers — the third child, the little girl, six months old, she is my child."

" You fool, you! "

" Don't say that, Thomas. You should be just, even if you are angry, to her and to — why shouldn't it be my child? And as for

Aline, she isn't in the least worthless, and you ought not to say she is. She is not at all promiscuous; she broke with Consul Holm on my account, and he has much more money than I have. That's how decent she is. No, Thomas, you simply can't understand what a splendid creature she is – and *healthy* – she is as *healthy* – ! " He repeated the word, and held up one hand before his face with the fingers crooked, in the same gesture as when he used to tell about " Maria " and the depravity of London. " You should see her teeth when she laughs. I've never found any other teeth to compare with them, not in Valparaiso, or London, or anywhere else in the world. I'll never forget the evening I first met her, in the oyster-room, at Uhlich's. She was living with Consul Holm then. Well, I told her a story or so, and was a bit friendly; and when I went home with her afterwards – well, Thomas, that's a different sort of feeling from the one you have when you do a good stroke of business! But you don't like to hear about such things – I can see that already – and anyhow, it's over with. I'm saying good-bye to her, though I shall keep in touch with her on account of the child. I'll pay up everything I owe in Hamburg, and shut up shop. I can't go on. I've talked with Mother, and she is willing to give me the five thousand thaler to start with, so I can put things in order; and I hope you will agree to it, for it is much better to say quite simply that Christian Buddenbrook is winding up his business and going abroad, than for me to make a failure. You think so too, don't you? I intend to go to London again, Thomas, and take a position. It isn't good for me to be independent – I can see that more and more. The responsibility – whereas in a situation one just goes home quite care-free, at the end of the day. And I liked living in London. Do you object? "

During this exposition, the Consul had turned his back on his brother, and stood with his hands in his pockets, describing figures on the floor with his foot.

" Very good, go to London," he said, shortly, and without turning more than half-way toward his brother, he passed into the living-room.

But Christian followed him. He went up to Gerda, who sat there alone, reading, and put out his hand.

" Good night, Gerda. Well, Gerda, I'm off for London. Yes, it's remarkable how one gets tossed about hither and yon. Now it's again into the unknown, into a great city, you know, where one meets an adventure at every third step, and sees so much of life. Strange – do you know the feeling? One gets it here – sort of in the pit of the stomach – it's very odd."

CHAPTER III

James Möllendorpf, the oldest of the merchant senators, died in a grotesque and horrible way. The instinct of self-preservation became very weak in this diabetic old man; and in the last years of his life he fell a victim to a passion for cakes and pastries. Dr. Grabow, as the Möllendorpf family physician, had protested energetically, and the distressed relatives employed gentle constraint to keep the head of the family from committing suicide with sweet bake-stuffs. But the old Senator, mental wreck as he was, rented a room somewhere, in some convenient street, like Little Groping Alley, or Angelswick, or Behind-the-Wall – a little hole of a room, whither he would secretly betake himself to consume sweets. And there they found his lifeless body, the mouth still full of half-masticated cake, the crumbs upon his coat and upon the wretched table. A mortal stroke had supervened, and put a stop to slow dissolution.

The horrid details of the death were kept as much as possible from the family, but they flew about the town, and were discussed at length on the Bourse, in the club, and at the Harmony, in all the business offices, in the Assembly of Burgesses – likewise at all the balls, dinners, and evening parties, for the death occurred in February of the year '62, and the season was in full swing. Even the Frau Consul's friends talked about it, on the Jerusalem evenings, in the pauses of Lea Gerhardt's reading aloud; the little Sunday-school children discussed it in awesome whispers as they crossed the Buddenbrook entry; and Herr Stuht, in Bell-Founders' Street, went into ample detail over it with his wife, who moved in the highest circles.

But interest could not long remain concentrated upon the past. And even with the first rumour of the old man's death, the great question had at once sprung up: who was to succeed him?

What suspense, what subterranean activity! A stranger, intent on the sights of the mediaeval town, would have noticed nothing; but beneath the surface there was unimaginable bustle and commotion, as one firm and unassailable honest conviction after another was exploded; and slowly, slowly the while, divergent views approached each other! Passions are stirred, Ambition and Vanity wrestle together in silence. Dead and buried hopes spring once more to life – and again are blasted. Old Kurz, the merchant, in Bakers' Alley, who gets three or four votes at every election, will sit quaking at home on the fatal day, and listen to the shouting, but he will not be elected this time either. He will continue to take his walks abroad, displaying outwardly his usual mingling of civic pride and self-satisfaction: but he will bear down with him into the grave the secret chagrin of never having been elected Senator.

James Möllendorpf's death was discussed at the Buddenbrook Thursday dinner-table; and Frau Permaneder, after the proper expressions of sympathy, began to let her tongue play upon her upper lip and look across artfully at her brother. The Buddenbrook ladies marked the look. They exchanged piercing glances, and with one accord shut their eyes and their lips tightly together. The Consul had, for a second, responded to the sly smile his sister gave him, and then given the talk another turn. He knew that the thought which Tony hugged to her breast in secret was being spoken in the street.

Names were suggested and rejected, others came up and were sifted out. Henning Kurz in Bakers' Alley was too old. They needed new blood. Consul Huneus, the lumber dealer, whose millions would have weighted the scale heavily in his favour, was constitutionally ineligible, as his brother already sat in the Senate. Consul Eduard Kistenmaker, the wine dealer, and Consul Hermann Hagenström were names that kept their places on the list. But from the very first was heard the name of Thomas Buddenbrook; and as election day approached, it grew constantly plainer that he and Hermann Hagenström were the favoured candidates.

Hermann Hagenström had his admirers and hangers-on – there was no doubt of that. His zeal in public affairs, the spectacular rise of the firm of Strunck and Hagenström, the showy house the Consul kept, the luxurious life he led, the pâtés-de-foie-gras he ate for breakfast – all these could not fail to make an impression. This large, rather over-stout man with the short, full, reddish beard and the snub nose coming down flat on his upper lip, this man whose grandfather nobody knew, not even himself, and whose father had made himself socially impossible by a rich but doubtful marriage; this man had become a brother-in-law of the Huneus' and the Möllendorpfs, had ranged his name alongside those of the five or six reigning families in the town, and was undeniably a remarkable and a respected figure. The novel and therewith the attractive element in his personality – that which singled him out for a leading position in the eyes of many – was its liberal and tolerant strain. His light, large way of making money and spending it again differed fundamentally from the patient, persistent toil and the inherited principles of his fellow merchants. This man stood on his own feet, free from the fetters of tradition and ancestral piety; and all the old ways were foreign to him. His house was not one of the ancient patrician mansions, built with senseless waste of space, in tall white galleries mounting above a stone-paved ground floor. His home on Sand Street, the southern extension of Broad Street, was a modern dwelling, not conforming to any set style of architecture, with a simple painted façade, but furnished inside with every luxury and planned with the cleverest economy of space. Recently, on the occasion of one of his large evening parties, he had invited a prima donna from the government theatre, to sing after dinner to his guests – among them his witty, art-loving brother – and had paid her an enormous fee for her services. Hermann Hagenström was not the man to vote in the Assembly for the application of large sums of money to preserve and restore the town's mediaeval monuments. But it was a fact that he was the first, absolutely the first man in town to light his house and his offices with gas. Yes, if Consul Hagenström could be said to represent any tradition whatever, it was the free, progressive, tolerant, unprejudiced habit of thought which he had inherited from his father, old Hinrich – and on this was based all the admiration people undoubtedly felt for him.

Thomas Buddenbrook's prestige was of a different kind. People honoured in him not only his own personality, but the personalities of his father, grandfather, and great-grandfather as well: quite apart from his own business and public achievement, he was the representative of a hundred years of honourable tradition. And the easy, charming way, indeed, with which he carried the family standard made no small part of his success. What distinguished him, even among his professional fellow citizens, was an unusual degree of formal culture, which, wherever he went, aroused both wonder and respect in about equal degrees.

On Thursdays at the Buddenbrooks', the coming election received only brief and passing comment in the presence of the Consul. Whenever it was mentioned, the old Frau Consul discreetly averted her light eyes. But Frau Permaneder, now and then, could not refrain from displaying her astonishing knowledge of the Constitution. She had gone very thoroughly into the decrees touching the election of a member of the Senate, precisely as once she thoroughly informed herself on the laws governing divorce. She talked about voting chambers, ballots, and electors, she weighed all the possible eventualities, she could recite verbatim and glibly the oath taken by the voters. She spoke of the "free and frank discussion" which the Constitution ordains must be held over each name upon the list of candidates, and vivaciously wished she might be present when Hermann Hagenström's character was being pulled to pieces! A moment later she leaned over and began to count the prune-pits on her brother's dessert-plate: tinker, tailor, soldier, sailor – finishing triumphantly with "senator" when she came to the last pit. But after dinner she could not hold in any longer. She took her brother's arm and drew him into the bow-window.

"Oh, Tom! *Tom!* Suppose you are really elected – if our coat-of-arms is put up in the Senate-chamber at the Town Hall I shall just die of joy, I know I shall. I shall fall dead at the news – you'll see!"

"Now, Tony dear! Have a little self-control, a little dignity, I beg of you. You are not usually lacking in dignity. Am I going around like Henning Kurz? We amount to something even without the 'Senator.' And I hope you won't die, whichever way it turns out!"

And the agitations, the consultations, the struggles of opinion took their course. Consul Peter Döhlman, the rake with a business now entirely ruined, which existed only in name, and the twenty-seven-year-old daughter whose inheritance he was eating up, played his part by attending two dinners, one given by Thomas Buddenbrook and the other by Hermann Hagenström, and both times addressing his host, in his loud, resounding voice, as "Senator." But Siegismund Gosch, old Gosch the broker, went about like a raging lion, and engaged to throttle anybody, out of hand, who wasn't minded to vote for Consul Buddenbrook.

"Consul Buddenbrook, gentlemen – ah, there's a man for you! I stood at his father's side in the '48, when, with a word, he tamed the unleashed fury of the mob. His father, and his father's father before him, would have been Senator were there any justice on this earth!"

But at bottom it was not so much Consul Buddenbrook himself whose personality fired Gosch's soul to its innermost depths. It was rather the young Frau Consul, Gerda Arnoldsen. Not that the broker had ever exchanged a word with her. He did not belong to her circle of wealthy merchant families, nor sit at their tables, nor pay visits to them. But, as we have seen, Gerda Buddenbrook had but to arrive in the town to be singled out by the roving fancy of the sinister broker, ever on the look-out for the unusual. With unerring instinct he divined that this figure was calculated to add content to his unsatisfied existence, and he made himself the slave of one who had scarcely ever heard his name. Since then he encompassed in his reveries this nervous, exceedingly reserved lady, to whom he had not even been presented: he lifted his Jesuit hat to her, on the street, to her great surprise, and treated her to a pantomime of cringing treachery, gloating over her the while in his thoughts as a tiger might over his trainer. This dull existence would afford him no chance of committing atrocities for this woman's sake – ah, if it only would, with what devilish indifference would he answer for them! Its stupid conventions prevented him from raising her, by deeds of blood and horror, to an imperial throne! – And thus, nothing was left but for him to go to the Town Hall and cast his vote in favour of her furiously respected husband – and, perhaps, one day, to dedicate to her his forthcoming transition of Lope de Vega.

CHAPTER IV

Every vacant seat in the Senate must, according to the Constitution, be filled within four weeks. Three of them have passed, and this is election-day — a day of thaw, at the end of February.

It is about one o'clock, and people are thronging into Broad Street. They are thronging before the Town Hall, with its ornamental glazed-brick façade, its pointed towers and turrets mounting toward a whitish grey sky, its covered steps supported on outstanding columns, its pointed arcades, through which there is a glimpse of the market place and the fountain. The crowd stands steadfastly in the dirty slush that melts beneath their feet; they look into each other's faces and then straight ahead again, and crane their necks. For beyond that portal, in the Council Room, in fourteen armchairs arranged in a semicircle sit the electors, who have been chosen from the Senate and the Assembly and await the proposals of the voting chambers.

The affair has spun itself out. It appears that the debate in the chambers will not die down; the struggle is so bitter that up to now not one single unanimous choice has been put before the Council — otherwise the Burgomaster would at once announce an election. Extraordinary! Rumours — nobody knows whence, nobody knows how — come from within the building and circulate in the street. Perhaps Herr Kaspersen, the elder of the two beadles, who always refers to himself as a " servant of the State," is standing inside there and telling what he hears, out of the corner of his mouth, through his shut teeth, with his eyes turned the other way! The story goes that proposals have been laid before the sitting, but that each of the three chambers has turned in a different name: namely Hagenström, Kistenmaker, and Buddenbrook. A secret ballot must now be taken, with ballot-papers — it is to be hoped that it will show a clear plurality! For people without overshoes are suffering, and stamping their feet to warm them.

The waiting crowd is made up of all sorts and conditions. There are sea-faring characters, with bare tattoed necks and their hands in the pockets of their sailor trousers; grain porters with their incomparably respectable countenances, and their blouses and knee-breeches of black glazed calico; drivers who have clambered down from their wagons of piled-up sacks, and stand whip in hand to wait for the decision; servant-maids in neckerchiefs, aprons and thick striped petticoats with little white caps perched on the backs of their heads and market-baskets hanging on their bare arms; fish and vegetable women with their flat straw baskets – even a couple of pretty farm girls with Dutch caps, short skirts, and long flowing sleeves coming out from their gaily-embroidered stay-bodies. Mingled among these, burghers, shop-keepers who have come out hatless from neighbouring shops to exchange their views, sprucely-dressed young men who are apprentices in the business of their fathers or their fathers' friends – and schoolboys with satchels and bundles of books.

Two labourers with bristling sailor beards, stand chewing their tobacco; behind them is an excited lady, craning her neck this way and that to get a glimpse of the Town Hall between their powerful shoulders. She wears a long evening cloak trimmed with brown fur, which she holds together from the inside with both hands. Her face is well covered with a thick brown veil. She shifts her feet about in the melting snow.

" Gawd! Kurz bain't gettin' it this time, nuther, be he? " says the one labourer to the other.

" Naw, ye mutton-head, 'tis certain he bain't. There's no more talk o' him. Th' votin's between Hagenström, Buddenbrook, 'n' Kistenmaker. 'Tis all about they, – now."

" 'Tis whether which one o' th' three be ahead o' the others, eh? "

" So 'tis; yes, they do say so."

" Then I'm minded they'll be choosin' Hagenström."

" Eh, smarty – so they'll be choosin' Hagenström? Ye can tell that to yer grandmother! " And therewith he spits his tobacco-juice on the ground close to his own feet, the crowd being too dense to admit of a trajectory. He takes hold of his trousers in both hands and pulls them up higher under his belt, and goes on: " Hagenström, he's a great pig – he be so fat he can't breathe through his own nose! If so be it's all o'er wi' Kurz then I'm fer Buddenbrook. 'Tis a very shrewd chap."

" So 'tis, so 'tis. But Hagenström, he's got the money."

" That bain't the question – 'tis no matter o' riches."

" 'n' then this Buddenbrook – he be so devilish fine wi' his cuffs 'n' his silk tie 'n' his stickin'-out moustaches; hast seen him walk? He hops along like a bird."

"Ye ninny, that bain't the question, no more'n th' other."

"They say his sister've put away two men a'ready." The lady in the fur cloak trembles visibly.

"Eh, that soart o' thing – what do we know about it? Likely the Consul he couldn't help it hisself."

The lady in the veil thinks to herself, "He couldn't, indeed! Thank God for that," and presses her hands together, inside her cloak.

"'n' then," adds the Buddenbrook partisan, "didn't the Burgomaster his own self stan' godfeyther to his son? Can't ye tell somethin' by that?"

"Yes, can't you indeed?" thinks the lady. "Thank heaven, that did do some good." She starts. A fresh rumour from the Town Hall, running zig-zag through the crowd, has reached her ears. The balloting, it seems, has not been decisive. Eduard Kistenmaker, indeed, has received fewer votes than the other two candidates, and his name has been dropped. But the struggle goes on between Buddenbrook and Hagenström. A sapient citizen remarks that if the voting continues to be even, it will be necessary to appoint five arbitrators.

A voice, down in front at the entrance steps, shouts suddenly: "Heine Seehas is 'lected – 'rah for Heine Seehas!" Heine Seehas, be it known, is an habitual drunkard, who peddles hot bread on a little wagon through the streets. Everybody roars with laughter, and stands on tip-toe to see the wag who is responsible for the joke. The lady in the veil is seized with a nervous giggle; her shoulders shake for a moment, and then give a shrug which expresses as plainly as words: "Is this the time for tom-foolery like that?" She collects herself again, and stares with intensity between the two labourers at the Town Hall. But almost at the same moment her hands slip from her cloak, so that it opens in front, her figure relaxes, her shoulders droop, she stands there entirely crushed.

Hagenström! – The word seems to have come from nobody knows where – down from the sky, or up from the earth. It is everywhere at once. There is no contradiction. So it is decided. Hagenström! Hagenström it is, then. One may as well go home. The lady in the veil might have known. It was ever thus. She will go home – she feels the tears rising in her throat.

This state of things has lasted a second or so, when there occurs a shouting and a backward jostling of the throng. It runs through the whole assemblage, as those in front press back those behind, and at the same time something red appears in the doorway. It is the coats of the beadles Kaspersen and Uhlefeldt. They are in full-dress uniform, with white riding breeches, three-cornered hats, yellow gauntlet gloves, and short dress swords. They appear side by side, and make their way through the crowd, which falls back before them.

They move like fate: silent, resolved, inexorable, not looking to right or left, with gaze directed toward the ground. They take, according to instructions, the route marked out by the election. And it is *not* in the direction of Sand Street! They have turned to the right – they are going down Broad Street!

The lady in the veil cannot believe her eyes. However, all about her, people are seeing just what she sees; they are pushing on after the beadles, and saying to each other: " It isn't Hagenström, it's Buddenbrook! " And a group of gentlemen emerge from the portal, in excited conversation, and hurry with rapid steps down Broad Street, to be the first to offer congratulations.

Then the lady holds her cloak together and runs for it. She runs, indeed, as seldom lady runs. Her veil blows up, revealing her flushed face – no matter for that; and one of her furred goloshes keeps flapping open in the sloppy snow and hindering her frightfully: yet she outruns them all! She gains the house at the corner of Bakers' Street, she rings the alarm-bell at the vestibule-door – fire, murder, thieves! – she shouts at the maid who opens: " They're coming, Kathrin, they're coming," takes the stairs, and storms into the living-room. Her brother himself sits there, certainly a little pale. He puts down his paper and makes a gesture, almost as if to ward her off. But she puts her arms about him, and repeats: " They're coming, Tom, they're coming! You are the man – and Hermann Hagenström is out! "

That was Friday. On the following day, Senator Buddenbrook stood in the Council Hall, in the seat of the deceased James Möllendorpf, and in the presence of the City Fathers there assembled, and the Delegation of Burgesses, he took the oath: " I will conscientiously perform the duties of my office, strive with all my power for the good of the State, faithfully obey the Constitution, honourably pursue the public weal, and in the discharge of my office, regard neither my own advantage nor that of my relatives and friends. I will support the laws of the State and do justice on all alike, whether rich or poor. In all things where secrecy is needful, I will not speak, and especially will I not reveal what is given me to keep silent. So help me God! "

CHAPTER V

OUR desires and our performance are conditioned by certain needs of our nervous systems which are very hard to define in words. What people called Thomas Buddenbrook's "vanity" — his care for his personal appearance, his extravagant dressing — was at bottom not vanity but something else entirely. It was, originally, no more than the effort of a man of action to be certain, from head to toe, of the adequacy and correctness of his bearing. But the demands made by himself and by others upon his talents and his capacities were constantly increased. He was overwhelmed by public and private affairs. When the Senate sat to appoint its committees, one of the main departments, the administration of the taxes, fell to his lot. But tolls, railways, and other administrative business claimed his time as well; and he presided at hundreds of committees that called into play all the capacities he possessed: he had to summon every ounce of his flexibility, his foresight, his power to charm, in order not to wound the sensibilities of his elders, to defer constantly to them, and yet to keep the reins in his own hands. If his so-called vanity notably increased at the same time, if he felt a greater and greater need to refresh himself bodily, to renew himself, to change his clothing several times a day, all this meant simply that Thomas Buddenbrook, though he was barely thirty-seven years old, was losing his elasticity, was wearing himself out fast.

When good Dr. Grabow begged him to relax a little, he answered, "Oh, my dear Doctor, I haven't reached that point yet!" By which he meant that he still had an interminable deal of work to do before he arrived at the goal and could settle back to enjoy himself. The truth was, he hardly believed himself in such a condition. Yet it drove him on, it left him no peace. Even when he seemed to rest, as he sat with the paper after dinner, a thousand ideas whirled about in his brain, while the veins stood out on his temples, and he twisted the ends of his moustaches with a certain still intensity of passion. He concentrated with equal violence whether the subject of his thought was a business manœuvre, a public speech, or a decision to renew his entire stock of body linen, in order to be sure that he had enough, for a while, at least.

If such wholesale buying afforded him passing relief and satisfaction, he could indulge himself in it without scruple, for his business at this time was as brilliant as ever it had been in his grandfather's day. The repute of the firm grew, not only in the town but round about, and throughout the whole community he continued to be held in ever greater regard. His talents were admitted on all hands, with admiration or envy as the case might be; while he himself wrestled ceaselessly, at times despairingly, to evolve an order and method of work which should enable him to overtake the flights of his own restless imagination.

Thus, when, in the summer of 1863, Senator Buddenbrook went about with his mind full of plans for the building of a great new house, it was not arrogance which impelled him. He was driven by his own inability to be quiet – which his fellow-burghers would have been right in ascribing to his " vanity " – for it was another manifestation of the same thing. To make a new home, and a radical change in his outward life; to pack up, to re-install himself afresh, to weed out all the accumulations of bygone years and set aside everything old or superfluous: all this, even in imagination, gave him feelings of freshness, newness, spotlessness, stimulation. All of which he must have craved indeed, for he attacked the plan with great enthusiasm, and already had his eye on a suitable location.

There was a property of considerable extent at the lower end of Fishers' Lane. The house, grey with age, in bad repair, was offered for sale on the death of its owner, an ancient spinster, the relic of a forgotten family, who had dwelt there alone. On this piece of land the Senator thought to build his house; and he surveyed it with a speculative eye when he passed the spot on his way to the harbour. The neighbourhood was pleasant enough – good burgher-houses, the most modest among them being the narrow little façade opposite, with a small flower-shop on the ground floor.

He threw himself into the affair. He made a rough estimate of the expense involved, and though the sum he fixed provisionally was by no means a small one, he felt he could compass it without undue effort. But then he would suddenly have the thought that the whole thing was a senseless folly, and confess to himself that his present house had plenty of room for himself, his wife, their child, and their servants. But the half-conscious cravings were stronger; and in the desire to have them strengthened and justified from outside, he first revealed his plan to his sister.

"Well, Tony, what do you say to it? The whole house is a sort of band-box, isn't it – and the winding stair is really a joke. It isn't quite the thing, is it? and now that you've had me made Senator – in a word, don't you think I owe it to myself?"

Ah, in the eyes of Madame Permaneder, what was there he did not owe to himself? She was full of practical enthusiasm. She crossed her arms on her breast and walked up and down with her shoulders raised and her head in the air.

"Of course you do, Tom; goodness gracious, yes! What possible objection could there be? And when you have married an Arnoldsen, with a hundred thousand thaler to boot – I'm very proud to be the first you've told it to. It was lovely of you. And if you do do it, Tom, why, you must do it well, that's what I say. It must be grand."

"H'm, well, yes, I agree with you. I'm willing to spend something on it. I'll have Voigt, and we'll go over the plans together. Voigt has a great deal of taste."

The second opinion which Thomas called in was Gerda's. She praised the idea unreservedly. The confusion of moving would not be pleasant, but the prospect of a large music-room with good acoustic properties impressed her most happily. As for the old Frau Consul, she was quite prepared to think of the new house as a logical consequence of all the other blessings which had fallen to her lot, and to give thanks to God therefor, accordingly. Since the birth of the heir, and the recent election, she gave freer expression to her motherly pride, and had a way of saying "my son, the Senator," which the Broad Street Buddenbrooks found most offensive.

These aging spinsters felt that all too little shadow set off the sunshine through which Thomas's outward life ran its brilliant course. It was no great consolation – at the Thursday family gatherings – to pour contempt on poor, good-natured Clothilde. As for Christian – Christian, through the good offices of Mr. Richardson, his former chief, had found a situation in London, whence he had lately telegraphed a fantastic desire to marry Fräulein Puvogel, an idea upon which his mother had firmly set her foot – Christian now belonged, quite simply, to Jacob Kröger's class, and was, as it were, a dead issue. They consoled themselves, to some extent, with the little weaknesses of the old Frau Consul and Frau Permaneder. They would bring the conversation round to the subject of coiffures: the Frau Consul was capable of saying, in the blandest way, that she always wore "her" hair very simply, whereas it was plain to any one gifted by God with intelligence, and certainly to the Misses Buddenbrook, that the immutable red-blonde hair under the old lady's cap could no longer by any stretch be called " her " hair. Still more gratifying was it to get Cousin Tony started on the subject of those nefarious persons who had formerly had an influence on her life. Teary Trietschke! Grünlich! Permaneder! Hagenström! – Tony, when she was egged on to it, would utter these names into the air like so many little trumpetings of disgust, with her shoulders well up. They had a sweet sound in the ears of the daughters of Uncle Gotthold.

They could not dissimulate, and they would accept no responsibility for omitting to say that little Johann was frightfully slow about learning to walk and talk. They were really quite right: it was an admitted fact that Hanno – this was the nickname adopted by the Frau Senator for her son – at a time when he was able to call all the members of his family by name with fair correctness, was incapable of pronouncing the names Friederike, Henriette, and Pfiffi so that any one could understand what he said. And at fifteen months he had not taken a single step alone. The Misses Buddenbrook, shaking their heads pessimistically, declared that the child would be halt and tongue-tied to the end of his days.

They later admitted the error of their gloomy prophecy; but nobody, in fact, denied that Hanno was a little backward. His early infancy was a struggle for life, and his family was in constant anxiety. At birth he had been too feeble to cry out; and soon after the christening a three-day attack of cholera-infantum was almost enough to still for ever the little heart set pumping, in the first place, with such difficulty. But he survived; and good Dr. Grabow did his best, by the most painstaking care and nourishment, to strengthen him for the difficult period of teething. The first tiny white point had barely pricked through the gum, when the child was attacked by convulsions, which repeated themselves with greater and greater violence, until again the worst was to be feared. Once more the old doctor speechlessly pressed the parents' hands. The child lay in profound exhaustion, and the vacant look in the shadowy eyes indicated an affection of the brain. The end seemed almost to be wished for.

But Hanno regained some little strength, consciousness returned; and though the crisis which he had survived greatly hindered his progress in walking and talking, there was no longer any immediate danger to be feared.

The child was slender of limb, and rather tall for his age. His hair, pale brown and very soft, began to grow rapidly, and fell waving over the shoulders of his full, pinafore-like frocks. The family likenesses were abundantly clear, even now. From the first he possessed the Buddenbrook hand, broad, a little too short, but finely articulated, and his nose was precisely the nose of his father and great-grandfather, though the nostrils would probably remain more delicate. But the whole lower part of his face, longish and narrow, was neither Buddenbrook nor Kröger, but from the mother's side of the house. This was true of the mouth in particular, which, when closed, began very early to wear an anxious, woebegone expression that later matched the look of his strange, gold-brown, blue-shadowed eyes.

So he began to live: brooded over by his father's reserved tenderness, clothed and nurtured under his mother's watchful eye; prayed over by Aunt Antonie, presented with tops and hobby-horses by the Frau Consul and Uncle Justus; and when his charming little perambulator appeared on the streets, it was looked after with interest and expectation. Madame Decho, the stately nurse, had attended the child up to now; but it had been settled that when they moved into the new house, not she, but Ida Jungmann, should move in with them, and the latter's place with the old Frau Consul be filled by somebody else.

Senator Buddenbrook carried out his plan. He had no difficulty in obtaining title to the property in Fishers' Lane. The Broad Street house was turned over to Gosch the broker, who dramatically declared himself prepared to assume the task of disposing of it. Stephan Kistenmaker, who had a growing family, and, with his brother Eduard, made good money in the wine business, bought it at once. Herr Voigt undertook the new building, and soon there was a clean plan to unroll before the eyes of the family on Thursday afternoons, when they could, in fancy, see the façade already before them: an imposing brick façade with sandstone caryatides supporting the bow-window, and a flat roof, of which Clothilde remarked, in her pleasant drawl, that one might drink afternoon coffee there. The Senator planned to transfer the business offices to his new building, which would, of course, leave empty the ground floor of the house in Meng Street. But here also things turned out well: for it appeared that the City Fire Insurance Company wanted to rent the rooms by the month for their offices — which was quickly arranged.

Autumn came, and the grey walls crumbled to heaps of rubbish, and Thomas Buddenbrook's new house rose above its roomy cellars, while winter set in and slowly waned again. In all the town there was no pleasanter topic of conversation. It was "tip-top" – it was the finest dwelling-house far and wide. But it must cost like the deuce – the old Consul would never have spent money so recklessly. Thus the neighbours, the middle-class dwellers in the gabled houses, looking out at the workmen on the scaffoldings, enjoying the sight of the rising walls, and speculating on the date of the carpenters' feast.

It came at length, and was celebrated with due circumstance. Up on the flat-topped roof an old master mason made the festal speech and flung the champagne bottle over his shoulder, while the tremendous wreath, woven of roses, green garlands, and gay-coloured leaves, swayed between standards, heavily in the breeze. The workmen's feast was held at a neighbouring inn, at long tables, with beer, sandwiches, and cigars; and Senator Buddenbrook and his wife and his little son on Madame Decho's arm, walked the narrow space between the tables and bowed his thanks at the cheers they gave him.

When they got outside, they put little Hanno back into his carriage, and Thomas and Gerda crossed the road to have another look at the red façade with the white caryatides. They stood before the flower-shop with the narrow door and the poor little show-window, in which only a few pots of bulbs stood on a green glass slab. Iwersen, the proprietor, a blond giant of a man, in woollen jacket, was in the doorway with his wife. She was of a quite different build, slender and delicate, with a dark, southern-looking face. She held a four- or five-year-old boy by one hand, while with the other she was pushing a little carriage back and forth, in which a younger child lay asleep; and she was plainly expecting a third blessing.

Iwersen made a low, awkward bow; his wife, continuing to push the little carriage back and forth, looked calmly and observantly at the Frau Senator with her narrow black eyes, as the lady approached them on her husband's arm.

Thomas paused and pointed with his walking-stick at the great garland far above them.

"You did a good job, Iwersen," said he.

"No, Herr Sen'tor. That's the wife's work. She's the one fer these affairs."

"Oh," said the Senator, raised his head with a little jerk, and gave, for a second, a clear friendly look straight into Frau Iwersen's face. Then, without adding a word, he courteously waved his hand, and they moved on their way.

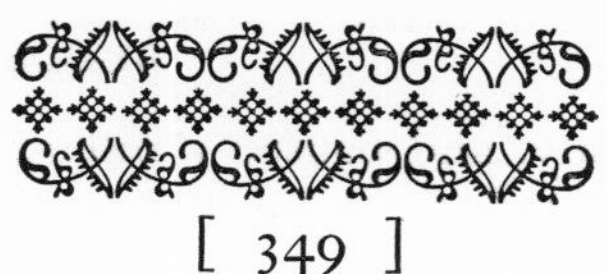

CHAPTER VI

ONE Sunday at the beginning of July – Senator Buddenbrook had moved some four weeks before – Frau Permaneder appeared at her brother's house toward evening. She crossed the cool ground floor, paved with flags and decorated with reliefs by Thorwaldsen, whence there was a door leading into the bureau; she rang at the vestibule door – it could be opened from the kitchen by pressing on a rubber bulb – and entered the spacious lobby, where, at the foot of the steps, stood the bear presented by Tiburtius and Clara. Here she learned from Anton that the Senator was still at work.

"Very good, Anton," she said. "I will go to him."

Yet she did not go at once into the office, but passed the door that led into it and stood at the bottom of the splendid staircase, which as far as the first storey had a cast-iron balustrade, but at the distance of the second storey became a wide pillared balcony in white and gold, with a great gilt chandelier hanging down from the skylight's dizzy height.

"Very elegant," said Frau Permaneder, softly, in a tone of great satisfaction, gazing up into this spacious magnificence. To her it meant, quite simply, the power, the brilliance, and the triumph of the Buddenbrook family. But now it occurred to her that she was not, in fact, come upon a very cheerful errand, and she slowly turned away and passed through the door into the office.

Thomas sat there quite alone, in his place by the window, writing a letter. He glanced up, raised an eyebrow, and put out his hand to his sister.

"'Evening, Tony. What's the good word?"

"Oh, nothing very good, Tom. Oh, your staircase – it's just *too* splendid! Why are you sitting here writing in the dark?"

"It was a pressing letter. Well – nothing very good, eh? Come into the garden, a little. It is pleasanter out there."

As they crossed the entry, a violin adagio came trillingly down from the storey above.

"Listen," said Tony, and paused a moment. "Gerda is playing. How heavenly! What a woman! She isn't a woman, she's a fairy. How is Hanno, Tom?"

"Just having his supper, with Jungmann. Too bad he is so slow about walking –"

"Oh, that will come, Tom, that will come. Are you pleased with Ida?"

"Why not?"

They crossed the flags at the back, leaving the kitchen on the right, went through a glass door and up two steps into the lovely, scented flower-garden.

"Well?" the Senator asked.

It was warm and still. The fragrance from the neat beds and borders hung in the evening air, and the fountain, surrounded by tall pale purple iris, sent its stream gently plashing heavenward, where the first stars began to gleam. In the background, an open flight of steps flanked by low obelisks, led up to a gravelled terrace, with an open wooden pavilion, a closed marquee, and some garden chairs. On the left hand was the property wall between them and the next garden; on the right the side wall of the next house was covered with a wooden trellis intended for climbing plants. There were a few currant and gooseberry bushes at the sides of the terrace steps, but there was only one tree, a large, gnarled walnut by the left-hand wall.

"The thing is this," answered Frau Permaneder, with some hesitation, as the brother and sister began to pace the gravel path of the fore part of the garden. "Tiburtius has written –"

"Clara?" questioned Thomas. "Please don't make a long story of it."

"Yes. Tom. She is in bed; she is very bad – the doctor is afraid of tuberculosis – of the brain. – I can hardly speak the words. Here is the letter Tiburtius wrote me, and enclosed another for Mother, which we are to give her when we have prepared her a little. It tells the same story. And there is this second enclosure, to Mother, from Clara herself – written in pencil, in a shaky hand. And Tiburtius wrote that she herself said they were the last she should write, for it seems the sad thing is she makes no effort to live. She was always longing for Heaven –" finished Frau Permaneder, and wiped her eyes.

The Senator walked at her side, his hands behind his back, his head bowed.

"You are so quiet, Tom. But you are right – what is there to say? Just now, too, when Christian lies ill in Hamburg –"

For this was, in fact, the state of things. Christian's "misery" in the left side had increased so much of late that it had become actual pain, severe enough to make him forget all smaller woes. He was quite helpless, and had written to his mother from London that he was coming home, for her to take care of him. He quit his situation in London and started off, but at Hamburg had been obliged to take to his bed; the doctor diagnosed his ailment as rheumatism of the joints, and he had been removed from his hotel to a hospital. Any further journey was for the time impossible. There he lay, and dictated to his attendant letters that betrayed extreme depression.

"Yes," said the Senator, quietly. "It seems as if one thing just followed on another.

She put her arm for an instant across his shoulders.

"But *you* mustn't give way, Tom. This is no time for you to be down-hearted. You need all your courage – "

"Yes, God knows I need it."

"What do you mean, Tom? Tell me, why were you so quiet Thursday afternoon at dinner, if I may ask? "

"Oh – business, my child. I had to sell no very small quantity of grain not very advantageously – or, rather, I had to sell a large quantity very much at a loss."

"Well, that happens, Tom. You sell at a loss to-day, and to-morrow you make it good again. To get discouraged over a thing of that kind – "

"Wrong, Tony," he said, and shook his head. "My courage does not go down to zero because I have a piece of bad luck. It's the other way on. I believe in that, and events show it."

"But what is the matter with it, then? " she asked, surprised and alarmed. "One would think you have enough to make you happy, Tom. Clara is alive, and with God's help she will get better. And as for everything else – here we are, walking about, in your own garden, and it all smells so sweet – and yonder is your house, a dream of a house – Hermann Hagenström's is a dog-kennel beside it! And you have done all that – "

"Yes, it is almost too beautiful, Tony. I'll tell you – it is too new. It jars on me a little – perhaps that is what is the matter with me. It may be responsible for the bad mood that comes over me and spoils everything. I looked forward immensely to all this; but the anticipation was the best part of it – it always is. Everything gets done too slowly – so when it is finished the pleasure is already gone."

"The pleasure is gone, Tom? At your age? "

"A man is as young, or as old, as he feels. And when one gets one's wish too late, or works too hard for it, it comes already weighted with all sorts of small vexatious drawbacks – with all the dust of reality upon it, that one did not reckon with in fancy. It is so irritating – so *irritating* – "

"Oh yes. – But what do you mean by 'as old as you feel'?"

"Why, Tony – it is a mood, certainly. It may pass. But just now I feel older than I am. I have business cares. And at the Directors' meeting of the Buchen Railway yesterday, Consul Hagenström simply talked me down, refuted my contentions, nearly made me appear ridiculous. I feel that could not have happened to me before. It is as though something had begun to slip – as though I haven't the firm grip I had on events. – What is success? It is an inner, and indescribable force, resourcefulness, power of vision; a consciousness that I am, by my mere existence, exerting pressure on the movement of life about me. It is my belief in the adaptability of life to my own ends. Fortune and success lie with ourselves. We must hold them firmly – deep within us. For as soon as something begins to slip, to relax, to get tired, *within us*, then everything without us will rebel and struggle to withdraw from our influence. One thing follows another, blow after blow – and the man is finished. Often and often, in these days, I have thought of a Turkish proverb; it says, 'When the house is finished, death comes.' It doesn't need to be death. But the decline, the falling-off, the beginning of the end. You know, Tony," he went on, in a still lower voice, putting his arm underneath his sister's, "when Hanno was christened, you said: 'It looks as if quite a new life would dawn for us all!' I can still hear you say it, and I thought then that you were right, for I was elected Senator, and was fortunate in my business, and this house seemed to spring up out of the ground. But the 'Senator' and this house are superficial after all. I know, from life and from history, something you have not thought of: often, the outward and visible material signs and symbols of happiness and success only show themselves when the process of decline has already set in. The outer manifestations take time – like the light of that star up there, which may in reality be already quenched, when it looks to us to be shining its brightest."

He ceased to speak, and they walked for a while in silence, while the fountain gently murmured, and a whispering sounded from the top of the walnut tree. Then Frau Permaneder breathed such a heavy sigh that it sounded like a sob.

"How sadly you talk, Tom. You never spoke so sadly before.

But it is good to speak out, and it will help you to put all that kind of thoughts out of your mind."

"Yes, Tony, I must try to do that, I know, as well as I can. And now give me the enclosures from Clara and the Pastor. It will be best, won't it, for me to take over the matter, and speak to-morrow morning with Mother? Poor Mother! If it is really tuberculosis, one may as well give up hope."

CHAPTER VII

"You don't even ask me? You go right over my head?"

"I have done as I had to do."

"You have acted like a distracted person, in a perfectly unreasonable way.

"Reason is not the highest thing on earth."

"Please don't make phrases. The question is one of the most ordinary justice, which you have most astonishingly ignored."

"Let me suggest to you, my son, that you yourself are ignoring the duty and respect which you owe to your mother."

"And I answer you, my dear Mother, by telling you that I have never for a moment forgotten the respect I owe you; but that my attributes as a son became void when I took my father's place as head of the family and of the firm."

"I desire you to be silent, Thomas!"

"No, I will not be silent, so long as you fail to realize the extent of your own weakness and folly."

"I have a right to dispose of my own property as I choose!"

"Within the limits of justice and reason."

"I could never have believed you would have the heart to wound me like this!"

"And I could never have believed that my own Mother would slap me in the face!"

"Tom! Why, Tom!" Frau Permaneder's anguished voice got itself a hearing at last. She sat at the window of the landscape-room, wringing her hands, while her brother paced up and down in a state of high excitement, and the Frau Consul, beside herself with angry grief, sat on the sofa, leaning with one hand on its upholstered arm, while the other struck the table to emphasize her words. All three wore mourning for Clara, who was now no longer of this earth; and all three were pale and excited.

What was going on? Something amazing, something dreadful, something at which the very actors in the scene themselves stood aghast and incredulous. A quarrel, an embittered disagreement between mother and son!

It was a sultry August afternoon. Only ten days after the Senator had gently prepared his mother and given her the letters from Clara and Tiburtius, the blow fell, and he had the harder task of breaking to the old lady the news of death itself. He travelled to Riga for the funeral, and returned with his brother-in-law, who spent a few days with the family of his deceased wife, and also visited Christian in the hospital at Hamburg. And now, two days after the Pastor had departed for home, the Frau Consul, with obvious hesitation, made a certain revelation to her son.

"One hundred and twenty-seven thousand, five hundred marks current," cried he, and shook his clasped hands in front of him. "If it were the dowry, even! If he wanted to keep the eighty thousand marks! Though, considering there's no heir, even that – ! But to promise him Clara's whole inheritance, right over my head! Without saying aye, yes, or no!"

"Thomas, for our blessed Lord's sake, do me some sort of justice, at least. Could I act otherwise? Tell me, could I? She who has been taken from us, and is now with God, she wrote me from her death-bed, with faltering hand, a pencilled letter. 'Mother,' she wrote, 'we shall see each other no more on this earth, and these are, I know, my dying words to you. With my last conscious thoughts, I appeal to you for my husband. God gave us no children; but when you follow me, let what would have been mine if I had lived go to him to enjoy during his lifetime. Mother, it is my last request – my dying prayer. You will not refuse it.' – No, Thomas, I did not refuse it – I could not. I sent a despatch to her, and she died in peace." The Frau Consul wept violently.

"And you never told me a syllable. Everybody conceals things from me, and acts without my authority," repeated the Senator.

"Yes, Thomas, I have kept silent. For I felt I *must* fulfil the last wish of my dying child, and I knew you would have tried to prevent me!"

"Yes! By God, I would have!"

"You would have had no right to, for three of my children would have been on my side."

"I think my opinion has enough weight to balance that of two women and a degenerate fool."

"You speak of your brother and sisters as heartlessly as you do to me."

"Clara was a pious, ignorant woman, Mother. And Tony is a child – and, anyhow, she knew nothing about the affair at all until now – or she might have talked at the wrong time, eh? And Christian? Oh, he got Christian's consent, did Tiburtius! Who would have thought it of him? Do you know now, or don't you grasp it yet – what he is, this ingenious pastor? He is a rogue, and a fortune-hunter! "

" Sons-in-law are always rogues," said Frau Permaneder, in a hollow voice.

" He is a fortune-hunter! What does he do? He travels to Hamburg, and sits down by Christian's bed. He talks to him – ' Yes,' says Christian, ' yes, Tiburtius, God bless you! Have you any idea of the pain I suffer in my left side? ' – Oh, the idiots, the scoundrels! They joined hands against me! " And the Senator, perfectly beside himself, leaned against the wrought-iron fire-screen and pressed his clenched hands to his temples.

This paroxysm of anger was out of proportion to the circumstances. No, it was not the hundred and twenty-seven thousand marks that had brought him to this unprecedented state of rage. It was rather that his irritated senses connected this case with the series of rebuffs and misfortunes which had lately attended him in both public and private business. Nothing went well any more. Nothing turned out as he intended it should. And now, had it come to this, that in the house of his fathers they " went over his head " in matters of the highest importance? That a pastor from Riga could thus bamboozle him behind his back? He could have prevented it if he had only been told! But events had taken their course without him. It was this which he felt could not have happened earlier – would not have dared to happen earlier! Again his faith tottered – his faith in himself, his luck, his power, his future. And it was nothing but his own inward weakness and despair that broke out in this scene before mother and sister.

Frau Permaneder stood up and embraced her brother. " Tom," she said, " do control yourself. Try to be calm. You will make yourself ill. Are things so very bad? Tiburtius doesn't need to live so very long, perhaps, and the money would come back after he dies. And if you want it to, it can be altered – can it not be altered, Mamma? "

The Frau Consul answered only with sobs.

" Oh, no, no," said the Consul, pulling himself together, and making a weak gesture of dissent. " Let it be as it is. Do you think I would carry it into court and sue my own mother, and add a public scandal to the family one? It may go as it is," he concluded, and walked lifelessly to the glass door, where he paused and stood.

" But you need not imagine," he said in a suppressed voice, " that things are going so brilliantly with us. Tony lost eighty thousand marks, and Christian, beside the setting up of fifty thousand that he has run through with, has already had thirty thousand in advance, and will need more, as he is not earning anything, and will have to take a cure at Öynhausen. And now Clara's dowry is permanently lost, and her whole inheritance besides for an indefinite period. And business is poor; it seems to have gone to the devil precisely since the time when I spent more than a hundred thousand marks on my house. No, things are not going well in a family where there are such scenes as this to-day. Let me tell you one thing; if Father were alive, if he were here in this room, he would fold his hands and commend us to the mercy of God."

CHAPTER VIII

WARS and rumours of war, billeting and bustle! Prussian officers tread the parquetry floors of Senator Buddenbrook's bel-étage, kiss the hand of the lady of the house, and frequent the club with Christian, who is back from Öynhausen. In Meng Street Mamsell Severin, Riekchen Severin, the Frau Consul's new companion, helps the maids to drag piles of mattresses into the old garden-house, which is full of soldiers.

Confusion, disorder, and suspense reign. Troops march off through the gate, new ones come in. They overrun the town; they eat, sleep, fill the ears of the citizens with the noise of rolling drums, commands, and trumpet calls — and march off again. Royal princes are fêted, entry follows entry. Then quiet again — and suspense.

In the late autumn and winter the victorious troops return. Again they are billeted in the town for a time, are mustered out and go home — to the great relief of the cheering citizens. Peace comes — the brief peace, heavy with destiny, of the year 1865.

And between two wars, little Johann played. Unconscious and tranquil, with his soft curling hair and voluminous pinafore frocks, he played in the garden by the fountain, or in the little gallery partitioned off for his use by a pillared railing from the vestibule of the second storey — played the plays of his four and a half years — those plays whose meaning and charm no grown person can possibly grasp: which need no more than a few pebbles, or a stick of wood with a dandelion for a helmet, since they command the pure, powerful, glowing, untaught and unintimidated fancy of those blissful years before life touches us, when neither duty nor remorse dares to lay upon us a finger's weight, when we may see, hear, laugh, dream, and feel amazement, when the world yet makes upon us not one single demand; when the impatience of those whom we should like so much to love does not yet torment us for evidence of our ability to succeed in the impending struggle. Ah, only a little while, and that struggle will be upon us — and they will do their best to bend us to their will and cut us to their pattern, to exercise us, to lengthen us, to shorten us, to corrupt us. . . .

Great things happened while little Hanno played. The war flamed up, and its fortunes swayed this way and that, then inclined to the side of the victors; and Hanno Buddenbrook's native city, which had shrewdly stuck with Prussia, looked on not without satisfaction at wealthy Frankfort, which had to pay with her independence for her faith in Austria.

But with the failure in July of a large firm of Frankfort wholesale dealers, immediately before the armistice, the firm of Johann Buddenbrook lost at one fell swoop the round sum of twenty thousand thaler.

PART EIGHT

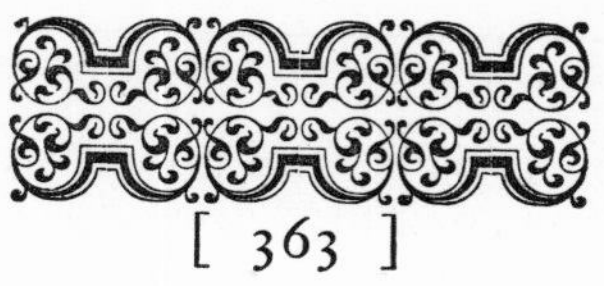

CHAPTER I

When Herr Hugo Weinschenk – in his buttoned-up frock-coat, with his drooping lower lip and his narrow black moustaches, which grew, in the most masculine way imaginable, right into the corners of his mouth; with both his fists held out in front of him, and making little motions with his elbows at about the height of his waist – when Herr Hugo Weinschenk, now for some time Director of the City Fire Insurance Company, crossed the great entry in Meng Street and passed, with a swinging, pompous stride, from his front to his back office, he gave an impressive impersonation of an energetic and prosperous man.

And Erica Grünlich, on the other hand, was now twenty years old: a tall, blooming girl, fresh-coloured and pretty, full of health and strength. If chance took her up or down the stairs just as Herr Weinschenk passed that way – and chance did this not seldom – the Director took off his top-hat, displaying his short black hair, which was already greying at the temples, minced rather more than ever at the waist of his frockcoat, and greeted the young girl with an admiring glance from his bold and roving brown eye. Whereat Erica ran away, sat down somewhere in a window, and wept for hours out of sheer helpless confusion.

Fräulein Grünlich had grown up under Therese Weichbrodt's care and correction: her thoughts did not fly far afield. She wept over Herr Weinschenk's top-hat, the way he raised his eyebrows at sight of her and let them fall; over his regal bearing and his balancing fists. Her mother, Frau Permaneder, saw further.

Her daughter's future had troubled her for years; for Erica was at a disadvantage compared with other young girls of her age. Frau Permaneder not only did not go into society, she was actually at war with it. The conviction that the " best people " thought slightingly of her because of her two divorces, had become almost a fixed idea; and she read contempt and aversion where probably there was only indifference. Consul Hermann Hagenström, for instance, simple and liberal-minded man that he was, would very likely have been perfectly glad to greet her on the street; his money had only increased his joviality and good nature. But she stared, with her head flung back, past his " goose-liver-paté " face, which, to use her own strong language, she " hated like the plague " — and her look, of course, distinctly forbade him. So Erica grew up outside her uncle's social circle; she frequented no balls, and had small chance of meeting eligible young gentlemen.

Yet it was Frau Antonie's most ardent hope, especially after she herself had " failed in business," as she said, that her daughter might realize her own unfulfilled dream of a happy and advantageous marriage, which should redound to the glory of the family and sink the mother's failure in final oblivion. Tony longed for this beyond everything, and chiefly now for her brother's sake, who had latterly shown so little optimism, as a sign to him that the luck of the family was not yet lost, that they were by no means " at the end of their rope." Her second dowry, the eighteen thousand thaler so magnanimously returned by Herr Permaneder, lay waiting for Erica; and directly Frau Antonie's practiced glance marked the budding tenderness between her daughter and the Director, she began to trouble Heaven with a prayer that Herr Weinschenk might be led to visit them.

He was. He appeared in the first storey, where he was received by the three ladies, mother, daughter, and granddaughter, talked for ten minutes, and promised to return another day for coffee and more leisurely conversation.

This too came to pass, and the acquaintance progressed. The Director was a Silesian by birth. His old father, in fact, still lived in Silesia; but the family seemed not to come into consideration, Hugo being, evidently, a " self-made man." He had the self-consciousness of such men: a not quite native, rather insecure, mistrustful, exaggerated air. His grammar was not perfect, and his conversation was distinctly clumsy. And his countrified frock coat had shiny spots; his cuffs, with large jet cuff-buttons, were not quite fresh; and the nail on the middle finger of his left hand had been crushed in some accident, and was shrivelled and blackened. The impression, on the whole, was rather unpleasing; yet it did not prevent Hugo Weinschenk from being a highly worthy young man, industrious and energetic, with a yearly salary of twelve thousand marks current; nor from being, in Erica Grünlich's eyes, handsome to boot.

Frau Permaneder quickly looked him over and summed him up. She talked freely with her mother and the Senator. It was clear to her that here was a case of two interests meeting and complementing each other. Director Weinschenk was, like Erica, devoid of every social connection: the two were thus, in a manner, marked out for each other – it was plainly the hand of God himself. If the Director, who was nearing the forties, his hair already sprinkled with grey, desired to found a family appropriate to his station and connections, here was an opening for him into one of the best circles in town, calculated to advance him in his calling and consolidate his position. As for Erica's welfare, Frau Permaneder could feel confident that at least her own lot would be out of the question. Herr Weinschenk had not the faintest resemblance to Herr Permaneder; and he was differentiated from Bendix Grünlich by his position as an old-established official with a fixed salary – which, of course, did not preclude a further career.

In a word, much good will was shown on both sides. Herr Weinschenk's visits followed each other in quick succession, and by January – January of the year 1867 – he permitted himself to make a brief and manly offer for Erica Grünlich's hand.

From now on he belonged to the family. He came on children's day, and was received civilly by the relatives of his betrothed. He must soon have seen that he did not fit very well; but he concealed the fact under an increased assurance of manner, while the Frau Consul, Uncle Justus, and the Senator – though hardly the Broad Street Buddenbrooks – practised a tactful complaisance toward the socially awkward, hard-working official.

And tact was needed. For pauses would come at the family table, when Director Weinschenk tried to make conversation by asking if " orange marmalade " was a " pudden "; when he gave out the opinion that Romeo and Juliet was a piece by Schiller; when his manner with Erica's cheek or arm became too roguish. He uttered his views frankly and cheerfully, rubbing his hands like a man whose mind is free from care, and leaning back sidewise against the arm of his chair. Some one always needed to fill in the pause by a sprightly or diverting remark.

He got on best with the Senator, who knew how to steer a safe course between politics and business. His relations with Gerda Buddenbrook were hopeless. This lady's personality put him off to such a degree that he was incapable of finding anything to talk about with her for two minutes on end. The fact that she played the violin made a strong impression upon him; and he finally confined himself, on each Thursday afternoon encounter, to the jovial enquiry, " Well, how's the fiddle? " After the third time, however, the Frau Senator refrained from reply.

Christian, on the other hand, used to look at his new relative down his nose, and the next day imitate him and his conversation with full details. The second son of the deceased Consul Buddenbrook had been relieved of his rheumatism in Öynhausen; but a certain stiffness of the joints was left, as well as the periodic misery in the left side, where all the nerves were too short, and sundry other ills to which he was heir, as difficulty in breathing and swallowing, irregularity of the heart action, and a tendency to paralysis – or at least to a fear of it. He did not look like a man at the end of the thirties. His head was entirely bald except for vestiges of reddish hair at the back of the neck and on the temples; and his small round roving eyes lay deeper than ever in their sockets. And his great bony nose and his lean, sallow cheeks were startlingly prominent above his heavy drooping red moustaches. His trousers, of beautiful and lasting English stuff, flapped about his crooked emaciated legs.

He had come back once more to his mother's house, and had a room on the corridor of the first storey. But he spent more of his time at the club than in Meng Street, for life there was not made any too pleasant for him. Riekchen Severin, Ida Jungmann's successor, who now reigned over the Frau Consul's household and managed the servants, had a peasant's instinct for hard facts. She was a thick-set country-bred creature, with coarse lips and fat red cheeks. She perceived directly that it was not worth while to put herself out for this idle story-teller, who was silly and ill by turns, whom his brother, the Senator – the real head of the family – ignored with lifted eyebrows. So she quite calmly neglected Christian's wants. "Gracious, Herr Buddenbrook," she would say, "you needn't think as I've got time for the likes of you!" Christian would look at her with his nose all wrinkled up, as if to say "Aren't you ashamed of yourself?" and go his stiff-kneed way.

"Do you think," he said to Tony, "that I have a candle to go to bed by? Very seldom. I generally take a match." The sum his mother could allow him was small. "Hard times," he would say. "Yes, things were different once. Why, what do you suppose? Sometimes I've had to borrow money for tooth-powder!"

"Christian!" cried Frau Permaneder. "How undignified! And going to bed with a match!" She was shocked and outraged in her deepest sensibilities – but that did not mend matters.

The tooth-powder money Christian borrowed from his old friend Andreas Gieseke, Doctor of Civil and Criminal Jurisprudence. He was fortunate in this friendship, and it did him credit; for Dr. Gieseke, though as much of a rake as Christian, knew how to keep his dignity. He had been elected Senator the preceding winter, for Dr. Överdieck had sunk gently to his long rest, and Dr.

Langhals sat in his place. His elevation did not affect Andreas Gieseke's mode of life. Since his marriage with Fräulein Huneus, he had acquired a spacious house in the centre of the town; but as everybody knew, he also owned a certain comfortable little vine-clad villa in the suburb of St. Gertrude, which was charmingly furnished, and occupied quite alone by a still young and uncommonly pretty person of unknown origin. Above the house-door, in ornamental gilt lettering, was the word "Quisisana," by which name the retired little dwelling was known throughout the town, where they pronounced it with a very soft *s* and a very broad *a*. Christian Buddenbrook, as Senator Gieseke's best friend, had obtained entry into Quisisana, and been successful there, as formerly with Aline Puvogel in Hamburg, and on other occasions in London, Valparaiso, and sundry other parts of the world. He "told a few stories," and was "a little friendly"; and now he visited the little vine-clad house on the same footing as Senator Gieseke himself. Whether this happened with the latter's knowledge and consent, is of course doubtful. What is certain is, that Christian found there, without money and without price, the same friendly relaxation as Dr. Gieseke, who, however, had to pay for the same with his wife's money.

A short time after the betrothal of Hugo Weinschenk and Erica Grünlich, the Director proposed to his relative that he should enter the Insurance office; and Christian actually worked for two weeks in the service of the Company. But the misery in his side began to get worse, and his other, indefinable ills as well; and the Director proved to be a domineering superior, who did not hesitate, on the occasion of a little misunderstanding, to call his relative a booby. So Christian felt constrained to leave this post too.

Madame Permaneder, at this period of the family's history, was in such a joyful mood that her happiness found vent in shrewd observations about life: how, when all was said and done, it had its good side. Truly, she bloomed anew in these weeks; and their invigorating activity, the manifold plans, the search for suitable quarters, and the feverish preoccupation with furnishings brought back with such force the memories of her first betrothal that she could not but feel young again – young and boundlessly hopeful. Much of the graceful high spirits of girlhood returned to her ways, and movements; indeed, she profaned the mood of one entire Jerusalem evening by such uncontrollable hilarity that even Lea Gerhardt let the book of her ancestor fall in her lap and stared about the room with the great, innocent, startled eyes of the deaf.

Erica was not to be parted from her mother. The Director

agreed — nay, it was even his wish, — that Frau Antonie should live with the Weinschenks, at least at first, and help the inexperienced Erica with her housekeeping. And it was precisely this which called up in her the most priceless feeling, as though no Bendix Grünlich or Alois Permaneder had ever existed, and all the trials, disappointments, and sufferings of her life were as nothing, and she might begin anew and with fresh hopes. She bade Erica be grateful to God, who bestowed upon her the one man of her desire, whereas the mother had been obliged to offer up her first and dearest choice on the altar of duty and reason. It was Erica's name which, with a hand trembling with joy, she inscribed in the family book next the Director's. But she, Tony Buddenbrook, was the real bride. It was she who might once more ransack furniture and upholstery shops and test hangings and carpets with a practised hand; she who once more found and rented a truly "elegant" apartment. It was she who was once more to leave the pious and roomy parental mansion and cease to be a divorced wife; she who might once more lift her head and begin a new life, calculated to arouse general remark and enhance the prestige of the family. Even — was it a dream? — dressing-gowns appeared upon the horizon: two dressing-gowns, for Erica and herself, of soft, woven stuff, with close rows of velvet trimming from neck to hem!

The weeks fled by — the last weeks of Erica Grünlich's maidenhood. The young pair had made calls in only a few houses; for the Director, a serious and preoccupied man, with no social experience, intended to devote what leisure he had to intimate domesticity. There was a betrothal dinner in the great salon of the house in Fishers' Lane, at which, besides Thomas and Gerda, there were present the bridal pair and Henriette, Friederike and Pfiffi Buddenbrook, and some close friends of the Senator; and the Director continually pinched the bare shoulders of his fiancée, rather to the disgust of the other guests. And the wedding day drew near.

The marriage was solemnized in the columned hall, as on that other occasion when it was Frau Grünlich who wore the myrtle. Frau Stuht from Bell-Founders' Street, the same who moved in the best circles, helped to arrange the folds of the bride's white satin gown and pin on the decorations. The Senator gave away the bride, supported by Christian's friend Senator Gieseke, and two school friends of Erica's acted as bridesmaids. Director Hugo Weinschenk looked imposing and manly, and only trod once on Erica's flowing veil on the way to the improvised altar. Pastor Pringsheim held his hands clasped beneath his chin, and performed the service with his accustomed air of sweet exaltation; and everything went off with dignity and according to rule. When the rings were exchanged, and the deep and the treble " yes " sounded in the hush (both a trifle husky), Frau Permaneder, overpowered by the past, the present, and the future, burst into audible sobs: just the unthinking, unembarrassed tears of her childhood. And the sisters Buddenbrook – Pfiffi, in honour of the day, was wearing a gold chain to her pince-nez – smiled a little sourly, as always on such occasions. But Mademoiselle Weichbrodt, who had grown shorter with the lengthening years, and had the oval brooch with the miniature of her mother around her thin neck – Sesemi said, with the disproportionate solemnity which hides deep emotion: " Be happy, you good che-ild! "

Followed a banquet, as solemn as solid, beneath the eyes of the white Olympians, looking down composedly from their blue background. As it drew toward its end, the newly wedded pair disappeared, to begin their wedding journey, which was to include visits to several large cities. All this was at the middle of April; and in the next two weeks, Frau Permaneder, assisted by the upholsterer Jacobs, accomplished one of her masterpieces: she moved into and settled the spacious first storey which she had rented in a house halfway down Baker Alley. There, in a bower of flowers, she welcomed the married pair on their return.

And thus began Tony Buddenbrook's third marriage.

Yes, this was really the right way to put it. The Senator himself, one Thursday afternoon when the Weinschenks were not present, had called it that, and Frau Permaneder quite relished the joke. All the cares of the new household fell upon her, but she reaped her reward in pride and pleasure. One day she happened to meet on the street Frau Consul Julchen Möllendorpf, born Hagenström, into whose face she looked with a challenging, triumphant glance; it actually dawned upon Frau Möllendorpf that she had better speak first, and she did. Tony waxed so important in her pride and joy, when she showed off the new house to visiting relatives, that little Erica, beside her, seemed but a guest herself.

Frau Antonie displayed the house to their guests, the train of her morning gown dragging behind her, her shoulders up and her head thrown back, carrying on her arm the key-basket with its bow of satin ribbon. She displayed the furniture, the hangings, the translucent porcelain, the gleaming silver, the large oil paintings. These last had been purchased by the Director, and were nearly all still-lifes of edibles or nude figures of women, for such was Hugo Weinschenk's taste. Tony's every movement seemed to say: "See, I have managed all this for the third time in my life! It is almost as fine as Grünlich's, and much finer than Permaneder's!"

The old Frau Consul came, in a black and grey striped silk, giving out a discreet odour of patchouli. She surveyed everything with her pale, calm eyes and, without any loud expressions of admiration, professed herself pleased with the effect. The Senator came, with his wife and child; he and Gerda hugely enjoyed Tony's blissful self-satisfaction, and with difficulty prevented her from killing her adored little Johann with currant bread and port wine. The Misses Buddenbrook came, and were unanimously of opinion that it was all very fine – of course, being modest people themselves, they would not care to live in it. Poor, lean, grey, patient, hungry Clothilde came, submitted to the usual teasing, and drank four cups of coffee, praising everything the while, in her usual friendly drawl. Even Christian appeared now and then, when there was nobody at the club, drank a little glass of Benedictine, and talked about a project he had of opening an agency for champagne and brandy. He knew the business, and it was a light, agreeable job, in which a man could be his own master, write now and then in a note-book, and make thirty thaler by turning over his hand. Then he borrowed a little money from Frau Permaneder to buy a bouquet for the leading lady at the theatre; came, by God knows what train of thought, to Maria and the depravity in London; and then lighted upon the story of the mangy dog that travelled all the way from Valparaiso to San Francisco in a hand-satchel. By this time he was in full swing, and narrated with such gusto, verve, and irresistible drollery that he would have held a large audience spell-bound.

He narrated like one inspired; he possessed the gift of tongues. He narrated in English, Spanish, low German, and Hamburgese; he depicted stabbing affrays in Chile and pickpocketings in Whitechapel. He drew upon his repertory of comic songs, and half sung, half recited, with incomparable pantomime and highly suggestive gesture:

"I sauntered out one day,
In an idle sort o' way,
And chanced to see a maid, ahead o' me.
  She'd such a charmin' air,
Her – behind – was French, I'd swear,
  And she wore her 'at as rakish as could be.
I says, 'My pretty dear,
  Since you an' I are 'ere,

Perhaps you'd take me arm and walk along?'
She turned her pretty 'ead,
And looked – at me – and said,
'You just get on, my lad, and hold your tongue!'"

From this he went off on an account of a performance at the Renz Circus, in Hamburg, and reproduced a turn by a troupe of English vaudeville artists, in such a way that you felt you were actually present. There was the usual hubbub behind the curtain, shouts of "Open the door, will you!" quarrels with the ring-master; and then, in a broad, lugubrious English-German, a whole string of stories: the one about the man who swallowed a mouse in his sleep, and went to the vet., who advised him to swallow a cat; and the one about "my grandmother – lively old girl, she was" – who, on her way to the railway station, encounters all sorts of adventures, ending with the train pulling out of the station in front of the nose of the "lively old girl." And then Christian broke off with a triumphant "Orchestra!" and made as if he had just waked up and was very surprised that no music was forthcoming.

But, quite suddenly, he stopped. His face changed, his motions relaxed. His little deep round eyes began to stray moodily about; he rubbed his left side with his hand, and seemed to be listening to uncanny sounds within himself. He drank another glass of liqueur, which relieved him a little. Then he tried to tell another story, but broke down in a fit of depression.

Frau Permaneder, who in these days was uncommonly prone to laugh and had enjoyed the performance hugely, accompanied her brother to the door, in rather a prankish mood. "Adieu, Herr Agent," said she. "Minnesinger – Ninnysinger! Old goose! Come again soon!" She laughed full-throatedly behind him and went back into her house.

But Christian did not mind. He did not even hear her, so deep was he in thought. "Well," he said to himself, "I'll go over to Quisisana for a bit." His hat a little awry, leaning on his stick with the nun's bust for a handle, he went slowly and stiffly down the steps.

CHAPTER II

In the spring of 1868, one evening towards ten o'clock, Frau Permaneder entered the first story of her brother's house. Senator Buddenbrook sat alone in the living-room, which was done in olive-green rep, with a large round centre-table and a great gas-lamp hanging down over it from the ceiling. He had the *Berlin Financial Gazette* spread out in front of him on the table, and was reading it, with a cigarette held between the first and second fingers of his left hand, and a gold pince-nez on his nose – he had now for some time been obliged to use glasses for reading. He heard his sister's footsteps as she passed through the dining-room, took off his glasses, and peered into the darkness until Tony appeared between the portières and in the circle of light from the lamp.

"Oh, it is you? How are you? Back from Pöppenrade? How are your friends?"

"Evening, Tom. Thanks, Armgard is very well. Are you here alone?"

"Yes; I'm glad you have come. I ate my dinner all alone to-night like the Pope. I don't count Mamsell Jungmann, because she is always popping up to look after Hanno. Gerda is at the Casino. Christian fetched her, to hear Tamayo play the violin."

"Bless and save us – as Mother says. – Yes, I've noticed lately that Gerda and Christian get on quite well together."

"Yes, I have too. Since he came back for good, she seems to have taken to him. She sits and listens to him when he tells about his troubles – dear me, I suppose he entertains her. She said to me lately: 'There is nothing of the burgher about Christian, Thomas – he is even less of a burgher than you are, yourself!'"

"Burgher, Tom? What did she mean? Why, it seems to me there is no better burgher on top of the earth than you are!"

"Oh, well – she didn't mean it just in that sense. Take off your things and sit down a while, my child. How splendid you look! The country air did you good."

"I'm in very good form," she said, as she took off her mantle and the hood with lilac silk ribbons and sat down with dignity in an easy-chair by the table. " My sleep and my digestion both improved very much in this short time. The fresh milk, and the farm sausages and hams – one thrives like the cattle and the crops. And the honey, Tom, I have always considered honey one of the very best of foods. A pure nature product – one knows just what one's eating. Yes, it was really very sweet of Armgard to remember an old boarding-school friendship and send me the invitation. Herr von Maiboom was very polite, too. They urged me to stay a couple of weeks longer, but I know Erica is rather helpless without me, especially now, with little Elisabeth – "

" How is the child? "

" Doing nicely, Tom. She is really not bad at all, for four months, even if Henriette and Friederike and Pfiffi did say she wouldn't live."

" And Weinschenk? How does he like being a father? I never see him except on Thursdays – "

" Oh, he is just the same. You know he is a very good, hard-working man, and in a way a model husband; he never stops in anywhere, but comes straight home from the office and spends all his free time with us. But – you see, Tom – we can speak quite openly, just between ourselves – he requires Erica to be always lively, always laughing and talking, because when he comes home tired and worried from the office, he needs cheering up, and his wife must amuse him and divert him."

" Idiot! " murmured the Senator.

" What? Well, the bad thing about it is, that Erica is a little bit inclined to be melancholy. She must get it from me, Tom. Sometimes she is very serious and quiet and thoughtful; and then he scolds and grumbles and complains, and really, to tell the truth, is not at all sympathetic. You can't help seeing that he is a man of no family, and never enjoyed what one would call a refined bringing-up. To be quite frank – a few days before I went to Pöppenrade, he threw the lid of the soup-tureen on the floor and broke it, because the soup was too salt."

" How charming! "

" Oh, no, it wasn't, not at all! But we must not judge. God knows, we are all weak creatures – and a good, capable, industrious man like that – Heaven forbid! No, Tom, a rough shell with a sound kernel inside is not the worst thing in this life. I've just come from something far sadder than that, I can tell you! Armgard wept bitterly, when she was alone with me – "

" You don't say! Is Herr von Maiboom – ? "

" Yes, Tom – that is what I wanted to tell you. We sit here

visiting, but I really came to-night on a serious and important errand."

"Well, what is the trouble with Herr von Maiboom?"

"He is a very charming man, Ralf von Maiboom, Thomas; but he is very wild – a hail-fellow-well-met with everybody. He gambles in Rostock, and he gambles in Warnemünde, and his debts are like the sands of the sea. Nobody could believe it, just living a couple of weeks at Pöppenrade. The house is lovely, everything looks flourishing, there is milk and sausage and ham and all that, in great abundance. So it is hard to measure the actual situation. But their affairs are in frightful disorder – Armgard confessed it to me, with heart-breaking sobs."

"Very sad."

"You may well say so. But, as I had already suspected, it turned out that I was not invited over there just for the sake of my *beaux yeux*."

"How so?"

"I will tell you, Tom. Herr von Maiboom needs a large sum of money immediately. He knew the old friendship between his wife and me, and he knew that I am your sister. So, in his extremity, he put his wife up to it, and she put me up to it. – You understand?"

The Senator passed his finger-tips across his hair and screwed up his face a little.

"I think so," he said. "Your serious and important business evidently concerns an advance on the Pöppenrade harvest – if I am not mistaken. But you have come to the wrong man, I think, you and your friends. In the first place, I have never done any business with Herr von Maiboom, and this would be a rather strange way to begin. In the second place – though, in the past, Grandfather, Father, and I myself have made advances on occasion to the landed gentry, it was always when they offered a certain security, either personally or through their connections. But to judge from the way you have just characterized Herr von Maiboom and his prospects, I should say there can be no security in his case."

"You are mistaken, Tom. I have let you have your say, but you are mistaken. It is not a question of an advance, at all. Maiboom has to have thirty-five thousand marks current –"

"Heavens and earth!"

"– five-and-thirty thousand marks current, to be paid within two weeks. The knife is at his throat – to be plain, he has to sell at once, immediately."

"In the blade – oh, the poor chap!" The Senator shook his

head as he stood, playing with his pince-nez on the tablecloth. " That is a rather unheard-of thing for our sort of business," he went on. " I have heard of such things, mostly in Hesse, where a few of the landed gentry are in the hands of the Jews. Who knows what sort of cut-throat it is that has poor Herr von Maiboom in his clutches? "

" Jews? Cut-throats? " cried Frau Permaneder, astonished beyond measure. " But it's *you* we are talking about, Tom! "

Thomas Buddenbrook suddenly threw down his pince-nez on the table so that it slid along on top of the newspaper, and turned toward his sister with a jerk.

" Me? " he said, but only with his lips, for he made no sound. Then he added aloud: " Go to bed, Tony. You are tired out."

" Why, Tom, that is what Ida Jungmann used to say to us, when we were just beginning to have a good time. But I assure you I was never wider awake in my life than now, coming over here in the dead of night to make Armgard's offer to you – or rather, indirectly, Ralf von Maiboom's – "

" And I will forgive you for making a proposal which is the product of your naïveté and the Maibooms' helplessness."

" Helplessness? Naïveté, Thomas? I don't understand you – I am very far from understanding you. You are offered an opportunity to do a good deed, and at the same time the best stroke of business you ever did in your life – "

" Oh, my darling child, you are talking the sheerest nonsense," cried the Senator, throwing himself back impatiently in his chair. " I beg your pardon, but you make me angry with your ridiculous innocence. Can't you understand that you are asking me to do something discreditable, to engage in underhand manœuvres? Why should I go fishing in troubled waters? Why should I fleece this poor land-owner? Why should I take advantage of his necessity to do him out of a year's harvest at a usurious profit to myself? "

" Oh, is that the way you look at it! " said Frau Permaneder, quite taken aback and thoughtful. But she recovered in a moment and went on: " But it is not at all necessary to look at it like that, Tom. How are you forcing him, when it is he who comes to you? He needs the money, and would like the matter arranged in a friendly way, and under the rose. That is why he traced out the connection between us, and invited me to visit."

" In short, he has made a mistake in his calculations about me and the character of my firm. I have my own traditions. We have been in business a hundred years without touching that sort of transaction, and I have no idea of beginning at this late day."

"Certainly, Tom, you have your traditions, and nobody respects them more than I do. And I know Father would not have done it – God forbid! Who says he would? But, silly as I am, I know enough to know that you are quite a different sort of man from Father, and since you took over the business it has been different from what it was before. That is because you were young and had enterprise and brains. But lately I am afraid you have let yourself get discouraged by this or that piece of bad luck. And if you are no longer having the same success you once did, it is because you have been too cautious and conscientious, and let slip your chances for good *coups* when you had them – "

"Oh, my dear child, stop, please; you irritate me!" said the Senator sharply, and turned away. "Let us change the subject."

"Yes, you are vexed, Tom, I can see it. You were from the beginning, and I have kept on, on purpose, to show you you are wrong to feel yourself insulted. But I know the real reason why you are vexed: it is because you are not so firmly decided not to touch the business. I know I am silly; but I have noticed about myself – and about other people too – that we are most likely to get angry and excited in our opposition to some idea when we ourselves are not quite certain of our own position, and are inwardly tempted to take the other side."

"Very fine," said the Senator, bit his cigarette-holder, and was silent.

"Fine? No, it's very simple – one of the simplest things life has taught me. But let it go, Tom. I won't urge you. Don't imagine that I think I could persuade you – I know I don't know enough. I'm only a silly female. It's a pity. Well, never mind. – It interested me very much. On the one hand I was shocked and upset about the Maibooms, but on the other I was pleased for you. I said to myself: 'Tom has been going about lately feeling very down in the mouth. He used to complain, but now he does not even complain any more. He has been losing money, and times are poor – and all that just now, when God has been good to me, and I am feeling happier than I have for a long time.' So I thought, 'This would be something for him: a stroke of luck, a good *coup*. It would offset a good deal of misfortune, and show people that luck is still on the side of the firm of Johann Buddenbrook.' And if you had undertaken it, I should have been so proud to have been the means – for you know it has always been my dream and my one desire, to be of some good to the family name. – Well, never mind. It is settled now. What I feel vexed about is that Maiboom has to sell, in any case, and if he looks around in the town here, he will find a purchaser — and it will be that rascal Hermann Hagenström! "

" Oh, yes — he probably would not refuse it," the Senator said bitterly; and Frau Permaneder answered, three times, one after the other: " You see, you see, you see! "

Thomas Buddenbrook suddenly began to shake his head and laugh angrily.

" We are silly. We sit here and work ourselves up — at least, you do — over something that is neither here nor there. So far as I know, I have not even asked what the thing is about — what Herr von Maiboom actually has to sell. I do not know Pöppenrade."

" Oh, you would have had to go there," she said eagerly. " It's not far from here to Rostock — and from there it is no distance at all. And as for what he has to sell — Pöppenrade is a large estate, I know for a fact that it grows more than a thousand sacks of wheat. But I don't know details. About rye, oats, or barley, there might be five hundred sacks of them, more or less. Everything is of the best, I can say that. But I can't give you any figures, I am such a goose, Tom. You would have to go over."

A pause ensued.

"No, it is not worth wasting words over," the Senator said decidedly. He folded his pince-nez and put it into his pocket, buttoned up his coat, and began to walk up and down the room with firm and rapid strides, which studiously betrayed no sign that he was giving the subject any further consideration.

He paused by the table and turned toward his sister, drumming lightly on the surface with his bent forefinger as he said: " I'll tell you a little story, my dear Tony, which will illustrate my attitude toward this affair. I know your weakness for the nobility, and the Mecklenburg nobility in particular — please don't mind if one of these gentry gets rapped a bit. You know, there is now and then one among them who doesn't treat the merchant classes with any great respect, though perfectly aware that he can't do without them. Such a man is too much inclined to lay stress on the superiority — to a certain extent undeniable — of the producer over the middleman. In short, he sometimes acts as if the merchant were like a peddling Jew to whom one sells old clothes, quite conscious that one is being overreached. I flatter myself that in my dealings with these gentry I have not usually made the impression of a morally inferior exploiter; to tell the truth, the boot has sometimes been on the other foot — I've run across men who were far less scrupulous than I am! But in one case, it only needed a single bold stroke to bring me into social relations. The man was the lord of Gross-Poggendorf, of whom you have surely heard. I had considerable dealings with him some while back: Count Strelitz, a very smart-appearing man, with a square eye-glass (I could never make out why he did not cut himself), patent-leather top-boots, and a riding-whip with a gold handle. He had a way of looking down at me from a great height, with his eyes half shut and his mouth half open. My first visit to him was very telling. We had had some correspondence. I drove over, and was ushered by a servant into the study, where Count Strelitz was sitting at his writing-table. He returns my bow, half gets up, finishes the last lines of a letter; then he turns to me and begins to talk business, looking over the top of my head. I lean on the sofa-table, cross my arms and my legs, and enjoy myself. I stand five minutes talking. After another five minutes, I sit down on the table and swing my leg. We get on with our business, and at the end of fifteen minutes he says to me, very graciously, 'won't you sit down?' 'Beg pardon?' I say. 'Oh, don't mention it – I've been sitting for some time!'"

"Did you say that? Really?" cried Frau Permaneder, enchanted. She had straightway forgotten all that had gone before, and lived for the moment entirely in the anecdote.

"'I've been sitting for some time' – oh, that is too good!"

"Well, and I assure you that the Count altered his tune at once. He shook hands when I came, and asked me to sit down – in the course of time we became very friendly. But I have told you this in order to ask you if you think I should have the right, or the courage, or the inner self-confidence to behave in the same way to Herr von Maiboom if, when we met to discuss the bargain, he were to forget to offer me a chair?"

Frau Permaneder was silent. "Good," she said then, and got up. "You may be right; and, as I said, I'm not going to press you. You know what you must do and what leave undone, and that's an end of it. If you only feel that I spoke in good part – you do, don't you? All right. Good night, Tom. Or – no, wait – I must go and say 'How do you do' to the good Ida and give Hanno a little kiss. I'll look in again on my way out." With that she went.

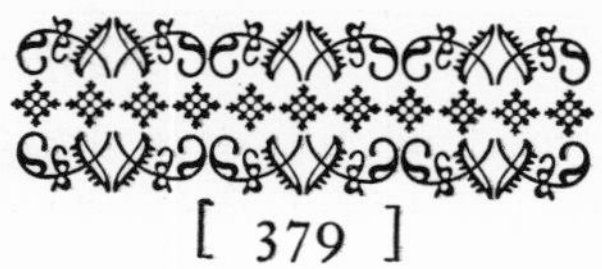

CHAPTER III

SHE mounted the stairs to the second storey, left the little balcony on her right, went along the white-and-gold balustrade and through an ante-chamber, the door of which stood open on the corridor, and from which a second exit to the left led into the Senator's dressing-room. Here she softly turned the handle of the door opposite and went in.

It was an unusually large chamber, the windows of which were draped with flowered curtains. The walls were rather bare: aside from a large black-framed engraving above Ida's bed, representing Giacomo Meyerbeer surrounded by the characters in his operas, there was nothing but a few English coloured prints of children with yellow hair and little red frocks, pinned to the window hangings. Ida Jungmann sat at the large extension-table in the middle of the room, darning Hanno's stockings. The faithful Prussian was now at the beginning of the fifties. She had begun early to grow grey, but her hair had never become quite white, having remained a mixture of black and grey; her erect bony figure was as sturdy, and her brown eyes as bright, clear, and unwearied as twenty years ago.

"Well, Ida, you good soul," said Frau Permaneder, in a low but lively voice, for her brother's little story had put her in good spirits, "and how are you, you old stand-by, you?"

"What's that, Tony—stand-by, is it? And how do you come to be here so late?"

"I've been with my brother—on pressing business. Unfortunately, it didn't turn out.—Is he asleep?" she asked, and gestured with her chin toward the little bed on the left wall, its head close to the door that led into the parents' sleeping chamber.

"Sh-h!" said Ida. "Yes, he is asleep." Frau Permaneder went on her tip-toes toward the little bed, cautiously raised the curtain, and bent to look down at her sleeping nephew's face.

The small Johann Buddenbrook lay on his back, his little face, in its frame of long light-brown hair, turned toward the room. He was breathing softly but audibly into the pillow. Only the fingers showed beneath the too long, too wide sleeves of his nightgown: one of his hands lay on his breast, the other on the coverlet, with the bent fingers jerking slightly now and then. The half-parted lips moved a little too, as if forming words. From time to time a pained expression mounted over the little face, beginning with a trembling of the chin, making the lips and the delicate nostrils quiver and the muscles of the narrow forehead contract. The long dark eyelashes did not hide the blue shadows that lay in the corners of the eyes.

"He is dreaming," said Frau Permaneder, moved.

She bent over the child and gently kissed his slumbering cheek; then she composed the curtains and went back to the table, where Ida, in the golden light from the lamp, drew a fresh stocking over her darning-ball, looked at the hole, and began to fill it in.

"You are darning, Ida – funny, I can't imagine you doing anything else."

"Yes, yes, Tony. The boy tears everything, now he has begun to go to school."

"But he is such a quiet, gentle child."

"Ye-s, he is. But even so – "

"Does he like going to school? "

"Oh, no-o, Tony. He would far rather have gone on here with me. And I should have liked it better too. The masters haven't known him since he was a baby, the way I have – they don't know how to take him, when they are teaching him. It is often hard for him to pay attention, and he gets tired so easily – "

"Poor darling! Have they whipped him yet? "

"No, indeed. Sakes alive, how could they have the heart, if the boy once looked at them – ? "

"How was it the first time he went? Did he cry? "

"Yes, indeed, he did. He cries so easily – not loud, but sort of to himself. And he held your brother by the coat and begged to be allowed to stop at home – "

"Oh, my brother took him, did he? – Yes, that is a hard moment, Ida. I remember it like yesterday. I *howled*. I do assure you. I howled like a chained-up dog; I felt dreadfully. And why? Because I had had such a good time at home. I noticed at once that all the children from the nice houses wept, and the others not at all – they just stared and grinned at us. – Goodness, what is the matter with him, Ida? "

She turned in alarm toward the little bed, where a cry had interrupted her chatter. It was a frightened cry, and it repeated itself in an even more anguished tone the next minute; and then three, four, five times more, one after another. " Oh, oh, *oh!* " It became a loud, desperate protest against something which he saw or which was happening to him. The next moment little Johann sat upright in bed, stammering incomprehensibly, and staring with wide-open, strange golden-brown eyes into a world which he, and he alone, could see.

" That's nothing," said Ida. " It is the *pavor*. It is sometimes much worse than that." She put her work down calmly and crossed the room, with her long heavy stride, to Hanno's bed. She spoke to him in a low, quieting voice, laid him down, and covered him again.

" Oh, I see — the *pavor*," repeated Frau Permaneder. " What will he do now? Will he wake up? "

But Hanno did not waken at all, though his eyes were wide and staring, and his lips still moved.

" 'In my — little — garden — go —,' "

said Hanno, mumblingly,

" 'All — my — onions — water — ' "

" He is saying his piece," explained Ida Jungmann, shaking her head. " There, there, little darling — go to sleep now."

" 'Little man stands — stands there —
He begins — to — sneeze — ' "

He sighed. Suddenly his face changed, his eyes half closed; he moved his head back and forth on the pillow and said in a low, plaintive sing-song:

" 'The moon it shines,
The baby cries,
The clock strikes twelve,
God help all suff'ring folk to close their eyes.' "

But with the words came so deep a sob that tears rolled out from under his lashes and down his cheeks and wakened him. He put his arms around Ida, looked about him with tear-wet eyes, murmured something in a satisfied tone about " Aunt Tony," turned himself a little in his bed, and then went quietly off to sleep.

" How very strange," said Frau Permaneder, as Ida sat down at the table once more. " What was all that? "

" They are in his reader," answered Fraulein Jungmann. " It says underneath 'The Boys' Magic Horn.' They are all rather queer. He has been having to learn them, and he talks a great deal about that one with the little man. Do you know it? It is really rather frightening. It is a little dwarf that gets into everything: eats up the broth and breaks the pot, steals the wood, stops the spinning-wheel, teases everybody — and then, at the end, he asks to be prayed for! It touched the child very much. He has thought about it day in and day out; and two or three times he said: 'You know, Ida, he doesn't do that to be wicked, but only because he is unhappy, and it only makes him more unhappy still. . . . But if one prays for him, then he does not need to do it any more!' Even to-night, when his Mama kissed him good night before she went to the concert, he asked her to 'pray for the little man.'"

"And did he pray too?"

"Not aloud, but probably to himself. — He hasn't said much about the other poem — it is called 'The Nursery Clock' — he has only wept. He weeps so easy, poor little lad, and it is so hard for him to stop."

"But what is there so sad about it?"

"How do I know? He has never been able to say any more than the beginning of it, the part that makes him cry in his sleep. And that about the waggoner, who gets up at three from his bed of straw — that always made him weep too."

Frau Permaneder laughed emotionally, and then looked serious.

"I'll tell you, Ida, it's no good. It isn't good for him to feel everything so much. 'The waggoner gets up at three from his bed of straw' — why, of course he does! That's why he is a waggoner. I can see already that the child takes everything too much to heart — it consumes him, I feel sure. We must speak seriously with Grabow. But there, that is just what it is," she went on, folding her arms, putting her head on one side, and tapping the floor nervously with her foot. "Grabow is getting old; and aside from that, good as he is — and he really is a very good man, a perfect angel — so far as his skill is concerned, I have no such great opinion of it, Ida, and may God forgive me if I am wrong. Take this nervousness of Hanno's, his starting up at night and having such frights in his sleep. Grabow knows what it is, and all he does is to tell us the Latin name of it — *pavor nocturnus*. Dear knows, that is very enlightening, of course! No, he is a dear good man, and a great friend of the family and all that — but he is no great light. An important man looks different — he shows when he is young that there is something in him. Grabow lived through the '48. He was a young man then. Do you imagine he was the least bit thrilled over it — over freedom and justice, and the downfall of privilege and arbitrary power? He is a cultivated man; but I am convinced that the unheard-of laws concerning the press and the universities did not interest him in the least. He has never behaved even the least little bit wild, never jumped over the traces. He has always had just the same long, mild face, and always prescribed pigeon and French bread, and when anything is serious, a teaspoon of tincture of althaea. – Good night, Ida. No, I think there are other doctors in the world! Too bad I have missed Gerda. Yes, thanks, there is a light in the corridor. Good night."

When Frau Permaneder opened the dining-room door in passing, to call a good night to her brother in the living-room, she saw that the whole storey was lighted up, and that Thomas was walking up and down with his hands behind his back.

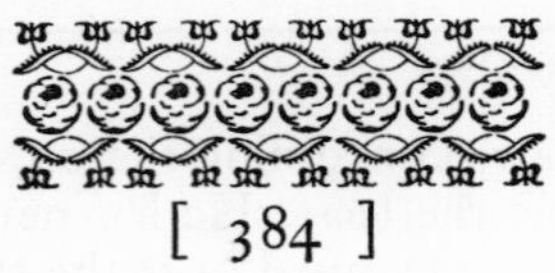

CHAPTER IV

The Senator, when he was alone again, sat down at the table, took out his glasses, and tried to resume his reading. But in a few minutes his eyes had roved from the printed page, and he sat for a long time without changing his position, gazing straight ahead of him between the portières into the darkness of the salon.

His face, when he was alone, changed so that it was hardly recognizable. The muscles of his mouth and cheeks, otherwise obedient to his will, relaxed and became flabby. Like a mask the look of vigour, alertness, and amiability, which now for a long time had been preserved only by constant effort, fell from his face, and betrayed an anguished weariness instead. The tired, worried eyes gazed at objects without seeing them; they became red and watery. He made no effort to deceive even himself; and of all the dull, confused, rambling thoughts that filled his mind he clung to only one: the single, despairing thought that Thomas Buddenbrook, at forty-three years, was an old, worn-out man.

He rubbed his hand over his eyes and forehead, drawing a long, deep breath, mechanically lighted another cigarette, though he knew they were bad for him, and continued to gaze through the smoke-haze into the darkness. What a contrast between that relaxed and suffering face and the elegant, almost military style of his hair and beard! the stiffened and perfumed moustaches, the meticulously shaven cheeks and chin, and the careful hair-dressing which sedulously hid a beginning thinness. The hair ran back in two longish bays from the delicate temples, with a narrow parting on top; over the ears it was not long and waving, but kept short-cut now, in order not to betray how grey it had grown. He himself felt the change and knew it could not have escaped the eyes of others: the contrast between his active, elastic movements and the dull pallor of his face.

Not that he was in reality less of an important and indispensable personage than he always had been. His friends said, and his enemies could not deny, that Senator Buddenbrook was the Burgomaster's right hand: Burgomaster Langhals was even more emphatic on that point than his predecessor Överdieck had been. But the firm of Johann Buddenbrook was no longer what it had been – this seemed to be common property, so much so that Herr Stuht discussed it with his wife over their bacon broth – and Thomas Buddenbrook groaned over the fact.

At the same time, it was true that he himself was mainly responsible. He was still a rich man, and none of the losses he had suffered, even the severe one of the year '66, had seriously undermined the existence of the firm. But the notion that his luck and his consequence had fled, based though it was more upon inward feelings than upon outward facts, brought him to a state of lowness and suspicion. He entertained, of course, as before, and set before his guests the normal and expected number of courses. But, as never before, he began to cling to money and, in his private life, to save in small and petty ways. He had a hundred times regretted the building of his new house, which he felt had brought him nothing but bad luck. The summer holidays were given up, and the little city garden had to take the place of mountains or seashore. The family meals were, by his express and emphatic command, of such simplicity as to seem absurd by contrast with the lofty, splendid dining-room, with its extent of parquetry floors and its imposing oak furniture. For a long time now, there had been dessert only on Sundays. His own appearance was as elegant as ever; but the old servant, Anton, carried to the kitchen the news that the master only changed his shirt now every *other* day, as the washing was too hard on the fine linen. He knew more than that. He knew that he was to be dismissed. Gerda protested: three servants were few enough to do the work of so large a house as it should be done. But it was no use: old Anton, who had so long sat on the box when Thomas Buddenbrook drove down to the Senate, was sent away with a suitable present.

Such decrees as these were in harmony with the joyless state of affairs in the firm. That fresh enterprising spirit with which young Thomas Buddenbrook had taken up the reins – that was all gone, now; and his partner, Herr Friedrich Wilhelm Marcus – who, with his small capital, could not have had a prepondering influence in any case – was by nature lacking in initiative.

Herr Marcus' pedantry had so increased in the course of years that it had become a distinct eccentricity. It took him a quarter of an hour of stroking his moustaches, casting side-glances, and giving little coughs, just to cut his cigar and put the tip in his pocket-book. Evenings, when the gas-light made every corner of the office as bright as day, he still used a tallow candle on his own desk. Every half-hour he would get up and go to the tap and put water on his head. One morning there had been an empty sack untidily left under his desk. He took it for a cat and began to shoo it out with loud imprecations, to the joy of the office staff. No, he was not the man to give any quickening impulse to the business in the face of his partner's present lassitude. Mortification and a sort of desperate irritation often seized upon the Senator: as now, when he sat and stared wearily into the darkness, bringing home to himself the petty retail transactions and the pennywise policies to which the firm of Johann Buddenbrook had lately sunk.

But, after all, was it not best thus? Misfortune too has its time, he thought. Is it not better, while it holds sway, to keep oneself still, to wait in quiet and assemble one's inner powers? Why must this proposition come up just now, to shake him untimely out of his canny resignation and make him a prey to doubts and suspicions? Was the time come? Was this a sign? Should he feel encouraged to stand up and strike a blow? He had refused with all the decisiveness he could put into his voice, to think of the proposition; but had that settled it? It seemed not, since here he sat and brooded over it. "We are most likely to get angry in our opposition to some idea when we ourselves are not quite certain of our own position." A deucedly sly little person, Tony was!

What had he answered her? He had spoken very impressively, he recollected, about "underhand manœuvres," "fishing in troubled waters," "fleecing the poor land-owner," "usury," and so on. Very fine! But really one might ask if this were just the right time for so many large words. Consul Hermann Hagenström would not have thought of them, and would not have used them. Was he, Thomas Buddenbrook, a man of action, a business man – or was he a finicking dreamer?

Yes, that was the question. It had always been, as far back as he could remember, the question. Life was harsh: and business, with its ruthless unsentimentality, was an epitome of life. Did Thomas Buddenbrook, like his father, stand firmly on his two feet, in face of this hard practicality of life? Often enough, even far back in the past, he had seen reason to doubt it. Often enough, from his youth onwards, he had sternly brought his feelings into line. To inflict punishment, to take punishment, and not to think of it as punishment, but as something to be taken for granted – should he never completely learn that lesson?

He recalled the catastrophe of the year 1866, and the inexpressibly painful emotions which had then overpowered him. He had lost a large sum of money in the affair – but that had not been the unbearable thing about it. For the first time in his career he had fully and personally experienced the ruthless brutality of business life and seen how all better, gentler, and kindlier sentiments creep away and hid themselves before the one raw, naked, dominating instinct of self-preservation. He had seen that when one suffers a misfortune in business, one is met by one's friends – and one's best friends – not with sympathy, not with compassion, but with suspicion – cold, cruel, hostile suspicion. But he had known all this before; why should he be surprised at it? And in stronger and hardier hours he had blushed for his own weakness, for his own distress and sleepless nights, for his revulsion and disgust at the hateful and shameless harshness of life!

How foolish all that was! How ridiculous such feelings had been! How could he entertain them? – unless, indeed, he were a feeble visionary and not a practical business man at all! Ah, how many times had he asked himself that question? And how many times had he answered it: in strong and purposeful hours with one answer, in weak and discouraged ones with another! But he was too shrewd and too honest not to admit, after all, that he was a mixture of both.

All his life, he had made the impression on others of a practical man of action. But in so far as he legitimately passed for one – he, with his fondness for quotations from Goethe – was it not because he deliberately set out to do so? He had been successful in the past, but was that not because of the enthusiasm and impetus drawn from reflection? And if he were now discouraged, if his powers were lamed – God grant it was only for a time – was not his depression the natural consequence of the conflict that went on within himself? Whether his father, grandfather, and great-grandfather would have bought the Pöppenrade harvest in the blade was not the point after all. The thing was that they were practical men, more naturally, more vigorously, more impeccably practical than he was himself.

He was seized by a great unrest, by a need for movement, space, and light. He shoved back his chair, went into the salon, and lighted several burners of the chandelier over the centre-table. He stood there, pulling slowly and spasmodically at the long ends of his moustaches and vacantly gazing about the luxurious room. Together with the living-room it occupied the whole front of the house; it had light, ornate furniture and looked like a music-room, with the great grand piano, Gerda's violin-case, the étagère with music books, the carved music-stand, and the bas-reliefs of singing cupids over the doors. The bow-window was filled with palms.

Senator Buddenbrook stood for two or three minutes motionless. Then he went back through the living-room into the dining-room and made light there also. He stopped at the sideboard and poured a glass of water, either to be doing something or to quiet his heart. Then he moved quickly on through the house, lighting up as he went. The smoking-room was furnished in dark colours and wainscoted. He absently opened the door of the cigar cabinet and shut it again, and at the table lifted the lid of a little oak box which had playing-cards, score-cards, and other such things in it. He let some of the bone counters glide through his fingers with a rattling sound, clapped the lid shut, and began again to walk up and down.

A little room with a small stained-glass window opened into the smoking-room. It was empty except for some small light serving-tables of the kind which fit one within another. On one of them a liqueur cabinet stood. From here one entered the dining-room, with its great extent of parquetry flooring and its four high windows, hung with wine-coloured curtains, looking out into the garden. It also occupied the whole breadth of the house. It was furnished by two low, heavy sofas, covered with the same wine-coloured material as the curtains, and by a number of high-backed chairs standing stiffly along the walls. Behind the fire-screen was a chimney-place, its artificial coals covered with shining red paper to make them look glowing. On the marble mantel-shelf in front of the mirror stood two towering Chinese vases.

The whole storey was now lighted by the flame of single gas-jets, and looked like a party the moment after the last guest is gone. The Senator measured the room throughout its length, and then stood at one of the windows and looked down into the garden.

The moon stood high and small between fleecy clouds, and the little fountain splashed in the stillness on the overhanging boughs of the walnut tree. Thomas looked down on the pavilion which enclosed his view, on the little glistening white terrace with the two obelisks, the regular gravel paths, and the freshly turned earth of the neat borders and beds. But this whole minute and punctilious symmetry, far from soothing him, only made him feel the more exasperated. He held the catch of the window, leaned his forehead on it, and gave rein to his tormenting thoughts again.

What was he coming to? He thought of a remark he had let fall to his sister – something he had felt vexed with himself the next minute for saying, it seemed so unnecessary. He was speaking of Count Strelitz and the landed aristocracy, and he had expressed the view that the producer had a social advantage over the middleman. What was the point of that? It might be true and it might not; but was he, Thomas Buddenbrook, called upon to express such ideas – was he called upon to even think them? Should he have been able to explain to the satisfaction of his father, his grandfather – or any of his fellow townsmen – how he came to be expressing, or indulging in, such thoughts? A man who stands firm and confident in his own calling, whatever it may be, recognizes only it, understands only it, values only it.

Then he suddenly felt the blood rushing to his face as he recalled another memory, from farther back in the past. He saw himself and his brother Christian, walking around the garden of the Meng Street house, involved in a quarrel – one of those painful, regrettable, heated discussions. Christian, with artless indiscretion, had made a highly undesirable, a compromising remark, which a number of people had heard; and Thomas, furiously angry, irritated to the last degree, had called him to account. At bottom, Christian had said, at bottom every business man was a rascal. Well! was that foolish and trifling remark, in point of fact, so different from what he himself had just said to his sister? He had been furiously angry then, had protested violently – but what was it that sly little Tony said? "When we ourselves are not quite certain of our own position . . ."

"No," said the Senator, suddenly, aloud, lifted his head with a jerk, and let go the window fastening. He fairly pushed himself away from it. "That settles it," he said. He coughed, for the sound of his own voice in the emptiness made him feel unpleasant. He turned and began to walk quickly through all the rooms, his hands behind his back and his head bowed.

"That settles it," he repeated. "It will have to settle it. I am wasting time, I am sinking into a morass, I'm getting worse than Christian." It was something to be glad of, at least, that he was in no doubt where he stood. It lay, then, in his own hands to apply the corrective. Relentlessly. Let us see, now – let us see – what sort of offer was it they had made? The Pöppenrade harvest, in the blade? "I will do it!" he said in a passionate whisper, even stretching out one hand and shaking the forefinger. "I will do it!"

It would be, he supposed, what one would call a *coup:* an opportunity to double a capital of, say, forty thousand marks current — though that was probably an exaggeration. — Yes, it was a sign — a signal to him that he should rouse himself! It was the first step, the beginning, that counted; and the risk connected with it was a sort of offset to his moral scruples. If it succeeded, then he was himself again, then he would venture once more, then he would know how to hold fortune and influence fast within his grip.

No, Messrs. Strunck and Hagenström would not be able to profit by this occasion, unfortunately for them. There was another firm in the place, which, thanks to personal connections, had the upper hand. In fact, the personal was here the decisive factor. It was no ordinary business, to be carried out in the ordinary way. Coming through Tony, as it had, it bore more the character of a private transaction, and would need to be carried out with discretion and tact. Hermann Hagenström would hardly have been the man for the job. He, Thomas Buddenbrook, as a business man, was taking advantage of the market — and he would, by God, when he sold, know how to do the same. On the other hand, he was doing the hard-pressed land-owner a favour which he was called upon to do, by reason of Tony's connection with the Maibooms. The thing to do was to write, to write this evening — not on the business paper with the firm name, but on his own personal letter-paper with "Senator Buddenbrook" stamped across it. He would write in a courteous tone and ask if a visit in the next few days would be agreeable. But it was a difficult business, none the less — slippery ground, upon which one needed to move with care. — Well, so much the better for him.

His step grew quicker, his breathing deeper. He sat down a moment, sprang up again, and began roaming about through all the rooms. He thought it all out again; he thought about Herr Marcus, Hermann Hagenström, Christian, and Tony; he saw the golden harvests of Pöppenrade wave in the breeze, and dreamed of the upward bound the old firm would take after this coup; scornfully repulsed all his scruples and hesitations, put out his hand and said "I'll do it!"

Frau Permaneder opened the door and called out "Good-bye!" He answered her without knowing it. Gerda said good-night to Christian at the house door and came upstairs, her strange deep-set eyes wearing the expression that music always gave them. The

Senator stopped mechanically in his walk, asked mechanically about the concert and the Spanish virtuoso, and said he was ready to go to bed.

But he did not go. He took up his wanderings again. He thought about the sacks of wheat and rye and oats and barley which should fill the lofts of the Lion, the Walrus, the Oak, and the Linden; he thought about the price he intended to ask – of course it should not be an extravagant price. He went softly at midnight down into the counting-house and, by the light of Herr Marcus' tallow candle, wrote a letter to Herr von Maiboom of Pöppenrade – a letter which, as he read it through, his head feeling feverish and heavy, he thought was the best and most tactful he had ever written.

That was the night of May 27. The next day he indicated to his sister, treating the affair in a light, semi-humorous way, that he had thought it all over and decided that he could not just refuse Herr von Maiboom out of hand and leave him at the mercy of the nearest swindler. On the thirtieth of May he went to Rostock, whence he drove in a hired wagon out to the country.

His mood for the next few days was of the best, his step elastic and free, his manners easy. He teased Clothilde, laughed heartily at Christian, joked with Tony, and played with Hanno in the little gallery for a whole hour on Sunday, helping him to hoist up miniature sacks of grain into a little brick-red granary, and imitating the hollow, drawling shouts of the workmen. And at the Burgesses' meeting of the third of June he made a speech on the most tiresome subject in the world, something connected with taxation, which was so brilliant and witty that everybody agreed with it unanimously, and Consul Hagenström, who had opposed him, became almost a laughing-stock.

CHAPTER V

WAS it forgetfulness, or was it intention, which would have made Senator Buddenbrook pass over in silence a certain fact, had not his sister Tony, the devotee of the family papers, announced it to all the world: the fact, namely, that in those documents the founding of the firm of Johann Buddenbrook was ascribed to the date of the 7th of July, 1768, the hundredth anniversary of which was now at hand?

Thomas seemed almost disturbed when Tony, in a moving voice, called his attention to the fact. His good mood had not lasted. All too soon he had fallen silent again, more silent than before. He would leave the office in the midst of work, seized with unrest, and roam about the garden, sometimes pausing as if he felt confined in his movements, sighing, and covering his eyes with his hand. He said nothing, gave his feelings no vent – to whom should he speak, then? When he told his partner of the Pöppenrade matter, Herr Marcus had for the first time in his life been angry with him, and had washed his hands of the whole affair. But Thomas betrayed himself to his sister Tony, when they said good-bye on the street one Thursday evening, and she alluded to the Pöppenrade harvest. He gave her hand a single quick squeeze, and added passionately " Oh, Tony, if I had only sold it already! " He broke off abruptly, and they parted, leaving Frau Permaneder dismayed and anxious. The sudden hand-pressure had something despairing, the low words betrayed pent-up feeling. But when Tony, as chance offered, tried to come back to the subject, he wrapped himself in silence, the more forbidding because of his inward mortification over having given way – his inward bitterness at being, as he felt, feeble and inadequate to the situation in hand.

He said now, slowly and fretfully: " Oh, my dear child, I wish we might ignore the whole affair! "

" Ignore it, Tom? Impossible! Unthinkable! Do you think you could suppress the fact? Do you imagine the whole town would forget the meaning of the day? "

"I don't say it is possible – I only say I wish it were. It is pleasant to celebrate the past, when one is gratified with the present and the future. It is agreeable to think of one's forefathers when one feels at one with them and conscious of having acted as they would have done. If the jubilee came at a better time – but just now, I feel small inclination to celebrate it."

"You must not talk like that, Tom. You don't mean it; you know perfectly that it would be a shame to let the hundredth anniversary of the firm of Johann Buddenbrook go by without a sign or a sound of rejoicing. You are a little nervous now, and I know why, though there is really no reason for it. But when the day comes, you will be as moved as all the rest of us."

She was right; the day could not be passed over in silence. It was not long before a notice appeared in the papers, calling attention to the coming anniversary and giving a detailed history of the old and estimable firm – but it was really hardly necessary. In the family, Justus Kröger was the first to mention the approaching event, on the Thursday afternoon; and Frau Permaneder saw to it that the venerable leather portfolio was solemnly brought out after dessert was cleared away, and the whole family, by way of foretaste, perused the dates and events in the life of the first Johann Buddenbrook, Hanno's great-great-grandfather: when he had varioloid and when genuine smallpox, when he fell out of the third-storey window on to the floor of the drying-house, and when he had fever and delirium – she read all that aloud with pious fervour. Not content with that, she must go back into the 16th century, to the oldest Buddenbrook of whom there was knowledge, to the one who was Councillor in Grabau, and the Rostock tailor who had been "very well off" and had so many children, living and dead. "What a splendid man!" she cried; and began to rummage through yellow papers and read letters and poems aloud.

On the morning of the seventh of July, Herr Wenzel was naturally the first with his congratulations.

"Well, Herr Sen'ter, many happy returns!" he said, gesturing freely with razor and strop in his red hands. "A hundred years! And nearly half of it, I may say, I have been shaving in the respected family – oh, yes, one goes through a deal with the family, when one sees the head of it the first thing in the morning! The deceased Herr Consul was always the most talkative in the morning, too: 'Wenzel,' he would ask me, 'Wenzel, what do you think about the rye? Should I sell or do you think it will go up again?'"

"Yes, Wenzel, and I cannot think of these years without you, either. Your calling, as I've often said to you, has a certain charm about it. When you have made your rounds, you are wiser than anybody: you have had the heads of nearly all the great houses under your hand, and know the mood of each one. All the others can envy you that, for it is really valuable information."

"'s a good bit of truth in that, Herr Sen'ter. But what about the Herr Sen'ter's own mood, if I may be so bold to ask? Herr Sen'ter's looking a trifle pale again this morning."

"Am I? Well, I have a headache – and so far as I can see, it will get worse before it gets better, for I suspect they'll put a good deal of strain on it to-day."

"I'm afraid so, Herr Sen'ter. The interest is great – the interest is very great. Just look out o' window when I've done with you. Hosts of flags! And down at the bottom of the Street the 'Wullenwewer' and the 'Friederike Överdieck' with all their pennons flying."

"Well, let's be quick, then, Wenzel; there's no time to lose, evidently."

The Senator did not don his office jacket, as he usually did of a morning, but put on at once a black cutaway coat with a white waistcoat and light-coloured trousers. There would certainly be visits. He gave a last glance in the mirror, a last pressure of the tongs to his moustache, and turned with a little sigh to go. The dance was beginning. If only the day were all over! Would he have a single minute to himself, a single minute to relax the muscles of his face? All day long he should certainly have to receive, with tact and dignity, the congratulations of a host of people, find just the right word and just the right tone for everybody, be serious, hearty, ironic, jocose, and respectful by turns; and from afternoon late into the night there would be the dinner at the Ratskeller.

It was not true that his head ached. He was only tired. Already, though he had just risen, with his nerves refreshed by sleep, he felt his old, indefinable burden upon him. Why had he said his head ached – as though he always had a bad conscience where his own health was concerned? Why? Why? However, there was no time now to brood over the question.

He went into the dining-room, where Gerda met him gaily. She too was already arrayed to meet their guests, in a plaid skirt, a white blouse, and a thin silk zouave jacket over it, the colour of her heavy hair. She smiled and showed her white teeth, so large and regular, whiter than her white face; her eyes, those close-set, enigmatic brown eyes, were smiling too, to-day.

"I've been up for hours – you can tell from that how excited I am," she said, "and how hearty my congratulations are."

"Well, well! So the hundred years make an impression on you too?"

"Tremendous. But perhaps it is only the excitement of the celebration. What a day! Look at that, for instance." She pointed to the breakfast-table, all garlanded with garden flowers. "That is Fräulein Jungmann's work. But you are mistaken if you think you can drink tea now. The family is in the drawing-room already, waiting to make a presentation – something in which I too have had a share. Listen, Thomas. This is, of course, only the beginning of a stream of callers. At first I can stand it, but at about midday I shall have to withdraw, I am sure. The barometer has fallen a little, but the sky is still the most staring blue. It makes the flags look lovely, of course, and the whole town is flagged – but it will be frightfully hot. Come into the salon. Breakfast must wait. You should have been up before. Now the first excitement will have to come on an empty stomach."

The Frau Consul, Christian, Clothilde, Ida Jungmann, Frau Permaneder, and Hanno were assembled in the salon, the last two supporting, not without difficulty, the family present, a great commemorative tablet. The Frau Consul, deeply moved, embraced her eldest-born.

"This is a wonderful day, my dear son – a wonderful day," she repeated. "We must thank God unceasingly, with all our hearts, for His mercies – for all His mercies." She wept.

The Senator was attacked by weakness in her embrace. He felt as though something within him freed itself and flew away. His lips trembled. An overwhelming need possessed him to lay his head upon his mother's breast, to close his eyes in her arms, to breathe in the delicate perfume that rose from the soft silk of her gown, to lie there at rest, seeing nothing more, saying nothing more. He kissed her and stood erect, putting out his hand to his brother, who greeted him with the absent-minded embarrassment which was his usual bearing on such occasions. Clothilde drawled out something kindly. Ida Jungmann confined herself to making a deep bow, while she played with the silver watch-chain on her flat bosom.

"Come here, Tom," said Frau Permaneder uncertainly. "We can't hold it any longer, can we, Hanno?" She was holding it almost alone, for Hanno's little arms were not much help; and she looked, what with her enthusiasm and her effort, like an enraptured martyr. Her eyes were moist, her cheeks burned, and her tongue played, with a mixture of mischief and nervousness, on her upper lip.

"Here I am," said the Senator. "What in the world is this? Come, let me have it; we'll lean it against the wall." He propped it up next to the piano and stood looking at it, surrounded by the family.

In a large, heavy frame of carved nut-wood were the portraits of the four owners of the firm, under glass. There was the founder, Johann Buddenbrook, taken from an old oil painting – a tall, grave old gentleman, with his lips firmly closed, looking severe and determined above his lace jabot. There was the broad and jovial countenance of Johann Buddenbrook, the friend of Jean Jacques Hoffstede. There was Consul Johann Buddenbrook, in a stiff choker collar, with his wide, wrinkled mouth and large aquiline nose, his eyes full of religious fervour. And finally there was Thomas Buddenbrook himself, as a somewhat younger man. The four portraits were divided by conventionalized blades of wheat, heavily gilded, and beneath, likewise in figures of brilliant gilt, the dates 1768–1868. Above the whole, in the tall, Gothic hand of him who had left it to his descendants, was the quotation: "My son, attend with zeal, to thy business by day; but do none that hinders thee from thy sleep at night."

The Senator, his hands behind his back gazed for a long time at the tablet.

"Yes, yes," he said abruptly, and his tone was rather mocking, "an undisturbed night's rest is a very good thing." Then, seriously, if perhaps a little perfunctorily, "Thank you very much, my dear family. It is indeed a most thoughtful and beautiful gift. What do you think – where shall we put it? Shall we hang it in my private office?"

"Yes, Tom, over the desk in your office," answered Frau Permaneder, and embraced her brother. Then she drew him into the bow-window and pointed.

Under a deep blue sky, the two-coloured flag floated above all the houses, right down Fishers' Lane, from Broad Street to the wharf, where the "Wullenwewer" and the "Friederike Överdieck" lay under full flag, in their owner's honour.

"The whole town is the same," said Frau Permaneder, and her voice trembled. "I've been out and about already. Even the Hagenströms have a flag. They couldn't do otherwise. – I'd smash in their window!" He smiled, and they went back to the table together. "And here are the telegrams, Tom, the first ones to come – the personal ones, of course; the others have been sent to the office." They opened a few of the dispatches: from the family in Hamburg, from the Frankfort Buddenbrooks, from Herr Arnoldsen in Amsterdam, from Jürgen Kröger in Wismar. Suddenly Frau Permaneder flushed deeply.

"He is a good man, in his way," she said, and pushed across to her brother the telegram she had just opened: it was signed Permaneder.

"But time is passing," said the Senator, and looked at his watch. "I'd like my tea. Will you come in with me? The house will be like a bee-hive after a while."

His wife, who had given a sign to Ida Jungmann, held him back. "Just a moment, Thomas. You know Hanno has to go to his lessons. He wants to say a poem to you first. Come here, Hanno. And now, just as if no one else were here – you remember? Don't be excited."

It was the summer holidays, of course, but little Hanno had private lessons in arithmetic, in order to keep up with his class. Somewhere out in the suburb of St. Gertrude, in a little ill-smelling room, a man in a red beard, with dirty fingernails, was waiting to discipline him in the detested "tables." But first he was to recite to Papa a poem painfully learned by heart, with Ida Jungmann's help, in the little balcony on the second floor.

He leaned against the piano, in his blue sailor suit with the white V front and the wide linen collar with a big sailor's knot coming out beneath. His thin legs were crossed, his body and head a little inclined in an attitude of shy, unconscious grace. Two or three weeks before, his hair had been cut, as not only his fellow pupils, but the master as well, had laughed at it; but his head was still covered with soft abundant ringlets, growing down over the forehead and temples. His eyelids drooped, so that the long brown lashes lay over the deep blue shadows; and his closed lips were a little wry.

He knew well what would happen. He would begin to cry, would not be able to finish for crying; and his heart would contract, as it did on Sundays in St. Mary's, when Herr Pfühl played on the organ in a certain piercingly solemn way. It always turned out that he wept when they wanted him to do something – when they examined him and tried to find out what he knew, as Papa so loved to do. If only Mamma had not spoken of getting excited! She meant to be encouraging, but he felt it was a mistake. There they stood, and looked at him. They expected, and feared, that he would break down – so how was it possible *not* to? He lifted his lashes and sought Ida's eyes. She was playing with her watch-chain, and nodded to him in her usual honest, crabbed way. He would have liked to cling to her and have her take him away; to hear nothing but her low, soothing voice, saying "There, little Hanno, be quiet, you need not say it."

"Well, my son, let us hear it," said the Senator, shortly. He had sat down in an easy-chair by the table and was waiting. He did not smile – he seldom did on such occasions. Very serious, with one eyebrow lifted, he measured little Hanno with cold and scrutinizing glance.

Hanno straightened up. He rubbed one hand over the piano's polished surface, gave a shy look at the company, and, somewhat emboldened by the gentle looks of Grandmamma and Aunt Tony, brought out, in a low, almost a hard voice: "'The Shepherd's Sunday Hymn,' by Uhland."

"Oh, my dear child, not like that," called out the Senator. "Don't stick there by the piano and cross your hands on your tummy like that! Stand up! Speak out! That's the first thing. Here, stand here between the curtains. Now, hold your head up – let your arms hang down quietly at your sides."

Hanno took up his position on the threshold of the living-room and let his arms hang down. Obediently he raised his head, but his eyes – the lashes drooped so low that they were invisible. They were probably already swimming in tears.

"'This is the day of our –'"

he began, very low. His father's voice sounded loud by contrast when he interrupted: "One begins with a bow, my son. And then, much louder. Begin again, please: 'Shepherd's Sunday Hymn' –"

It was cruel. The Senator was probably aware that he was robbing the child of the last remnant of his self-control. But the boy should not let himself be robbed. He should have more manliness by now. "'Shepherd's Sunday Hymn,'" he repeated encouragingly, remorselessly.

But it was all up with Hanno. His head sank on his breast, and the small, blue-veined right hand tugged spasmodically at the brocaded portière.

"'I stand alone on the vacant plain,'"

he said, but could get no further. The mood of the verse possessed him. An overmastering self-pity took away his voice, and the tears could not be kept back: they rolled out from beneath his lashes. Suddenly the thought came into his mind: if he were only ill, a little ill, as on those nights when he lay in bed with a slight fever and sore throat, and Ida came and gave him a drink, and put a compress on his head, and was kind – He put his head down on the arm with which he clung to the portière, and sobbed.

"Well," said the Senator, harshly, "there is no pleasure in that." He stood up, irritated. "What are you crying about? Though it is certainly a good enough reason for tears, that you haven't the courage to do anything, even for the sake of giving me a little pleasure! Are you a little girl? What will become of you if you go on like that? Will you always be drowning yourself in tears, every time you have to speak to people?"

"I never *will* speak to people, never!" thought Hanno in despair.

"Think it over till this afternoon," finished the Senator, and went into the dining-room. Ida Jungmann knelt by her fledgling and dried his eyes, and spoke to him, half consoling, half reproachful.

The Senator breakfasted hurriedly, and the Frau Consul, Tony, Clothilde, and Christian meanwhile took their leave. They were to dine with Gerda, as likewise were the Krögers, the Weinschenks, and the three Misses Buddenbrook from Broad Street, while the Senator, willy-nilly, must be present at the dinner in the Ratskeller. He hoped to leave in time to see his family again at his own house.

Sitting at the be-garlanded table, he drank his hot tea out of a saucer, hurriedly ate an egg, and on the steps took two or three puffs of a cigarette. Grobleben, wearing his woollen scarf in defiance of the July heat, with a boot over his left forearm and the polish-brush in his right, a long drop pendent from his nose, came from the garden into the front entry and accosted his master at the foot of the stairs, where the brown bear stood with his tray.

"Many happy returns, Herr Sen'ter, many happy – 'n' one is rich 'n' great, 'n' t'other's pore –"

"Yes, yes, Grobleben, you're right, that's just how it is!" And the Senator slipped a piece of money into the hand with the brush, and crossed the entry into the anteroom of the office. In the office the cashier came up to him, a tall man with honest, faithful eyes, to convey, in carefully selected phrases, the good wishes of the staff. The Senator thanked him in a few words, and went on to his place by the window. He had hardly opened his letters and glanced into the morning paper lying there ready for him, when a knock came on the door leading into the front entry, and the first visitors appeared with their congratulations.

It was a delegation of granary labourers, who came straddling in like bears, the corners of their mouths drawn down with befitting solemnity and their caps in their hands. Their spokesman spat tobacco-juice on the floor, pulled up his trousers, and talked in great excitement about "a hun'erd year" and "many more hun'erd year." The Senator proposed to them a considerable increase in their pay for the week, and dismissed them. The office staff of the revenue department came in a body to congratulate their chief. As they left, they met in the doorway a number of sailors, with two pilots at the head, from the "Wullenwewer" and the "Friederike Överdieck," the two ships belonging to the firm which happened at the time to be in port. Then there was a deputation of grain-porters, in black blouses, knee-breeches, and top-hats. And single citizens, too, were announced from time to time: Herr Stuht from Bell-Founders' Street came, with a black coat over his flannel shirt, and Iwersen the florist, and sundry other neighbours. There was an old postman, with watery eyes, ear-rings, and a white beard – an ancient oddity whom the Senator used to salute on the street and call him Herr Postmaster: he came, stood in the doorway, and cried out "Ah bain't come fer *that*, Herr Sen'ter! Ah knows as iverybody gits summat as comes here to-day, but ah bain't come fer that, an' so ah tells ye!" He received his piece of money with gratitude, none the less. There was simply no end to it. At half past ten the servant came from the house to announce that the Frau Senator was receiving guests in the salon.

Thomas Buddenbrook left his office and hurried upstairs. At the door of the salon he paused a moment for a glance into the mirror to order his cravat, and to refresh himself with a whiff of the eau-de-cologne on his handkerchief. His body was wet with perspiration, but his face was pale, his hands and feet cold. The reception in the office had nearly used him up already. He drew a long breath and entered the sunlit room, to be greeted at once by Consul Huneus, the lumber dealer and multi-millionaire, his wife, their daughter, and the latter's husband, Senator Dr. Gieseke. These had all driven in from Travemünde, like many others of the first families of the town, who were spending July in a cure which they interrupted only for the Buddenbrook jubilee.

They had not been sitting for three minutes in the elegant armchairs of the salon when Consul Överdieck, son of the deceased Burgomaster, and his wife, who was a Kistenmaker, were announced. When Consul Huneus made his adieux, his place was taken by his brother, who had a million less money than he, but made up for it by being a senator.

Now the ball was open. The tall white door, with the relief of the singing cupids above it, was scarcely closed for a moment; there was a constant view from within of the great staircase, upon which the light streamed down from the skylight far above, and of the stairs themselves, full of guests either entering or taking their leave. But the salon was spacious, the guests lingered in groups to talk, and the number of those who came was for some time far greater than the number of those who went away. Soon the maid-servant gave up opening and shutting the door that led into the salon and left it wide open, so that the guests stood in the corridor as well. There was the drone and buzz of conversation in masculine and feminine voices, there were handshakings, bows, jests, and loud, jolly laughter, which reverberated among the columns of the staircase and echoed from the great glass panes of the skylight. Senator Buddenbrook stood by turns at the top of the stairs and in the bow-window, receiving the congratulations, which were sometimes mere formal murmurs and sometimes loud and hearty expressions of good will. Burgomaster Dr. Langhals, a heavily built man of elegant appearance, with a shaven chin nestling in a white neck-cloth, short grey mutton-chops, and a languid diplomatic air, was received with general marks of respect. Consul Eduard Kistenmaker the wine-merchant, his wife, who was a Möllendorpf, and his brother and partner Stephan, Senator Buddenbrook's loyal friend and supporter, with his wife, the rudely healthy daughter of a landed proprietor, arrive and pay their respects. The widowed Frau Senator Möllendorpf sits throned in the centre of the sofa in the salon, while her children, Consul August Möllendorpf and his wife Julchen, born Hagenström, mingle with the crowd. Consul Hermann Hagenström supports his considerable weight on the balustrade, breathes heavily into his red beard, and talks with Senator Dr. Cremer, the Chief of Police, whose brown beard, mixed with grey, frames a smiling face expressive of a sort of gentle slyness. State Attorney Moritz Hagenström, smiling and showing his defective teeth, is there with his beautiful wife, the former Fräulein Puttfarken of Hamburg. Good old Dr. Grabow may be seen pressing Senator Buddenbrook's hand for a moment in both of his, to be displaced next moment by Contractor Voigt. Pastor Pringsheim, in secular garb, only betraying his dignity by the length of his frock coat, comes up the steps with outstretched arms and a beaming face. And Herr Friedrich Wilhelm Marcus is present, of course. Those gentlemen who come as delegates from any body such as the Senate, the Board of Trade, or the Assembly of Burgesses, appear in frock coats. It is half-past eleven. The heat is intense. The lady of the house withdrew a quarter of an hour ago.

Suddenly there is a hubbub below the vestibule door, a stamping and shuffling of feet, as of many people entering together; and a ringing, noisy voice echoes through the whole house. Everybody rushes to the landing, blocks up the doors to the salon, the dining-room, and the smoking-room, and peers down. Below is a group of fifteen or twenty men with musical instruments, headed by a gentleman in a brown wig, with a grey nautical beard and yellow artificial teeth, which he shows when he talks. What is happening? It is Consul Peter Döhlmann, of course: he is bringing the band from the theatre, and mounts the stairs in triumph, swinging a packet of programmes in his hand!

The serenade in honour of the hundredth anniversary of the firm of Johann Buddenbrook begins: in these impossible conditions, with the notes all running together, the chords drowning each other, the loud grunting and snarling of the big bass trumpet heard above everything else. It begins with " Now let us all thank God," goes over into the adaptation of Offenbach's " La Belle Hélène," and winds up with a *pot-pourri* of folk-songs — quite an extensive programme! And a pretty idea of Döhlmann's! They congratulate him on it; and nobody feels inclined to break up until the concert is finished. They stand or sit in the salon and the corridor; they listen and talk.

Thomas Buddenbrook stood with Stephan Kistenmaker, Senator Dr. Gieseke, and Contractor Voigt, beyond the staircase, near the open door of the smoking-room and the flight of stairs up to the second storey. He leaned against the wall, now and then contributing a word to the conversation, and for the rest looking out into space across the balustrade. It was hotter than ever, and more oppressive; but it would probably rain. To judge from the shadows that drove across the skylight there must be clouds in the sky. They were so many and moved so rapidly that the changeful, flickering light on the staircase came in time to hurt the eyes. Every other minute the brilliance of the gilt chandelier and the brass instruments below was quenched, to blaze out the next minute as before. Once the shadows lasted a little longer, and six or seven times something fell with a slight crackling sound upon the panes of the skylight — hail-stones, no doubt. Then the sunlight streamed down again.

There is a mood of depression in which everything that would ordinarily irritate us and call up a healthy reaction, merely weighs us down with a nameless, heavy burden of dull chagrin. Thus Thomas brooded over the break-down of little Johann, over the feelings which the whole celebration aroused in him, and still more over those which he would have liked to feel but could not. He sought again and again to pull himself together, to clear his countenance, to tell himself that this was a great day which was bound to heighten and exhilarate his mood. And indeed the noise which the band was making, the buzz of voices, the sight of all these people gathered in his honour, did shake his nerves; did, together with his memories of the past and of his father, give rise in him to a sort of weak emotionalism. But a sense of the ridiculous, of the disagreeable, hung over it all—the trumpery music, spoiled by the bad acoustics, the banal company chattering about dinners and the stock market—and this very mingling of emotion and disgust heightened his inward sense of exhaustion and despair.

At a quarter after twelve, when the musical program was drawing to a close, an incident occurred which in no wise interfered with the prevailing good feeling, but which obliged the master of the house to leave his guests for a short time. It was of a business nature. At a pause in the music the youngest apprentice in the firm appeared, coming up the great staircase, overcome with embarrassment at sight of so many people. He was a little, stunted fellow; and he drew his red face down as far as possible between his shoulders and swung one long, thin arm violently back and forth to show that he was perfectly at his ease. In the other hand he had a telegram. He mounted the steps, looking everywhere for his master, and when he had discovered him he passed with blushes and murmured excuses through the crowds that blocked his way.

His blushes were superfluous—nobody saw him. Without looking at him or breaking off their talk, they slightly made way, and they hardly noticed when he gave his telegram to the Senator, with a scrape, and the latter turned a little away from Kistenmaker, Voigt, and Gieseke to read it. Nearly all the telegrams that came to-day were messages of congratulation; still, during business hours, they had to be delivered at once.

The corridor made a bend at the point where the stairs mounted to the second storey, and then went on to the back stairs, where there was another, a side entrance into the dining-room. Opposite the stairs was the shaft of the dumb-waiter, and at this point there was a sizable table, where the maids usually polished the silver. The Senator paused here, turned his back to the apprentice, and opened the despatch.

Suddenly his eyes opened so wide that any one seeing him would have started in astonishment, and he gave a deep, gasping intake of breath which dried his throat and made him cough.

He tried to say " Very well," but his voice was inaudible in the clamour behind him. " Very well," he repeated; but the second word was only a whisper.

As his master did not move or turn round or make any sign, the hump-backed apprentice shifted from one foot to the other, then made his outlandish scrape again and went down the back stairs.

Senator Buddenbrook still stood at the table. His hands, holding the despatch, hung weakly down in front of him; he breathed in difficult, short breaths through his mouth; his body swayed back and forth, and he shook his head meaninglessly, as if stunned. " That little bit of hail," he said, " that little bit of hail." He repeated it stupidly. But gradually his breathing grew longer and quieter, the movement of his body less; his half-shut eyes clouded over with a weary, broken expression, and he turned around, slowly nodding his head, opened the door into the dining-room, and went in. With bent head he crossed the wide polished floor and sat down on one of the dark red sofas by the window. Here it was quiet and cool. The sound of the fountain came up from the garden, and a fly buzzed on the pane. There was only a dull murmur from the front of the house.

He laid his weary head on the cushion and closed his eyes. " That's good, that's good," he muttered, half aloud, drawing a deep breath of relief and satisfaction, " Oh, that *is* good! "

He lay five minutes thus, with limbs relaxed and a look of peace upon his face. Then he sat up, folded the telegram, put it in his breast pocket, and rose to rejoin his guests.

But in the same minute he sank back with a disgusted groan upon the sofa. The music – it was beginning again; an idiotic racket, meant to be a galop, with the drum and cymbals marking a rhythm in which the other instruments all joined either ahead of or behind time; a naïve, insistent, intolerable hullabaloo of snarling, crashing, and feebly piping noises, punctuated by the silly tootling of the piccolo.

CHAPTER VI

" OH, Bach, Sebastian Bach, dear lady! " cried Edmund Pfühl, Herr Edmund Pfühl, the organist of St. Mary's, as he strode up and down the salon with great activity, while Gerda, smiling, her head on her hand, sat at the piano; and Hanno listened from a big chair, his hands clasped round his knees. " Certainly, as you say, it was he through whom the victory was achieved by harmony over counterpoint. He invented modern harmony, assuredly. But how? Need I tell you how? By progressive development of the contrapuntal style – you know it as well as I do. Harmony? Ah, no! By no means. Counterpoint, my dear lady, counterpoint! Whither, I ask you, would experiments in harmony have led? While I have breath to speak, I will warn you against mere experiments in harmony! "

His zeal as he spoke was great, and he gave it free rein, for he felt at home in the house. Every Wednesday afternoon there appeared on the threshold his bulky, square, high-shouldered figure, in a coffee-coloured coat, whereof the skirts hung down over his knees. While awaiting his partner, he would open lovingly the Bechstein grand piano, arrange the violin parts on the stand, and then prelude a little, softly and artistically, with his head sunk, in high contentment, on one shoulder.

An astonishing growth of hair, a wilderness of tight little curls, red-brown mixed with grey, made his head look big and heavy, though it was poised easily upon a long neck with an extremely large Adam's apple that showed above his low collar. The straight, bunchy moustaches, of the same colour as the hair, were more prominent than the small snub nose. His eyes were brown and bright, with puffs of flesh beneath them; when he played they looked as though their gaze passed through whatever was in their way and rested on the other side. His face was not striking, but it had at least the stamp of a strong and lively intelligence. His eyelids were usually half drooped, and he had a way of relaxing his lower jaw without opening his mouth, which gave him a flabby, resigned expression like that sometimes seen on the face of a sleeping person.

The softness of his outward seeming, however, contrasted strongly with the actual strength and self-respect of his character. Edmund Pfühl was an organist of no small repute, whose reputation for contrapuntal learning was not confined within the walls of his native town. His little book on Church Music was recommended for private study in several conservatories, and his fugues and chorals were played now and then where an organ sounded to the glory of God. These compositions, as well as the voluntaries he played on Sundays at Saint Mary's, were flawless, impeccable, full of the relentless, severe logicality of the *Strenge Satz.* Such beauty as they had was not of this earth, and made no appeal to the ordinary layman's human feeling. What spoke in them, what gloriously triumphed in them, was a technique amounting to an ascetic religion, a technique elevated to a lofty sacrament, to an absolute end in itself. Edmund Pfühl had small use for the pleasant and the agreeable, and spoke of melody, it must be confessed, in slighting terms. But he was no dry pedant, notwithstanding. He would utter the name of Palestrina in the most dogmatic, awe-inspiring tone. But even while he made his instrument give out a succession of archaistic virtuosities, his face would be all aglow with feeling, with rapt enthusiasm, and his gaze would rest upon the distance as though he saw there the ultimate logicality of all events, issuing in reality. This was the musician's look; vague and vacant precisely because it abode in the kingdom of a purer, profounder, more absolute logic than that which shapes our verbal conceptions and thoughts.

His hands were large and soft, apparently boneless, and covered with freckles. His voice, when he greeted Gerda Buddenbrook, was low and hollow, as though a bite were stuck in his throat: "Good morning, honoured lady!"

He rose a little from his seat, bowed, and respectfully took the hand she offered, while with his own left he struck the fifths on the piano, so firmly and clear that she seized her Stradivarius and began to tune the strings with practised ear.

"The G minor concerto of Bach, Herr Pfühl. The whole adagio still goes badly, I think."

And the organist began to play. But hardly were the first chords struck, when it invariably happened that the corridor door would open gently, and without a sound little Johann would steal across the carpet to an easy-chair, where he would sit, his hands clasped round his knees, motionless, and listen to the music and the conversation.

"Well, Hanno, so you want a little taste of music, do you?"

said Gerda in a pause, and looked at her son with her shadowy eyes, in which the music had kindled a soft radiance.

Then he would stand up and put out his hand to Herr Pfühl with a silent bow, and Herr Pfühl would stroke with gentle affection the soft light-brown hair that hung gracefully about brow and temples.

"Listen, now my child," he would say, with mild impressiveness; and the boy would look at the Adam's apple that went up and down as the organist spoke, and then go back to his place with his quick, light steps, as though he could hardly wait for the music to begin again.

They played a movement of Haydn, some pages of Mozart, a sonata of Beethoven. Then, while Gerda was picking out some music, with her violin under her arm, a surprising thing happened: Herr Pfühl, Edmund Pfühl, organist at St. Mary's, glided over from his easy interlude into music of an extraordinary style; while a sort of shame-faced enjoyment showed upon his absent countenance. A burgeoning and blooming, a weaving and singing rose beneath his fingers; then, softly and dreamily at first, but ever clearer and clearer, there emerged in artistic counterpoint the ancestral, grandiose, magnificent march motif—a mounting to a climax, a complication, a transition; and at the resolution of the dominant the violin chimed in, fortissimo. It was the overture to *Die Meistersinger*.

Gerda Buddenbrook was an impassioned Wagnerite. But Herr Pfühl was an equally impassioned opponent—so much so that in the beginning she had despaired of winning him over.

On the day when she first laid some piano arrangements from *Tristan* on the music-rack, he played some twenty-five beats and then sprung up from the music-stool to stride up and down the room with disgust painted upon his face.

"I cannot play that, my dear lady! I am your most devoted servant—but I cannot. That is not music—believe me! I have always flattered myself I knew something about music—but this is chaos! This is demagogy, blasphemy, insanity, madness! It is a perfumed fog, shot through with lightning! It is the end of all honesty in art. I will not play it!" And with the words he had thrown himself again on the stool, and with his Adam's apple working furiously up and down, with coughs and sighs, had accomplished another twenty-five beats. But then he shut the piano and cried out:

"Oh, fie, fie! No, this is going too far. Forgive me, dear lady, if I speak frankly what I feel. You have honoured me for years, and paid me for my services; and I am a man of modest means. But I must lay down my office, I assure you, if you drive me to it by asking me to play these atrocities! Look, the child sits there listening – would you then utterly corrupt his soul? "

But let him gesture as furiously as he would, she brought him over – slowly, by easy stages, by persistent playing and persuasion.

" Pfühl," she would say, " be reasonable, take the thing calmly. You are put off by his original use of harmony. Beethoven seems to you so pure, clear, and natural, by contrast. But remember how Beethoven himself affronted his contemporaries, who were brought up in the old way. And Bach – why, good Heavens, you know how he was reproached for his want of melody and clearness! You talk about honesty – but what do you mean by honesty in art? Is it not the antithesis of hedonism? And, if so, then that is what you have here. Just as much as in Bach. I tell you, Pfühl, this music is less foreign to your inner self than you think! "

" It is all juggling and sophistry – begging your pardon," he grumbled. But she was right, after all: the music was not so impossible as he thought at first. He never, it is true, quite reconciled himself to *Tristan,* though he eventually carried out Gerda's wish and made a very clever arrangement of the Liebestod for violin and piano. He was first won over by certain parts of *Die Meistersinger;* and slowly a love for this new art began to stir within him. He would not confess it – he was himself aghast at the fact, and would pettishly deny it when the subject was mentioned. But after the old masters had had their due, Gerda no longer needed to urge him to respond to a more complex demand upon his virtuosity; with an expression of shame-faced pleasure, he would glide into the weaving harmonies of the *Leit-motiv.* After the music, however, there would be a long explanation of the relation of this style of music to that of the *Strenge Satz;* and one day Herr Pfühl admitted that, while not personally interested in the theme, he saw himself obliged to add a chapter to his book on Church Music, the subject of which would be the application of the old key-system to the church- and folk-music of Richard Wagner.

Hanno sat quite still, his small hands clasped round his knees, his mouth, as usual, a little twisted as his tongue felt out the hole in a back tooth. He watched his mother and Herr Pfühl with large quiet eyes; and thus, so early, he became aware of music as an extraordinarily serious, important, and profound thing in life. He understood only now and then what they were saying, and the music itself was mostly far above his childish understanding. Yet he came again, and sat absorbed for hours – a feat which surely faith, love, and reverence alone enabled him to perform.

When only seven, he began to repeat with one hand on the piano certain combinations of sound that made an impression on him. His mother watched him smiling, improved his chords, and showed him how certain tones would be necessary to carry one chord over into another. And his ear confirmed what she told him.

After Gerda Buddenbrook had watched her son a little, she decided that he must have piano lessons.

"I hardly think," she told Herr Pfühl, "that he is suited for solo work; and on the whole I am glad, for it has its bad side apart from the dependence of the soloist upon his accompanist, which can be very serious too; – if I did not have you, for instance! – there is always the danger of yielding to more or less complete virtuosity. You see, I know whereof I speak. I tell you frankly that, for the soloist, a high degree of ability is only the first step. The concentration on the tone and phrasing of the treble, which reduces the whole polyphony to something vague and indefinite in the consciousness, must surely spoil the feeling for harmony – unless the person is more than usually gifted – and the memory as well, which is most difficult to correct later on. I love my violin, and I have accomplished a good deal with it; but to tell the truth, I place the piano higher. What I mean is this: familiarity with the piano, as a means of summarizing the richest and most varied structures, as an incomparable instrument for musical reproduction, means for me a clearer, more intimate and comprehensive intercourse with music. Listen, Pfühl. I would like to have you take him, if you will be so good. I know there are two or three people here in the town who give lessons – women, I think. But they are simply piano-teachers. You know what I mean. I feel that it matters so little whether one is trained upon an instrument, and so much whether one knows something about music. I depend upon you. And you will see, you will succeed with him. He has the Buddenbrook hand. The Buddenbrooks can all strike the ninths and tenths – only they have never set any store by it," she concluded, laughing. And Herr Pfühl declared himself ready to undertake the lessons.

From now on, he came on Mondays as well as Wednesdays, and gave little Hanno lessons, while Gerda sat beside them. He went at it in an unusual way, for he felt that he owed more to his pupil's dumb and passionate zeal than merely to employ it in playing the piano a little. The first elementary difficulties were hardly got over when he began to theorize, in a simple way, with graphic illustrations, and to give his pupil the foundations of the theory of harmony. And Hanno understood. For it was all only a confirmation of what he had always known.

As far as possible, Herr Pfühl took into consideration the eager ambition of the child. He spent much thought upon the problem, how best to lighten the material load that weighed down the wings of his fancy. He did not demand too much finger dexterity or practice of scales. What he had in mind, and soon achieved, was a clear and lively grasp of the key system on Hanno's part, an inward, comprehensive understanding of its relationships, out of which would come, at no distant day, the quick eye for possible combinations, the intuitive mastery over the piano, which would lead to improvisation and composition. He appreciated with a touching delicacy of feeling the spiritual needs of this young pupil, who had already heard so much, and directed it toward the acquisition of a serious style. He would not disillusionize the deep solemnity of his mood by making him practise commonplaces. He gave him chorals to play, and pointed out the laws controlling the development of one chord into another.

Gerda, sitting with her embroidery or her book, just beyond the portières, followed the course of the lessons.

"You outstrip all my expectations," she told Herr Pfühl, later on. "But are you not going too fast? Aren't you getting too far ahead? Your method seems to me eminently creative – he has already begun to try to improvise a little. But if the method is beyond him, if he hasn't enough gift, he will learn absolutely nothing."

"He has enough gift," Herr Pfühl said, and nodded. "Sometimes I look into his eyes, and see so much lying there – but he holds his mouth tight shut. In later life, when his mouth will probably be shut even tighter, he must have some kind of outlet – a way of speaking – "

She looked at him – at this square-built musician with the red-brown hair, the pouches under the eyes, the bushy moustaches, and the inordinate Adam's apple – and then she put out her hand and said: "Thank you, Pfühl. You mean well by him. And who knows, yet, how much you are doing for him?"

Hanno's feeling for his teacher was one of boundless gratitude and devotion. At school he sat heavy and hopeless, unable, despite strenuous coaching, to understand his tables. But he grasped without effort all that Herr Pfühl told him, and made it his own – if he could make more his own that which he had already owned before. Edmund Pfühl, like a stout angel in a tail-coat, took him in his arms every Monday afternoon and transported him above all his daily misery, into the mild, sweet, grave, consoling kingdom of sound.

The lessons sometimes took place at Herr Pfühl's own house, a roomy old gabled dwelling full of cool passages and crannies, in which the organist lived alone with an elderly housekeeper. Sometimes, too, little Buddenbrook was allowed to sit up with the organist at the Sunday service in St. Mary's – which was quite a different matter from stopping below with the other people, in the nave. High above the congregation, high above Pastor Pringsheim in his pulpit, the two sat alone, in the midst of a mighty tempest of rolling sound, which at once set them free from the earth and dominated them by its own power; and Hanno was sometimes blissfully permitted to help his master control the stops.

When the choral was finished, Herr Pfühl would slowly lift his fingers from the keyboard, so that only the bass and the fundamental would still be heard, in lingering solemnity; and after a meaningful pause, the well-modulated voice of Pastor Pringsheim would rise up from under the sounding-board in the pulpit. Then it happened not infrequently that Herr Pfühl would, quite simply, begin to make fun of the preacher: his artificial enunciation, his long, exaggerated vowels, his sighs, his crude transitions from sanctity to gloom. Hanno would laugh too, softly but with heartfelt glee; for those two up there were both of the opinion – which neither of them expressed – that the sermon was silly twaddle, and that the real service consisted in that which the Pastor and his congregation regarded merely as a devotional accessory: namely, the music.

Herr Pfühl, in fact, had a constant grievance in the small understanding there was for his accomplishments down there among the Senators, Consuls, citizens, and their families. And thus, he liked to have his small pupil by him, to whom he could point out the extraordinary difficulties of the passages he had just played. He performed marvels of technique. He had composed a melody which was just the same read forward or backward, and based upon it a fugue which was to be played "crab-fashion." But after performing this wonder: "Nobody knows the difference," he said, and folded his hands in his lap with a dreary look, shaking his head hopelessly. While Pastor Pringsheim was delivering his sermon, he whispered to Hanno: "That was a crab-fashion imitation, Johann. You don't know what that is yet. It is the imitation of a theme composed backward instead of forward – a very, very difficult thing. Later on, I will show you what an imitation in the *Strenge Satz* involves. As for the ' crab,' I would never ask you to try that. It isn't necessary. But do not believe those who tell you that such things are trifles, without any musical value. You will find the crab in musicians of all ages. But exercises like that are the scorn of the mediocre and the superficial musician. Humility, Hanno, *humility* – is the feeling one should have. Don't forget it."

On his eighth birthday, April 15th, 1869, Hanno played before the assembled family a fantasy of his own composition. It was a simple affair, a motif entirely of his own invention, which he had slightly developed. When he showed it to Herr Pfühl, the organist, of course, had some criticism to make.

" What sort of theatrical ending is that, Johann? It doesn't go with the rest of it. In the beginning it is all pretty good; but why do you suddenly fall from B major into the six-four chord on the fourth note with a minor third? These are tricks; and you tremolo here, too – where did you pick that up? I know, of course: you have been listening when I played certain things for your mother. Change the end, child: then it will be quite a clean little piece of work."

But it appeared that Hanno laid the greatest stress precisely on this minor chord and this finale; and his mother was so very pleased with it that it remained as it was. She took her violin and played the upper part, and varied it with runs in demi-semi-quavers. That sounded gorgeous: Hanno kissed her out of sheer happiness, and they played it together to the family on the 15th of April.

The Frau Consul, Frau Permaneder, Christian, Clothilde, Herr and Frau Consul Kröger, Herr and Frau Director Weinschenk, the Broad Street Buddenbrooks, and Therese Weichbrodt were all bidden to dinner at four o'clock, with the Senator and his wife, in honour of Hanno's birthday; and now they sat in the salon and looked at the child, perched on the music-stool in his sailor suit, and at the elegant, foreign appearance his mother made as she played a wonderful cantilena on the G string, and then, with profound virtuosity, developed a stream of purling, foaming cadences. The silver on the end of her bow gleamed in the gaslight.

Hanno was pale with excitement, and had hardly eaten any dinner. But now he forgot all else in his absorbed devotion to his task, which would, alas, be all over in ten minutes! The little melody he had invented was more harmonic than rhythmic in its structure; there was an extraordinary contrast between the simple primitive material which the child had at his command, and the impressive, impassioned, almost over-refined method with which that material was employed. He brought out each leading note with a forward inclination of the little head; he sat far forward on the music-stool, and strove by the use of both pedals to give each new harmony an emotional value. In truth, when Hanno concentrated upon an effect, the result was likely to be emotional rather than merely sentimental. He gave every simple harmonic device a special and mysterious significance by means of retardation and accentuation; his surprising skill in effects was displayed in each chord, each new harmony, by a suddenly introduced pianissimo. And he sat with lifted eyebrows, swaying back and forth with the whole upper part of his body. Then came the finale, Hanno's beloved finale, which crowned the elevated simplicity of the whole piece. Soft and clear as a bell sounded the E minor chord, tremolo pianissimo, amid the purling, flowing notes of the violin. It swelled, it broadened, it slowly, slowly rose: suddenly, in the forte, he introduced the discord C sharp, which led back to the original key, and the Stradivarius ornamented it with its welling and singing. He dwelt on the dissonance until it became fortissimo. But he denied himself and his audience the resolution; he kept it back. What would it be, this resolution, this enchanting, satisfying absorption into the B major chord? A joy beyond compare, a gratification of overpowering sweetness! Peace! Bliss! The kingdom of Heaven: only not yet—not yet! A moment more of striving, hesitation, suspense, that must become well-nigh intolerable in order to heighten the ultimate moment of joy.—Once more—a last, a final tasting of this striving and yearning, this craving of the entire being, this last forcing of the will to deny oneself the fulfilment and the conclusion, in the knowledge that joy, when it comes, lasts only for the moment. The whole upper part of Hanno's little body straightened, his eyes grew larger, his closed lips trembled, he breathed short, spasmodic breaths through his nose. At last, at last, joy would no longer be denied. It came, it poured over him; he resisted no more. His muscles relaxed, his head sank weakly on his shoulder, his eyes closed, and a pathetic, almost an anguished smile of speechless rapture hovered about his mouth; while his tremolo, among the rippling and rustling runs from the violin, to which he now added runs in the bass, glided over into B major, swelled up suddenly into forte, and after one brief, resounding burst, broke off.

It was impossible that all the effect which this had upon Hanno should pass over into his audience. Frau Permaneder, for instance, had not the slightest idea what it was all about. But she had seen the child's smile, the rhythm of his body, the beloved little head swaying enraptured from side to side – and the sight had penetrated to the depths of her easily moved nature.

"How the child can play! Oh, how he can play!" she cried, hurrying to him half-weeping and folding him in her arms. "Gerda, Tom, he will be a Meyerbeer, a Mozart, a –" As no third name of equal significance occurred to her, she confined herself to showering kisses on her nephew, who sat there, still quite exhausted, with an absent look in his eyes.

"That's enough, Tony," the Senator said softly. "Please don't put such ideas into the child's head."

CHAPTER VII

THOMAS BUDDENBROOK was, in his heart, far from pleased with the development of little Johann.

Long ago he had led Gerda Arnoldsen to the altar, and all the Philistines had shaken their heads. He had felt strong and bold enough then to display a distinguished taste without harming his position as a citizen. But now, the long-awaited heir, who showed so many physical traits of the paternal inheritance – did he, after all, belong entirely to the mother's side? He had hoped that one day his son would take up the work of the father's lifetime in his stronger, more fortunate hands, and carry it forward. But now it almost seemed that the son was hostile, not only to the surroundings and the life in which his lot was cast, but even to his father as well.

Gerda's violin-playing had always added to her strange eyes, which he loved, to her heavy, dark-red hair and her whole exotic appearance, one charm the more. But now that he saw how her passion for music, strange to his own nature, utterly, even at this early age, possessed the child, he felt in it a hostile force that came between him and his son, of whom his hopes would make a Buddenbrook – a strong and practical-minded man, with definite impulses after power and conquest. In his present irritable state it seemed to him that this hostile force was making him a stranger in his own house.

He could not, himself, approach any nearer to the music practised by Gerda and her friend Herr Pfühl; Gerda herself, exclusive and impatient where her art was concerned, made it cruelly hard for him.

Never had he dreamed that music was so essentially foreign to his family as now it seemed. His grandfather had enjoyed playing the flute, and he himself always listened with pleasure to melodies that possessed a graceful charm, a lively swing, or a tender melancholy. But if he happened to express his liking for any such composition, Gerda would be sure to shrug her shoulders and say with a pitying smile, "How can you, my friend? A thing like that, without any musical value whatever!"

He hated this "musical value." It was a phrase which had no meaning for him save a certain chilling arrogance. It drove him on, in Hanno's presence, to self-assertion. More than once he remonstrated angrily, "This constant harping on musical values, my dear, strikes me as rather tasteless and opinionated." To which she rejoined: "Thomas, once for all, you will never understand anything about music as an art, and, intelligent as you are, you will never see that it is more than an after-dinner pleasure and a feast for the ears. In every other field you have a perception of the banal – in music not. But it is the test of musical comprehension. What pleases you in music? A sort of insipid optimism, which, if you met with it in literature, would make you throw down the book with an angry or sarcastic comment. Easy gratification of each unformed wish, prompt satisfaction before the will is even roused – that is what pretty music is like – and it is like nothing else in the world. It is mere flabby idealism."

He understood her; that is, he understood what she said. But he could not follow her: could not comprehend why melodies which touched or stirred him were cheap and worthless, while compositions which left him cold and bewildered possessed the highest musical value. He stood before a temple from whose threshold Gerda sternly waved him back – and he watched while she and the child vanished within.

He betrayed none of his grief over this estrangement, though the gulf seemed to widen between him and his little son. The idea of suing for his child's favour seemed frightful to him. During the day he had small time to spare; at meals he treated him with a friendly cordiality that had at times a tonic severity. "Well, comrade," he would say, giving him a tap or two on the back of the head and seating himself opposite his wife, "well, and how are you? Studying? And playing the piano, eh? Good! But not too much piano, else you won't want to do your task, and then you won't go up at Easter." Not a muscle betrayed the anxious suspence with which he waited to see how Hanno took his greeting and what his reply would be. Nothing revealed his painful inward shrinking when the child merely gave him a shy glance of the gold-brown, shadowy eyes – a glance that did not even reach his father's face – and bent again over his plate.

It was monstrous for him to brood over this childish awkwardness. It was his fatherly duty to occupy himself a little with the child: so, while the plates were changed, he would examine him and try to stimulate his sense for facts. How many inhabitants were there in the town? What streets led from the Trave to the upper town? What were the names of the granaries that belonged to the firm? Out with it, now; speak up! But Hanno was silent. Not with any idea of wounding or annoying his father! But these inhabitants, these streets and granaries, which were normally a matter of complete indifference to him, became positively hateful when they were made the subject of an examination. However lively he was beforehand, however gaily he had laughed and talked with his father, his mood would go down to zero at the first symptom of an examination, and his resistance would collapse entirely. His eyes would cloud over, his mouth take on a despondent droop, and he would be possessed by a feeling of profound regret at the thoughtlessness of Papa, who surely knew that such tests came to nothing and only spoiled the whole meal for everybody! With eyes swimming in tears he looked down at his plate. Ida would nudge him and whisper to him: the streets, the granaries. Oh, that was all useless, perfectly useless. She did not understand. He did know the names – at least some of them. It would have been easy to do what Papa asked – if only he were not possessed and prevented by an overpowering sadness! A severe word from his father and a tap with the fork against the knife rest brought him to himself with a start. He cast a glance at his mother and Ida and tried to speak. But the first syllables were already drowned in sobs. "That's enough," shouted the Senator, angrily. "Keep still – you needn't tell me! You can sit there dumb and silly all the rest of your life!" And the meal would be finished in uncomfortable silence.

When the Senator felt troubled about Hanno's passionate preoccupation with his music, it was this dreaminess, this weeping, this total lack of freshness and energy, that he fixed upon.

All his life the boy had been delicate. His teeth had been particularly bad, and had been the cause of many painful illnesses and difficulties. It had nearly cost him his life to cut his first set; the gums showed a constant tendency to inflammation, and there were abscesses, which Mamsell Jungmann used to open with a needle at the proper time. Now his second teeth were beginning to come in, and the suffering was even greater. He had almost more pain than he could bear, and he spent many sleepless, feverish nights. His teeth, when they came, were as white and beautiful as his mother's; but they were soft and brittle, and crowded each other out of shape when they came in; so that little Hanno was obliged, for the correction of all these evils, to make the acquaintance early in life of a very dreadful man – no less than Herr Brecht, the dentist, in Mill Street.

Even this man's name was significant: it suggested the frightful sensation in Hanno's jaw when the roots of a tooth were pulled, lifted, and wrenched out; the sound of it made Hanno's heart contract, just as it did when he cowered in an easy-chair in Herr Brecht's waiting-room, with the faithful Jungmann sitting opposite, and looked at the pictures in a magazine, while he breathed in the sharp-smelling air of the room and waited for the dentist to open the door of the operating-room, with his polite and horrible " Won't you come in, please? "

This operating-room possessed one strange attraction, a gorgeous parrot with venomous little eyes, which sat in a brass cage in the corner and was called, for unknown reasons, Josephus. He used to say " Sit down; one moment, please," in a voice like an old fish-wife's; and though the hideous circumstances made this sound like mockery, yet Hanno felt for the bird a curious mixture of fear and affection. Imagine – a parrot, a big, bright-coloured bird, that could talk and was called Josephus! He was like something out of an enchanted forest; like Grimm's fairy tales, which Ida read aloud to him. And when Herr Brecht opened the door, his invitation was repeated by Josephus in such a way that somehow Hanno was laughing when he went into the operating-room and sat down in the queer big chair by the window, next the treadle machine.

Herr Brecht looked a good deal like Josephus. His nose was of the same shape, above his grizzled moustaches. The bad thing about him was that he was nervous, and dreaded the tortures he was obliged to inflict. " We must proceed to extraction, Fräulein," he would say, growing pale. Hanno himself was in a pale cold sweat, with staring eyes, incapable of protesting or running away; in short, in much the same condition as a condemned criminal. He saw Herr Brecht, with the forceps in his sleeve, bend over him, and noticed that little beads were standing out on his bald brow, and that his mouth was twisted. When it was all over, and Hanno, pale and trembling, spat blood into the blue basin at his side, Herr Brecht too had to sit down, and wipe his forehead and take a drink of water.

They assured little Johann that this man would do him good and save him suffering in the end. But when Hanno weighed his present pains against the positive good that had accrued from them, he felt that the former far outweighed the latter; and he regarded these visits to Mill Street as so much unnecessary torture. They removed four beautiful white molars which had just come in, to make room for the wisdom teeth expected later: this required four weeks of visits, in order not to subject the boy to too great a strain. It was a fearful time! – a long drawn-out martyrdom, in which dread of the next visit began before the last one, with its attendant exhaustion, was fairly over. When the last tooth was drawn, Hanno was quite worn out, and was ill in bed for a week.

This trouble with his teeth affected not only his spirits but also the functioning of all his other organs. What he could not chew he did not digest, and there came attacks of gastric fever, accompanied by fitful heart action, according as the heart was either weakened or too strongly stimulated. And there were spells of giddiness, while the *pavor nocturnus*, that strange affliction beloved of Dr. Grabow, continued unabated. Hardly a night passed that little Johann did not start up in bed, wringing his hands with every mark of unbearable anguish, and crying out piteously for help, as though some one were trying to choke him or some other awful thing were happening. In the morning he had forgotten it all. Dr. Grabow's treatment consisted of giving fruit-juice before the child went to bed; which had absolutely no effect.

The physical arrests and the pains which Hanno suffered made him old for his age; he was what is called precocious; and though this was not very obvious, being restrained in him, as it were, by his own unconscious good taste, still it expressed itself at times in the form of a melancholy superiority. "How are you, Hanno?" somebody would ask: his grandmother or one of the Broad Street Buddenbrooks. A little resigned curl of the lip, or a shrug of the shoulders in their blue sailor suit, would be the only answer.

"Do you like to go to school?"

"No," answered Hanno, with quiet candour – he did not consider it worth while to try to tell a lie in such cases.

"No? But one has to learn writing, reading, arithmetic –"

"And so on," said little Johann.

No, he did not like going to school – the old monastic school with its cloisters and vaulted classrooms. He was hampered by his illnesses, and often absent-minded, for his thoughts would linger among his harmonic combinations, or upon the still unravelled marvel of some piece which he had heard his mother and Herr Pfühl playing; and all this did not help him on in the sciences. These lower classes were taught by assistant masters and seminarists, for whom he entertained mingled feelings: a dread of possible future punishments and a secret contempt for their social inferiority, their spiritual limitations, and their physical unkemptness. Herr Tietge, a little grey man in a greasy black coat, who had taught in the school even in the time of the deceased Marcellus Stengel; who squinted abominably and sought to remedy this defect by wearing glasses as thick and round as a ship's port-holes — Herr Tietge told little Johann how quick and industrious his father had been at figures. Herr Tietge had severe fits of coughing, and spat all over the floor of his platform.

Hanno had, among his schoolmates, no intimates save one. But this single bond was very close, even from his earliest school days. His friend was a child of aristocratic birth but neglected appearance, a certain Count Mölln, whose first name was Kai.

Kai was a lad of about Hanno's height, dressed not in a sailor suit, but in shabby clothes of uncertain colour, with here and there a button missing, and a great patch in the seat. His arms were too long for the sleeves of his coat, and his hands seemed impregnated with dust and earth to a permanent grey colour; but they were unusually narrow and elegant, with long fingers and tapering nails. His head was to match: neglected, uncombed, and none too clean, but endowed by nature with all the marks of pure and noble birth. The carelessly parted hair, reddish-blond in colour, waved back from a white brow, and a pair of light blue eyes gleamed bright and keen from beneath. The cheek bones were slightly prominent: while the nose, with its delicate nostrils and slightly aquiline curve, and the mouth, with its short upper lip, were already quite unmistakable and characteristic.

Hanno Buddenbrook had seen the little count once or twice, even before they met at school, when he took his walks with Ida northward from the Castle Gate. Some distance outside the town, nearly as far as the first outlying village, lay a small farm, a tiny, almost valueless property without even a name. The passer-by got the impression of a dunghill, a quantity of chickens, a dog-hut, and a wretched, kennel-like building with a sloping red roof. This was the manor-house, and therein dwelt Kai's father, Count Eberhard Mölln.

He was an eccentric, hardly ever seen by anybody, busy on his dunghill with his dogs, his chickens, and his vegetable-patch: a large man in top-boots, with a green frieze jacket. He had a bald head and a huge grey beard like the tail of a turnip; he carried a riding-whip in his hand, though he had no horse to his name, and wore a monocle stuck into his eye under the bushy eyebrow. Except him and his son, there was no Count Mölln in all the length and breadth of the land any more: the various branches of a once rich, proud, and powerful family had gradually withered off, until now there was only an aunt, with whom Kai's father was not on terms. She wrote romances for the family story-papers, under a dashing pseudonym. The story was told of Count Eberhard that when he first withdrew to his little farm, he devised a means of protecting himself from the importunities of peddlers, beggars, and busy-bodies. He put up a sign which read: " Here lives Count Mölln. He wants nothing, buys nothing, and gives nothing away." When the sign had served its purpose, he removed it.

Motherless – for the Countess had died when her child was born, and the housework was done by an elderly female – little Kai grew up like a wild animal, among the dogs and chickens; and here Hanno Buddenbrook had looked at him shyly from a distance, as he leaped like a rabbit among the cabbages, romped with the dogs, and frightened the fowls by turning somersaults.

They met again in the schoolroom, where Hanno probably felt again his first alarm at the little Count's unkempt exterior. But not for long. A sure instinct had led him to pay no heed to the outward negligence; had shown him instead the white brow, the delicate mouth, the finely shaped blue eyes, which looked with a sort of resentful hostility into his own; and Hanno felt sympathy for this one alone among all his fellows. But he would never, by himself, have taken the first steps; he was too timid for that. Without the ruthless impetuosity of little Kai they might have remained strangers, after all. The passionate rapidity of his approach even frightened Hanno, at first. The neglected little count sued for the favour of the quiet, elegantly dressed Hanno with a fiery, aggressive masculinity impossible to resist. Kai could not, it is true, help Hanno with his lessons. His untamed spirits were as hostile to the " tables " as was little Buddenbrook's dreamy abstractedness. But he gave him everything he had: glass bullets, wooden tops, even a broken lead pistol which was his dearest treasure. During the recess he told him about his home and the puppies and chickens, and walked with him at midday as far as he dared, though Ida Jungmann, with a packet of sandwiches, was always waiting for her fledgling at the school gate. It was from Ida that Kai heard little Buddenbrook's nickname; he took it up, and never called him henceforth by anything else.

One day he demanded that Hanno, instead of going to the Millwall, should take a walk with him to his father's house to see the baby guinea-pigs. Fräulein Jungmann finally yielded to the teasing of the two children. They strolled out to the noble domain, viewed the dunghill, the vegetables, the fowls, dogs, and guinea-pigs, and even went into the house, where in a long low room on the ground floor, Count Eberhard sat in defiant isolation, reading at a clumsy table. He asked crossly what they wanted.

Ida Jungmann could not be brought to repeat the visit. She insisted that, if the two children wished to be together, Kai could visit Hanno instead. So for the first time, with honest admiration, but no trace of shyness, Kai entered Hanno's beautiful home. After that he went often. Soon nothing but the deep winter snows prevented him from making the long way back again for the sake of a few hours with his friend.

They sat in the large play-room in the second storey and did their lessons together. There were long sums that covered both sides of the slate with additions, subtractions, multiplications, and divisions, and had to come out to zero in the end; otherwise there was a mistake, and they must hunt and hunt till they had found the little beast and exterminated him. Then they had to study grammar, and learn the rules of comparison, and write down very neat, tidy examples underneath. Thus: " Horn is transparent, glass is more transparent, light is most transparent." They took their exercise-books and conned sentences like the following: " I received a letter, saying that he felt aggrieved because he believed that you had deceived him." The fell intent of this sentence, so full of pitfalls, was that you should write *ei* where you ought to write *ie*, and contrariwise. They had, in fact, done that very thing, and now it must be corrected. But when all was finished they might put their books aside and sit on the window-ledge while Ida read to them.

The good soul read about Cinderella, about the prince who could not shiver and shake, about Rumpelstiltskin, about Rapunzel and the Frog Prince – in her deep, patient voice, her eyes half-shut, for she knew the stories by heart, she had read them so often. She wet her finger and turned the page automatically.

But after a while Kai, who possessed the constant craving to do something himself, to have some effect on his surroundings, would close the book and begin to tell stories himself. It was a good idea, for they knew all the printed ones, and Ida needed a rest sometimes, too. Kai's stories were short and simple at first, but they expanded and grew bolder and more complicated with time. The interesting thing about them was that they never stood quite in the air, but were based upon a reality which he presented in a new and mysterious light. Hanno particularly liked the one about the wicked enchanter who tortured all human beings by his malignant art; who had captured a beautiful prince named Josephus and turned him into a green-and-red parrot, which he kept in a gilded cage. But in a far distant land the chosen hero was growing up, who should one day fearlessly advance at the head of an invincible army of dogs, chickens, and guinea-pigs and slay the base enchanter with a single sword-thrust, and deliver all the world – in particular, Hanno Buddenbrook – from his clutches. Then Josephus would be restored to his proper form and return to his kingdom, in which Kai and Hanno would be appointed to high offices.

Senator Buddenbrook saw the two friends together now and then, as he passed the door of the play-room. He had nothing against the intimacy, for it was clear that the two lads did each other good. Hanno gentled, tamed, and ennobled Kai, who loved him tenderly, admired his white hands, and, for his sake, let Ida Jungmann wash his own with soap and a nail-brush. And if Hanno could absorb some of his friend's wild energy and spirits, it would be welcome, for the Senator realized keenly the constant feminine influence that surrounded the boy, and knew that it was not the best means for developing his manly qualities.

The faithful devotion of the good Ida could not be repaid with gold. She had been in the family now for more than thirty years. She had cared for the previous generations with self-abnegation; but Hanno she carried in her arms, lapped him in tender care, and loved him to idolatry. She had a naïve, unshakable belief in his privileged station in life, which sometimes went to the length of absurdity. In whatever touched him she showed a surprising, even an unpleasant effrontery. Suppose, for instance, she took him with her to buy cakes at the pastry-shop: she would poke among the sweets on the counter and select a piece for Hanno, which she would coolly hand him without paying for it – the man should feel himself honoured, indeed! And before a crowded show-window she would ask the people in front, in her west-Prussian dialect, pleasantly enough, but with decision, to make a place for her charge. He was so uncommon in her eyes that she felt there was hardly another child in the world worthy to touch him. In little Kai's case, the mutual preference of the two children had been too strong for her. Possibly she was a little taken by his name, too. But if other children came up to them on the Mill-wall, as she sat with Hanno on a bench, Fräulein Jungmann would get up almost at once, make some excuse or other – it was late, or there was a draught – and take her charge away. The pretexts she gave to little Johann would have led him to believe that all his contemporaries were either scrofulous or full of " evil humours," and that he himself was a solitary exception; which did not tend to increase his already deficient confidence and ease of manner.

Senator Buddenbrook did not know all the details; but he saw enough to convince him that his son's development was not taking the desired course. If he could only take his upbringing in his own hands, and mould his spirit by daily and hourly contact! But he had not the time. He perceived the lamentable failure of his occasional efforts: he knew they only strained the relations between father and son. In his mind was a picture which he longed to reproduce: it was a picture of Hanno's great-grandfather, whom he himself had known as a boy: a clear-sighted man, jovial, simple, sturdy, humorous – why could not little Johann grow up like that? If only he could suppress or forbid the music, which was surely not good for the lad's physical development, absorbed his powers, and took his mind from the practical affairs of life! That dreamy nature – did it not almost, at times, border on irresponsibility?

One day, some three quarters of an hour before dinner, Hanno had gone down alone to the first storey. He had practised for a long time on the piano, and now was idling about in the living-room. He half lay, half sat, on the chaise-longue, tying and untying his sailor's knot, and his eyes, roving aimlessly about, caught sight of an open portfolio on his mother's nut-wood writing-table. It was the leather case with the family papers. He rested his elbow on the sofa-cushion, and his chin in his hand, and looked at the things for a while from a distance. Papa must have had them out after second breakfast, and left them there because he was not finished with them. Some of the papers were sticking in the portfolio, some loose sheets lying outside were weighted with a metal ruler, and the large gilt-edged notebook with the motley paper lay there open.

Hanno slipped idly down from the sofa and went to the writing-table. The book was open at the Buddenbrook family tree, set forth in the hand of his various forbears, including his father; complete, with rubrics, parentheses, and plainly marked dates. Kneeling with one knee on the desk-chair, leaning his head with its soft waves of brown hair on the palm of his hand, Hanno looked at the manuscript sidewise, carelessly critical, a little contemptuous, and supremely indifferent, letting his free hand toy with Mamma's gold-and-ebony pen. His eyes roved all over these names, masculine and feminine, some of them in queer old-fashioned writing with great flourishes, written in faded yellow or thick black ink, to which little grains of sand were sticking. At the very bottom, in Papa's small, neat handwriting that ran so fast over the page, he read his own name, under that of his parents: Justus, Johann, Kasper, born April 15, 1861. He liked looking at it. He straightened up a little, and took the ruler and pen, still rather idly; let his eye travel once more over the whole genealogical host; then, with absent care, mechanically and dreamily, he made with the gold pen a beautiful, clean double line diagonally across the entire page, the upper one heavier than the lower, just as he had been taught to embellish the page of his arithmetic book. He looked at his work with his head on one side, and then moved away.

After dinner the Senator called him up and surveyed him with his eyebrows drawn together.

"What is this? Where did it come from? Did you do it?"

Hanno had to think a minute, whether he really had done it; and then he answered "Yes."

"What for? What is the matter with you? Answer me! What possessed you, to do such a mischievous thing?" cried the Senator, and struck Hanno's cheek lightly with the rolled-up notebook.

And little Johann stammered, retreating, with his hand to his cheek, "I thought – I thought – there was nothing else coming."

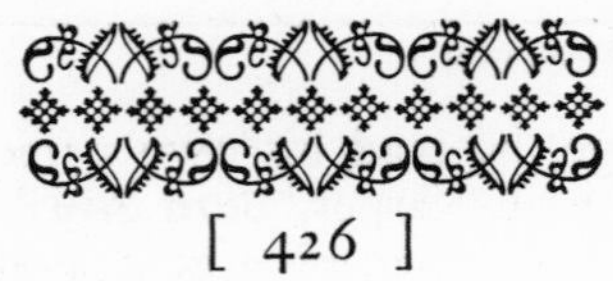

CHAPTER VIII

Nowadays, when the family gathered at table on Thursdays, under the calmly smiling gaze of the immortals on the walls, they had a new and serious theme. It called out on the faces of the female Buddenbrooks, at least the Broad Street ones, an expression of cold restraint. But it highly excited Frau Permaneder, as her manner and gestures betrayed. She tossed back her head, stretched out her arms before her, or flung them above her head as she talked; and her voice showed by turns anger and dismay, passionate opposition and deep feeling. She would pass over from the particular to the general, and talk in her throaty voice about wicked people, interrupting herself with the little cough that was due to poor digestion. Or she would utter little trumpetings of disgust: Teary Trietschke, Grünlich, Permaneder! A new name had now been added to these, and she pronounced it in a tone of indescribable scorn and hatred: " The District Attorney! "

But when Director Hugo Weinschenk entered – late, as usual, for he was overwhelmed with work; balancing his two fists and weaving about more than ever at the waist of his frock-coat – and sat down at table, his lower lip hanging down with its impudent expression under his moustaches, then the conversation would come to a full stop, and heavy silence would brood over the table until the Senator came to the rescue by asking the Director how his affair was going on – as if it were an ordinary business dealing.

Hugo Weinschenk would answer that things were going very well, very well indeed, they could not go otherwise; and then he would blithely change the subject. He was much more sprightly than he used to be; there was a certain lack of restraint in his roving eye, and he would ask ever so many times about Gerda Buddenbrook's fiddle without getting any reply. He talked freely and gaily – only it was a pity his flow of spirits prevented him from guarding his tongue; for he now and then told anecdotes which were not at all suited to the company. One, in particular, was about a wet-nurse who prejudiced the health of her charge by the fact that she suffered from flatulence. Too late, or not at all, he remarked that his wife was flushing rosy red, that Thomas, the Frau Consul and Gerda were sitting like statues, and the Misses Buddenbrook exchanging glances that were fairly boring holes in each other. Even Riekchen Severin was looking insulted at the bottom of the table, and old Consul Kröger was the single one of the company who gave even a subdued snort.

What was the trouble with Director Weinschenk? This industrious, solid citizen with the rough exterior and no social graces, who devoted himself with an obstinate sense of duty to his work alone – this man was supposed to have been guilty, not once but repeatedly, of a serious fault: he was accused of, he had been indicted for, performing a business manœuvre which was not only questionable, but directly dishonest and criminal. There would be a trial, the outcome of which was not easy to guess. What was he accused of? It was this: certain fires of considerable extent had taken place in different localities, which would have cost his company large sums of money. Director Weinschenk was accused of having received private information of such accidents through his agents, and then, in wrongful possession of this information, of having transferred the back insurance to another firm, thus saving his own the loss. The matter was now in the hands of the State Attorney, Dr. Moritz Hagenström.

"Thomas," said the Frau Consul in private to her son, "please explain it to me. I do not understand. What do you make of the affair?"

"Why, my dear Mother," he answered, "what is there to say? It does not look as though things were quite as they should be – unfortunately. It seems unlikely to me that Weinschenk is as guilty as people think. In the modern style of doing business, there is a thing they call usance. And usance – well, imagine a sort of manœuvre, not exactly open and above-board, something that looks dishonest to the man in the street, yet perhaps quite customary and taken for granted in the business world: that is usance. The boundary line between usance and actual dishonesty is extremely hard to draw. Well – if Weinschenk has done anything he shouldn't, he has probably done no more than a good many of his colleagues who will not get caught. But – I don't see much chance of his being cleared. Perhaps in a larger city he might be, but here everything depends on cliques and personal motives. He should have borne that in mind in selecting his lawyer. It is true that we have no really eminent lawyer in the whole town, nobody with superior oratorical talent, who knows all the ropes and is versed in dubious transactions. All our jurists hang together; they have family connections, in many cases; they eat together; they work together, and they are accustomed to considering each other. In my opinion, it would have been clever to take a town lawyer. But what did Weinschenk do? He thought it necessary – and this in itself makes his innocence look doubtful – to get a lawyer from Berlin, a Dr. Breslauer, who is a regular rake, an accomplished orator and up to all the tricks of the trade. He has the reputation of having got so-and-so many dishonest bankrupts off scot-free. He will conduct this affair with the same cleverness – for a consideration. But will it do any good? I can see already that our town lawyers will band together to fight him tooth and nail, and that Dr. Hagenström's hearers will already be prepossessed in his favour. As for the witnesses: well, Weinschenk's own staff won't be any too friendly to him, I'm afraid. What we indulgently call his rough exterior – he would call it that, himself, too – has not made him many friends. In short, Mother, I am looking forward to trouble. It will be a pity for Erica, if it turns out badly; but I feel most for Tony. You see, she is quite right in saying that Hagenström is glad of the chance. The thing concerns all of us, and the disgrace will fall on us too; for Weinschenk belongs to the family and eats at our table. As far as I am concerned, I can manage. I know what I have to do: in public, I shall act as if I had nothing whatever to do with the affair. I will not go to the trial – although I am sorry not to, for Breslauer is sure to be interesting. And in general I must behave with complete indifference, to protect myself from the imputation of wanting to use my influence. But Tony? I don't like to think what a sad business a conviction will be for her. She protests vehemently against envious intrigues and calumniators and all that; but what really moves her is her anxiety lest, after all her other troubles, she may see her daughter's honourable position lost as well. It is the last blow. She will protest her belief in Weinschenk's innocence the more loudly the more she is forced to doubt it. Well, he may be innocent, after all. We can only wait and see, Mother, and be very tactful with him and Tony and Erica. But I'm afraid – "

It was under these circumstances that the Christmas feast drew near, to which little Hanno was counting the days, with a beating heart and the help of a calendar manufactured by Ida Jungmann, with a Christmas tree on the last leaf.

The signs of festivity increased. Ever since the first Sunday in Advent a great gaily coloured picture of a certain Ruprecht had been hanging on the wall in grandmama's dining-room. And one morning Hanno found his covers and the rug beside his bed sprinkled with gold tinsel. A few days later, as papa was lying with his newspaper on the living-room sofa, and Hanno was reading " The Witch of Endor " out of Gerock's " Palm Leaves," an " old man " was announced. This had happened every year since Hanno was a baby – and yet was always a surprise. They asked him in, this " old man," and he came shuffling along in a big coat with the fur side out, sprinkled with bits of cotton-wool and tinsel. He wore a fur cap, and his face had black smudges on it, and his beard was long and white. The beard and the big, bushy eyebrows were also sprinkled with tinsel. He explained – as he did every year – in a harsh voice, that *this* sack (on his left shoulder) was for good children, who said their prayers (it contained apples and gilded nuts); but that *this* sack (on his right shoulder) was for naughty children. The " old man " was, of course, Ruprecht; perhaps not actually the real Ruprecht – it might even be Wenzel the barber, dressed up in Papa's coat turned fur side out – but it was as much Ruprecht as possible. Hanno, greatly impressed, said Our Father for him, as he had last year – both times interrupting himself now and again with a little nervous sob – and was permitted to put his hand into the sack for good children, which the " old man " forgot to take away.

The holidays came, and there was not much trouble over the report, which had to be presented for Papa to read, even at Christmas-time. The great dining-room was closed and mysterious, and there were marzipan and ginger-bread to eat – and in the streets, Christmas had already come. Snow fell, the weather was frosty, and on the sharp clear air were borne the notes of the barrel-organ, for the Italians, with their velvet jackets and their black moustaches, had arrived for the Christmas feast. The shop-windows were gay with toys and goodies; the booths for the Christmas fair had been erected in the market-place; and wherever you went you breathed in the fresh, spicy odour of the Christmas trees set out for sale.

The evening of the twenty-third came at last, and with it the present-giving in the house in Fishers' Lane. This was attended by the family only – it was a sort of dress rehearsal for the Christmas Eve party given by the Frau Consul in Meng Street. She clung to the old customs, and reserved the twenty-fourth for a celebration to which the whole family group was bidden; which, accordingly, in the late afternoon, assembled in the landscape-room.

The old lady, flushed of cheek, and with feverish eyes, arrayed in a heavy black-and-grey striped silk that gave out a faint scent of patchouli, received her guests as they entered, and embraced them silently, her gold bracelets tinkling. She was strangely excited this evening – "Why, Mother, you're fairly trembling," the Senator said when he came in with Gerda and Hanno. "Everything will go off very easily." But she only whispered, kissing all three of them, "For Jesus Christ's sake – and my blessed Jean's."

Indeed, the whole consecrated programme instituted by the deceased Consul had to be carried out to the smallest detail; and the poor lady fluttered about, driven by her sense of responsibility for the fitting accomplishment of the evening's performance, which must be pervaded with a deep and fervent joy. She went restlessly back and forth, from the pillared hall where the choir-boys from St. Mary's were already assembled, to the dining-room, where Riekchen Severin was putting the finishing touches to the tree and the tableful of presents, to the corridor full of shrinking old people – the "poor" who were to share in the presents – and back into the landscape-room, where she rebuked every unnecessary word or sound with one of her mild sidelong glances. It was so still that the sound of a distant hand-organ, faint and clear like a toy music-box, came across to them through the snowy streets. Some twenty persons or more were sitting or standing about in the room; yet it was stiller than a church – so still that, as the Senator cautiously whispered to Uncle Justus, it reminded one more of a funeral!

There was really no danger that the solemnity of the feast would be rudely broken in upon by youthful high spirits. A glance showed that almost all the persons in the room were arrived at an age when the forms of expression are already long ago fixed. Senator Thomas Buddenbrook, whose pallor gave the lie to his alert, energetic, humorous expression; Gerda, his wife, leaning back in her chair, the gleaming, blue-ringed eyes in her pale face gazing fixedly at the crystal prisms in the chandelier; his sister, Frau Permaneder; his cousin, Jürgen Kröger, a quiet, neatly-dressed official; Friederike, Henriette, and Pfiffi, the first two more long and lean, the third smaller and plumper than ever, but all three wearing their stereotyped expression, their sharp, spiteful smile at everything and everybody, as though they were perpetually saying "Really – it seems incredible!" Lastly, there was poor, ashen-grey Clothilde, whose thoughts were probably fixed upon the coming meal. – Every one of these persons was past forty. The hostess herself, her brother Justus and his wife, and little Therese Weichbrodt were all well past sixty; while old Frau Consul Buddenbrook, Uncle Gotthold's widow, born Stüwing, as well as Madame Kethelsen, now, alas almost entirely deaf, were already in the seventies.

Erica Weinschenk was the only person present in the bloom of youth; she was much younger than her husband, whose cropped, greying head stood out against the idyllic landscape behind him. When her eyes – the light blue eyes of Herr Grünlich – rested upon him, you could see how her full bosom rose and fell without a sound, and how she was beset with anxious, bewildered thoughts about usance and book-keeping, witnesses, prosecuting attorneys, defence, and judges. Thoughts like these, un-Christmaslike though they were, troubled everybody in the room. They all felt uncanny at the presence in their midst of a member of the family who was actually accused of an offence against the law, the civic weal, and business probity, and who would probably be visited by shame and imprisonment. Here was a Christmas family party at the Buddenbrooks' – with an accused man in the circle! Frau Permaneder's dignity became majestic, and the smile of the Misses Buddenbrook more and more pointed.

And what of the children, the scant posterity upon whom rested the family hopes? Were they conscious too of the slightly uncanny atmosphere? The state of mind of the little Elisabeth could not be fathomed. She sat on her bonne's lap in a frock trimmed by Frau Permaneder with satin bows, folded her small hands into fists, sucked her tongue, and stared straight ahead of her. Now and then she would utter a brief sound, like a grunt, and the nurse would rock her a little on her arm. But Hanno sat still on his footstool at his mother's knee and stared up, like her, into the chandelier.

Christian was missing – where was he? At the last minute they noticed his absence. The Frau Consul's characteristic gesture, from the corner of her mouth up to her temple, as though putting back a refractory hair, became frequent and feverish. She gave an order to Mamsell Severin, and the spinster went out through the hall, past the choir-boys and the "poor" and down the corridor to Christian's room, where she knocked on the door.

Christian appeared straightway; he limped casually into the landscape-room, rubbing his bald brow. "Good gracious, children," he said, "I nearly forgot the party!"

"You nearly forgot –" his mother repeated, and stiffened.

"Yes, I really forgot it was Christmas. I was reading a book of travel, about South America. – Dear me, I've seen such a lot of

Christmases! " he added, and was about to launch out upon a description of a Christmas in a fifth-rate variety theatre in London – when all at once the church-like hush of the room began to work upon him, and he moved on tip-toe to his place, wrinkling up his nose.

" Rejoice, O Daughter of Zion! " sang the choir-boys. They had previously been indulging in such audible practical jokes that the Senator had to get up and stand in the doorway to inspire respect. But now they sang beautifully. The clear treble, sustained by the deeper voices, soared up in pure, exultant, glorifying tones, bearing all hearts along with them: softening the smiles of the spinsters, making the old folk look in upon themselves and back upon the past; easing the hearts of those still in the midst of life's tribulations, and helping them to forget for a little while.

Hanno unclasped his hands from about his knees. He looked very pale, and cold, played with the fringe of his stool, and twisted his tongue about among his teeth. He had to draw a deep breath every little while, for his heart contracted with a joy almost painful at the exquisite bell-like purity of the chorale. The white folding doors were still tightly closed, but the spicy poignant odour drifted through the cracks and whetted one's appetite for the wonder within. Each year with throbbing pulses he awaited this vision of ineffable, unearthly splendour. What would there be for him, in there? What he had wished for, of course; there was always that – unless he had been persuaded out of it beforehand. The theatre, then, the long-desired toy theatre, would spring at him as the door opened, and show him the way to his place. This was the suggestion which had stood heavily underlined at the top of his list, ever since he had seen *Fidelio;* indeed, since then, it had been almost his single thought.

He had been taken to the opera as compensation for a particularly painful visit to Herr Brecht; sitting beside his mother, in the dress circle, he had followed breathless a performance of *Fidelio*, and since that time he had heard nothing, seen nothing, thought of nothing but opera, and a passion for the theatre filled him and almost kept him sleepless. He looked enviously at people like Uncle Christian, who was known as a regular frequenter and might go every night if he liked: Consul Döhlmann, Gosch the broker – how could they endure the joy of seeing it every night? He himself would ask no more than to look once a week into the hall, before the performance: hear the voices of the instruments being tuned, and gaze for a while at the curtain! For he loved it all, the seats, the musicians, the drop-curtain – even the smell of gas.

Would his theatre be large? What sort of curtain would it have? A tiny hole must be cut in it at once – there was a peep-hole in the curtain at the theatre. Had Grandmamma, or rather had Mamsell Severin – for Grandmamma could not see to everything herself – been able to find all the necessary scenery for *Fidelio?* He determined to shut himself up to-morrow and give a performance all by himself, and already in fancy he heard his little figures singing: for he was approaching the theatre by way of his music.

"Exult, Jerusalem!" finished the choir; and their voices, following one another in fugue form, united joyously in the last syllable. The clear accord died away; deep silence reigned in the pillared hall and the landscape-room. The elders looked down, oppressed by the pause; only Director Weinschenk's eyes roved boldly about, and Frau Permaneder coughed her dry cough, which she could not suppress. Now the Frau Consul moved slowly to the table and sat among her family. She turned up the lamp and took in her hands the great Bible with its edges of faded gold-leaf. She stuck her glasses on her nose, unfastened the two great leather hasps of the book, opened it to the place where there was a book-mark, took a sip of *eau sucrée*, and began to read, from the yellowed page with the large print, the Christmas chapter.

She read the old familiar words with a simple, heart-felt accent that sounded clear and moving in the pious hush. "'And to men good-will,'" she finished, and from the pillared hall came a trio of voices: "Holy night, peaceful night!" The family in the landscape-room joined in. They did so cautiously, for most of them were unmusical, as a tone now and then betrayed. But that in no wise impaired the effect of the old hymn. Frau Permaneder sang with trembling lips; it sounded sweetest and most touching to the heart of her who had a troubled life behind her, and looked back upon it in the brief peace of this holy hour. Madame Kethelsen wept softly, but comprehended nothing.

Now the Frau Consul rose. She grasped the hands of her grandson Johann and her granddaughter Elisabeth, and proceeded through the room. The elders of the family fell in behind, and the younger brought up the rear; the servants and poor joined in from the hall; and so they marched, singing with one accord "Oh, Evergreen" – Uncle Christian sang "Oh, Everblue," and made the children laugh by lifting up his legs like a jumping-jack –

through the wide-open, lofty folding doors, and straight into Paradise.

The whole great room was filled with the fragrance of slightly singed evergreen twigs and glowing with light from countless tiny flames. The sky-blue hangings with the white figures on them added to the brilliance. There stood the mighty tree, between the dark red window-curtains, towering nearly to the ceiling, decorated with silver tinsel and large white lilies, with a shining angel at the top and the manger at the foot. Its candles twinkled in the general flood of light like far-off stars. And a row of tiny trees, also full of stars and hung with comfits, stood on the long white table, laden with presents, that stretched from the window to the door. All the gas-brackets on the wall were lighted too, and thick candles burned in all four of the gilded candelabra in the corners of the room. Large objects, too large to stand upon the table, were arranged upon the floor, and two smaller tables, likewise adorned with tiny trees and covered with gifts for the servants and the poor, stood on either side of the door.

Dazzled by the light and the unfamiliar look of the room, they marched once around it, singing, filed past the manger where lay the little wax figure of the Christ-child, and then moved to their places and stood silent.

Hanno was quite dazed. His fevered glance had soon sought out the theatre, which, as it stood there upon the table, seemed larger and grander than anything he had dared to dream of. But his place had been changed – it was now opposite to where he had stood last year, and this made him doubtful whether the theatre was really his. And on the floor beneath it was something else, a large, mysterious something, which had surely not been on his list; a piece of furniture, that looked like a commode – could it be meant for him?

"Come here, my dear child," said the Frau Consul, "and look at this." She lifted the lid. "I know you like to play chorals. Herr Pfühl will show you how. You must tread all the time, sometimes more and sometimes less; and then, not lift up the hands, but change the fingers so, *peu à peu*."

It was a harmonium – a pretty little thing of polished brown wood, with metal handles at the sides, gay bellows worked with a treadle, and a neat revolving stool. Hanno struck a chord. A soft organ tone released itself and made the others look up from their presents. He hugged his grandmother, who pressed him tenderly to her, and then left him to receive the thanks of her other guests.

He turned to his theatre. The harmonium was an overpowering dream – which just now he had no time to indulge. There was a superfluity of joy; and he lost sight of single gifts in trying to see and notice everything at once. Ah, here was the prompter's box, a shell-shaped one, and a beautiful red and gold curtain rolled up and down behind it. The stage was set for the last act of *Fidelio*. The poor prisoners stood with folded hands. Don Pizarro, in enormous puffed sleeves, was striking a permanent and awesome attitude, and the minister, in black velvet, approached from behind with hasty strides, to turn all to happiness. It was just as in the theatre, only almost more beautiful. The Jubilee chorus, the finale, echoed in Hanno's ears, and he sat down at the harmonium to play a fragment which stuck in his memory. But he got up again, almost at once, to take up the book he had wished for, a mythology, in a red binding with a gold Pallas Athene on the cover. He ate some of the sweetmeats from his plate full of marzipan, gingerbread, and other goodies, looked through various small articles like writing utensils and school-bag – and for the moment forgot everything else, to examine a penholder with a tiny glass bulb on it: when you held this up to your eye, you saw, like magic, a broad Swiss landscape.

Mamsell Severin and the maid passed tea and biscuits; and while Hanno dipped and ate, he had time to look about. Every one stood talking and laughing; they all showed each other their presents and admired the presents of others. Objects of porcelain, silver, gold, nickel, wood, silk, cloth, and every other conceivable material lay on the table. Huge loaves of decorated gingerbread, alternating with loaves of marzipan, stood in long rows, still moist and fresh. All the presents made by Frau Permaneder were decorated with huge satin bows.

Now and then some one came up to little Johann, put an arm across his shoulders, and looked at his presents with the overdone, cynical admiration which people manufacture for the treasures of children. Uncle Christian was the only person who did not display this grown-up arrogance. He sauntered over to his nephew's place, with a diamond ring on his finger, a present from his mother; and his pleasure in the toy theatre was as unaffected as Hanno's own.

"By George, that's fine," he said, letting the curtain up and down, and stepping back for a view of the scenery. "Did you ask for it? Oh, so you did ask for it!" he suddenly said after a pause, during which his eyes had roved about the room as though he were full of unquiet thoughts. "Why did you ask for it?

What made you think of it? Have you been in the theatre? *Fidelio*, eh? Yes, they give that well. And you want to imitate it, do you? Do opera yourself, eh? Did it make such an impression on you? Listen, son – take my advice: don't think too much about such things – theatre, and that sort of thing. It's no good. Believe your old uncle. I've always spent too much time on them, and that is why I haven't come to much good. I've made great mistakes, you know."

Thus he held forth to his nephew, while Hanno looked up at him curiously. He paused, and his bony, emaciated face cleared up as he regarded the little theatre. Then he suddenly moved forward one of the figures on the stage, and sang, in a cracked and hollow tremolo, "Ha, what terrible transgression!" He sat down on the piano-stool, which he shoved up in front of the theatre, and began to give a performance, singing all the rôles and the accompaniment as well, and gesticulating furiously. The family gathered at his back, laughed, nodded their heads, and enjoyed it immensely. As for Hanno, his pleasure was profound. Christian broke off, after a while, very abruptly. His face clouded, he rubbed his hand over his skull and down his left side, and turned to his audience with his nose wrinkled and his face quite drawn.

"There it is again," he said. "I never have a little fun without having to pay for it. It is not an ordinary pain, you know, it is a misery, down all this left side, because the nerves are too short."

But his relatives took his complaints as little seriously as they had his entertainment. They hardly answered him, but indifferently dispersed, leaving Christian sitting before the little theatre in silence. He blinked rapidly for a bit and then got up.

"No, child," said he, stroking Hanno's head: "amuse yourself with it, but not too much, you know: don't neglect your work for it, do you hear? I have made a great many mistakes. – I think I'll go over to the club for a while," he said to the elders. "They are celebrating there to-day, too. Good-bye for the present." And he went off across the hall, on his stiff, crooked legs.

They had all eaten the midday meal earlier than usual to-day, and been hungry for the tea and biscuits. But they had scarcely finished when great crystal bowls were handed round full of a yellow, grainy substance which turned out to be almond cream. It was a mixture of eggs, ground almonds, and rose-water, tasting perfectly delicious; but if you ate even a tiny spoonful too much, the result was an attack of indigestion. However, the company was not restrained by fear of consequences – even though Frau Consul begged them to "leave a little corner for supper." Clothilde, in particular, performed miracles with the almond cream, and lapped it up like so much porridge, with heart-felt gratitude. There was also wine jelly in glasses, and English plum-cake. Gradually they all moved over to the landscape-room, where they sat with their plates round the table.

Hanno remained alone in the dining-room. Little Elisabeth Weinschenk had already been taken home; but he was to stop up for supper, for the first time in his life. The servants and the poor folk had had their presents and gone; Ida Jungmann was chattering with Riekchen Severin in the hall – although generally, as a governess, she preserved a proper distance between herself and the Frau Consul's maid. – The lights of the great tree were burnt down and extinguished, the manger was in darkness. But a few candles still burned on the small trees, and now and then a twig came within reach of the flame and crackled up, increasing the pungent smell in the room. Every breath of air that stirred the trees stirred the pieces of tinsel too, and made them give out a delicate metallic whisper. It was still enough to hear the hand-organ again, sounding through the frosty air from a distant street.

Hanno abandoned himself to the enjoyment of the Christmas sounds and smells. He propped his head on his hand and read in his mythology book, munching mechanically the while, because that was proper to the day: marzipan, sweet-meats, almond cream, and plum-cake; until the chest-oppression caused by an over-loaded stomach mingled with the sweet excitation of the evening and gave him a feeling of pensive felicity. He read about the struggles of Zeus before he arrived at the headship of the gods; and every now and then he listened into the other room, where they were going at length into the future of poor Aunt Clothilde.

Clothilde, on this evening, was far and away the happiest of them all. A smile lighted up her colourless face as she received congratulations and teasing from all sides; her voice even broke now and then out of joyful emotion. She had at last been made a member of the Order of St. John. The Senator had succeeded by subterranean methods in getting her admitted, not without some private grumblings about nepotism, on the part of certain gentlemen. Now the family all discussed the excellent institution, which was similar to the homes in Mecklenburg, Dobberthien, and Ribnitz, for ladies from noble families. The object of these establishments was the suitable care of portionless women from old and worthy families. Poor Clothilde was now assured of a small but certain income, which would increase with the years, and finally, when she had succeeded to the highest class, would secure her a decent home in the cloister itself.

Little Hanno stopped awhile with the grown-ups, but soon strayed back to the dining-room, which displayed a new charm now that the brilliant light did not fairly dazzle one with its splendours. It was an extraordinary pleasure to roam about there, as if on a half-darkened stage after the performance, and see a little behind the scenes. He touched the lilies on the big fir-tree, with their golden stamens; handled the tiny figures of people and animals in the manger, found the candles that lighted the transparency for the star of Bethlehem over the stable; lifted up the long cloth that covered the present-table, and saw quantities of wrapping-paper and pasteboard boxes stacked beneath.

The conversation in the landscape-room was growing less and less agreeable. Inevitably, irresistibly, it had arrived at the one dismal theme which had been in everybody's mind, but which they had thus far avoided, as a tribute to the festal evening. Hugo Weinschenk himself dilated upon it, with a wild levity of manner and gesture. He explained certain details of the procedure — the examination of witnesses had now been interrupted by the Christmas recess — condemned the very obvious bias of the President, Dr. Philander, and poured scorn on the attitude which the Public Prosecutor, Dr. Hagenström, thought it proper to assume toward himself and the witnesses for the defence. Breslauer had succeeded in drawing the sting of several of his most slanderous remarks; and he had assured the Director that, for the present, there need be no fear of a conviction. The Senator threw in a question now and then, out of courtesy; and Frau Permaneder, sitting on the sofa with elevated shoulders, would utter fearful imprecations against Dr. Moritz Hagenström. But the others were silent: so profoundly silent that the Director at length fell silent too. For little Hanno, over in the dining-room, the time sped by on angels' wings; but in the landscape-room there reigned an oppressive silence, which dragged on till Christian came back from the club, where he had celebrated Christmas with the bachelors and good fellows.

The cold stump of a cigar hung between his lips, and his haggard cheeks were flushed. He came through the dining-room and said, as he entered the landscape-room, "Well, children, the tree was simply gorgeous. Weinschenk, we ought to have had Breslauer come to see it. He has never seen anything like it, I am sure."

He encountered one of his mother's quiet, reproachful side-glances, and returned it with an easy, unembarrassed questioning look. At nine o'clock the party sat down to supper.

It was laid, as always on these occasions, in the pillared hall. The Frau Consul recited the ancient grace with sincere conviction:

> "Come, Lord Jesus, be our guest,
> And bless the bread thou gavest us"

— to which, as usual on the holy evening, she added a brief prayer, the substance of which was an admonition to remember those who, on this blessed night, did not fare so well as the Buddenbrook family. This accomplished, they all sat down with good consciences to a lengthy repast, beginning with carp and butter sauce and old Rhine wine.

The Senator put two fish-scales into his pocket, to help him save money during the coming year. Christian, however, ruefully remarked that he hadn't much faith in the prescription; and Consul Kröger had no need of it. His pittance had long since been invested securely, beyond the reach of fluctuations in the exchange. The old man sat as far away as possible from his wife, to whom he hardly ever spoke nowadays. She persisted in sending money to Jacob, who was still roaming about, nobody knew where, unless his mother did. Uncle Justus scowled forbiddingly when the conversation, with the advent of the second course, turned upon the absent members of the family, and he saw the foolish mother wipe her eyes. They spoke of the Frankfort Buddenbrooks and the Duchamps in Hamburg, and of Pastor Tiburtius in Riga, too, without any ill-will. And the Senator and his sister touched glasses in silence to the health of Messrs. Grünlich and Permaneder — for, after all, did they not in a sense belong to the family too?

The turkey, stuffed with chestnuts, raisins, and apples, was universally praised. They compared it with other years, and decided that this one was the largest for a long time. With the turkey came roast potatoes and two kinds of compote, and each dish held enough to satisfy the appetite of a family all by itself. The old red wine came from the firm of Möllendorpf.

Little Johann sat between his parents and choked down with difficulty a small piece of white meat with stuffing. He could not begin to compete with Aunt Tilda, and he felt tired and out of sorts. But it was a great thing none the less to be dining with the grown-ups, and to have one of the beautiful little rolls with poppy-seed in his elaborately folded serviette, and three wine-glasses in front of his place. He usually drank out of the little gold mug which Uncle Justus gave him. But when the red, white, and brown meringues appeared, and Uncle Justus poured some oily, yellow

Greek wine into the smallest of the three glasses, his appetite revived. He ate a whole red ice, then half a white one, then a little piece of the chocolate, his teeth hurting horribly all the while. Then he sipped his sweet wine gingerly and listened to Uncle Christian, who had begun to talk.

He told about the Christmas celebration at the club, which had been very jolly, it seemed. " Good God! " he said, just as if he were about to relate the story of Johnny Thunderstorm, " those fellows drank Swedish punch just like water."

" Ugh! " said the Frau Consul shortly, and cast down her eyes.

But he paid no heed. His eyes began to wander – and thought and memory became so vivid that they flickered like shadows across his haggard face.

" Do any of you know," he asked, " how it feels to drink too much Swedish punch? I don't mean getting drunk: I mean the feeling you have the next day – the after-effects. They are very queer and unpleasant; yes, queer and unpleasant at the same time."

" Reason enough for describing them," said the Senator.

" *Assez*, Christian. That does not interest us in the least," said the Frau Consul. But he paid no attention. It was his peculiarity that at such times nothing made any impression on him. He was silent awhile, and then it seemed that the thing which moved him was ripe for speech.

" You go about feeling ghastly," he said, turning to his brother and wrinkling up his nose. " Headache, and upset stomach – oh, well, you have that with other things, too. But you feel *filthy* " – here he rubbed his hands together, his face entirely distorted. " You wash your hands, but it does no good; they feel dirty and clammy, and there is grease under the nails. You take a bath: no good, your whole body is sticky and unclean. You itch all over, and you feel disgusted with yourself. Do you know the feeling, Thomas? you do know it, don't you? "

" Yes, yes," said the Senator, making a gesture of repulsion with his hand. But Christian's extraordinary tactlessness had so increased with the years that he never perceived how unpleasant he was making himself to the company, nor how out of place his conversation was in these surroundings and on this evening. He continued to describe the evil effects of too much Swedish punch; and when he felt that he had exhausted the subject, he gradually subsided.

Before they arrived at the butter and cheese, the Frau Consul found occasion for another little speech to her family. If, she said, not quite everything in the course of the years had gone as we, in our short-sightedness, desired, there remained such manifold blessings as should fill our hearts with gratitude and love. For it was precisely this mingling of trials with blessings which showed that God never lifted his hand from the family, but ever guided its destinies according to His wise design, which we might not seek to question. And now, with hopeful hearts, we might drink together to the family health and to its future — that future when all the old and elderly of the present company would be laid to rest; and to the children, to whom the Christmas feast most properly belonged.

As Director Weinschenk's small daughter was no longer present, little Johann had to make the round of the table alone and drink severally with all the company, from Grandmamma to Mamsell Severin. When he came to his father, the Senator touched the child's glass with his and gently lifted Hanno's chin to look into his eyes. But his son did not meet his glance: the long, gold-brown lashes lay deep, deep upon the delicate bluish shadows beneath his eyes.

Therese Weichbrodt took his head in both her hands, kissed him explosively on both cheeks, and said with such a hearty emphasis that surely God must have heeded it, "Be happy, you good che-ild!"

An hour later Hanno lay in his little bed, which now stood in the ante-chamber next to the Senator's dressing-room. He lay on his back, out of regard for his stomach, which was feeling far from pleasant over all the things he had put into it that evening. Ida came out of her room in her dressing-gown, waving a glass about in circles in the air in order to dissolve its contents. He drank the carbonate of soda down quickly, made a wry face, and fell back again.

"I think I'll just have to give it all up, Ida," he said.

"Oh, nonsense, Hanno. Just lie still on your back. You see, now: who was it kept making signs to you to stop eating, and who was it that wouldn't do it?"

"Well, perhaps I'll be all right. When will the things come, Ida?"

"To-morrow morning, first thing, my dearie."

"I wish they were here — I wish I had them now."

"Yes, yes, my dearie — but just have a good sleep now." She kissed him, put out the light, and went away.

He lay quietly, giving himself up to the operation of the soda he had taken. But before his eyes gleamed the dazzling brilliance of the Christmas tree. He saw his theatre and his harmonium, and his book of mythology; he heard the choir-boys singing in the distance: " Rejoice, Jerusalem! " Everything sparkled and glittered. His head felt dull and feverish; his heart, affected by the rebellious stomach, beat strong and irregularly. He lay for long, in a condition of mingled discomfort, excitement, and reminiscent bliss, and could not fall asleep.

Next day there would be a third Christmas party, at Fräulein Weichbrodt's. He looked forward to it as to a comic performance in the theatre. Therese Weichbrodt had given up her *pensionnat* in the past year. Madame Kethelsen now occupied the first storey of the house on the Mill Brink, and she herself the ground floor, and there they lived alone. The burden of her deformed little body grew heavier with the years, and she concluded, with Christian humility and submission, that the end was not far off. For some years now she had believed that each Christmas was her last; and she strove with all the powers at her command to give a departing brilliance to the feast that was held in her small overheated rooms. Her means were very narrow, and she gave away each year a part of her possessions to swell the heap of gifts under the tree: knick-knacks, paper-weights, emery-bags, needle-cushions, glass vases, and fragments of her library, miscellaneous books of every shape and size. Books like " The Secret Journal of a Student of Himself," Hebel's " Alemannian Poems," Krummacher's " Parables " — Hanno had once received an edition of the " Pensées de Blaise Pascal," in such tiny print that it had to be read with a glass.

Bishop flowed in streams, and Sesemi's ginger-bread was very spicy. But Fräulein Weichbrodt abandoned herself with such trembling emotion to the joys of each Christmas party that none of them ever went off without a mishap. There was always some small catastrophe or other to make the guests laugh and enhance the silent fervour of the hostess' mien. A jug of bishop would be upset and overwhelm everything in a spicy, sticky red flood. Or the decorated tree would topple off its wooden support just as they solemnly entered the room. Hanno fell asleep with the mishap of the previous year before his eyes. It had happened just before the gifts were given out. Therese Weichbrodt had read the Christmas chapter, in such impressive accents that all the vowels got inextricably commingled, and then retreated before her guests to the door, where she made a little speech. She stood upon the threshold, humped and tiny, her old hands clasped before her childish bosom, the green silk cap-ribbons falling over her fragile shoulders. Above her head, over the door, was a transparency, garlanded with evergreen, that said " Glory to God in the Highest." And Sesemi spoke of God's mercy; she mentioned that this was her last Christmas, and ended by reminding them that the words of the apostle commended them all to joy – wherewith she trembled from head to foot, so much did her whole poor little body share in her emotions. " Rejoice! " said she, laying her head on one side and nodding violently: " and again I say unto you, rejoice! " But at this moment the whole transparency, with a puffing, crackling, spitting noise, went up in flames, and Mademoiselle Weichbrodt gave a little shriek and a side-spring of unexpected picturesqueness and agility, and got herself out of the way of the rain of flying sparks.

As Hanno recalled the leap which the old spinster performed, he giggled nervously for several minutes into his pillow.

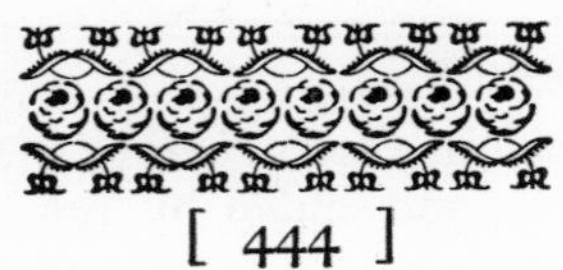

CHAPTER IX

FRAU PERMANEDER was going along Broad Street in a great hurry. There was something abandoned about her air: she showed almost none of the impressive bearing usual to her on the street. Hunted and harassed, in almost violent haste, she had as it were been able to save only a remnant of her dignity — like a beaten king who gathers what is left of his army about him to seek safety in the arms of flight.

She looked pitiable indeed. Her upper lip, that arched upper lip that had always done its share to give charm to her face, was quivering now, and the eyes were large with apprehension. They were very bright and stared fixedly ahead of her, as though they too were hurrying onward. Her hair came in disorder from under her close hat, and her face showed the pale yellow tint which it always had when her digestion took a turn for the worse.

Her digestion was obviously worse in these days. The family noticed that on Thursdays. And no matter how hard every one tried to keep off the rocks, the conversation always made straight for them and stuck there: on the subject of Hugo Weinschenk's trial. Frau Permaneder herself led up to it. She would call on God and her fellow men to tell her how Public Prosecutor Moritz Hagenström could sleep of nights. For her part, she could not understand it — she never would! Her agitation increased with every word. "Thank you, I can't eat," she would say, and push away her plate. She would elevate her shoulders, toss her head, and in the height of her passion fall back upon the practice, acquired in her Munich years, of taking nothing but beer, cold Bavarian beer, poured into an empty stomach, the nerves of which were in rebellion and would revenge themselves bitterly. Toward the end of the meal she always had to get up and go down to the garden or the court, where she suffered the most dreadful fits of nausea, leaning upon Ida Jungmann or Riekchen Severin. Her stomach would finally relieve itself of its contents, and contract with spasms of pain, which sometimes lasted for minutes and would continue at intervals for a long time.

It was about three in the afternoon, a windy, rainy January day. Frau Permaneder turned the corner at Fishers' Lane and hurried down the steep declivity to her brother's house. After a hasty knock she went from the court straight into the bureau, her eye flying across the desks to where the Senator sat in his seat by the window. She made such an imploring motion with her head that he put down his pen without more ado and went to her.

"Well?" he said, one eyebrow lifted.

"A moment, Thomas—it's very pressing; there's no time to waste."

He opened the baize door of his private office, closed it behind him when they were both inside, and looked at his sister inquiringly.

"Tom," she said, her voice quavering, wringing her hands inside her muff, "you must give it to us—lay it out for us—you will, won't you?—the money for the bond, I mean. We haven't it—where should we get twenty-five thousand marks from, I should like to know? You will get them back—you'll get them back all too soon, I'm afraid. You understand—the thing is this: in short, they have reached a point where Hagenström demands immediate arrest or else a bond of twenty-five thousand marks. And Weinschenk will give you his word not to stir from the spot—"

"Has it really come to that?" the Senator said, shaking his head.

"Yes, they have succeeded in getting that far, the villains!" Frau Permaneder sank upon the sofa with an impotent sob. "And they will go on; they will go on to the end, Tom."

"Tony," he said, and sat down sidewise by his mahogany desk, crossing one leg over the other and leaning his head on his hand, "tell me straight out, do you still have faith in his innocence?"

She sobbed once or twice before she answered, hopelessly: "Oh, no, Tom. How could I? I've seen so much evil in the world. I haven't believed in it from the beginning, even, though I tried my very best. Life makes it so very hard, you know, to believe in any one's innocence. Oh, no—I've had doubts of his good conscience for a long time, and Erica has not known what to make of him—she confessed it to me, with tears—on account of his behaviour at home. We haven't talked about it, of course. He got ruder and ruder, and kept demanding all the time that Erica should be lively and divert his mind and make him forget his troubles. And he broke the dishes when she wasn't. You can't imagine what it was like, when he shut himself up evenings with his papers: when anybody knocked, you could hear him jump up and shout 'Who's there?'"

They were silent.

" But suppose he *is* guilty, Tom. Suppose he did do it," began Frau Permaneder afresh, and her voice gathered strength. " He wasn't working for his own pocket, but for the company – and then – good Heavens, in this life, people have to realize – there are other things to be taken into consideration. He married into our family – he is one of us, now. They can't just go and stick him into prison like that! "

He shrugged his shoulders.

" What are you shrugging your shoulders for, Tom? Do you mean that you are willing to sit down under the last and crowning insult these adventurers think they can offer us? We must do something! He mustn't be convicted! Aren't you the Burgomaster's right hand? My God, can't the Senate just pardon him if it likes? You know, before I came to you, I nearly went to Cremer, to get him – to implore him to intervene and take a stand in the matter – he is Chief of Police – "

" Oh, child, that is all just nonsense."

" Nonsense, Tom? And Erica? And the child? " said she, lifting up her muff, with her two imploring hands inside. She was still a moment, she let her arms fall, her chin began to quiver, and two great tears ran down from under her drooping lids. She added softly, " And me? "

" Oh, Tony, be brave," said the Senator. Her helplessness went through him. He pushed his chair up to hers and stroked her hair, in an effort to console her. " Everything isn't over, yet. Perhaps it will come out all right. Of course I will give you the money – that goes without saying – and Breslauer's very clever."

She shook her head, weeping.

" No, Tom, it will not come out all right. I've no hope that it will. They will convict him, and put him in prison – and then the hard time will come for Erica and me. Her dowry is gone: it all went to the setting-out, the furniture and pictures; we sha'n't get a quarter of it back by selling. And the salary was always spent. We never put a penny by. We will go back to Mother, if she will take us, until he is free. And then where can we go? We'll just have to sit on the rocks." She sobbed.

" On the rocks? "

" Oh, that's just an expression – a figure. What I mean is, it won't turn out all right. I've had too much to bear – I don't know how I came to deserve it all – but I can't hope any more. Erica will be like me – with Grünlich and Permaneder. But now you can see just how it is – and how it all comes over you! Could I help it? Could any one help it, I ask you, Tom? " she repeated drearily, and looked at him with her tear-swimming eyes. "Everything I've ever undertaken has gone wrong and turned to misfortune – and I've meant everything so well. God knows I have! And now this too – This is the last straw – the very last."

She wept, leaning on the arm which he gently put about her: wept over her ruined life and the quenching of this last hope.

A week later, Herr Director Hugo Weinschenk was sentenced to three and a half years' imprisonment, and arrested at once.

There was a very large crowd at the final session. Lawyer Breslauer of Berlin made a speech for the defence the like of which had never been heard before. Gosch the broker went about for weeks afterwards bursting with enthusiasm for the masterly pathos and irony it displayed. Christian Buddenbrook heard it too, and afterward got behind a table at the club, with a pile of newspapers in front of him, and reproduced the whole speech. At home he declared that jurisprudence was the finest profession there was, and he thought it would just have suited him. The Public Prosecutor himself, Dr. Moritz Hagenström, who was a great connoisseur, said in private that the speech had been a genuine treat to him. But the famous advocate's talents did not prevent his colleagues from thumping him on the back and telling him he had not pulled the wool over their eyes.

The necessary sale followed upon the disappearance of the Director; and when it was over, people in town began gradually to forget about Hugo Weinschenk. But the Misses Buddenbrook, sitting on Thursday at the family table, declared that they had known the first moment, from the man's eyes, that he was not straight, that his conscience was bad, and that there would be trouble in the end. Certain considerations, which they wished now they had not regarded, had led them to suppress these painful observations.

PART NINE

CHAPTER I

SENATOR BUDDENBROOK followed the two gentlemen, old Dr. Grabow and young Dr. Langhals, out of the Frau Consul's bedchamber into the breakfast-room and closed the door.

"May I ask you to give me a moment, gentlemen?" he said, and led them up the steps, through the corridor, and into the landscape-room, where, on account of the raw, damp weather, the stove was already burning. "You will understand my anxiety," he said. "Sit down and tell me something reassuring, if possible."

"Zounds, my dear Senator," answered Dr. Grabow, leaning back comfortably, his chin in his neck-cloth, his hat-brim propped in both hands against his stomach. Dr. Langhals put his top-hat down on the carpet beside him and regarded his hands, which were exceptionally small and covered with hair. He was a heavy dark man with a pointed beard, a pompadour hair-cut, beautiful eyes, and a vain expression.

"There is positively no reason for serious disquiet at present," Dr. Grabow went on. "When we take into consideration our honoured patient's powers of resistance – my word, I think, as an old and tried councillor, I ought to know what that resistance is – it is simply astonishing, for her years, I must say."

"Yes, precisely: for her years," said the Senator, uneasily, twisting his moustaches.

"I don't say," went on Dr. Grabow, in his gentle voice, "that your dear Mother will be walking out to-morrow. You can tell that by looking at her, of course. There is no denying that the inflammation has taken a disappointing turn in the last twenty-four hours. The chill yesterday afternoon did not please me at all, and to-day there is actually pain in the side. And some fever – oh, nothing to speak of, but still – In short, my dear Senator, we shall probably have to reckon with the troublesome fact that the lung is slightly affected."

"Inflammation of the lungs then?" asked the Senator, and looked from one physician to the other.

"Yes – pneumonia," said Dr. Langhals, with a solemn and correct bow.

" A slight inflammation, however, and confined to the right side," answered the family physician. " We will do our best to localize it."

" Then there is ground for serious concern, after all? " The Senator sat quite still and looked the speaker full in the face.

" Concern – oh, we must be concerned to limit the affection. We must ease the cough, and go at the fever energetically. The quinine will see to that. And by the by, my dear Senator, let me warn you against feeling alarm over single symptoms, you know. If the difficulty in breathing increases, or there should be a little delirium in the night, or a good deal of discharge to-morrow – a sort of rusty-looking mucous, with a little blood in it – well, all that is to be expected, entirely regular and normal. Do reassure dear Madame Permaneder on this point too – she is nursing the patient with such devotion. – How is she feeling? I quite forgot to ask how she has been, in the last few days."

" She is about as usual," the Senator said. " I have not heard of anything new. She is not taking much thought for her own condition, these days – "

" Of course, of course. And, apropos: your sister needs rest, especially at night, and Mamsell Severin has not time to give her all the rest she needs. What about a nurse, my dear Senator? Why not have one of our good Grey Sisters, in whom you feel such an interest? The Mother Superior would be glad to send you one."

" You consider it necessary? "

" I am only suggesting it. The sisters are invaluable – their experience and calmness are always so soothing to the patient, especially in an illness like this, where there is a succession of disquieting symptoms. Well – let me repeat, no anxiety, my dear Senator. And we shall see, we shall see. We will have another talk this evening."

" Positively," said Dr. Langhals, took his hat and got up, with his colleague. But the Senator had not finished: he had another question, another test to make.

" Gentlemen," he said, " one word more. My brother Christian is a nervous man. He cannot stand much. Do you advise me to send him word? Should I suggest to him to come home? "

" Your brother Christian is not in town? "

" No, he is in Hamburg – for a short time, on business, I understand."

Dr. Grabow gave his colleague a glance. Then he laughingly shook the Senator's hand and said, " Well, we'll let him attend to his business in peace. No use upsetting him unnecessarily. If any change comes which seems to make it advisable, to quiet the patient, or to raise her spirits – well, there is plenty of time still, plenty of time."

The gentlemen traversed the pillared hall and stood on the steps awhile, talking about other matters: politics, and the agitations and changes due to the war just then ended.

"Well, good times will be coming now, eh, Herr Senator? Money in the country, and fresh confidence everywhere."

And the Senator partially agreed with him. He said that the grain trade with Russia had been greatly stimulated since the outbreak of war, and mentioned the dimensions to which the import trade in oats had attained – though the profit, it was true, had been very unevenly divided.

The physicians took their leave, and Senator Buddenbrook turned to go back to the sick-room. He revolved what Dr. Grabow had said. He had spoken with reserve – he gave the impression of avoiding anything definite. The single plain word was "inflammation of the lungs"; which became no more reassuring after Dr. Langhals added the scientific terminology. Pneumonia – at the Frau Consul's age. The fact that there were two physicians coming and going was in itself disquieting. Grabow had arranged that very unobtrusively. He intended to retire before long, and as young Dr. Langhals would then be taking over the practice, he, Dr. Grabow, would be pleased if he might bring him in now and again.

When the Senator entered the darkened room, his mien appeared alert and his bearing energetic. He was used to hiding his cares and weariness under an air of calmness and poise; and the mask glided over his features as he opened the door, almost as though by a single act of will.

Frau Permaneder sat by the high bed, the hangings of which were thrust back, and held her mother's hand. The old lady was propped up on pillows. She turned her head as her son came in, and looked searchingly with her pale blue eyes into his face – a look of calm self-control, yet of deliberate insistence. Coming as it did, slightly sidewise, there was almost something sinister about it, too. Two red spots stood out upon the pallor of her cheeks, but there were no signs of weakness or exhaustion. The old lady was very wide awake, more so in fact than those around her – for, after all, she was the person most concerned. And she mistrusted this illness; she was not at all disposed to lie down and let it have its own way.

"What did they say, Thomas?" she asked in a brisk, decided

voice which made her cough directly. She tried to keep the cough behind her closed lips, but it burst out and made her put her hand to her side.

"They said," answered the Senator, when the spasm was over, stroking her hand, "they said that our dear, good mother will be up again in a few days. The wretched cough is responsible for your lying here. The lung is of course slightly affected – it is not exactly inflammation," he hastened to say, as he saw her narrowing gaze, "but even if it were, that needn't necessarily be so bad. It might be much worse," he finished. "In short, the lung is somewhat irritated, and they may be right – where is Mamsell Severin?"

"Gone to the chemist's," said Frau Permaneder.

"Yes, you see. She has gone to the chemist's again, and you look as though you might go to sleep any minute, Tony. No, it isn't good enough. If only for a day or so, we should have a nurse in, don't you think so? I will find out if my Mother Superior up at the Grey Sisters has any one free."

"Thomas," said the Frau Consul, this time in a more cautious voice, so as not to let loose another cough, "believe me, you cause a good deal of feeling by your protection of the Catholic order against the black Protestant Sisters. You have shown the Catholics a distinct preference. Pastor Pringsheim complained to me about it very strenuously a little time ago."

"Well, he needn't. I am convinced that the Grey Sisters are more faithful, devoted, and self-sacrificing than the Black ones are. The Protestants aren't the real thing. They all marry the first chance they get. They are worldly, egotistical, and ordinary, while the Grey Sisters are perfectly disinterested. I am sure they are much nearer Heaven. And they are better for us for the very reason that they owe me some gratitude. What should we have done without Sister Leandra when Hanno had convulsions? I only hope she is free!"

And Sister Leandra came. She put down her cloak and little handbag, took off the grey veil which she wore on the street over her white one, and went softly about her work, in her gentle, friendly way, the rosary at her waist clicking as she moved. She remained a day and a night with the querulous, not always patient sufferer, and then withdrew, almost apologetic over the human weakness that enforced a little repose. She was replaced by another sister, but came back again after she had slept.

The Frau Consul required constant attendance at her bedside. The worse her condition grew, the more she bent all her thoughts and all her energies upon her illness, for which she felt a naïve hatred. Nearly all her life she had been a woman of the world, with a quiet, native, and permanent love of life and good living. Yet she had filled her latter years with piety and charitable deeds: largely out of loyalty toward her dead husband, but also, perhaps, by reason of an unconscious impulse which bade her make her peace with Heaven for her own strong vitality, and induce it to grant her a gentle death despite the tenacious clutch she had always had on life. But the gentle death was not to be hers. Despite many a sore trial, her form was quite unbowed, her eyes still clear. She still loved to set a good table, to dress well and richly, to ignore events that were unpleasant, and to share with complacency in the high regard that was everywhere felt for her son. And now this illness, this inflammation of the lungs, had attacked her erect form without any previous warning, without any preparation to soften the blow. There had been no spiritual anticipation, none of that mining and sapping of the forces which slowly, painfully estranges us from life and rouses in us the sweet longing for a better world, for the end, for peace. No, the old Frau Consul, despite the spiritual courses of her latter years, felt scarce prepared to die; and she was filled with agony of spirit at the thought that if this were indeed the end, then this illness, of itself, in awful haste, in the last hour, must, with bodily torments, break down her spirit and bring her to surrender.

She prayed much; but almost more she watched, as often as she was conscious, over her own condition: felt her pulse, took her temperature, and fought her cough. But the pulse was poor, the temperature mounted after falling a little, and she passed from chills to fever and delirium; her cough increased, bringing up a blood-impregnated mucous, and she was alarmed by the difficulty she had in breathing. It was accounted for by the fact that now not only a lobe of the right lung, but the whole right lung, was affected, with even distinct traces of a process in the left, which Dr. Langhals, looking at his nails, called hepatization, and about which Dr. Grabow said nothing at all. The fever wasted the patient relentlessly. The digestion failed. Slowly, inexorably, the decline of strength went on.

She followed it. She took eagerly, whenever she could, the concentrated nourishment which they gave her. She knew the hours for her medicines better than the nurse; and she was so absorbed in watching the progress of her case that she hardly spoke to any one but the physicians, and displayed actual interest only when talking with them. Callers had been admitted in the beginning, and the old ladies of her social circle, pastors' wives and members of the Jerusalem evenings, came to see her; but she received them with apathy and soon dismissed them. Her relatives felt the difference in the old lady's greeting: it was almost disdainful, as though she were saying to them: "You can't do anything for me." Even when little Hanno came, in a good hour, she only stroked his cheek and turned away. Her manner said more plainly than words: "Children, you are all very good – but – perhaps – I may be dying!" She received the two physicians, on the other hand, with very lively interest, and went into the details of her condition.

One day the Gerhardt ladies appeared, the descendants of Paul Gerhardt. They came in their mantles, with their flat shepherdess hats and their provision-baskets, from visiting the poor, and could not be prevented from seeing their sick friend. They were left alone with her, and God only knows what they said as they sat at her bedside. But when they departed, their eyes and their faces were more gentle, more radiant, more blissfully remote than ever; while the Frau Consul lay within, with just such eyes and just such an expression, quite still, quite peaceful, more peaceful than ever before; her breath came very softly and at long intervals, and she was visibly declining from weakness to weakness. Frau Permaneder murmured a strong word in the wake of the Gerhardt ladies, and sent at once for the physicians. The two gentlemen had barely entered the sick-chamber when a surprising alteration took place in the patient. She stirred, she moved, she almost sat up. The sight of her trusted and faithful professional advisers brought her back to earth at a bound. She put out her hands to them and began: "Welcome, gentlemen. To-day, in the course of the day –"

The illness had attacked both lungs – of that there was no more room for doubt.

"Yes, my dear Senator," Dr. Grabow said, and took Thomas Buddenbrook by the hand, "it is now both lungs – we have not been able to prevent it. That is always serious, you know as well as I do. I should not attempt to deceive you. No matter what the age of the patient, the condition is serious; and if you ask me again to-day whether in my opinion your brother should be written to – or perhaps a telegram would be better – I should hesitate to deter you from it. How is he, by the way? A good fellow, Christian; I've always liked him immensely. – But for Heaven's sake, my dear Senator, don't draw any exaggerated conclusions from what I say. There is no immediate danger – I am foolish to take the word in my mouth! But still – under the circumstances, you know, one must reckon with the unexpected. We are very well satisfied with your mother as a patient. She helps all she can, she doesn't leave us in the lurch; no, on my word, she is an incomparable patient! So there is still great hope, my dear sir. And we must hope for the best."

But there is a moment when hope becomes something artificial and insincere. There is a change in the patient. He alters — there is something strange about him — he is not as he was in life. He speaks, but we do not know how to reply: what he says is strange, it seems to cut off his retreat back to life, it condemns him to death. And when that moment comes, even if he is our dearest upon this earth, we do not know how to wish him back. If we could bid him arise and walk, he would be as frightful as one risen from his coffin.

Dreadful symptoms of the coming dissolution showed themselves, even though the organs, still in command of a tenacious will, continued to function. It had now been weeks since Frau Consul first took to her bed with a cold; and she began to have bed sores. They would not heal, and grew worse and worse. She could not sleep, because of pain, coughing and shortness of breath, and also because she herself clung to consciousness with all her might. Only for minutes at a time did she lose herself in fever; but now she began, even when she was conscious, to talk to people who had long been dead. One afternoon, in the twilight, she said suddenly, in a loud, fervent, anxious voice, " Yes, my dear Jean, I am coming! " And the immediacy of the reply was such that one almost thought to hear the voice of the deceased Consul calling her.

Christian arrived. He came from Hamburg, where he had been, he said, on business. He only stopped a short time in the sick-room, and left it, his eyes roving wildly, rubbing his forehead, and saying " It's frightful — it's frightful — I can't stand it any longer."

Pastor Pringsheim came, measured Sister Leandra with a chilling glance, and prayed with a beautifully modulated voice at the bedside.

Then came the brief " lightening ": the flickering up of the dying flame. The fever slackened; there was a deceptive return of strength, and a few plain, hopeful words, that brought tears of joy to the eyes of the watchers at the bedside.

" Children, we shall keep her; you'll see, we shall keep her after all! " cried Thomas Buddenbrook. " She will be with us next Christmas! "

But even in the next night, shortly after Gerda and her husband had gone to bed, they were summoned back to Meng Street by Frau Permaneder, for the mother was struggling with death. A cold rain was falling, and a high wind drove it against the windowpanes.

The bed-chamber, as the Senator and his wife entered it, was lighted by two sconces burning on the table; and both physicians were present. Christian too had been summoned from his room, and sat with his back to the bed and his forehead bowed in his hands. They had sent for the dying woman's brother, Justus Kröger, and he would shortly be here. Frau Permaneder and Erica were sobbing softly at the foot of the bed. Sister Leandra and Mamsell Severin had nothing more to do, and stood gazing in sadness on the face of the dying.

The Frau Consul lay on her back, supported by a quantity of pillows. With both her blue-veined hands, once so beautiful, now so emaciated, she ceaselessly stroked the coverlet in trembling haste. Her head in the white nightcap moved from side to side with dreadful regularity. Her lips were drawn inward, and opened and closed with a snap at every tortured effort to breathe, while the sunken eyes roved back and forth or rested with an envious look on those who stood about her bed, up and dressed and able to breathe. They were alive, they belonged to life; but they could help her no more than this, to make the sacrifice that consisted in watching her die. . . . And the night wore on, without any change.

"How long can it go on, like this?" asked Thomas Buddenbrook, in a low tone, drawing Dr. Grabow away to the bottom of the room, while Dr. Langhals was undertaking some sort of injection to give relief to the patient. Frau Permaneder, her handkerchief in her hand, followed her brother.

"I can't tell, my dear Senator," answered Dr. Grabow. "Your dear mother may be released in the next few minutes, or she may live for hours. It is a process of strangulation: an oedema — "

"I know," said Frau Permaneder, and nodded while the tears ran down her cheeks. "It often happens in cases of inflammation of the lungs — a sort of watery fluid forms, and when it gets very bad the patient cannot breathe any more. Yes, I know."

The Senator, his hands folded, looked over at the bed.

"How frightfully she must suffer," he whispered.

"No," Dr. Grabow said, just as softly, but in a tone of authority, while his long, mild countenance wrinkled more than ever. "That is a mistake, my dear friend, believe me. The consciousness is very clouded. These are largely reflex motions which you see; depend upon it." And Thomas answered: "God grant it" – but a child could have seen from the Frau Consul's eyes that she was entirely conscious and realized everything.

They took their places again. Consul Kröger came and sat bowed over his cane at the bedside, with reddened eyelids.

The movements of the patient increased. This body, delivered over to death, was possessed by a terrible unrest, an unspeakable craving, an abandonment of helplessness, from head to foot. The pathetic, imploring eyes now closed with the rustling movement of the head from side to side, now opened with a heart-breaking expression, so wide that the little veins of the eyeballs stood out blood-red. And she was still conscious!

A little after three, Christian got up. "I can't stand it any more," he said, and went out, limping, and supporting himself on the furniture on his way to the door. Erica Weinschenk and Mamsell Severin had fallen asleep to the monotonous sound of the raucous breathing, and sat rosy with slumber on their chairs.

About four it grew much worse. They lifted the patient and wiped the perspiration from her brow. Her breathing threatened to stop altogether. "Let me sleep," she managed to say. "Give me a sleeping-draught." Alas, they could give her nothing to make her sleep.

Suddenly she began again to reply to voices which the others could not hear. "Yes, Jean, not much longer now." And then, "Yes, dear Clara, I am coming."

The struggle began afresh. Was this a wrestling with death? Ah, no, for it had become a wrestling with life for death, on the part of the dying woman. "I want –," she panted, "I want – I cannot – let me sleep! Have mercy, gentlemen – let me sleep!"

Frau Permaneder sobbed aloud as she listened, and Thomas groaned softly, clutching his head a moment with both hands. But the physicians knew their duty: they were obliged, under all circumstances, to preserve life just as long as possible; and a narcotic would have effected an unresisting and immediate giving-up of the ghost. Doctors were not made to bring death into the world, but to preserve life at any cost. There was a religious and moral basis for this law, which they had known once, though they did not have it in mind at the moment. So they strengthened the heart action by various devices, and even improved the breathing by causing the patient to retch.

By five the struggle was at its height. The Frau Consul, erect in convulsions, with staring eyes, thrust wildly about her with her arms as though trying to clutch after some support or to reach the hands which she felt stretching toward her. She was answering constantly in every direction to voices which she alone heard, and which evidently became more numerous and urgent. Not only her dead husband and daughter, but her parents, parents-in-law, and other relatives who had passed before her into death, seemed to summon her; and she called them all by name – though the names were some of them not familiar to her children. "Yes," she cried, " yes, I am coming now – at once – a moment – I cannot – oh, let me sleep! "

At half-past five there was a moment of quiet. And then over her aged and distorted features there passed a look of ineffable joy, a profound and quivering tenderness; like lightning she stretched up her arms and cried out, with an immediate suddenness swift as a blow, so that one felt there was not a second's space between what she heard and what she answered, with an expression of absolute submission and a boundless and fervid devotion: " Here I am! " and parted.

They were all amazed. What was it? Who had called her? To whose summons had she responded thus instantly?

Some one drew back the curtains and put out the candles, and Dr. Grabow gently closed the eyes of the dead.

They all shivered in the autumn dawn that filled the room with its sallow light. Sister Leandra covered the mirror of the toilet table with a cloth.

CHAPTER II

THROUGH the open door Frau Permaneder could be seen praying in the chamber of death. She knelt there alone, at a chair near the bed, with her mourning garments flowing about her on the floor. While she prayed, her hands folded before her on the seat of the chair, she could hear her brother and sister-in-law in the breakfast-room, where they stood and waited for the prayer to come to an end. But she did not hurry on that account. She finished, coughed her usual little dry cough, gathered her gown about her, and rose from the chair, then moved toward her relatives with a perfectly dignified bearing in which there was no trace of confusion.

" Thomas," she said, with a note of asperity in her voice, " it strikes me, that as far as Severin is concerned, our blessed mother was cherishing a viper in her bosom."

" What makes you think that? "

" I am perfectly furious with her. I shall try to behave with dignity, but – has the woman any right to disturb us at this solemn moment by her common ways? "

" What has she been doing? "

" Well in the first place, she is outrageously greedy. She goes to the wardrobe and takes out Mother's silk gowns, folds them over her arm, and starts to retire. ' Why, Riekchen,' I say, ' what are you doing with those? ' ' Frau Consul promised me.' ' My dear Severin! ' I say, and show her, in a perfectly ladylike way, what I think of her unseemly haste. Do you think it did any good? She took not only the silk gowns, but a bundle of underwear as well, and went out. I can't come to blows with her, can I? And it isn't Severin alone. There are wash-baskets full of stuff going out of the house. The servants divide up things before my face – Severin has the keys to the cupboards. I said to her: ' Fräulein Severin, I shall be much obliged for the keys.' And she told me, in good set terms, that I've nothing to say to her, she's not in my service, I didn't engage her, and she will keep the keys until she leaves! "

" Have you the keys to the silver-chest? Good. Let the rest go. That sort of thing is inevitable when a household breaks up, especially when the rule has been rather lax already. I don't want to make any scenes. The linen is old and worn. We can see what there is there. Have you the lists? Good. We'll have a look at them."

They went into the bed-chamber and stood a while in silence by the bed; Frau Antonie removed the white cloth from the face of the dead. The Frau Consul was arrayed in the silk garment in which she would that afternoon lie upon her bier in the hall. Twenty-eight hours had passed since she drew her last breath. The mouth and chin, without the false teeth, looked sunken and senile, and the pointed chin projected sharply. All three tried their best to recognize their mother's face in this sunken countenance before them, with its eyelids inexorably closed. But under the old lady's Sunday cap there showed, as in life, the smooth, reddish-brown wig over which the Misses Buddenbrook had so often made merry. Flowers were strewn on the coverlet.

"The most beautiful wreaths have come," said Frau Permaneder. "From all the families in town, simply from everybody. I had everything carried up to the corridor. You must look at them afterwards, Gerda and Tom. They are heart-breakingly lovely."

"How are they progressing down in the hall?" asked the Senator.

"They will soon be done. Tom. Jacobs has taken the greatest pains. And the —" she choked down a sob — "the coffin has come. But you must take off your things, my dears," she went on, carefully replacing the white cloth over the face of the dead. "It is cold in here, but there is a little fire in the breakfast-room. Let me help you, Gerda. Such an elegant mantle, one must be careful with it. Let me give you a kiss — you know I love you, even if you have always despised me. No, I won't make your hair untidy when I take off your hat — Your lovely hair! Such hair Mother had too, when she was young. She was never so splendid as you are, but there was a time, and since I was born, too, when she was really beautiful. How true it is, isn't it, what your old Grobleben always says: we must all return to earth at last: such a simple man, too. Here, Tom. These are the most important lists."

They returned to the next room and sat down at the round table, while the Senator took up the paper, on which was a list of objects to be divided among the nearest heirs. Frau Permaneder's eyes never left her brother's face, and her own wore a strained, excited look. There was something in her mind, a question hard to put, upon which, nevertheless, all her thoughts were bent, and which must, in the next few hours, come up for discussion.

"I think," said the Senator, "we may as well keep to the usual rule, that presents go back; so — "

His wife interrupted him.

"Pardon me, Thomas. It seems to me — where is Christian?"

"Oh, goodness, yes, Christian!" cried Frau Permaneder. "We've forgotten him!"

She went to ring the bell. But at the same moment Christian opened the door. He entered rather quickly, closed it behind him with a slight bang, and stood there frowning, his little deep round eyes not resting on anybody, but rolling from side to side. His mouth opened and shut under the bushy red moustaches. His mood seemed irritated and defiant.

"I heard you were here," he said. "If the things are to be talked about, it is proper that I should be told."

"We were just about to call you," the Senator said indifferently. "Sit down."

His eyes rested, as he spoke, on the white studs in Christian's shirt. He himself was in irreproachable mourning: a black cloth coat, blinding white shirt set off at the collar with a black tie, and black studs instead of the gold ones he usually wore. Christian saw his glance. He drew up a chair to the table and sat down, saying as he did so, with a gesture toward his shirt, "I know I have on white studs. I haven't got round to buying black — or rather, I haven't bothered. In the last few years I've seen times when I had to borrow money for tooth-powder, and go to bed by the light of a match. I don't know that I am altogether and entirely to blame. Anyhow, there are other things in the world more important than black studs. I don't set much store by appearances — I never have."

Gerda looked at him as he spoke, and now she gave a little laugh. The Senator remarked: "I doubt if you could bear out the truth of the last statement."

"No? Perhaps you know better than I do, Thomas. I say I don't set much store by them. I've seen too much of the world, and lived with too many different sorts of men, with too many different ways, to care what — and anyhow, I am a grown man" — his voice grew suddenly loud — "I am forty-three years old, and my own master and in a position to warn everybody not to mix in my affairs."

The Senator was quite astonished. "It seems to me you have something on your mind, my friend," he said. "As far as the studs go, I haven't so much as mentioned them, if my memory serves me. Wear whatever mourning you choose, or none at all if that pleases you; but don't imagine you make any impression on me with your cheap broadmindedness — "

" I am not trying to make an impression on you."

" Tom — Christian! " said Frau Permaneder. " Don't let us have any hard words — not to-day — when in the next room — Just go on, Thomas. Presents are to be returned? That is only right."

And Thomas went on. He began with the large things, and wrote down for himself the articles he could use in his own house: the candelabra in the dining-room, the great carved chest that stood in the downstairs entry. Frau Permaneder paid extraordinarily close attention. No matter what the article was, the future possession of which was at the moment in question, she would say with an incomparable air, " Oh, well, I'm willing to take it " — as if the whole world owed her thanks for her act of self-sacrifice. She accepted for herself, her daughter, and her granddaughter far and away the largest share of the furnishings.

Christian had some pieces of furniture, an Empire table-clock and the harmonium. He seemed satisfied enough. But when they came to dividing the table-linen and silver and the sets of dishes, he displayed, to the great astonishment of the others, an eagerness that was almost avidity.

" What about me? " he would say. " I must ask you not to forget me, please."

" Who is forgetting you? Look: I've put a whole tea-service and a silver tray down to you. I've taken the gilt Sunday service, as we are probably the only ones who would have a use for it."

" I'm willing to take the every-day onion pattern," said Frau Permaneder.

" And what about me? " cried Christian. He was possessed now by that excitement which sometimes seized him and sat so extraordinarily on his haggard cheek. " I certainly want a share in the dishes. And how many forks and spoons do I get? Almost none at all, it seems to me."

" But, my dear man, what do you want of them? You have no use for them at all. I don't understand. It is better the things should continue in the family — "

" But suppose I say I want them — if only in remembrance of Mother," Christian cried defiantly.

To which the Senator impatiently replied, " I don't feel much like making jokes; but am I to judge from your words that you would like to put a soup-tureen on your chest of drawers and keep it there in memory of Mother? Please don't get the idea that we want to cheat you out of your share. If you get less of the effects, you will get more elsewhere. The same is true of the linen."

"I don't want the money. I want the linen and dishes."

"Whatever for?"

Christian's reply to this was one that made Gerda Buddenbrook turn and gaze at him with an enigmatic expression in her eyes. The Senator hastily donned his pince-nez to look the better, and Frau Permaneder simply folded her hands. He said: "Well, I am thinking of getting married, sooner or later."

He said this rather low and quickly, with a short gesture, as though he were tossing something to his brother across the table. Then he leaned back, avoiding their eyes, looking surly, defiant, and yet extremely embarrassed. There was a long pause. At last the Senator broke it by saying:

"I must say, Christian, your ideas come rather late. That is, of course, if this really is anything serious, and not the same kind of thing you proposed to Mother a while ago."

"My intentions have remained what they were," Christian said. He did not look at anybody or change his expression.

"That is impossible, I should think. Were you waiting for Mother's death—?"

"I had that amount of consideration, yes. You seem to think, Thomas, that you have a monopoly of all the tact and feeling in the world—"

"I don't know what justifies you in making remarks like that. And, moreover, I must admire the extent of your consideration. On the day after Mother's death, you propose to display your lack of filial feeling by—"

"Only because the subject came up. But the point is that now Mother cannot be affected by any step I may take—no more today than she would be a year from now. Good Lord, Thomas, Mother couldn't have any actual *right*—but I saw it from her point of view, and had consideration for that, as long as she lived. She was an old woman, a woman of a past generation, with different views about life—"

"I can only say that I concur with her absolutely in this particular view."

"I cannot be bothered about that."

"But you will be bothered about it, my dear sir."

Christian looked at him.

"No," he shouted. "I won't! I can't do it. Suppose I tell you I can't? I must know what I have to do, mustn't I? I am a grown man—"

" You don't in the least know what you have to do. Your being what you call a grown man is only very external."

" I know very well what I have to do. In the first place, I have to act like a man of honour! You don't know how the thing stands. With Tony and Gerda here we can't really talk – but I have already told you I have responsibilities – The last child, little Gisela – "

" I know nothing about any little Gisela – and I don't care to. I am perfectly convinced they are making a fool of you. In any case, what sort of responsibility can you have toward a person like the one you have in mind – other than the legal one, which you can perform as before – ? "

" Person, Thomas, *person?* You are making a mistake about her. Aline – "

" Silence! " roared Senator Buddenbrook in a voice like thunder. The two brothers glared across the table into each other's faces. Thomas was pale and trembling with scorn; the rims of Christian's deep little eyes had got suddenly red, his mouth and eyes spread wide open, his lean cheeks seemed nothing but hollows, and a pair of red patches showed just under the cheek-bones. Gerda looked rather disdainfully from one to the other, and Tony wrung her hands, imploring – " Tom, Christian! And Mother lying there in the next room! "

" You have no sense of shame," went on the Senator. " How can you bring yourself – what must it cost you – to mention that name, on this spot, under these circumstances? You have a lack of feeling that amounts to a disease! "

" Will you tell me why I should not mention Aline's name? " Christian was so beside himself that Gerda looked at him with increasing intentness. " I do mention it, as you hear, Thomas; I intend to marry her – for I have a longing for a home, and for peace and quiet – and I insist – you hear the word I use – I insist that you keep out of my affairs. I am free. I am my own master! "

" Oh, you fool, you! When you hear the will read, you will see just how much you are your own master! You won't get the chance to squander Mother's inheritance as you have run through with the thirty thousand marks already! I have been made the guardian of your affairs, and I will see to it that you never get your hands on more than a monthly sum at a time – that I swear! "

" Well, you know better than I who it was that instigated Mother to make such a will! But I am surprised, very much so, that Mother did not give the office to somebody that had a little more brotherly feeling for me than you have." Christian no longer knew what he was saying; he leaned over the table, knocking on it all the while with his knuckle, glaring up, red-eyed, his moustaches bristling, at his brother, who, on his side, stood looking down at him, pale, and with half-closed lids.

Christian went on, and his voice was hollow and rasping. " Your heart is full of coldness and ill-will toward me, all the while. As far back as I can remember I have felt cold in your presence – you freeze me with a perfect stream of icy contempt. You may think that is a strange expression, but what I feel is just like that. You repulse me, just by looking at me – and you hardly ever even so much as look at me. How have you got a right to treat me like that? You are a man too, you have your own weaknesses. You have always been a better son to our parents; but if you really stood so much closer to them than I do, you might have absorbed a little of their Christian charity. If you have no brotherly love to spare for me, you might have had some Christlike love. But you are entirely without affection. You never came near me in the hospital, when I lay there and suffered with rheumatism – "

" I have more serious things to think about than your illnesses. And my own health – "

" Oh, come, Thomas, your health is magnificent. You wouldn't be sitting here for what you are, if your health weren't far and away better than mine."

" I may be perhaps worse off than you are! "

" Worse than I am – come, that's too much! Gerda, Tony! He says he is worse off than I am. Perhaps it was you that came near dying, in Hamburg, of rheumatism. Perhaps you have had to endure torments in your left side, perfectly indescribable torments, for every little trifling irregularity! Perhaps all your nerves are short on the left side! All the authorities say that is what is the matter with me. Perhaps it happens to you that you come into your room when it is getting dark and see a man sitting on the sofa, nodding at you, when there is no man there? "

" Christian! " Frau Permaneder burst out in horror. " What are you saying? And, my God! what are you quarrelling about? Is it an honour for one to be worse off than the other? If it were, Gerda and I might have something to say, too. – And with Mother lying in there! How can you? "

" Don't you realize, you fool," cried Thomas Buddenbrook, in a passion, " that all these horrors are the consequence and effect of your vices, your idleness, and your self-tormenting? Go to work! Stop petting your condition and talking about it! If you do go crazy – and I tell you plainly I don't think it at all unlikely

– I shan't be able to shed a tear; for it will be entirely your own fault."

"No, and when I die you won't shed any tears either."

"You won't die," said the Senator bitingly.

"I shan't die? Very good, I shan't die, then. We'll see who dies first. Work! Suppose I can't work? My God! I can't do the same thing long at a time! It kills me. If you have been able to, and are able to, thank God for it, but don't sit in judgment on others, for it isn't a virtue. God gives strength to one, and not to another. But that is the way you are made, Thomas. You are self-righteous. Oh, wait, that is not what I am going to say, nor what I accuse you of. I don't know where to begin, and however much I can say is only a millionth part of the feeling I have in my heart against you. You have made a position for yourself in life; and there you stand, and push everything away which might possibly disturb your equilibrium for a moment – for your equilibrium is the most precious thing in the world to you. But it isn't the most precious thing in life, Thomas – no, before God, it is not. You are an egotist, that is what you are. I am still fond of you, even when you are angry, and tread on me, and thunder me down. But when you get silent: when somebody says something and you are suddenly dumb, and withdraw yourself, quite elegant and remote, and repulse people like a wall and leave the other fellow to his shame, without any chance of justifying himself – ! Yes, you are without pity, without love, without humility. – Oh," he cried, and stretched both arms in front of him, palms outward, as though pushing everything away from him, "Oh, how sick I am of all this tact and propriety, this poise and refinement – sick to death of it!"

The outburst was so genuine, so heart-felt, it sounded so full of loathing and satiety, that it was actually crushing. Thomas shrank a little and looked down in front of him, weary and without a word.

At last he said, and his voice had a ring of feeling, "I have become what I am because I did not want to become what you are. If I have inwardly shrunk from you, it has been because I needed to guard myself – your being, and your existence, are a danger to me – that is the truth."

There was another pause, and then he went on, in a crisper tone: "Well, we have wandered far away from the subject. You have read me a lecture on my character – a somewhat muddled lecture, with a grain of truth in it. But we are not talking about me, but about you. You are thinking of marrying; and I should like to convince you that it is impossible for you to carry out your plan. In the first place, the interest I shall be able to pay you on your capital will not be a very encouraging sum — "

" Aline has put some away."

The Senator swallowed, and controlled himself. " You mean you would mingle your mother's inheritance with the — savings of this lady? "

" Yes. I want a home, and somebody who will be sympathetic when I am ill. And we suit each other very well. We are both rather damaged goods, so to speak — "

" And you intend, further, to adopt the existing children and legitimize them? "

" Yes."

" So that after your death your inheritance would pass to them? " As the Senator said this, Frau Permaneder laid her hand on his arm and murmured adjuringly, " Thomas! Mother is lying in the next room! "

" Yes," answered Christian. " That would be the way it would be."

" Well, you shan't do it, then," shouted the Senator, and sprang up. Christian got behind his chair, which he clutched with one hand. His chin went down on his breast; he looked apprehensive as well as angry.

" You shan't do it," repeated Thomas, almost senseless with anger; pale, trembling, jerking convulsively. " As long as I am alive it won't happen. I swear it — so take care! There's enough money gone already, what with bad luck and foolishness and rascality, without your throwing a quarter of Mother's inheritance into this creature's lap — and her bastards' — and that after another quarter has been snapped up by Tiburtius! You've brought enough disgrace on the family already, without bringing us home a courtesan for a sister-in-law, and giving our name to her children. I forbid it, do you hear? I forbid it! " he shouted, in a voice that made the room ring, and Frau Permaneder squeeze herself weeping into the corner of the sofa. " And I advise you not to attempt to defy me! Up to now I have only despised you and ignored you: but if you try any tricks, if you bring the worse to the worst, we'll see who will come out ahead! You can look out for yourself! I shan't have any mercy! I'll have you declared incompetent, I'll get you shut up, I'll ruin you — I'll ruin you, you understand? "

" And I tell *you* — " Thus it all began over again, and went on and on: a battle of words, destructive, futile, lamentable, without any purpose other than to insult, to wound, to cut one another to the quick. Christian came back to his brother's character and cited examples of Thomas's egotism – painful anecdotes out of the distant past, which he, Christian, had never forgotten, but carried about with him to feed his bitterness. And the Senator retorted with scorn, and with threats which he regretted a moment later. Gerda leaned her head on her hand and watched them, with an expression in her eyes impossible to read. Frau Permaneder repeated over and over again, in her despair: "And Mother lying there in the next room!"

Christian, who at the end had been walking up and down in the room, at last forsook the field.

"Very good, we shall see!" he shouted. With his eyes red, his moustaches ruffled, his handkerchief in his hand, his coat wide open, hot and beside himself, he went out of the door and slammed it behind him.

In the sudden stillness the Senator stood for a moment upright and gazed after his brother. Then he sat down without a word and took up the papers jerkily. He went curtly through the remaining business, then leaned back and twisted his moustaches through his fingers, lost in thought.

Frau Permaneder's anxiety made her heart beat loudly. The question, the great question, could now not be put off any longer. It must come up, and he must answer; but was her brother now in a mood to be governed by gentleness and filial piety? Alas, she feared not.

"And – Tom –," she began, looking down into her lap, and then up, as she made a timid effort to read his thoughts. "The furniture – you have taken everything into consideration of course – the things that belong to us, I mean to Erica and me and the little one, they remain here with us? In short, the house – what about it?" she finished, and furtively wrung her hands.

The Senator did not answer at once. He went on for a while twisting his moustaches and drearily meditating. Then he drew a deep breath and sat up.

"The house?" he said. "Of course it belongs to all of us, to you and me, and Christian – and, queerly enough, to Pastor Tiburtius too. I can't decide anything about it by myself. I have to get your consent. But obviously the thing to do is to sell as soon as possible," he concluded, shrugging his shoulders. Yet something crossed his face, after all, as though he were startled by his own words.

Frau Permaneder's head sank deep on her breasts; her hands stopped pressing themselves together; she relaxed all over.

"Our consent," she repeated after a pause, sadly, and rather bitterly as well. "Dear me, Tom, you know you will do whatever you think best — the rest of us are not likely to withhold our consent for long. But if we might put in a word — to beg you," she went on, almost dully, but her lip was trembling too — "the house — Mother's house — the family home, in which we have all been so happy! We must sell it — ?"

The Senator shrugged his shoulders again. "Child, you will believe me when I tell you that I feel everything you can say, as much as you do yourself. But those are only our feelings; they aren't actual objections. What has to be done, remains the problem. Here we have this great piece of property — what shall we do with it? For years back, ever since Father's death, the whole back part has been going to pieces. A family of cats is living rent-free in the billiard-room, and you can't walk there for fear of going through the floor. Of course, if I did not have my house in Fishers' Lane — But I have, and what should I do with it? Do you think I might sell that instead? Tell me yourself, to whom? I should lose half the money I put into it. We have property enough, Tony; we have far too much, in fact. The granary buildings, and two great houses. The invested capital is out of all proportion to the value of the property. No, no, we must sell."

But Frau Permaneder was not listening. She was sitting bent over on the sofa, withdrawn into herself with her own thoughts.

"Our house," she murmured. "I remember the house-warming. We were no bigger than that. The whole family was there. And Uncle Hoffstede read a poem. It is in the family papers. I know it by heart. Venus Anadyomene. The landscape-room. The dining-hall! And strange people — !"

"Yes, Tony. They must have felt the same — the family of whom Grandfather bought the house. They had lost their money and had to give up their home, and they are all dead and gone now. Everything has its time. We ought to be grateful to God that we are better off than the Ratenkamps, and are not saying good-bye to the house under such sorry circumstances as theirs."

Sobs, long, painful sobs, interrupted him. Frau Permaneder so abandoned herself to her grief that she did not even dry the tears that ran down her cheeks. She sat bent over, and the warm drops fell unheeded upon the hands lying limp in her lap.

"Tom," said she, and there was a gentle, touching decision in her voice, which, a moment before her sobs had threatened to choke, "you can't understand how I feel at this hour — you cannot understand your sister's feelings! Things have not gone well with her in this life. — I have had everything to bear that fate could think of to inflict upon me. But I have borne it all without flinching, Tom: all my troubles with Grünlich and Permaneder and Weinschenk. For, however my life seemed to go awry, I was never quite lost. I had always a safe haven to fly to. Even this last time, when everything came to an end, when they took away Weinschenck to prison, 'Mother,' I said, 'may we come to you?' And she said, 'Yes, my children, come!' Do you remember, Tom, when we were little, and played war, there was always a little spot marked off for us to run to, where we could be safe and not be touched until we were rested again? Mother's house, this house, was my little spot, my refuge in life, Tom. And now – it must be sold –"

She leaned back, buried her face in her handkerchief, and wept unrestrainedly.

He drew down one of her hands and held it in his own.

"I know, dear Tony, I know it all. But we must be sensible. Our dear good Mother is gone. We cannot bring her back. And so – It is madness to keep the house as dead capital. Shall we turn it into a tenement-house? I know it is painful to think of strangers living here; but after all it is better you should *not* see it. You must take a nice, pretty little house or flat somewhere for yourself and your family – outside the Castle Gate, for example. Or would you rather stop on here and let out floors to different families? And you still have the family: Gerda and me, and the Buddenbrooks in Broad Street, and the Krögers, and Therese Weichbrodt, and Clothilde – that is, if Clothilde will condescend to associate with us, now that she's become a lady of the Order of St. John – it's so very exclusive, you know!"

She gave a sigh that was already partly a laugh, and mopped her eyes with her handkerchief, looking like a hurt child whom somebody is helping, with a jest, to forget its pain. Then she resolutely cleared her face and put herself to rights, tossing her head with the characteristic gesture and bringing her chin down on her breast.

"Yes, Tom," she said, and blinked with her tear-reddened eyes, "I'll be good now; I am already. You must forgive me – and you too, Gerda – for breaking down like that. But it may happen to any one, you know. It is a weakness. But, believe me, it is only outward. I am a woman steeled by misfortunes. And that about the dead capital is very convincing to me, Tom – I've enough intelligence to understand that much, anyhow. I can only repeat that you must do what you think best. You must think and act for us all; for Gerda and I are only women, and Christian – well, God help him, poor soul! We cannot oppose you, for whatever we could say would be only sentiment, not real objections, it is very plain. To whom will you sell it, Tom? Do you think it will go off right away? "

" Ah, child – how do I know? But I talked a little this morning with old Gosch the broker; he did not seem disinclined to undertake the business."

" That is a good idea, Tom. Siegismund Gosch has his weaknesses, of course. That thing about his translation from the Spanish – I can't remember the man's name, but it is very odd, one must admit. However, he was Father's friend, and he is an honest man through and through. – What shall you ask? A hundred thousand marks would be the least, I should think."

And " A hundred thousand marks would be the least, wouldn't it, Tom? " she was still asking, the door-knob in her hand, as the Senator and his wife went down the steps. Then she was alone, and stood there in the middle of the room with her hands clasped palms down in front of her, looking all around with large, helpless eyes. Her head, heavy with the weight of her thoughts, adorned with the little black lace cap, sank slowly, shaking all the while, deeper and deeper on one shoulder.

CHAPTER III

Little Johann was to go to take his farewell of his grandmother's mortal remains. His father so arranged it, and, though Hanno was afraid, he made not a syllable of objection. At table, the day after the Frau Consul's dying struggle, the Senator, in his son's presence and apparently with design, had commented harshly upon the conduct of Uncle Christian, who had slipped away and gone to bed when the patient's suffering was at its height. "That was his nerves, Thomas," Gerda had answered. But with a glance at Hanno, which had not escaped the child, the Senator had severely retorted that an excuse was not in place. The agony of their departed mother had been so sore that one had felt ashamed even to be sitting there free from pain – not to mention entertaining the cowardly thought of trying to escape any suffering of mind called up by the sight. From which, Hanno had gathered that it would not be safe to object to the visit to the open coffin.

The room looked as strange to him as it had at Christmas, when, on the day before the funeral, between his father and his mother, he entered it from the hall. There was a half-circle of potted plants, arranged alternately with high silver candelabra; and against the dark green leaves gleamed from a black pedestal the marble copy of Thorwaldsen's Christ, which belonged in the corridor outside. Black crape hangings fluttered everywhere in the draught, hiding the sky-blue tapestries and the smiling immortals who had looked down from these walls upon so many festive dinner-tables. Little Johann stood beside the bier among his black-clad relatives. He had a broad mourning band on his own sailor suit, and his senses felt misty with the scent from countless bouquets and wreaths – and with another odour that came wafted now and then on a current of air, and smelled strange, yet somehow familiar.

He stood beside the bier and looked at the motionless white figure stretched out there severe and solemn, amid white satin. This was not Grandmamma. There was her Sunday cap with the white silk ribbons, and her red-brown hair beneath it. But the pinched nose was not hers, nor the drawn lips, nor the sharp chin, nor the yellow, translucent hands, whose coldness and stiffness one could see. This was a wax-doll – to dress it up and lay it out like that seemed rather horrible. He looked across to the landscape-room, as though the real Grandmamma might appear there the next minute. But she did not come: she was dead. Death had turned her for ever into this wax figure that kept its lids and lips so forbiddingly closed.

He stood resting on his left leg, the right knee bent, balancing lightly on the toe, and clutched his sailor knot with one hand, the other hanging down. He held his head on one side, the curly light-brown locks swaying over the temples, and looked with his gold-brown, blue-encircled eyes in brooding repugnance upon the face of the dead. His breath came long and shuddering, for he kept expecting that strange, puzzling odour which all the scent of the flowers sometimes failed to disguise. When the odour came, and he perceived it, he drew his brows still more together, his lip trembled, and the long sigh which he gave was so like a tearless sob that Frau Permaneder bent over and kissed him and took him away.

And after the Senator and his wife, and Frau Permaneder and Erica, had received for long hours the condolences of the entire town, Elisabeth Buddenbrook, born Kröger, was consigned to earth. The out-of-town families, from Hamburg and Frankfort, came to the funeral and, for the last time, received hospitality in Meng Street. And the hosts of the sympathizers filled the hall and the landscape-room, the corridor and the pillared hall; and Pastor Pringsheim of St. Mary's, erect among burning tapers at the head of the coffin, turning his face up to heaven, his hands folded beneath his chin, preached the funeral sermon.

He praised in resounding tones the qualities of the departed: he praised her refinement and humility, her piety and cheer, her mildness and her charity. He spoke of the Jerusalem evenings and the Sunday-school; he gilded with matchless oratory the whole long rich and happy earthly course of her who had left them; and when he came to the end, since the word " end " needed some sort of qualifying adjective, he spoke of her " peaceful end."

Frau Permaneder was quite aware of the dignity, the representative bearing, which she owed to herself and the community in this hour. She, her daughter Erica, and her granddaughter Elisabeth occupied the most conspicuous places of honour, close to the pastor at the head of the coffin; while Thomas, Gerda, Clothilde, and little Johann, as likewise old Consul Kröger, who had a chair to sit in, were content, as were the relatives of the second class, to occupy less prominent places. Frau Permaneder stood there, very erect, her shoulders elevated, her black-bordered handkerchief between her folded hands; and her pride in the chief rôle which it fell to her lot to perform was so great as sometimes entirely to obscure her grief. Conscious of being the focus of all eyes, she kept her own discreetly cast down; yet now and again she could not resist letting them stray over the assembly, in which she noted the presence of Julchen Möllendorpf, born Hagenström, and her husband. Yes, they had all had to come: Möllendorpfs, Kistenmakers, Langhals, Överdiecks – before Tony Buddenbrook left her parental roof for ever, they had all gathered here, to offer her, despite Grünlich, despite Permaneder, despite Hugo Weinschenk, their sympathy and condolences.

Pastor Pringsheim's sermon went on, turning the knife in the wound that death had made: he caused each person present to remember his own dead, he knew how to make tears flow where none would have flowed of themselves – and for this the weeping ones were grateful to him. When he mentioned the Jerusalem evenings, all the old friends of the dead began to sob – excepting Madame Kethelsen, who did not hear a word he said, but stared straight before her with the remote air of the deaf, and the Gerhardt sisters, the descendants of Paul, who stood hand in hand in a corner, their eyes glowing. They were glad for the death of their friend, and could have envied her but that envy and unkindness were foreign to their natures.

Poor Mademoiselle Weichbrodt blew her nose all the time, with a short, emphatic sound. The Misses Buddenbrook did not weep. It was not their habit. Their bearing, less angular than usual, expressed a mild satisfaction with the impartial justice of death.

Pastor Pringsheim's last "amen" resounded, and the four bearers, in their black three-cornered hats, their black cloaks billowing out behind them with the swiftness of their advance, came softly in and put their hands upon the coffin. They were four lackeys, known to everybody, who were engaged to hand the heavy dishes at every large dinner in the best circles, and who drank Möllendorpf's claret out of the carafes, between the courses. But, also, they were indispensable at every funeral of the first or second class, being of large experience in this kind of work. They knew that the harshness of this moment, when the coffin was laid hold upon by strange hands and borne away from the survivors, must be ameliorated by tact and swiftness. Their movements were quick, agile, and noiseless; hardly had any one time to be sensible of the pain of the situation, before they had lifted the burden from the bier to their shoulders, and the flower-covered casket swayed away smoothly and with decorum through the pillared hall.

The ladies pressed tenderly about Frau Permaneder and her daughter to offer their sympathy. They took her hand and murmured, with drooping eyes, precisely no more and no less than what on such occasions must be murmured; while the gentlemen made ready to go down to the carriages.

Then came, in a long, black procession, the slow drive through the grey, misty streets out through the Burg Thor, along the leafless avenue in a cold driving rain, to the cemetery, where the funeral march sounded behind half-bare shrubbery on the edge of the little grove, and the great sandstone cross marked the Buddenbrook family lot. The stone lid of the grave, carven with the family arms, lay close to the black hole framed in dripping greens.

A place had been prepared down below for the new-comer. In the last few days, the Senator had supervised the work of pushing aside the remains of a few early Buddenbrooks. The music sounded, the coffin swayed on the ropes above the open depth of masonry; with a gentle commotion it glided down. Pastor Pringsheim, who had put on pulse-warmers, began to speak afresh, his voice ringing fervid and emotional above the open grave. He bent over the grave and spoke to the dead, calling her by her full name, and blessed her with the sign of the cross. His voice ceased; all the gentlemen held their top-hats in front of their faces with their black-gloved hands; and the sun came out a little. It had stopped raining, and into the sound of the single drops that fell from the trees and bushes there broke now and then the short, fine, questioning twitter of a bird.

All the gentlemen turned a moment to press the hands of the sons and brother of the dead once more.

Thomas Buddenbrook, as the others filed by, stood between his brother Christian and his uncle Justus. His thick dark woollen overcoat was dewed with fine silver drops. He had begun of late to grow a little stout, the single sign of age in his carefully preserved exterior, and his cheeks, behind the pointed protruding ends of his moustaches, looked rounder than they used; but it was a pale and sallow roundness, without blood or life. He held each man's hand a moment in his own, and his slightly reddened eyes looked them all, with weary politeness, in the face.

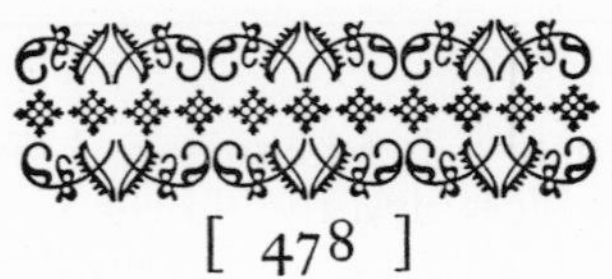

[478]

CHAPTER IV

A WEEK later there sat in Senator Buddenbrook's private office, in the leather chair beside the writing-desk, a little smooth-shaven old man with snow-white hair falling over his brow and temples. He sat in a crouching position, supporting both hands on the white top of his crutch-cane, and his pointed chin on his hands; while he directed at the Senator a look of such malevolence, such a crafty, penetrating glance, that one wondered why the latter did not avoid contact with such a man as this. But the Senator sat apparently at ease, leaning back in his chair, talking to this baleful apparition as to a harmless ordinary citizen. Broker Siegismund Gosch and the head of the firm of Johann Buddenbrook were discussing the price of the Meng Street house.

It took a long time. The offer of twenty-eight thousand thaler made by Herr Gosch seemed too low to the Senator, and the broker called heaven to witness that it would be an act of madness to add a single groschen to the sum. Thomas Buddenbrook spoke of the central position and unusual extent of the property; but Herr Gosch, with picturesque gestures, in low and sibilant tones, expatiated upon the criminal risk he would be running. He waxed almost poetic. Ha! Could his honoured friend tell him when, to whom, for how much, he would be able to get rid of the house again? How often, in the course of the century, would there be a demand for such a house? Perhaps his friend and patron could assure him that to-morrow, on the train from Buchen, there was arriving an Indian nabob who wished to establish himself in the Buddenbrook mansion? He, Siegismund Gosch, would have it on his hands, simply on his hands, and it would be the ruin of him. He would be a beaten man, his race would be run, his grave dug – yes, it would be dug – and, as the phrase enchanted him, he repeated it, and added something more about chattering apes and clods of earth falling upon the lid of his coffin.

But the Senator was not satisfied. He spoke of the ease with which the property could be divided, emphasized his responsibility toward his sister, and remained by the sum of thirty thousand thaler. After which he had to listen, with a mixture of enjoyment and impatience, to a rejoinder from Herr Gosch, which lasted some two hours, during which the broker sounded, as it were, all the registers of his character. He played two rôles at once: first, the hypocritical villain, with a sweet voice, his head on one side, and a smile of open-hearted simplicity. Stretching out his large, white hand, with the long, trembling fingers, he said " Agree, my dear young patron: eighty-four thousand marks – it is the offer of an honest old man." But a child could have seen that this was all lies and treachery – a deceiving mask, behind which the man's deep villainy peeped forth.

Thomas Buddenbrook finally declared that he must take time to think, and that in any case he must consult his sister, before he accepted the twenty-eight thousand thaler – which was unlikely. Then he turned the conversation to indifferent topics and asked Herr Gosch about business and his health.

Things were going badly with Herr Gosch. He made a fine, sweeping gesture to wave away the imputation that he was a prosperous man. The burdens of old age approached, they were at hand even now; as aforesaid, his grave was dug. He could not even carry his glass of grog to his lips without spilling half of it, his arm trembled so like the devil. It did no good to curse. The will no longer availed. And yet – ! He had his life behind him – not such a poor life, after all. He had looked at the world with his eyes open. Revolutions had thundered by, their waves had beat upon his heart – so to speak. Ha! Those were other times, when he had stood at the side of Consul Johann Buddenbrook, the Senator's father, at that historic sitting, and defied the fury of the raging mob. A frightful experience! No, his life had not been poor, either outwardly or inwardly. Hang it – he had been conscious of powers – and as the power is, so is the ideal – as Feuerbach says. And even now – even now, his soul was not impoverished, his heart was still young: it had never ceased, and would never cease, to be capable of great emotions, to live fervently in and for his ideals. They would go with him to his grave. – But were ideals, after all, meant to be realized? No, a thousand times no! We might long for the stars, but should we ever reach them? No, hope, not realization, was the most beautiful thing in life: " L'espérance, tout trompeuse qu'elle est, sert au moins à nous mener à la fin de la vie par un chemin agréable." La Rochefoucauld said that, and it was fine, wasn't it? Oh, yes, his honoured friend and patron, of course, did not need to console himself with that sort of thing. The waves of life had lifted him high on their shoulders, and fortune played about his brow. But for the lonely and submerged, who dreamed alone in the darkness –

Suddenly – " *You* are happy," he said, laying his hand on the Senator's knee, and looking up at him with swimming eyes. " Don't deny it – it would be sacrilege. You are happy. You hold fortune in your arms. You have reached out your strong arms and conquered her – your strong hands," he corrected himself, not liking the sound of " arms " twice so close together. He was silent, and the Senator's deprecating, patient reply went unheard. He seemed to be darkly dreaming for a moment; then he got up.

" We have been chatting," he said, " but we came together on business. Time is money. Let us not waste it in hesitation. Listen to me. Since it is you: since it is you, you understand – " here it almost looked as though Herr Gosch was about to give way again to another rhapsody; but he restrained himself. He made a wide, sweeping gesture, and cried: " Twenty-nine thousand thaler, eighty-seven thousand marks current, for your mother's house! Is it a bargain? " And Senator Buddenbrook agreed.

Frau Permaneder, of course, found the sum ridiculously small. Considering the memories that clung about it, she would have thought a million down no more than an honest price for their old home. But she rapidly adjusted herself – the more readily that her thoughts and efforts were soon taken up by plans for the future.

She rejoiced from the bottom of her heart over all the good furniture that had fallen to her share. And though there was no idea of bustling her away from under the parental roof, she plunged at once, with the greatest zest, into the business of finding and renting a new home. The leave-taking would be hard – the very thought of it brought tears to her eyes. But the prospect of a change was not without its own charm too. It was almost like another setting-out – the fourth one! And so again she looked at houses and visited Jacob's; again she bargained for portières and stair-carpets. And while she did all that, her heart beat faster – yes, even the heart of this old woman who was steeled by the misfortunes of life!

Weeks passed like this: four, five, six weeks. The first snow fell, the stoves crackled. Winter was here again; and the Buddenbrooks began to consider sadly what sort of Christmas feast they should have this year. But now something happened: something surprising and dramatic beyond all words, something that simply knocked you off your feet. Frau Permaneder paused in the midst of her business, like one paralyzed.

"Thomas," she said, "am I crazy? Is Gosch dreaming? It is too absurd, too outlandish – " She held her temples with both her hands. The Senator shrugged his shoulders.

"My dear child, nothing at all is decided yet. But there is the possibility – and if you think it over quietly, you will see that there is nothing so extraordinary about it, after all. It is a little startling, I admit. It gave me a start when Gosch first told me. But absurd? What makes it absurd?"

"I should die," said she. She sat down in a chair and stopped there without moving.

What was going on? Simply that a buyer had appeared for the house; or, rather, a possible purchaser showed a desire to go over it, with a view to negotiations. And this possible purchaser was – Hermann Hagenström, wholesale dealer and Consul for the Kingdom of Portugal.

When the first rumour reached Frau Permaneder, she was stunned, incredulous, incapable of grasping the idea. But when the rumour became concrete, when it actually took shape in the person of Consul Hermann Hagenström, standing, as it were, before the door, then she pulled herself together, and animation came back to her.

"This must not happen, Thomas. As long as I live, it must not happen. When one sells one's house, one is bound to look out for the sort of master it gets. Our Mother's house! Our house! The landscape-room!"

"But what stands in the way?"

"What stands in the way? Heavens, Thomas! Mountains stand in the way – or they ought to! But he doesn't see them, this fat man with the snub nose! He doesn't care about them. He has no delicacy and no feeling – he is like the beasts that perish. From time immemorial the Hagenströms and we have been rivals. Old Hinrich played Father and Grandfather some dirty tricks; and if Hermann hasn't tripped you up yet, it is only because he hasn't had a chance. When we were children, I boxed his ears in the open street, for very good reasons; and his precious little sister Julchen nearly scratched me to pieces for it. That was all childishness, then. But they have always looked on and enjoyed it whenever we had a piece of bad luck – and it was mostly I myself who gave them the pleasure. God willed it so. Whatever the Consul did to injure you or overreach you in a business way, that I can't speak of, Tom. You must know better than I. But the last straw was when Erica made a good marriage and he wormed around and wormed around until he managed to spoil it and get her husband shut up, through his brother, who is a cat! And now they have the nerve – "

"Listen, Tony. In the first place, we have nothing more to say in the matter. We made our bargain with Gosch, and he has the right to deal with whomever he likes. But there is a sort of irony about it, after all – "

"Irony? Well, if you like to call it that – but what I call it is a disgrace, a slap in the face; because that is just what it would be. You don't realize what it would be like, in the least. But it would mean to everybody that the Buddenbrook family are finished and done for: they clear out, and the Hagenströms squeeze into their place, rattlety-bang! No, Thomas, never will I consent to sit by while this goes on. I will never stir a finger in such baseness. Let him come here if he dares. I won't receive him, you may be sure of that. I will sit in my room with my daughter and my granddaughter, and turn the key in the door, and forbid him to enter. – That is just what I will do."

"I know, Tony, you will do what you think best; and you will probably consider well beforehand if it will be wise not to preserve the ordinary social forms. For of course you don't imagine that Consul Hagenström would feel wounded by your conduct? Not in the least, my child. It would neither please nor displease him – he would simply be mildly surprised, that is all. The trouble is, you imagine he has the same feelings toward you that you have toward him. That is a mistake, Tony. He does not hate us in the least. He doesn't hate anybody. He is highly successful and extremely good-natured. As I've told you more than ten times already, he would speak to you on the street with the utmost cordiality if you didn't put on such a belligerent air. I'm sure he is surprised at it – for two minutes; of course not enough to upset the equilibrium of a man to whom nobody can do any harm. What is it you reproach him with? Suppose he has outstripped me in business, and even now and then got ahead of me in some public affair? That only means he is a better business man and a cleverer politician than I am. – There's no reason at all for you to laugh in that scornful way. – But to come back to the house. The truth is, it has lost most of its old significance for us – that has gradually passed over to mine. I say this to console you in advance; on the other hand, it is plain why Consul Hagenström is thinking of buying. These people have come up in the world, their family is growing, they have married into the Möllendorpf family, and become equal to the best in money and position. But so far, there has been something lacking, the outward sign of their position, which they were evidently willing to do without: the historic consecration – the legitimization, so to speak. But now they seem to have made up their minds to have that too; and some of it they will get by moving into a house like this one. You wait and see: mark my words, the Consul will preserve everything as much as possible as it is, he will even keep the 'Dominus providebit' over the door – though, to do him justice, it hasn't been the Lord at all, but Hermann Hagenström himself, single-handed, that has put the family and the firm where they are!"

"Bravo, Tom! Oh, it does me good to hear you say something spiteful about them once in a while! That's really all I want! Oh, if I only had your head! Wouldn't I just give it to him! But there you stand – "

"You see, my head doesn't really do me much good."

"There you stand, I say, with that awful calmness, which I simply don't understand at all, and tell me how Hermann Hagenström does things. Ah, you may talk as you like, but you have a heart in your body, the same as I have myself, and I simply don't believe you feel as calm inside as you make out. All the things you say are nothing but your own efforts to console yourself."

"Now, Tony, you are getting pert. What I *do* is all you have anything to do with – what I think is my own affair."

"Tell me one thing, Tom: wouldn't it be like a nightmare to you?"

"Exactly."

"Like something you dreamed in a fever?"

"Why not?"

"Like the most ridiculous kind of farce?"

"There, there, now, that's enough!"

And Consul Hagenström appeared in Meng Street, accompanied by Herr Gosch, who held his Jesuit hat in his hand, crouched over like a conspirator, and peered past the maid into the landscape-room even while he handed her his card.

Hermann Hagenström looked the City man to the life: an imposing Stock Exchange figure, in a coat the fur of which seemed a foot long, standing open over an English winter suit of good fuzzy yellow-green tweed. He was so uncommonly fat that not only his chin, but the whole lower part of his face, was double – a fact which his full short-trimmed blond beard could not disguise. When he moved his forehead or eyebrows, deep folds came even in the smoothly shorn skin of his skull. His nose lay flatter upon his upper lip than ever, and breathed down into his moustaches.

Now and then his mouth had to come to the rescue and fly open for a deep breath. When it did this it always made a little smacking noise, as the tongue came away from the roof of his mouth.

Frau Permaneder coloured when she heard this once well-known sound. A vision of lemon buns with truffled sausage on top, almost threatened, for a moment, the stony dignity of her bearing. She sat on the sofa, her arms crossed and her shoulders lifted, in an exquisitely fitting black gown with flounces up to the waist, and a dainty mourning cap on her smooth hair. As the two gentlemen entered, she made a remark to her brother the Senator, in a calm, indifferent tone. He had not had the heart to leave her in the lurch at this hour; and he now walked to the middle of the room to meet their guests, while Tony remained on the sofa. He exchanged a hearty greeting with Herr Gosch and a correct and courteous one with the Consul; then Tony rose of her own accord, performed a measured bow to both of them at once, and, without any excess of zeal, associated herself with her brother's invitation to the two gentlemen to be seated.

They all sat down, and the Consul and the broker talked by turns for the next few minutes. Herr Gosch's voice was offensively obsequious as he begged them to pardon the intrusion on their privacy – you could hear a malign undercurrent in it none the less – but Herr Consul Hagenström was anxious to go through the house with a view to possible purchase. And the Consul, in a voice that again called up visions of lemon-bun and goose-liver, said the same thing in different words. Yes, in fact, this was the idea he had in mind and hoped to be able to carry out – provided the broker did not try to drive too hard a bargain with him, ha, ha! He did not doubt but the matter could be settled to the satisfaction of everybody concerned.

His manner was free and easy and like a man of the world's, which did not fail to make a certain impression on Madame Permaneder; the more so that he nearly always turned to her as he spoke. His tone was almost apologetic when he went into detail upon the grounds for his desire to purchase. "Room!" he said. "We need more room. My house in Sand Street – you wouldn't believe it, my dear madam, nor you, Herr Senator, but in fact, it is getting so small we can't turn round in it. I'm not speaking of company. It only takes the family, and the Huneus, and the Möllendorpfs and my brother Moritz's family, and there we are – in fact, packed in like sardines. So, then – well, why should we, you know!"

He spoke in an almost fretful tone, while manner and gestures expressed: " You see for yourselves, there's no reason why I should put up with that sort of thing, when there is plenty of money to do what we like! "

" I thought of waiting," he went on, " till Zerline and Bob should want a house. Then they could take mine, and I could find something larger for myself. But in fact – you know," he interrupted himself, " my daughter Zerline has been engaged to Bob, my brother the attorney's eldest, for years. The wedding won't be put off much longer – two years at most. They are young – so much the better. Well – in fact – why should I wait for them and let slip a good chance when it offers? There would be no sense in that."

Everybody agreed. The conversation paused for a while on the subject of the approaching wedding. Marriages – advantageous marriages – between first cousins were not uncommon in the town, and this one excited no disapproval. The plans of the young pair were inquired into – with reference to the wedding journey. They thought of going to the Riviera, to Nice and so on. That was what they seemed to want to do – and why shouldn't they, you know? The younger children were mentioned, and the Consul spoke of them with easy satisfaction, shrugging his shoulders. He himself had five children, and his brother Moritz had four sons and daughters. Yes, they were all flourishing, thanks. Why shouldn't they be, – you know? In fact, they were all very well. And he came back to the growing up of the family, and to their narrow quarters. " Yes, this is something else entirely," he said. " I've seen that already, on the way upstairs. This house is a pearl, certainly a pearl – if you can compare anything so large with anything so small, ha, ha! Why, even the hangings here – I own up to having had my eye on the hangings all the time I've been talking. A most charming room – in fact. When I think that you have passed all your life in these surroundings – in fact – "

" With some interruptions," said Frau Permaneder, in that extraordinarily throaty voice of which she sometimes availed herself.

" Oh, yes, interruptions," repeated the Consul, with a civil smile. Then he glanced at Senator Buddenbrook and the broker; and, as those gentlemen were in conversation together, he drew up his chair to Frau Permaneder's sofa and leaned toward her, so that she felt his heavy breathing close under her nose. Being too polite to turn away, she sat as stiff and erect as possible and looked down at him under her drooping lids. But he was quite unconscious of her discomfort.

" Let me see, my dear Madame Permaneder," he said. " Seems

to me we've done business together before now. In fact – what was it we were dickering over then? Sweetmeats, wasn't it, or tit-bits of some sort – and now a whole house! "

" I don't remember," said Frau Permaneder. She held her neck as stiff as she could, for his face was really disgustingly, indecently near.

" You don't remember? "

" No, really, I don't remember anything at all about sweetmeats. I have a sort of hazy recollection of lemon-buns, with sausage on top – some disgusting sort of school luncheon – I don't know whether it was yours or mine. We were all children then. – But this matter of the house is entirely Herr Gosch's affair. I have nothing to do with it."

She gave her brother a quick, grateful look, for he had seen her need and come to her rescue by asking if the gentlemen were ready to make the round of the house. They were quite ready, and took temporary leave of Frau Permaneder, expressing the hope of seeing her again when they had finished. The Senator led the two gentlemen out through the dining-room.

He took them upstairs and down, and showed them the rooms in the second storey as well as those on the corridor of the first, and the ground floor, including the kitchen and cellars. As the visit fell in business hours, they refrained from visiting the offices of the Insurance Company. But the new Director was mentioned, and Consul Hagenström declared him to be a very honest chap – a remark which was received by the Senator in silence.

They went through the garden, lying bare and wretched under half-melting snow, looked at the Portal, and returned to the laundry, in the front courtyard; and thence by the narrow paved walk that led between walls to the back courtyard with the oak-tree, and the " back building." Here there was nothing but old age, neglect, and dilapidation. Grass and moss grew between the paving-stones, the steps were in a state of advanced decay, and they could only look into the billiard-room without entering, – the floor was so bad – so the family of cats that lived there rent-free was not disturbed.

Consul Hagenström said very little – he was obviously planning. " Well, yes," he kept saying, as he looked and turned away, suggesting by his manner that in case he bought the house all this would of course be different. He stood, with the same air, on the ground-floor of the back building and looked up at the empty attic. " Yes, well," he repeated, and set in motion the thick, rotting cable with a rusty iron hook on the end that had been hanging there for years. Then he turned on his heel.

"Best thanks for your trouble, Herr Senator," he said. "We're at the end, I suppose." He scarcely uttered a word on the rapid return to the front building, or later when the two gentlemen paid their respects to Frau Permaneder in the landscape-room and the Senator accompanied them down the steps and across the entry. But hardly had they said good-bye and Consul Hagenström turned with his companion to walk down the street, when it was seen that a very lively conversation began at once between the two.

The Senator returned to the room where Frau Permaneder, with her severest manner, sat bolt upright in the window, knitting with two huge wooden needles a black worsted frock for her granddaughter Elisabeth, and now and then casting a glance into the gossip's glass. Thomas walked up and down a while in silence, with his hands in his trousers pockets.

"Yes, we have put it in the broker's hands," he said at length. "We must wait and see what comes of it. My opinion is that he will buy the whole property, live here in the front, and utilize the back part in some other way."

She did not look at him, or change her position, or cease to knit. On the contrary, the needles flew back and forth faster than ever.

"Oh, certainly – of course he'll buy it. He'll buy the whole thing," she said, and it was her throaty voice she used. "Why shouldn't he buy it – you know? In fact, there would be no sense in that at all!"

She raised her eyebrows and looked severely through her pince-nez – which she now used for sewing, but never managed to put on straight – at her knitting-needles. They flew like lightning round and round each other, clacking all the while.

Christmas came: the first Christmas without the Frau Consul. They spent the evening of the twenty-fourth at the Senator's house, without the old Krögers and without the Misses Buddenbrook; for the old children's day had now ceased to exist, and Thomas Buddenbrook did not feel like making presents to everybody who used to attend the Frau Consul's celebration. Only Frau Permaneder and Erica, with little Elisabeth, Christian, Clothilde, and Mademoiselle Weichbrodt, were invited. The latter insisted on holding the customary present-giving on the twenty-fifth, in her own stuffy little rooms, where it was attended with the usual mishap.

There was no troop of poor retainers to receive shoes and woollen underwear, and there were no choir-boys, when they assembled in Fishers' Lane on the twenty-fourth. They joined quite simply together in "Holy Night," and Therese Weichbrodt read the Christmas chapter instead of the Frau Senator, who did not particularly care for such things. Then they went through the suite of rooms into the hall, singing in a subdued way the first stanza of "O Evergreen."

There was no special ground for rejoicing. Nobody's face was beaming with joy, there was no lively conversation. What was there to talk about? They thought of the departed mother, discussed the sale of the house and the well-lighted apartment which Frau Permaneder had rented in a pleasant house outside Holsten Gate, with a view on the green square of Linden Place, and what would happen when Hugo Weinschenk came out of prison. At intervals little Johann played on the piano something which he had been learning with Herr Pfühl, or accompanied his mother, not faultlessly, but with a lovely singing tone, in a Mozart sonata. He was praised and kissed, but had to be taken off to bed by Ida Jungmann, for he was pale and tired on account of a recent stomach upset.

Even Christian was disinclined to talk or joke. After the violent altercation in the breakfast-room he had not let fall another syllable about getting married. He lived on in the old way, on terms with his brother which were not very honourable to himself. He made a brief effort, rolling his eyes about, to awaken sympathy in the company for the misery in his side; went early to the club; and came back to supper, which was held after the prescribed traditions. And then the Buddenbrooks had this Christmas too behind them, and were glad of it.

In the beginning of the year 1872, the household of the deceased Frau Consul was broken up. The servants went, and Frau Permaneder thanked God to see the last of Mamsell Severin, who had continued to question her authority in the most unpleasant manner, and now departed with the silk gowns and linen which she had accumulated. Furniture wagons stood before the door, and the old house was emptied of its contents. The great carved chest, the gilt candelabra, and the other things that had fallen to his share, the Senator took to his house in Fishers' Lane; Christian moved with his into a three-room bachelor apartment near the club; and the little Permaneder-Weinschenk family took possession with theirs of the well-lighted flat in Linden Place, which was after all not without some claims to elegance. It was a pretty little apartment, and the front door of it had a bright copper plate with the name A. Permaneder-Buddenbrook, Widow, in ornamental lettering.

The house in Meng Street was hardly emptied when a host of workmen appeared and began to tear down the back-building; the dust from the old mortar darkened the air. The property had passed into the hands of Consul Hermann Hagenström. He had set his heart upon it, and had outbid an offer which Siegismund Gosch received for it from Bremen. He immediately began to turn it to the best advantage, in the ingenious way for which he had been so long admired. In the spring he moved with his family into the front house, where he left everything almost untouched, save for the necessary renovations and certain very modern improvements. For instance, he had the old bell-pulls taken out and the house fitted throughout with electric bells. And hardly had the back-building been demolished when a new, neat, and airy structure rose in its place, which fronted on Bakers' Alley and was intended for shops and warehouses.

Frau Permaneder had frequently sworn to her brother that no power on earth could bring her ever to look at the parental home again. But it was hardly possible to carry out this threat. Her way sometimes led her of necessity past the shops which had been quickly and advantageously rented, and past the show-windows of the back-building, or the dignified gable front on the other side, where now, beneath the "Dominus Providebit," was to be read the name of Consul Hermann Hagenström. When she saw that, Frau Permaneder, on the open street, before ever so many people, simply began to weep aloud. She put back her head like a bird beginning to sing, pressed her handkerchief to her eyes, uttered a wail of mingled protest and lament, and, giving no heed to the passers-by or to the remonstrances of her daughter, gave her tears free vent.

They were the unashamed, refreshing tears of her childhood, which she still retained despite all the storms and shipwrecks of her life.

PART TEN

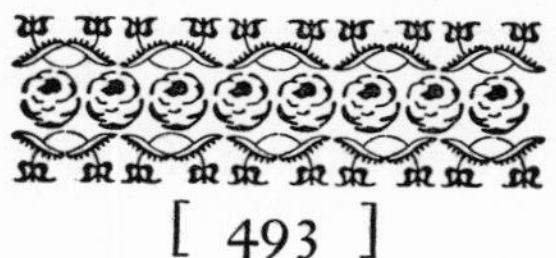

CHAPTER I

OFTEN, in an hour of depression, Thomas Buddenbrook asked himself what he was, or what there was about him to make him think even a little better of himself than he did of his honest, limited, provincial fellow-burghers. The imaginative grasp, the brave idealism of his youth was gone. To work at his play, to play at his work, to bend an ambition that was half-earnest, half-whimsical, toward the accomplishment of aims that even to himself possessed but a symbolic value – for such blithe scepticism and such an enlightened spirit of compromise, a great deal of vitality is necessary, as well as a sense of humour. And Thomas Buddenbrook felt inexpressibly weary and disgusted.

What there was in life for him to reach, he had reached. He was well aware that the high-water mark of his life – if that were a possible way to speak of such a commonplace, humdrum sort of existence – had long since passed.

As for money matters, his estate was much reduced and the business, in general, on the decline. Counting his mother's inheritance and his share of the Meng Street property, he was still worth more than six hundred thousand marks. But the working capital of the firm had lain fallow for years, under the penny wise policies of which the Senator had complained at the time of the affair of the Pöppenrade harvest. Since the blow he had then received, they had grown worse instead of better; until now, at a time when prospects were brighter than ever – when everybody was flushed with victory, the city had at last joined the Customs Union, and small retail firms all over the country were growing within a few years into large wholesale ones – the firm of Johann Buddenbrook rested on its oars and reaped no advantage from the favourable time. If the head of the firm were asked after his business, he would answer, with a deprecating wave of the hand, "Oh, it's not much good, these days." As a lively rival, a close friend of the Hagenströms, once put it, Thomas Buddenbrook's function on 'Change was now largely decorative! The jest had for its point a jeer at the Senator's carefully preserved and faultless exterior –

and it was received as a masterpiece of wit by his fellow-citizens.

Thus the Senator's services to the old firm were no longer what they had been in the time of his strength and enthusiasm; while his labours for the good of the community had at the same time reached a point where they were circumscribed by limitations from without. When he was elected to the Senate, in fact, he had reached those limitations. There were thereafter only places to keep, offices to hold, but nothing further that he could achieve: nothing but the present, the narrow reality; never any grandiose plans to be carried out in the future. He had, indeed, known how to make his position and his power mean more than others had made them mean in his place: even his enemies did not deny that he was "the Burgomaster's right hand." But Burgomaster himself Thomas Buddenbrook could never become. He was a merchant, not a professional man; he had not taken the classical course at the gymnasium, he was not a lawyer. He had always done a great deal of historical and literary reading in his spare time, and he was conscious of being superior to his circle in mind and understanding, in inward as well as outward culture; so he did not waste much time in lamenting the lack of external qualifications which made it impossible for him to succeed to the first place in his little community. "How foolish we were," he said to Stephan Kistenmaker – but he really only meant himself by "we" – "that we went into the office so young, and did not finish our schooling instead." And Stephan Kistenmaker answered: "You're right there. But how do you mean?"

The Senator now chiefly worked alone at the great mahogany writing-desk in his private office. No one could see him there when he leaned his head on his hand and brooded, with his eyes closed. But he preferred it, also, because the hair-splitting pedantries of Herr Marcus had become unendurable to him. The way the man for ever straightened his writing-materials and stroked his beard would in itself have driven Thomas Buddenbrook from his seat in the counting-room. The fussiness of the old man had increased with the years to a positive mania; but what made it intolerable to the Senator was the fact that of late he had begun to notice something of the same sort in himself. He, who had once so hated all smallness and pettiness, was developing a pedantry which seemed to him the outgrowth of anybody else's character rather than his own.

He was empty within. There was no stimulus, no absorbing task into which he could throw himself. But his nervous activity, his inability to be quiet, which was something entirely different from his father's natural and permanent fondness for work, had not lessened, but increased – it had indeed taken the upper hand and become his master. It was something artificial, a pressure on the nerves, a depressant, in fact, like the pungent little Russian cigarettes which he was perpetually smoking. This craving for activity had become a martyrdom; but it was dissipated in a host of trivialities. He was harassed by a thousand trifles, most of which had actually to do with the upkeep of his house and his wardrobe; small matters which he could not keep in his head, over which he procrastinated out of disgust, and upon which he spent an utterly disproportionate amount of time and thought.

What outsiders called his vanity had lately increased in a way of which he was himself ashamed, though he was without the power to shake off the habits he had formed. Nowadays it was nine o'clock before he appeared to Herr Wenzel, in his nightshirt, after hours of heavy, unrefreshing sleep; and quite an hour and a half later before he felt himself ready and panoplied to begin the day, and could descend to drink his tea in the first storey. His toilette was a ritual consisting of a succession of countless details which drove him half mad: from the cold douche in the bathroom to the last brushing of the last speck of dust off his coat, and the last pressure of the tongs on his moustache. But it would have been impossible for him to leave his dressing-room with the consciousness of having neglected a single one of these details, for fear he might lose thereby his sense of immaculate integrity – which, however, would be dissipated in the course of the next hour and have to be renewed again.

He saved in everything, so far as he could – without subjecting himself to gossip. But he did not save where his clothes were concerned – he still had them made by the best Hamburg tailor, and spared no expense in the care and replenishing of his wardrobe. A spacious cabinet, like another room, was built into the wall of his dressing-room; and here, on long rows of hooks, on wooden hangers, were coats, smoking jackets, frock-coats, evening clothes, clothes for all occasions, all seasons, and all grades of formality; the carefully creased trousers were arranged on chairs beneath. The top of his chest of drawers was covered with combs, brushes, and toilet preparations for hair and beard; while within it was the supply of body linen of all possible kinds, which was constantly changed, washed, worn out, and renewed.

He spent in this dressing-room not only the early hours of each morning, but also a long time before every dinner, every sitting of the Senate, every public appearance – in short, before every occasion on which he had to show himself among his fellow men – even before the daily dinner with his wife, little Johann, and Ida Jungmann. And when he left it, the fresh underwear on his body, the faultless elegance of his clothing, the smell of the brilliantine on his moustache, and the cool, astringent taste of the mouth-wash he used – all this gave him a feeling of satisfaction and adequacy, like that of an actor who has adjusted every detail of his costume and make-up and now steps out upon the stage. And, in truth, Thomas Buddenbrook's existence was no different from that of an actor – an actor whose life has become one long production, which, but for a few brief hours for relaxation, consumes him unceasingly. In the absence of any ardent objective interest, his inward impoverishment oppressed him almost without any relief, with a constant, dull chagrin; while he stubbornly clung to the determination to be worthily representative, to conceal his inward decline, and to preserve "the *dehors*" whatever it cost him. All this made of his life, his every word, his every motion, a constant irritating pretence.

And this state of things showed itself by peculiar symptoms and strange whims, which he observed with surprise and disgust. People who have no rôle to perform before the public, who do not conceive themselves as acting a part, but as standing unobserved to watch the performance of others, like to stand with the light at their backs. But Thomas Buddenbrook could not endure the feeling of standing in the shadow while the light streamed full upon the faces of those whom he wished to impress. He wanted his audience, before whom he was to act the rôle of a social light, a public orator, or a representative business man, to stand before him in a confused and shadowy mass while a blinding light played upon his own face. Only this gave him a feeling of separation and safety, an intoxicating sense of self-production, which was the atmosphere in which he achieved success. It had come to be the case that precisely this intoxication was the most bearable condition he knew. When he stood up at table, wine-glass in hand, to reply to a toast, with his charming manner, easy gestures, and witty turns of phrase, which struck unerringly home and released waves of merriment down the length of the table, then he might feel, as well as seem, the Thomas Buddenbrook of former days. It was much harder to keep the mastery over himself when he was sitting idle. For then his weariness and disgust rose up within him, clouded his eyes, relaxed his bearing and his facial muscles. At such times, he was possessed by one desire: to steal away, to be alone, to lie in silence, with his head resting on a cool pillow.

Frau Permaneder had dined that evening in Fishers' Lane. She was the only guest, for her daughter, who was to have gone, had visited her husband that afternoon in the prison, and felt, as she usually did, exhausted and incapable of further effort. So she had stayed at home.

Frau Antonie had spoken at table of the mental condition of her son-in-law, which, it appeared, was very bad; and the question arose whether one might not, with some hope of success, petition the Senate for a pardon. After dinner the three relatives sat in the living-room, at the round table beneath the great gas-lamp. The Frau Senator bent her lovely face over some embroidery, and the gas-light lit up gleams in her dark hair; Frau Permaneder, with careful fingers, fastened an enormous red satin bow on to a tiny yellow basket, intended as a birthday present for a friend. Her glasses were stuck absolutely awry and useless on her nose. The Senator sat with his legs crossed, partly turned away from the table, in a large upholstered easy-chair, reading the paper; he drew in the smoke of his Russian cigarette and let it out again in a light grey stream between his moustaches.

It was a warm summer Sunday evening. The lofty window was open, and the lifeless, rather damp air flowed into the room. From where they sat at the table they could look between the grey gables of intervening houses at the stars and the slowly moving clouds. There was still light in Iwersen's little flower-shop across the way. Further on in the quiet street a concertina was being played with a good many false notes, probably by the son of Dankwart the driver. But sometimes the street was noisy with a troop of sailors, singing, smoking, arm in arm, going, no doubt, from one doubtful waterside public-house to another still more doubtful one, and obviously in a jovial mood. Their rough voices and swinging tread would die off down a cross-street.

The Senator laid down his newspaper, put his glasses in his waistcoat pocket, and rubbed his hand over his eyes and forehead.

"Feeble – very feeble indeed, this paper," he said. "I always think when I read it of what Grandfather used to say about a dish that had no particular taste or consistency: it tastes as if you were hanging your tongue out of the window. One, two, three, and you've finished with the whole stupid thing."

"You are certainly right about that, Tom," said Frau Permaneder, letting fall her work and looking at her brother sidewise, past her glasses but not through them. "What is there in it? I've always said, ever since I was a mere slip of a girl, that this town paper is a wretched sheet! I read it too, of course, for want of a better one; but it isn't so very thrilling to hear that wholesale dealer Consul So-and-so is going to celebrate his silver wedding! We ought to read other papers: the *Königsberg Gazette*, or the *Rhenish Gazette;* then we'd – "

She interrupted herself. She had taken up the paper as she spoke, and let her eye run contemptuously down the columns. But her glance was arrested by a short notice of four or five lines, which she read through, clutching her eye-glasses, her mouth slowly opening. Then she uttered two shrieks, with the palms of her hands pressed against her cheeks, and her elbows held out straight.

" Oh, impossible – impossible! Imagine your not seeing that at all. It is frightful! Oh, *poor* Armgard! It had to come to her like that! "

Gerda had lifted her head from her work, and Thomas, startled, looked at his sister. Much upset, Frau Permaneder read the notice aloud, in a guttural, portentous tone. It came from Rostock, and it said that, the night before, Herr Ralf von Maiboom, owner of the Pöppenrade estate, had committed suicide by shooting himself with a revolver, in the study of the manor-house. " Pecuniary difficulties seem to have been the cause of the act. Herr von Maiboom leaves a wife and three children." She finished and let the paper fall in her lap, then leaned back and looked at her brother and sister with wide, piteous eyes.

Thomas Buddenbrook had turned away while he listened, and looked past his sister between the portières, into the dark salon.

" With a revolver? " he asked, after silence had reigned some two minutes. And then, after another pause, he said in a low voice, slowly and mockingly: " That is the nobility for you! "

Then he fell again to musing, and the rapidity with which he drew the ends of his moustaches through his fingers was in remarkable contrast to the vacant fixity of his gaze. He did not listen to the lamentations of his sister, or to her speculations on what poor Armgard would do now. Nor did he notice that Gerda, without turning her head in his direction, was fixing him with a searching and steady gaze from her close-set, blue-shadowed eyes.

CHAPTER II

THOMAS BUDDENBROOK did not contemplate the future of little Johann with the weary dejection which was now his settled mood when he thought about his own life and his own end. The family feeling which led him to cherish the past history of his house extended itself even more strongly into its future; and he was influenced, too, by the loving and expectant curiosity concentrated upon his son by his family and his friends and acquaintances, even by the Buddenbrook ladies in Broad Street. He said to himself that, however hopeless and thwarted he himself felt, he was still, wherever his son was concerned, capable of inexhaustible streams of energy, endurance, achievement, success – yes, that at this one spot his chilled and artificial life could still be warmed into a genuine and glowing warmth of hopes and fears and affections.

Perhaps, some day, it would be granted to him to look back upon his past from a quiet corner and watch the renascence of the old time, the time of Hanno's great-grandfather! Was such a hope, after all, entirely vain? He had felt that the music was his enemy; but it had almost begun to look as if it had no such important bearing upon the situation. Granted that the child's fondness for improvising, without notes, was evidence of a not quite common gift; in the systematic lessons with Herr Pfühl he had not showed by any means extraordinary progress. The preoccupation with music was no doubt due to his mother's influence; and it was not surprising that during his early years this influence had been preponderant. But the time was close at hand when it would be the father's turn to influence his son, to draw him over to his side, to neutralize the feminine influence by introducing a masculine one in its place. And the Senator determined not to let any such opportunities pass without improving them.

Hanno was now eleven years old. The preceding Easter, he had, by the skin of his teeth and by dint of two extra examinations in mathematics and geography, been passed into the fourth form – as had likewise his young friend Count Mölln. It had been settled that he should attend the mercantile side of the school –

for it went without saying that he would be a merchant and take over the family business. When his father asked him if he felt any inclination toward his future career, he answered yes — a simple, unadorned, embarrassed " yes," which the Senator tried to make a little more convincing by asking leading questions, but mostly without success.

If the Senator had had two sons, he would assuredly have allowed the second to go through the gymnasium and study. But the firm demanded a successor. And, besides, he was convinced he was doing the boy a kindness in relieving him of the unnecessary Greek. He was of opinion that the mercantile course was the easier to master, and that Hanno would therefore come through with greater credit and less strain if he took it, considering his defects — his slowness of comprehension, his absent, dreaming ways, and his physical delicacy, which often obliged him to be absent from school. If little Johann Buddenbrook were to achieve the position in life to which he was called, they must be mindful before everything else, by care and cherishing on the one hand, by sensible toughening on the other, to strengthen his far from robust constitution.

Hanno had grown sturdier in the past year; but, despite his blue sailor suit, he still looked a little strange in the playground of the school, by contrast with the blond Scandinavian type that predominated there. He now wore his brown hair parted on the side and brushed away from his white forehead. But it still inclined to fall in soft ringlets over the temples; and his eyes were as golden-brown as ever, and as veiled with their brown lashes. His legs, in long black stockings, and his arms, in the loose quilted blue sleeves of his suit, were small and soft like a girl's, and he had, like his mother, the blue shadows under his eyes. And still, in those eyes, especially when they gave a side glance, as they often did, there was that timid and defensive look; while the mouth closed with the old, woebegone expression which he had had even as a baby, or went slightly crooked when he explored the recesses of his mouth for a defective tooth. And there would come upon his face when he did this a look as if he were cold.

Dr. Langhals had now entirely taken over Dr. Grabow's practice and had become the Buddenbrook family physician. From him they learned the reason why the child's skin was so pale and his strength so inadequate. It seemed that Hanno's organism did not produce red corpuscles in sufficient number. But there was a remedy for this defect: cod-liver oil, which, accordingly, Dr. Langhals prescribed in great quantities: good, thick, greasy, yellow cod-liver oil, to be taken from a porcelain spoon twice a day. The Senator gave the order, and Ida Jungmann, with stern affection, saw it carried out. In the beginning, to be sure, Hanno threw up after each spoonful. His stomach seemed to have a prejudice against the good cod-liver oil. But he got used to it in the end — and if you held your breath and chewed a piece of rye bread immediately after, the nausea was not so severe.

His other troubles were all consequent upon this lack of red corpuscles, it appeared: secondary phenomena, Dr. Langhals called them, looking at his fingernails. But it was necessary to attack these other enemies ruthlessly. As for the teeth, for these Herr Brecht and his Josephus lived in Mill Street: to take care of them, to fill them; when necessary, to extract them. And for the digestion there was castor-oil, thick, clear castor-oil that slipped down your throat like a lizard, after which you smelled and tasted it for three days, sleeping and waking. Oh, why were all these remedies of such surpassing nastiness? One single time — Hanno had been rather ill, and his heart action had shown unusual irregularity — Dr. Langhals had with some misgiving prescribed a remedy which little Hanno had actually enjoyed, and which had done him a world of good. These were arsenic pills. But however much he asked to have the dose repeated — for he felt almost a yearning for these sweet, soothing little pills — Dr. Langhals never prescribed them again.

Castor-oil and cod-liver oil were excellent things. But Dr. Langhals was quite at one with the Senator in the view that they could not of themselves make a sound and sturdy citizen of little Johann if he did not do his part. There was gymnasium drill once a week in the summer, out on the Castle Field, where the youth of the city were given the opportunity to develop their strength and courage, their skill and presence of mind, under the guidance of Herr Fritsche, the drill-master. But to his father's annoyance, Hanno showed a distinct distaste for the manly sports — a silent, pronounced, almost haughty opposition. Why was it that he cared so little for playmates of his own class and age, with whom he would have to live, and was for ever sticking about with this little unwashed Kai, who was a good child, of course, but not precisely a proper friend for the future? Somehow or other a boy must know from the beginning how to gain the confidence and respect of his comrades, upon whose good opinion of him he will be dependent for the rest of his life! There were, on the other hand, the two sons of Consul Hagenström, two fine strapping boys, twelve and fourteen years old, strong and full of spirits, who instituted prizefights in the neighbouring woods, were the best gymnasts in the school, swam like otters, smoked cigars, and were ready for any devilry. They were popular, feared, and respected. Their cousins, the two sons of Dr. Moritz Hagenström, the State Attorney, were of a more delicate build, and gentler ways. They distinguished themselves in scholarship, and were model pupils: zealous, industrious, quiet, attentive, devoured by the ambition to bring home a report card marked "Number 1." They achieved their ambition, and were respected by their stupider and lazier colleagues. But – not to speak of his masters – what must his fellow-pupils think of Hanno, who was not only a very mediocre scholar, but a weakling into the bargain; who tried to get out of everything for which a scrap of courage, strength, skill, and energy were needed? When Senator Buddenbrook passed the little balcony on his way to his dressing-room, he would hear from Hanno's room, which was the middle one of the three on that floor since he had grown too large to sleep with Ida Jungmann, the notes of the harmonium, or the hushed and mysterious voice of Kai, Count Mölln telling a story.

Kai avoided the drill classes, because he detested the discipline which had to be observed there. "No, Hanno," he said, "I'm not going. Are you? Deuce take it! Anything that would be any fun is forbidden." Expressions like "deuce take it" he got from his father. Hanno answered: "If Herr Fritsche ever one single day smelled of anything but beer and sweat, I might consider it. Don't talk about it, Kai. Go on. Tell that one about the ring you got out of the bog – you didn't finish it." "Very good," said Kai. "But when I nod, then you must play." And he went on with his story.

If he was to be believed, he had once, on a warm evening, in a strange, unrecognizable region, slid down a slippery, immeasurable cliff, at the foot of which, by the flickering, livid light from will-o'-the-wisps, he saw a black marsh, from which silvery bubbles mounted with a hollow gurgling sound. One of these bubbles, which kept coming up near the bank, took the form of a ring when it burst; and he had succeeded in seizing it, after long and dangerous efforts – after which it burst no more, but remained in his grasp, a firm and solid ring, which he put on his finger. He rightly ascribed unusual powers to this ring; for by its help he climbed up the slippery cliff and saw, a little way off in the rosy mist, a black castle. It was guarded to the teeth, but he had forced an entrance, always by the help of the ring, and performed miracles of rescue and deliverance. All this Hanno accompanied with sweet chords on his harmonium. Sometimes, if the difficulties were not too great, these stories were acted in the marionette theatre, to musical accompaniment. But Hanno attended the drill class only on his father's express command – and then Kai went too.

It was the same with the skating in the wintertime, and with the bathing in summer at the wooden bathing establishment of Herr Asmussen, down on the river. "Bathing and swimming – let the boy have bathing and swimming – he must bathe and swim," Dr. Langhals had said. And the Senator was entirely of the same opinion. But Hanno had a reason for absenting himself from the bathing, as well as from the skating and the drill class. The two sons of Consul Hagenström, who took part in all such exercises with great skill and credit, singled Hanno out at once. And though they lived in his own grandmother's house, that fact did not prevent them from making his life miserable. They lost no opportunity of tormenting him. At drill they pinched him and derided him. They rolled him in the dirty snow at the ice-rink; and in the water they came up to him with horrid noises. Hanno did not try to escape. It would have been useless anyhow. He stood, with his girlish arms, up to his middle in the turbid water of the pool, which had large patches of duck-weed growing on it, and awaited his tormentors with a scowl – a dark look and twisted lips. They, sure of their prey, came on with long splashing strides. They had muscular arms, these two young Hagenströms, and they clutched him round his body and ducked him – ducked him a good long time, so that he swallowed rather a lot of the dirty water and gasped for breath a long time after. One single time he was a little avenged. One afternoon the two Hagenströms were holding him down under the water, when one of them suddenly gave a shriek of pain and fury and lifted his plump leg, from which drops of blood were oozing. Beside him rose the head of Kai, Count Mölln, who had somehow got hold of the price of admission, swum up invisible in the water, and bitten young Hagenström – bitten with all his teeth into his leg, like a furious little dog. His blue eyes flashed through the red-blond hair that hung down wet all over his face. He paid richly for the deed, did the little Count, and left the swimming-pool much the worse for the encounter. But Consul Hagenström's son limped perceptibly when he went home.

Nourishing remedies and physical exercise were the basis of the treatment calculated to turn Senator Buddenbrook's son into a strong and healthy lad. But no less painstakingly did the Senator strive to influence his mind and give him lively impressions of the practical world in which he was to live.

He began gradually to introduce him into the sphere of his future activities. He took him on business expeditions down to the harbour and let him stand by on the quay while he spoke to the dockers in a mixture of Danish and dialect or gave orders to the men who with hollow, long-drawn cries were hauling up the sacks to the granary floor. He took him into dark little warehouse offices to confer with superintendents. All this life of the harbours, ships, sheds, and granaries, where it smelled of butter, fish, seawater, tar, and greasy iron, had been to Thomas Buddenbrook from childhood up the most fascinating thing on earth. But his son gave no spontaneous expression of his own enchantment with the sight; and so the father was fain to arouse it in him. "What are the names of the boats that ply to Copenhagen? The *Naiad*, the *Halmstadt*, the *Friederike Överdieck* – why, if you know those, my son, at least that's something! You'll soon learn the others. Some of those people over there hauling up the grain have the same name as you – they were named after your grandfather, as you were. And their children are often named after me – or Mamma. We give them little presents every year. – Now this next granary – we don't stop at it; we go past and don't talk to the men; it is a rival business."

"Should you like to come, Hanno?" he said another time. "There is a ship of our line being launched to-day, and I shall christen it. Do you want to go?" And Hanno signified that he wanted to go. He went with his father, listened to his speech, and saw him break a bottle of champagne on the prow of the ship; saw how she glided down the ways, which had been smeared with green soap, and into the water.

On certain days of the year, as New Year's and Palm Sunday, when there were confirmations, Senator Buddenbrook drove out on a round of visits to particular houses in which he had social relations. His wife did not like these visits, and excused herself on the ground of headache and nervousness, so Hanno would be asked to go along in her place; and here, too, he signified his desire to go. He climbed into the carriage beside his father, and sat silent by his side in the reception-rooms, watching his easy, tactful, assured, and carefully graduated manner toward their hosts. He heard District Commander Colonel Herr von Rinnlingen tell his father how greatly he appreciated the honour of his visit, and saw how his father, in reply, put on an air of amiable depreciation and laid his arm an instant across the Colonel's shoulders. In another place the same remark was made, and he received it with quiet seriousness, and in a third with an ironically exaggerated compliment in return.

All this with a floridity of speech and gesture which he obviously liked to produce for the admiration of his son, and from which he promised himself the most edifying results.

But the little boy saw more than he should have seen; the shy, gold-brown, blue-shadowy eyes observed too well. He saw not only the unerring charm which his father exercised upon everybody: he saw as well, with strange and anguished penetration, how cruelly hard it was upon him. He saw how his father, paler and more silent after each visit, would lean back in his corner of the carriage with closed eyes and reddened eyelids; he realized with a sort of horror that on the threshold of the next house a mask would glide over his face, a galvanized activity take hold of the weary frame. Thus the visits, the social intercourse with one's kind, instead of giving little Johann, quite simply, the idea that one has practical interests in common with one's fellow men, which one looks after oneself, expecting others to do the same, appeared to him like an end in themselves; instead of straightforward and single-minded participation in the common business, he saw his father perform an artificial and complicated part, by dint of a fearful effort and an exaggerated, consuming virtuosity. And when he thought that some day he should be expected to perform the same part, under the gaze of the whole community, Hanno shut his eyes and shivered with rebellion and disgust.

Ah, that was not the effect Thomas Buddenbrook looked for from the influence of his own personality upon his son's! What he had hoped to do was to stimulate self-confidence in the boy, and a sense of the practical side of life. This was what he had in mind — and nothing else.

"You seem to enjoy good living, my boy," said he, when Hanno asked for a second portion of the sweet or a half-cup of coffee after dinner. "Well, then, you must become a merchant and earn a lot of money. Should you like to do that?" Little Johann said he would.

Sometimes when the family were invited to dinner, Aunt Antonie or Uncle Christian would begin to tease Aunt Clothilde and imitate her meek, drawling accents. Then little Johann, stimulated by the heavy red wine which they gave him, would ape his elders and make some remarks to Aunt Clothilde in the same vein. And then how Thomas Buddenbrook would laugh! He would give a loud, hearty, jovial roar, like a man put in high spirits by some unexpected piece of good luck, and join in on his son's side against poor Aunt Clothilde, though for his own part he had long since given up these witticisms at the expense of his poor relative. It was so easy, so safe, to tease poor, limited, modest, lean and hungry Clothilde, that, harmless though it was, he felt it rather beneath him. But he wished he did not, for it was the same story over again: too many considerations, too many scruples. Why must he be for ever opposing these scruples against the hard, practical affairs of life? Why could he never learn that it was possible to grasp a situation, to see around it, as it were, and still to turn it to one's own advantage without any feeling of shame? For precisely this, he said to himself, is the essence of a capacity for practical life!

And thus, how happy, how delighted, how hopeful he felt whenever he saw even the least small sign in little Johann of a capacity for practical life!

CHAPTER III

The extended summer trip which had once been customary with the Buddenbrooks had now been given up for some years. Indeed, when the Frau Senator, in the previous spring, had wished to make her old father in Amsterdam a visit and play a few duets with him, the Senator had given his consent rather curtly. But it had become the rule for Gerda, little Johann, and Fräulein Jungmann to spend the holidays at the Kurhouse, in Travemünde, for the sake of Hanno's health.

Summer holidays at the seashore! Did anybody really understand the joy of that? After the dragging monotony and worry of the endless school terms came four weeks of peaceful, care-free seclusion, full of the good smell of sea-weed and the whispering of the gentle surf. Four weeks! At the beginning it seemed endless; you could not believe that it would end; it was almost indelicate to suggest such a thing! Little Johann could not comprehend the crudity of a master who could say: "After the holidays we shall take up our work at —" this or that point! After the holidays! He appeared to be already rejoicing in the thought, this strange man in the shiny worsted suit! After the holidays! What a thought! And how far, far off in the grey distance lay everything that was on the other side of the holidays, on the other side of those four weeks!

The inspection of the school report, with its record of examinations well or badly got through, would be at last over, and the journey in the overcrowded carriage. Hanno would wake the first morning in his room at the Kurhouse, in one of the Swiss cottages that were united by a small gallery to the main building and the pastry-shop. He would have a vague feeling of happiness that mounted in his brain and made his heart contract. He would open his eyes and look with eager pleasure at the old-fashioned furniture of the cleanly little room. A moment of dazed and sleepy bliss: then he would be conscious that he was in Travemünde — for four immeasurable weeks in Travemünde. He did not stir. He lay on his back in the narrow yellow wooden bed, the linen of which was extremely thin and soft with age. He even shut his eyes again and felt his chest rising in deep, slow breaths of happy anticipation.

The room lay in yellow daylight that came in through the striped blind. Everything was still – Mamma and Ida Jungmann were asleep. Nothing was to be heard but a measured, peaceful sound which meant that the man was raking the gravelled paths of the Kurgarten below, and the buzzing of a fly that had got between the blind and the window and was storming the pane – you could see his shadow shooting about in long zigzag lines. Peace! Only the sound of the rake and the dull buzzing noise. This gently animated quiet filled little Johann with a priceless sensation: the feeling of quiet, well-cared-for, elegant repose which was the atmosphere of the resort, and which he loved better than anything else. Thank God, none of the shiny worsted coats who were the chosen representatives of grammar and the rule of three on this earth was in the least likely to come here – for here it was rather exclusive and expensive.

An access of joy made him spring up and run barefoot to the window. He put up the blind and unfastened the white-painted hook of the window; and as he opened it the fly escaped and flew away over the flower-beds and the gravelled paths. The music pavilion, standing in a half-circle of beech-trees opposite the main building, was still empty and quiet. The Leuchtenfield, which took its name from the lighthouse that stood on it, somewhere off to the right, stretched its extent of short sparse grass under the pale sky, to a point where the grass passed into a growth of tall, coarse water-plants; and then came the sand, with its rows of little wooden huts and tall wicker beach-chairs looking out to the sea. It lay there, the sea, in peaceful morning light, striped blue and green; and a steamer came in from Copenhagen, between the two red buoys that marked its course, and one did not need to know whether it was the *Naiad* or the *Friederike Överdieck*. Hanno Buddenbrook drew in a deep, quiet, blissful breath of the spicy air from the sea and greeted her tenderly, with a loving, speechless, grateful look.

Then the day began, the first of those paltry twenty-eight days, which seemed in the beginning like an eternity of bliss, and which flew by with such desperate haste after the first two or three. They breakfasted on the balcony or under the great chestnut tree near the children's playground, where the swing hung. Everything – the smell of the freshly washed table-cloth when the waiter shook it out, the tissue paper serviettes, the unaccustomed bread, the eggs they ate out of little metal cups, with ordinary spoons instead of bone ones like those at home — all this, and everything, enchanted little Johann.

And all that followed was so easy and care-free — such a wonderfully idle and protected life. There was the forenoon on the beach, while the Kurhouse band gave its morning programme; the lying and resting at the foot of the beach-chair, the delicious, dreamy play with the soft sand that did not make you dirty, while you let your eyes rove idly and lose themselves in the green and blue infinity beyond. There was the air that swept in from that infinity — strong, free, wild, gently sighing and deliciously scented; it seemed to enfold you round, to veil your hearing and make you pleasantly giddy, and blessedly submerge all consciousness of time and space. And the bathing here was a different affair altogether from that in Herr Asmussen's establishment. There was no duck-weed here, and the light green water foamed away in crystalline clearness when you stirred it up. Instead of a slimy wooden floor there was soft sand to caress the foot — and Consul Hagenström's sons were far away, in Norway or the Tyrol. The Consul loved to make an extended journey in the holidays, and — why shouldn't he?

A walk followed, to warm oneself up, along the beach to Seagull Rock or Ocean Temple, a little lunch by the beach-chair; then the time came to go up to one's room for an hour's rest, before making a toilette for the table-d'hôte. The table-d'hôte was very gay, for this was a good season at the baths, and the great dining-room was filled with acquaintances of the Buddenbrooks, Hamburg families, and even some Russians and English people. A black-clad gentleman sat at a tiny table and served the soup out of a silver tureen. There were four courses, and the food tasted nicer and more seasoned than that at home, and many people drank champagne. These were the single gentlemen who did not allow their business to keep them chained in town all the week, and who got up some little games of roulette after dinner: Consul Peter Döhlmann, who had left his daughter at home, and told such extremely funny stories that the ladies from Hamburg laughed till their sides ached and they begged him for mercy; Senator Dr. Cremer, the old Superintendent of Police; Uncle Christian, and his friend Dr. Gieseke, who was also without his family, and paid everything for Uncle Christian. After dinner, the grown-ups drank coffee under the awnings of the pastry-shop, and the band played, and Hanno sat on a chair close to the steps of the pavilion and listened unwearied. He was settled for the afternoon. There was a shooting-gallery in the Kurgarten, and at the right of the Swiss cottage were the stables, with horses and donkeys, and the cows whose foaming, fragrant milk one drank warm every evening. One could go walking in the little town or along the front; one could go out to the Prival in a boat and look for amber on the beach, or play croquet in the children's playground, or listen to Ida Jungmann reading aloud, sitting on a bench on the wooded hillside where hung the great bell for the table-d'hôte. But best of all was it to go back to the beach and sit in the twilight on the end of the breakwater, with your face turned to the open horizon. Great ships passed by, and you signalled them with your handkerchief; and you listened to the little waves slapping softly against the stones; and the whole space about you was filled with a soft and mighty sighing. It spoke so benignly to little Johann! it bade him close his eyes, it told him that all was well. But just then Ida would say, " Come, little Hanno. It's supper-time. We must go. If you were to sit here and go to sleep, you'd die." How calm his heart felt, how evenly it beat, after a visit to the sea! Then he had his supper in his room – for his mother ate later, down in the glass verandah – and drank milk or malt extract, and lay down in his little bed, between the soft old linen sheets, and almost at once sleep overcame him, and he slept, to the subdued rhythm of the evening concert and the regular pulsations of his quiet heart.

On Sunday the Senator appeared, with the other gentlemen who had stopped in town during the week, and remained until Monday morning. Ices and champagne were served at the table-d'hôte, and there were donkey-rides and sailing-parties out to the open sea. Still, little Johann did not care much for these Sundays. The peaceful isolation of the bathing-place was broken in upon. A crowd of townsfolk – good middle-class trippers, Ida Jungmann called them – populated the Kurgarten and crowded the beach, drank coffee and listened to the music. Hanno would have liked to stay in his room until these kill-joys in their Sunday clothes went away again. No, he was glad when everything returned to its regular course on Monday – and he felt relieved to feel his father's eyes no more upon him.

Two weeks had passed; and Hanno said to himself, and to every one who would listen to him, that there was still as much time left as the whole of the Michaelmas holidays amounted to. It consoled him to say this, but after all it was a specious consolation, for the crest of the holidays had been reached, and from now on they were going downhill – so quickly, so frightfully quickly, that he would have liked to cling to every moment, not to let it escape; to lengthen every breath he drew of the sea-air; to taste every second of his joy.

But the time went on, relentless: in rain and sun, sea-wind and land-wind, long spells of brooding warmth and endless noisy storms that could not get away out to sea and went on for ever so long. There were days on which the north-east wind filled the bay with dark green floods, covered the beach with seaweed, mussels, and jelly-fish, and threatened the bathing-huts. The turbid, heavy sea was covered far and wide with foam. The mighty waves came on in awful, awe-inspiring calm, and the under side of each was a sharp metallic green; then they crashed with an ear-splitting roar, hissing and thundering along the sand. There were other days when the west wind drove back the sea for a long distance, exposing a gently rolling beach and naked sand-banks everywhere, while the rain came down in torrents. Heaven, earth, and sea flowed into each other, and the driving wind carried the rain against the panes so that not drops but rivers flowed down, and made them impossible to see through. Then Hanno stayed in the salon of the Kurhouse and played on the little piano that was used to play waltzes and schottisches for the balls and was not so good for improvising on as the piano at home: still one could sometimes get amusing effects out of its muffled and clacking keys. And there were still other days, dreamy, blue, windless, broodingly warm, when the blue flies buzzed in the sun above the Leuchtenfield, and the sea lay silent and like a mirror, without stir or breath. When there were only three days left Hanno said to himself, and to everybody else, that the time remaining was just as long as Whitsuntide holiday; but, incontestable as this reckoning was, it did not convince even himself. He knew now that the man in the worsted coat was right, and that they would, in very truth, begin again where they had left off, and go on to this and that.

The laden carriage stood before the door. The day had come. Early in the morning Hanno had said good-bye to sea and strand. Now he said it to the waiters as they received their fees, to the music pavilion, the rose-beds, and the whole long summer as well. And amid the bows of the hotel servants the carriage drove off.

They passed the avenue that led to the little town, and rolled along the front. Ida Jungmann sat, white-haired, bright-eyed, and angular, opposite Hanno on the back seat, and he squeezed his head into the corner and looked past her out of the window. The morning sky was overcast; the Trave was full of little waves that hurried before the wind. Now and then rain-drops spattered the pane. At the farther end of the front, people sat before their house doors and mended nets; barefoot children ran past, and stared inquisitively at the occupants of the carriage. *They* did not need to go away!

As they left the last houses behind, Hanno bent forward once more to look after the lighthouse; then he leaned back and closed his eyes. " We'll come back again next year, darling," Ida Jungmann said in her grave, soothing voice. It needed only that to make Hanno's chin tremble and the tears run down beneath his long dark lashes.

His face and hands were brown from the sea air. But if his stay at the baths had been intended to harden him, to give him more resistance, more energy, more endurance, then it had failed of its purpose; and Hanno himself was aware of this lamentable fact. These four weeks of sheltered peace and adoration of the sea had not hardened him: they had made him softer than ever, more dreamy and more sensitive. He would be no better able to endure the rigours of Herr Tietge's class. The thought of the rules and history dates which he had to get by heart had not lost its power to make him shudder; he knew the feeling too well, and how he would fling them away in desperation and go to bed, and suffer next day the torments of the unprepared. And he would be exactly as much afraid of catastrophes at the recitation hour, of his enemies the Hagenströms, and of his father's injunctions not to be faint-hearted whatever else he was.

But he felt cheered a little by the fresh morning drive through flooded country roads, amid the twitterings of birds. He thought of seeing Kai again, and Herr Pfühl; of his music lessons, the piano and his harmonium. And as the morrow was Sunday, a whole day still intervened between him and the first lesson-hour. He could feel a few grains of sand from the beach, still inside his buttoned boot—how lovely! He would ask old Grobleben to leave them there. Let it all begin again—the worsted-coats, the Hagenströms, and the rest. He had what he had. When the waves of tribulation went over him once more he would think of the sea and of the Kurgarten, and of the sound made by the little waves, coming hither out of the mysterious slumbering distance. One single memory of the sound they made as they splashed against the breakwater could make him oppose an invincible front to all the pains and penalties of his life.

Then came the ferry, and Israelsdorfer Avenue, Jerusalem Hill, and the Castle Field, on the right side of which rose the walls of the prison where Uncle Weinschenk was. Then the carriage rolled along Castle Street and over the Koberg, crossed Broad Street, and braked down the steep decline of Fishers' Lane. There was the red house-front with the bow-window and the white caryatides; and as they went from the midday warmth of the street into the coolness of the stone-flagged entry the Senator, with his pen in his hand, came out of the office to greet them.

Slowly, slowly, with secret tears, little Johann learned to live without the sea; to lead an existence that was frightened and bored by turns; to keep out of the way of the Hagenströms; to console himself with Kai and Herr Pfühl and his music.

The Broad Street Buddenbrooks and Aunt Clothilde, directly they saw him again, asked him how he liked school after the holidays. They asked it teasingly, with that curiously superior and slighting air which grown people assume toward children, as if none of their affairs could possibly be worthy of serious consideration; but Hanno was proof against their questions.

Three or four days after the home-coming, Dr. Langhals, the family physician, appeared in Fishers' Lane to observe the results of the cure. He had a long consultation with the Frau Senator, and then Hanno was summoned and put, half undressed, through a long examination of his "status praesens," as Dr. Langhals called it, looking at his fingernails. He tested Hanno's heart action and measured his chest and his lamentable muscular development. He inquired particularly after all his functions, and lastly, with a hypodermic syringe, took a drop of blood from Hanno's slender arm to be tested at home. He seemed, in general, not very well satisfied.

"We've got rather brown," he said, putting his arm around Hanno as he stood before him. He arranged his small black-felled hand upon the boy's shoulder, and looked up at the Frau Senator and Ida Jungmann. "But we still look very down in the mouth."

"He is homesick for the sea," said Gerda Buddenbrook.

"Oh, so you like being there?" asked Dr. Langhals, looking with his shallow eyes into Hanno's face. Hanno coloured. What did Dr. Langhals mean by his question, to which he plainly expected an answer? A fantastic hope rose up in him, inspired by the belief that nothing was impossible to God – despite all the worsted-coated men there were in the world.

"Yes," he brought out, with his wide eyes full upon Dr. Langhals' face. But after all, it seemed, the physician had nothing particular in mind when he asked the question.

"Well, the effect of the bathing and the good air is bound to show itself in time," Dr. Langhals said. He tapped little Johann on the shoulder and then put him away, with a nod toward the

Frau Senator and Ida Jungmann – a superior, benevolent nod, the nod of the omniscient physician, used to have people hanging on his lips. He got up, and the consultation was at an end.

It was Aunt Antonie who best understood his yearning for the sea, and the wound in his heart that healed so slowly and was so likely to bleed afresh under the strain of everyday life. Aunt Antonie loved to hear him talk about Travemünde, and entered freely into his longings and enthusiasm.

" Yes, Hanno," she said, " the truth is the truth, and Travemünde is and always will be a beautiful spot. Till I go down to my grave I shall remember the weeks I spent there when I was a slip of a girl – and such a silly young girl! I lived with people I was fond of, and who seemed to care for me; I was a pretty young thing in those days, – though I'm an old woman now – and full of life and high spirits. They were splendid people, I can tell you, respectable and kind-hearted and straight-thinking; and they were cleverer and better educated, too, than any I've known since, and they had more enthusiasm. Yes, my life seemed very full when I lived with them, and I learned a great deal which I've never forgotten – information, beliefs, opinions, ways of looking at things. If other things hadn't interfered – as all sorts of things did, the way life does, you know – I might have learned a great deal more from them. Shall I tell you how silly I was in those days? I thought I could get the pretty star out of the jelly-fish, and I carried a quantity home with me and spread them in the sun on the balcony to dry. But when I looked at them again, of course there was nothing but a big wet spot, and a smell of rotten sea-weed."

CHAPTER IV

In the beginning of the year 1873 the Senate pardoned Hugo Weinschenk, and the former Director left prison, six months before his time was up.

Frau Permaneder, if she had told the truth, would have admitted that she was not so very glad. She had been living peacefully with her daughter and granddaughter in Linden Place, and had for society the house in Fishers' Lane and her friend Armgard von Maiboom, who had lived in the town since her husband's death. Frau Antonie had long been aware that there was no place for her outside the walls of her native city. She had her Munich memories, her weak digestion, and an increasing need of quiet and repose; and she felt not the least inclination to move to a large city of the united Fatherland, still less to migrate to another country.

"My dear child," she said to her daughter, "I must ask you something very serious. Do you still love your husband with your whole heart? Would you follow him with your child wherever he went in the wide world – as, unfortunately, it is not possible for him to remain here?"

And Frau Erica Weinschenk, amid tears that might have meant anything at all, replied just as dutifully as Tony herself, in similar circumstances, had once replied to the same question, in the villa outside Hamburg. So it was necessary to contemplate a parting in the near future.

On a day almost as dreadful as the day when he had been arrested, Frau Permaneder brought her son-in-law from the prison, in a closed carriage, to her house in Linden Place. And there he stayed, after he had greeted his wife and child in a dazed, helpless way, in the room that had been prepared for him, smoking from early to late, without going out, without even taking his meals with his family – a broken grey-haired man.

He had always had a very strong constitution, and the prison life could hardly have impaired his physical health. But his condition was, none the less, pitiable in the extreme. This man had in all probability done no more than his business colleagues did every day and thought nothing of; if he had not been caught, he would have gone on his way with head erect and conscience clear. Yet it was dreadful to see how his ruin as a citizen, the judicial correction, and the three years' imprisonment, had operated to break down his morale. His testimony before the court had been given with the most sincere conviction; and people who understood the technicalities of the case supported his contention that he had merely executed a bold manœuvre for the credit of his firm and himself — a manœuvre known in the business world as usance. The lawyers who had convicted him knew, in his opinion, nothing whatever about such things and lived in quite a different world. But their conviction, endorsed by the governing power of the state, had shattered his self-esteem to such a degree that he could not look anybody in the face. Gone was his elastic tread, the way he had of wriggling at the waist of his frock-coat and balancing with his fists and rolling his eyes about. Gone was the ignorant self-assurance with which he had delivered his uninformed opinions and put his questions. The change was such that his family shuddered at it — and indeed it was frightful to see such cowardice, dejection, and lack of self-respect.

Herr Hugo Weinschenk spent eight or ten days doing nothing but smoking: then he began to read the papers and write letters. The consequence of the letters was that after another eight or ten days he explained vaguely that there seemed to be a position for him in London, whither he wished to travel alone to arrange matters personally, and then to send for wife and child.

Accompanied by Erica, he drove to the station in a closed carriage and departed without having once seen any other members of the family.

Some days later a letter addressed to his wife arrived from Hamburg. It said that he had made up his mind not to send for his wife and child, or even to communicate with them, until such time as he could offer them a life fitting for them to live. And this letter was the very last sign of life from Hugo Weinschenk. No one from then henceforward heard anything from him. The experienced Frau Permaneder made several energetic attempts to get into touch with him, in order, as she importantly explained, to get evidence upon which to sue him for divorce on the ground of wilful desertion. But he was, and remained, missing. And thus it came about that Erica Weinschenk and her small daughter Elisabeth remained now, as before, with Erica's mother, in the light and airy apartment in Linden Place.

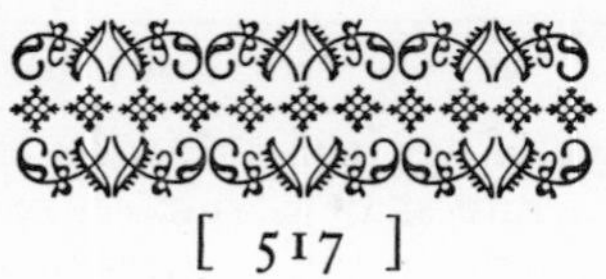

CHAPTER V

THE MARRIAGE of which little Johann had been the issue had never lost charm in the town as a subject for conversation. Since both of the parties to it were still felt to have something queer about them, the union itself must partake of that character of the strange and uncanny which they each possessed. To get behind it even a little, to look beneath the scanty outward facts to the bottom of this relation, seemed a difficult, but certainly a stimulating task. And in bedrooms and sitting-rooms, in clubs and casinos, yes, even on 'Change itself, people still talked about Gerda and Thomas Buddenbrook.

How had these two come to marry, and what sort of relationship was theirs? Everybody remembered the sudden resolve of Thomas Buddenbrook eighteen years ago, when he was thirty years old. "This one or no one," he had said. It must have been something of the same sort with Gerda, for it was well known that she had refused everybody up to her twenty-seventh year, and then forthwith lent an ear to this particular wooer. It must have been a love match, people said: they granted that the three hundred thousand thaler had probably not played much of a rôle. But of that which any ordinary person would call love, there was very little to be seen between the pair. They had displayed from the very beginning a correct, respectful politeness, quite extraordinary between husband and wife. And what was still more odd it seemed not to proceed out of any inner estrangement, but out of a peculiar, silent, deep mutual knowledge. This had not at all altered with the years. The one change due to the passage of time was an outward one. It was only this: that the difference in years began to make itself plainly visible.

When you saw them together you felt that here was a rapidly aging man, already a little heavy, with his young wife at his side. Thomas Buddenbrook was going off very much, and this despite the now almost laughable vanity by which he kept himself up. On the other hand, Gerda had scarcely altered in these eighteen years. She seemed to be, as it were, conserved in the nervous coldness which was the essence of her being. Her lovely dark red hair had kept its colour, the white skin its smooth texture, the figure its lofty aristocratic slimness. In the corners of her rather too small and close-set brown eyes were the same blue shadows. You could not trust those eyes. Their look was strange, and what was written in it impossible to decipher. This woman's personality was so cool, so reserved, so repressed, so distant, she showed so little human warmth for anything but her music – how could one help feeling a vague mistrust? People unearthed wise old saws on the subject of human nature and applied them to Senator Buddenbrook's wife. Still waters were known to run deep. Some people were slyer than foxes. And as they searched for an explanation, their limited imaginations soon led them to the theory that the lovely Gerda was deceiving her aging husband.

They watched, and before long they felt sure that Gerda's conduct, to put it mildly, passed the bounds of propriety in her relations with Herr Lieutenant von Throta.

Renée Maria von Throta came from the Rhineland. He was second lieutenant of one of the infantry battalions quartered in the town. The red collar of his uniform went well with his black hair, which he wore parted on the side and combed back in a high, thick curling crest from his white forehead. He looked big and strong enough, but was most unmilitary in speech and manner. He had a way of running one hand in between the buttons of his half-open undress coat and of sitting with his head supported on the back of his hand. His bows were devoid of military stiffness, and you could not hear his heels click together as he made them. And he had no more respect for his uniform than for ordinary clothes. Even the slim youthful moustaches that ran slantwise down to the corners of his mouth had neither point nor consistency; they only confirmed the unmartial impression he gave. The most remarkable thing about him was his eyes, so large, black, and extraordinarily brilliant that they seemed like glowing bottomless depths when he visited anything or anybody with his glance which was sparkling, ardent, or languishing by turns.

He had probably gone into the army against his will, or at least without any inclination for it; and despite his physique he was no good in the service. He was unregarded by his comrades, and shared but little in their interests – the interests and pleasures of young officers lately back from a victorious campaign. And they found him a disagreeable oddity, who did not care for horses or hunting or play or women. All his thoughts were bent on music. He was to be seen at all the concerts, with his languishing eyes and his lax, unmilitary, theatrical attitudes; on the other hand he despised the club and the casino and never went near them.

He made the duty calls which his position demanded; but the Buddenbrook house was the only one at which he visited — too much, people thought, and the Senator himself thought so too.

No one dreamed what went on in Thomas Buddenbrook. No one must guess. But it was just this keeping everybody in ignorance of his mortification, his hatred, his powerlessness, that was so cruelly hard! People were beginning to find him a little ludicrous; but perhaps their laugh would have turned to pity if they had even dimly suspected how much he was on his guard against their laughter! He had seen it coming long before, he had felt it beforehand, before any one else had such an idea in his head. His much-carped-at vanity had its source largely in this fear. He had been first to see, with dismay, the growing disparity between himself and his lovely wife, on whom the years had not laid a finger. And now, since the advent of Herr von Throta, he had to fight with the last remnant of his strength to dissimulate his own misgivings, in order that they might not make him a laughing-stock in the eyes of the community.

Gerda Buddenbrook and the eccentric young officer met each other, naturally, in the world of music. Herr von Throta played the piano, violin, viola, cello, and flute, and played them all unusually well. Often the Senator became aware of an impending visit when Herr von Throta's man passed the office-door with his master's cello-case on his back. Thomas Buddenbrook would sit at his desk and watch until he saw his wife's friend enter the house. Then, overhead in the salon, the harmonies would rise and surge like waves, with singing, lamenting, unearthly jubilation; would lift like clasped hands outstretched toward Heaven; would float in vague ecstasies; would sink and die away into sobbing, into night and silence. But they might roll and seethe, weep and exult, foam up and enfold each other, as unnaturally as they liked! They were not the worst. The worst, the actually torturing thing, was the silence. It would sometimes reign so long, so long, and so profoundly, above there in the salon, that it was impossible not to feel afraid of it. There would be no tread upon the ceiling, not even a chair would move — simply a soundless, speechless, deceiving, *secret* silence. Thomas Buddenbrook would sit there, and the torture was such that he sometimes softly groaned.

What was it that he feared? Once more people had seen Herr von Throta enter his house. And with their eyes he beheld the picture just as they saw it: Below, an aging man, worn out and crotchety, sat at his window in the office; above, his beautiful wife made music with her lover. *And not that alone.* Yes, that was the way the thing looked to them. He knew it. He was aware, too, that the word "lover" was not really descriptive of Herr von Throta. It would have been almost a relief if it were. If he could have understood and despised him as an empty-headed, ordinary youth who worked off his average endowment of high spirits in a little music, and thus beguiled the feminine heart! He tried to think of him like that. He tried to summon up the instincts of his father to meet the case: the instincts of the thrifty merchant against the frivolous, adventurous, unreliable military caste. He called Herr von Throta "the lieutenant," and tried to think of him as that; but in his heart he was conscious that the name was inappropriate.

What was it that Thomas Buddenbrook feared? Nothing – nothing to put a name to. If there had only been something tangible, some simple, brutal fact, something to defend himself against! He envied people the simplicity of their conceptions. For while he sat there in torments, with his head in his hands, he knew all too well that "betrayal," "adultery," were not words to describe the singing things, the abysmally silent things, that were happening up there.

He looked up sometimes at the grey gables, at the people passing by, at the jubilee present hanging above his desk with the portraits of his forefathers: he thought of the history of his house, and said to himself that this was all that was wanting: that his person should become a byword, his name and family life a scandal among the people. This was all that was lacking to set the crown upon the whole. And the thought, again, almost did him good, because it was a simple, comprehensible, normal thought, that one could think and express – quite another matter from this brooding over a mysterious disgrace, a blot upon his family 'scutcheon.

He could bear it no more. He shoved back his chair, left the office, and went upstairs. Whither should he go? Into the salon, to be greeted with unembarrassed slight condescension by Herr von Throta, to ask him to supper and be refused? For one of the worst features of the case was that the lieutenant avoided him, refused all official invitations from the head of the house, and confined himself to the free and private intercourse with its mistress.

Should he wait? Sit down somewhere, perhaps in the smoking-room, until the lieutenant went, and then go to Gerda and speak out, and call her to account? Ah, one did not speak out with Gerda, one did not call her to account. Why should one? Their alliance was based on mutual consideration, tact, and silence. To become a laughing-stock before her, too – no, surely he was not called upon to do that. To play the jealous hsuband would be to grant that outsiders were right, to proclaim a scandal, to cry it aloud. Was he jealous? Of whom? Of what? Alas, no! Jealousy – the word meant action: mistaken, crazy, wrong action, perhaps, but at least action, energetic, fearless, and conclusive. No, he only felt a slight anxiety, a harassing worry, over the whole thing.

He went into his dressing-room and bathed his face with eau-de-cologne. Then he descended to the music-room, determined to break the silence there, cost what it would. He laid his hand on the door-knob – but now the music struck up again with a stormy outburst of sound, and he shrank back.

One day in such an hour, he was leaning over the balcony of the second floor, looking down the well of the staircase. Everything was quite still. Little Johann came out of his room, down the gallery steps, and across the corridor, on his way to Ida Jungmann's room. He slipped along the wall with his book, and would have passed his father with lowered eyes, and a murmured greeting; but the Senator spoke to him.

"Well, Hanno, and what are you doing?"

"Studying my lessons, Papa. I am going to Ida, to have her hear my translation –"

"Well, and what do you have to-morrow?"

Hanno, still looking down, made an obvious effort to give a prompt, alert, and correct answer to the question. He swallowed once and said, "We have Cornelius Nepos, some accounts to copy, French grammar, the rivers of North America, German theme-correcting –"

He stopped and felt provoked with himself; he could not remember any more, and wished he had said *and* and let his voice fall, it sounded so abrupt and unfinished. "Nothing else," he said as decidedly as he could, without looking up. But his father did not seem to be listening. He held Hanno's free hand and played with it absently, unconsciously fingering the slim fingers.

And then Hanno heard something that had nothing to do with the lessons at all: his father's voice, in a tone he had never heard before, low, distressed, almost imploring: "Hanno – the lieutenant has been more than two hours with Mamma –"

Little Hanno opened wide his gold-brown eyes at the sound; and they looked, as never before, clear, large, and loving, straight into his father's face, with its reddened eyelids under the light brows, its white puffy cheeks and long stiff moustaches. God knows how much he understood. But one thing they both felt: in the long second when their eyes met, all constraint, coldness, and misunderstanding melted away. Hanno might fail his father in all that demanded vitality, energy and strength. But where fear and suffering were in question, there Thomas Buddenbrook could count on the devotion of his son. On that common ground they met as one.

He did not realize this – he tried not to realize it. In the days that followed, he urged Hanno on more sternly than ever to practical preparations for his future career. He tested his mental powers, pressed him to commit himself upon the subject of his calling, and grew irritated at every sign of rebellion or fatigue. For the truth was that Thomas Buddenbrook, at the age of forty-eight, began to feel that his days were numbered, and to reckon with his own approaching death.

His health had failed. Loss of appetite, sleeplessness, dizziness, and the chills to which he had always been subject forced him several times to call in Dr. Langhals. But he did not follow the doctor's orders. His will-power had grown flabby in these years of idleness or petty activity. He slept late in the morning, though every evening he made an angry resolve to rise early and take the prescribed walk before breakfast. Only two or three times did he actually carry out the resolve; and it was the same with everything else. And the constant effort to spur on his will, with the constant failure to do so, consumed his self-respect and made him a prey to despair. He never even tried to give up his cigarettes; he could not do without the pleasant narcotic effect; he had smoked them from his youth up. He told Dr. Langhals to his vapid face: "You see, Doctor, it is your duty to forbid me cigarettes – a very easy and agreeable duty. But I have to obey the order – that is my share, and you can look on at it. No, we will work together over my health; but I find the work unevenly divided – too much of yours falls to me. Don't laugh; it is no joke. One is so frightfully alone – well, I smoke. Will you have one?" He offered his case.

All his powers were on the decline. What strengthened in him was the conviction that it could not last long, that the end was close at hand. He suffered from strange apprehensive fancies. Sometimes at table it seemed to him that he was no longer sitting with his family, but hovering above them somewhere and looking down upon them from a great distance. "I am going to die," he said to himself. And he would call Hanno to him repeatedly and say: "My son, I may be taken away from you sooner than you think. And then you will be called upon to take my place. I was called upon very young myself. Can you understand that I am troubled by your indifference? Are you now resolved in your mind? Yes? Oh, ' yes ' is no answer! Again you won't answer me! What I ask you is, have you resolved, bravely and joyfully, to take up your burden? Do you imagine that you won't have to work, that you will have enough money without? You will have nothing, or very, very little; you will be thrown upon your own resources. If you want to live, and live well, you will have to work hard, harder even than I did."

But this was not all. It was not only the burden of his son's future, the future of his house, that weighed him down. There was another thought that took command, that mastered him and spurred on his weary thoughts. And it was this: As soon as he began to think of his mortal end not as an indefinite remote event, almost a contingency, but as something near and tangible for which it behoved him to prepare, he began to investigate himself, to examine his relations to death and questions of another world. And his earliest researches in this kind discovered in himself an irremediable unpreparedness.

His father had united with his hard practical sense a literal faith, a fanatic Bible-Christianity which his mother, in her latter years, had adhered to as well; but to himself it had always been rather repellent. The worldly scepticism of his grandfather had been more nearly his own attitude. But the comfortable superficiality of old Johann could not satisfy his metaphysical and spiritual needs, and he ended by finding in evolution the answer to all his questions about eternity and immortality. He said to himself that he had lived in his forbears and would live on in his descendants. And this line which he had taken coincided not only with his sense of family, his patrician self-consciousness, his ancestor-worship, as it were; it had also strengthened his ambitions and through them the whole course of his existence. But now, before the near and penetrating eye of death, it fell away; it was nothing, it gave him not one single hour of calm, of readiness for the end.

Thomas Buddenbrook had played now and then throughout his life with an inclination to Catholicism. But he was at bottom, none the less, the born Protestant: full of the true Protestant's passionate, relentless sense of personal responsibility. No, in the ultimate things there was, there could be, no help from outside, no mediation, no absolution, no soothing-syrup, no panacea. Each one of us, alone, unaided, of his own powers, must unravel the riddle before it was too late, must wring for himself a pious readiness before the hour of death, or else part in despair. Thomas Buddenbrook turned away, desperate and hopeless, from his only son, in whom he had once hoped to live on, renewed and strong, and began in fear and haste to seek for the truth which must somewhere exist for him.

It was high summer of the year 1874. Silvery, high-piled clouds drifted across the deep blue sky above the garden's dainty symmetry. The birds twittered in the boughs of the walnut tree, the fountain splashed among the irises, and the scent of the lilacs floated on the breeze, mingled, alas, with the smell of hot syrup from a sugar-factory nearby. To the astonishment of the staff, the Senator now often left his work during office hours, to pace up and down in the garden with his hands behind his back, or to work about, raking the gravel paths, tying up the rose-bushes, or dredging mud out of the fountain. His face, with its light eyebrows, seemed serious and attentive as he worked; but his thoughts travelled far away in the dark on their lonely, painful path.

Sometimes he seated himself on the little terrace, in the pavilion now entirely overgrown with green, and stared across the garden at the red brick rear wall of the house. The air was warm and sweet; it seemed as though the peaceful sounds about him strove to lull him to sleep. Weary of loneliness and silence and staring into space, he would close his eyes now and then, only to snatch them open and harshly frighten peace away. "I must think," he said, almost aloud. "I must arrange everything before it is too late."

He sat here one day, in the pavilion, in the little reed rocking-chair, and read for four hours, with growing absorption, in a book which had, partly by chance, come into his hands. After second breakfast, cigarette in mouth, he had unearthed it in the smoking-room, from behind some stately volumes in the corner of a bookcase, and recalled that he had bought it at a bargain one day years ago. It was a large volume, poorly printed on cheap paper and poorly sewed; the second part, only, of a famous philosophical system. He had brought it out with him into the garden, and now he turned the pages, profoundly interested.

He was filled with a great, surpassing satisfaction. It soothed him to see how a master-mind could lay hold on this strong, cruel, mocking thing called life and enforce it and condemn it. His was the gratification of the sufferer who has always had a bad conscience about his sufferings and concealed them from the gaze of a harsh, unsympathetic world, until suddenly, from the hand of an authority, he receives, as it were, justification and license for his suffering – justification before the world, this best of all possible worlds which the master-mind scornfully demonstrates to be the worst of all possible ones!

He did not understand it all. Principles and premises remained unclear, and his mind, unpractised in such reading, was not able to follow certain trains of thought. But this very alternation of vagueness and clarity, of dull incomprehension with sudden bursts of light, kept him enthralled and breathless, and the hours vanished without his looking up from his book or changing his position in his chair.

He had left some pages unread in the beginning of the book, and hurried on, clutching rapidly after the main thesis, reading only this or that section which held his attention. Then he struck on a comprehensive chapter and read it from beginning to end, his lips tightly closed and his brows drawn together with a concentration which had long been strange to him, completely withdrawn from the life about him. The chapter was called " On Death, and its Relation to our Personal Immortality."

Only a few lines remained when the servant came through the garden at four o'clock to call him to dinner. He nodded, read the remaining sentences, closed the book, and looked about him. He felt that his whole being had unaccountably expanded, and at the same time there clung about his senses a profound intoxication, a strange, sweet, vague allurement which somehow resembled the feelings of early love and longing. He put away the book in the drawer of the garden table. His hands were cold and unsteady, his head was burning, and he felt in it a strange pressure and strain, as though something were about to snap. He was not capable of consecutive thought.

What was this? He asked himself the question as he mounted the stairs and sat down to table with his family. What is it? Have I had a revelation? What has happened to me, Thomas Buddenbrook, Councillor of this government, head of the grain firm of Johann Buddenbrook? Was this message meant for me? Can I bear it? I don't know what it was: I only know it is too much for my poor brain.

He remained the rest of the day in this condition, this heavy lethargy and intoxication, overpowered by the heady draught he had drunk, incapable of thought. Evening came. His head was heavy, and since he could hold it up no longer, he went early to bed. He slept for three hours, more profoundly than ever before in his life. And, then, suddenly, abruptly, with a start, he awoke and felt as one feels on realizing, suddenly, a budding love in the heart.

He was alone in the large sleeping chamber; for Gerda slept

now in Ida Jungmann's room, and the latter had moved into one of the three balcony rooms to be nearer little Johann. It was dark, for the curtains of both high windows were tightly closed. He lay on his back, feeling the oppression of the stillness and of the heavy, warm air, and looked up into the darkness.

And behold, it was as though the darkness were rent from before his eyes, as if the whole wall of the night parted wide and disclosed an immeasurable, boundless prospect of light. "I shall live!" said Thomas Buddenbrook, almost aloud, and felt his breast shaken with inward sobs. "This is the revelation: that I shall live! For *it* will live — and that this *it* is not I is only an illusion, an error which death will make plain. This is it, this is it! Why?" But at this question the night closed in again upon him. He saw, he knew, he understood, no least particle more; he let himself sink deep in the pillows, quite blinded and exhausted by the morsel of truth which had been vouchsafed.

He lay still and waited fervently, feeling himself tempted to pray that it would come again and irradiate his darkness. And it came. With folded hands, not daring to move, he lay and looked.

What *was* Death? The answer came, not in poor, large-sounding words: he felt it within him, he possessed it. Death was a joy, so great, so deep that it could be dreamed of only in moments of revelation like the present. It was the return from an unspeakably painful wandering, the correction of a grave mistake, the loosening of chains, the opening of doors — it put right again a lamentable mischance.

End, dissolution! These were pitiable words, and thrice pitiable he who used them! What would end, what would dissolve? Why, this his body, this heavy, faulty, hateful incumbrance, which *prevented him from being something other and better*.

Was not every human being a mistake and a blunder? Was he not in painful arrest from the hour of his birth? Prison, prison, bonds and limitations everywhere! The human being stares hopelessly through the barred window of his personality at the high walls of outward circumstance, till Death comes and calls him home to freedom!

Individuality? — All, all that one is, can, and has, seems poor, grey, inadequate, wearisome; what one is not, can not, has not, that is what one looks at with a longing desire that becomes love because it fears to become hate.

I bear in myself the seed, the tendency, the possibility of all capacity and all achievement. Where should I be were I not here? Who, what, how could I be, if I were not I — if this my external self, my consciousness, did not cut me off from those who are not I? Organism! Blind, thoughtless, pitiful eruption of the urging will! Better, indeed, for the will to float free in spaceless, timeless night than for it to languish in prison, illumined by the feeble, flickering light of the intellect!

Have I hoped to live on in my son? In a personality yet more feeble, flickering, and timorous than my own? Blind, childish folly! What can my son do for me — what need have I of a son? Where shall I be when I am dead? Ah, it is so brilliantly clear, so overwhelmingly simple! I shall be in all those who have ever, do ever, or ever shall say " I " — *especially, however, in all those who say it most fully, potently, and gladly!*

Somewhere in the world a child is growing up, strong, well-grown, adequate, able to develop its powers, gifted, untroubled, pure, joyous, relentless, one of those beings whose glance heightens the joy of the joyous and drives the unhappy to despair. *He* is my son. He is I, myself, soon, soon; as soon as Death frees me from the wretched delusion that I am not he as well as myself.

Have I ever hated life — pure, strong, relentless life? Folly and misconception! I have but hated myself, because I could not bear it. I love you, I love you all, you blessed, and soon, soon, I shall cease to be cut off from you all by the narrow bonds of myself; soon will that in me which loves you be free and be in and with you — in and with you all.

He wept, he pressed his face into the pillows and wept, shaken through and through, lifted up in transports by a joy without compare for its exquisite sweetness. This it was which since yesterday had filled him as if with a heady, intoxicating draught, had worked in his heart in the darkness of the night and roused him like a budding love! And in so far as he could now understand and recognize — not in words and consecutive thoughts, but in sudden rapturous illuminations of his inmost being — he was already free, already actually released and free of all natural as well as artificial limitations. The walls of his native town, in which he had wilfully and consciously shut himself up, opened out; they opened and disclosed to his view the entire world, of which he had in his youth seen this or that small portion, and of which Death now promised him the whole. The deceptive perceptions of space, time and history, the preoccupation with a glorious historical continuity of life in the person of his own descendants, the dread of some future final dissolution and decomposition — all this his spirit now put aside. He was no longer prevented from grasping eternity. Nothing began, nothing left off. There was only an endless present; and that power in him which loved life with a love so exquisitely sweet and yearning – the power of which his person was only the unsuccessful expression – that power would always know how to find access to this present.

"I shall live," he whispered into his pillow. He wept, and in the next moment knew not why. His brain stood still, the vision was quenched. Suddenly there was nothing more – he lay in dumb darkness. "It will come back," he assured himself. And before sleep inexorably wrapped him round, he swore to himself never to let go this precious treasure, but to read and study, to learn its powers, and to make inalienably his own the whole conception of the universe out of which his vision sprang.

But that could not be. Even the next day, as he woke with a faint feeling of shame at the emotional extravagances of the night, he suspected that it would be hard to put these beautiful designs into practice.

He rose late and had to go at once to take part in the debate at an assembly of burgesses. Public business, the civic life that went on in the gabled narrow streets of this middle-sized trading city, consumed his energies once more. He still planned to take up the wonderful reading again where he had left it off. But he questioned of himself whether the events of that night had been anything firm and permanent; whether, when Death approached, they would be found to hold their ground.

His middle-class instincts rose against them – and his vanity, too: the fear of being eccentric, of playing a laughable rôle. Had he really seen these things? And did they really become him – him, Thomas Buddenbrook, head of the firm of Johann Buddenbrook?

He never succeeded in looking again into the precious volume – to say nothing of buying its other parts. His days were consumed by nervous pedantry: harassed by a thousand details, all of them unimportant, he was too weak-willed to arrive at a reasonable and fruitful arrangement of his time. Nearly two weeks after that memorable afternoon he gave it up – and ordered the maidservant to fetch the book from the drawer in the garden table and replace it in the bookcase.

And thus Thomas Buddenbrook, who had held his hands stretched imploringly upward toward the high ultimate truth, sank now weakly back to the images and conceptions of his childhood. He strove to call back that personal God, the Father of all human beings, who had sent a part of Himself upon earth to suffer and bleed for our sins, and who, on the final day, would come to judge the quick and the dead; at whose feet the justified, in the course of the eternity then beginning, would be recompensed for the sorrows they had borne in this vale of tears. Yes, he strove to subscribe to the whole confused unconvincing story, which required no intelligence, only obedient credulity; and which, when the last anguish came, would sustain one in a firm and childlike faith. — But would it, really?

Ah, even here there was no peace. This poor, well-nigh exhausted man, consumed with gnawing fears for the honour of his house, his wife, his child, his name, his family, this man who spent painful effort even to keep his body artificially erect and well-preserved — this poor man tortured himself for days with thoughts upon the moment and manner of death. How would it really be? Did the soul go to Heaven immediately after death, or did bliss first begin with the resurrection of the flesh? And, if so, where did the soul stay until that time? He did not remember ever having been taught this. Why had he not been told this important fact in school or in church? How was it justifiable for them to leave people in such uncertainty? He considered visiting Pastor Pringsheim and seeking advice and counsel; but he gave it up in the end for fear of being ridiculous.

And finally he gave it all up — he left it all to God. But having come to such an unsatisfactory ending of his attempts to set his spiritual affairs in order, he determined at least to spare no pains over his earthly ones, and to carry out a plan which he had long entertained.

One day little Johann heard his father tell his mother, as they drank their coffee in the living-room after the midday meal, that he expected Lawyer So-and-So to make his will. He really ought not to keep on putting it off. Later, in the afternoon, Hanno practised his music for an hour. When he went down the corridor after that, he met, coming up the stairs, his father and a gentleman in a long black overcoat.

"Hanno," said the Senator, curtly. And little Johann stopped, swallowed, and said quickly and softly: "Yes, Papa."

"I have some important business with this gentleman," his father went on. "Will you stand before the door into the smoking-room and take care that nobody — absolutely nobody, you understand — disturbs us?"

"Yes, Papa," said little Johann, and took up his post before the door, which closed after the two gentlemen.

He stood there, clutching his sailor's knot with one hand, felt with his tongue for a doubtful tooth, and listened to the earnest subdued voices which could be heard from inside. His head, with the curling light-brown hair, he held on one side, and his face with the frowning brows and blue-shadowed, gold-brown eyes, wore that same displeased and brooding look with which he had inhaled the odour of the flowers, and that other strange, yet half-familiar odour, by his grandmother's bier.

Ida Jungmann passed and said, "Well, little Hanno, why are you hanging about here?"

And the hump-backed apprentice came out of the office with a telegram, and asked for the Senator.

But, both times, little Johann put his arm in its blue sailor sleeve with the anchor on it horizontally across the door; both times he shook his head and said softly, after a pause, "No one may go in. Papa is making his will."

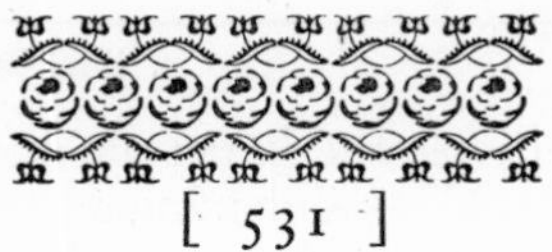

CHAPTER VI

In the autumn Dr. Langhals said, making play like a woman with his beautiful eyes: "It is the nerves, Senator; the nerves are to blame for everything. And once in a while the circulation is not what it should be. May I venture to make a suggestion? You need another little rest. These few Sundays by the sea, during the summer, haven't amounted to much, of course. It's the end of September, Travemünde is still open, there are still a few people there. Drive over, Senator, and sit on the beach a little. Two or three weeks will do you a great deal of good."

And Thomas Buddenbrook said "yes" and "amen." But when he told his family of the arrangement, Christian suggested going with him.

"I'll go with you, Thomas," he said, quite simply. "You don't mind, I suppose." And the Senator, though he did mind very much, said "yes" and "amen" to this arrangement as well.

Christian was now more than ever master of his own time. His fluctuating health had constrained him to give up his last undertaking, the champagne and spirit agency. The man who used to come and sit on his sofa and nod at him in the twilight had happily not recurred of late. But the misery in the side had, if anything, grown worse, and added to this was a whole list of other infirmities of which Christian kept the closest watch, and which he described in all companies, with his nose wrinkled up. He often suffered from that long-standing dread of paralysis of the tongue, throat, and œsophagus, even of the extremities and of the brain – of which there were no actual symptoms, but the fear in itself was almost worse. He told in detail how, one day when he was making tea, he had held the lighted match not over the spirit-lamp, but over the open bottle of methylated spirit instead; so that not only himself, but the people in his own and the adjacent buildings, nearly went up in flames. And he dwelt in particular detail, straining every resource he had at his command to make himself perfectly clear, upon a certain ghastly anomaly which he had of late observed in himself. It was this: that on certain days, i.e., under certain weather conditions, and in certain states of mind, he could not see an open window without having a horrible and inexplicable impulse to jump out. It was a mad and almost uncontrollable desire, a sort of desperate foolhardiness. The family were dining on Sunday in Fishers' Lane, and he described how he had to summon all his powers, and crawl on hands and knees to the window to shut it. At this point everybody shrieked; his audience rebelled, and would listen no more.

He told these and similar things with a certain horrible satisfaction. But the thing about himself which he did not know, which he never studied and described, but which none the less grew worse and worse, was his singular lack of tact. He told in the family circle anecdotes of such a nature that the club was the only possible place for them. And even his sense of personal modesty seemed to be breaking down. He was on friendly terms with his sister-in-law, Gerda. But when he displayed to her the beautiful weave and texture of his English socks, he did not stop at that, but rolled up his wide, checkered trouser-leg to far above the knee: "Look," he said, wrinkling his nose in distress: "Look how thin I'm getting. Isn't it striking and unusual?" And there he sat, sadly gazing at his crooked, bony leg and the gaunt knee visible through his white woollen drawers.

His mercantile activity then, was a thing of the past. But such hours as he did not spend at the club he liked to fill in with one sort of occupation or another; and he would proudly point out that he had never actually ceased to work. He extended his knowledge of languages and embarked upon a study of Chinese — though this was for the sake of acquiring knowledge, simply, with no practical purpose in view. He worked at it industriously for two weeks. He was also, just at this time, occupied with a project of enlarging an English-German dictionary which he had found inadequate. But he really needed a little change, and it would be better too for the Senator to have somebody with him; so he did not allow his business to keep him in town.

The two brothers drove out together to the sea along the turnpike, which was nothing but a puddle. The rain drummed on the carriage-top, and they hardly spoke. Christian's eyes roved hither and yon; he was as if listening to uncanny noises. Thomas sat muffled in his cloak, shivering, gazing with bloodshot eyes, his moustaches stiffly sticking out beyond his white cheeks. They drove up to the Kurhouse in the afternoon, their wheels grating in the wet gravel. Old Broker Gosch sat in the glass verandah, drinking rum punch. He stood up, whistling through his teeth, and they all sat down together to have a little something warm while the trunks were being carried up.

Herr Gosch was a late guest at the cure, and there were a few other people as well: an English family, a Dutch maiden lady, and a Hamburg bachelor, all of them presumably taking their rest before table-d'hôte, for it was like the grave everywhere but for the sound of the rain. Let them sleep! As for Herr Gosch, he was not in the habit of sleeping in the daytime. He was glad enough to get a few hours' sleep at night. He was far from well; he was taking a late cure for the benefit of this trembling which he suffered from in all his limbs. Hang it, he could hardly hold his glass of grog; and more often than not he could not write at all – so that the translation of Lope de Vega got on but slowly. He was in a very low mood indeed, and even his curses lacked relish. "Let it go hang!" was his constant phrase, which he repeated on every occasion and often on none at all.

And the Senator? How was he feeling? How long were the gentlemen thinking of stopping?

Oh, Dr. Langhals had sent him out on account of his nerves. He had obeyed orders, of course, despite the frightful weather – what doesn't one do out of fear of one's physician? He was really feeling more or less miserable, and they would probably remain till there was a little improvement.

"Yes, I'm pretty wretched too," said Christian, irritated at Thomas's speaking only of himself. He was about to fetch out his repertoire – the nodding man, the spirit-bottle, the open window – when the Senator interrupted him by going to engage the rooms.

The rain did not stop. It washed away the earth, it danced upon the sea, which was driven back by the southwest wind and left the beaches bare. Everything was shrouded in grey. The steamers went by like wraiths and vanished on the dim horizon.

They met the strange guests only at table. The Senator, in mackintosh and goloshes, went walking with Gosch; Christian drank Swedish punch with the barmaid in the pastry-shop.

Two or three times in the afternoon it looked as though the sun were coming out; and a few acquaintances from town appeared – people who enjoyed a holiday away from their families: Senator Dr. Gieseke, Christian's friend, and Consul Peter Döhlmann, who looked very ill indeed, and was killing himself with Hunyadi-Janos water. The gentlemen sat together in their overcoats, under the awnings of the pastry-shop, opposite the empty bandstand, drinking their coffee, digesting their five courses, and talking desultorily as they gazed over the empty garden.

The news of the town – the last high water, which had gone into the cellars and been so deep that in the lower part of the town people had to go about in boats; a fire in the dockyard sheds; a senatorial election – these were the topics of conversation. Alfred Lauritzen, of the firm of Stürmann & Lauritzen, tea, coffee, and spice merchants, had been elected, and Senator Buddenbrook had not approved of the choice. He sat smoking cigarettes, wrapped in his cloak, almost silent except for a few remarks on this particular subject. One thing was certain, he said, and that was that *he* had not voted for Herr Lauritzen. Lauritzen was an honest fellow and a good man of business. There was no doubt of that; but he was middle-class, respectable middle-class. His father had fished herrings out of the barrel and handed them across the counter to servant-maids with his own hands – and now they had in the Senate the proprietor of a retail business. His, Thomas Buddenbrook's grandfather had disowned his eldest son for " marrying a shop "; but that was in the good old days. " The standard is being lowered," he said. " The social level is not so high as it was; the Senate is being democratized, my dear Gieseke, and that is no good. Business ability is one thing – but it is not everything. In my view we should demand something more. Alfred Lauritzen, with his big feet and his boatswain's face – it is offensive to me to think of him in the Senate-house. It offends something in me, I don't know what. It goes against my sense of form – it is a piece of bad taste, in short."

Senator Gieseke demurred. He was rather piqued by this expression of opinion. After all, he himself was only the son of a Fire Commissioner. No, the labourer was worthy of his hire. That was what being a republican meant. " You ought not to smoke so much, Buddenbrook," he ended. " You won't get any sea air."

" I'll stop now," said Thomas Buddenbrook, flung away the end of his cigarette, and closed his eyes.

The conversation dragged on; the rain set in again and veiled the prospect. They began to talk about the latest town scandal – about P. Philipp Kassbaum, who had been falsifying bills of exchange and now sat behind locks and bars. No one felt outraged over the dishonesty: they spoke of it as an act of folly, laughed a bit, and shrugged their shoulders. Senator Dr. Gieseke said that the convicted man had not lost his spirits. He had asked for a mirror, it seemed, there being none in his cell. " I'll need a looking-glass," he was reported to have said: " I shall be here for some time." He had been, like Christian and Dr. Gieseke, a pupil of the lamented Marcellus Stengel.

They all laughed again at this, through their noses, without a sign of feeling. Siegismund Gosch ordered another grog in a tone of voice that was as good as saying, " What's the use of living? " Consul Döhlmann sent for a bottle of brandy. Christian felt inclined to more Swedish punch, so Dr. Gieseke ordered some for both of them. Before long Thomas Buddenbrook began to smoke again.

And the idle, cynical, indifferent talk went on, heavy with the food they had eaten, the wine they drank, and the damp that depressed their spirits. They talked about business, the business of each one of those present; but even this subject roused no great enthusiasm.

" Oh, there's nothing very good about mine," said Thomas Buddenbrook heavily, and leaned his head against the back of his chair with an air of disgust.

" Well, and you, Döhlmann," asked Senator Gieseke, and yawned. " You've been devoting yourself entirely to brandy, eh? "

" The chimney can't smoke, unless there's a fire," the Consul retorted. " I look into the office every few days. Short hairs are soon combed."

" And Strunck and Hagenström have all the business in their hands anyhow," the broker said morosely, with his elbows sprawled out on the table and his wicked old grey head in his hands.

" Oh, nothing can compete with a dung-heap, for smell," Döhlmann said, with a deliberately coarse pronunciation, which must have depressed everybody's spirits the more by its hopeless cynicism. " Well, and you, Buddenbrook – what are you doing now? Nothing, eh? "

" No," answered Christian, " I can't, any more." And without more ado, having perceived the mood of the hour, he proceeded to accentuate it. He began, his hat on one side, to talk about his Valparaiso office and Johnny Thunderstorm. " Well, in that heat – ' Good God! Work, Sir? No, Sir. As you see, Sir.' And they puffed their cigarette-smoke right in his face. Good God! " It was, as always, an incomparable expression of dissolute, impudent, lazy good-nature. His brother sat motionless.

Herr Gosch tried to lift his glass to his thin lips, put it back on the table again, cursing through his shut teeth, and struck the offending arm with his fist. Then he lifted the glass once more, and spilled half its contents, draining the remainder furiously at a gulp.

"Oh, you and your shaking, Gosch!" Peter Döhlmann exclaimed. "Why don't you just let yourself go, like me? I'll croak if I don't drink my bottle every day – I've got as far as that; and I'll croak if I do. How would you feel if you couldn't get rid of your dinner, not a single day – I mean, after you've got it in your stomach?" And he favoured them with some repulsive details of his condition, to which Christian listened with dreadful interest, wrinkling his nose as far as it could go and countering with a brief and forcible account of his "misery."

It rained harder than ever. It came straight down in sheets and filled the silence of the Kurgarten with its ceaseless, forlorn, and desolate murmur.

"Yes, life's pretty rotten," said Senator Gieseke. He had been drinking heavily.

"I'd just as lief quit," said Christian.

"Let it go hang," said Herr Gosch.

"There comes Fike Dahlbeck," said Senator Gieseke. The proprietress of the cow-stalls, a heavy, bold-faced woman in the forties, came by with a pail of milk and smiled at the gentlemen.

Senator Gieseke let his eyes rove after her.

"What a bosom," he said. Consul Döhlmann added a lewd witticism, with the result that all the gentlemen laughed once more, through their noses.

The waiter was summoned.

"I've finished the bottle, Schröder," said Consul Döhlmann. "May as well pay – we have to some time or other. You, Christian? Gieseke pays for you, eh?"

Senator Buddenbrook roused himself at this. He had been sitting there, hardly speaking, wrapped in his cloak, his hands in his lap and his cigarette in the corner of his mouth. Now he suddenly started up and said sharply, "Have you no money with you, Christian? Then I'll lend it to you."

They put up their umbrellas and emerged from their shelter to take a little stroll.

Frau Permaneder came out once in a while to see her brother. They would walk as far as Sea-Gull Rock or the little Ocean Temple; and here Tony Buddenbrook, for some reason or other, was always seized by a mood of vague excitement and rebellion. She would repeatedly emphasize the independence and equality of all human beings, summarily repudiate all distinctions of rank or class, use some very strong language on the subject or privilege and arbitrary power, and demand in set terms that merit should receive its just reward. And then she talked about her own life. She talked well, she entertained her brother capitally. This child of fortune, so long as she walked upon this earth, had never once needed to suppress an emotion, to choke down or swallow anything she felt. She had never received in silence either the blows or the caresses of fate. And whatever she had received, of joy or sorrow, she had straightway given forth again, in a flow of childish, self-important trivialities. Her digestion was not perfect, it is true. But her heart — ah, her heart was light, her spirit was free; freer than she herself comprehended. She was not consumed by the inexpressible. No sorrow weighed her down, or strove to speak but could not. And thus it was that her past left no mark upon her. She knew that she had led a troubled life — she knew it, that is, but at bottom she never believed in it herself. She recognized it as a fact, since everybody else believed it — and she utilized it to her own advantage, talking of it and making herself great with it in her own eyes and those of others. With outraged virtue and dignity she would call by name all those persons who had played havoc with her life and, in consequence, with the prestige of the Buddenbrook family; the list had grown long with time: Teary Trietschke! Grünlich! Permaneder! Tiburtius! Weinschenk! the Hagenströms! the State Attorney! Severin! — "What *filoux*, all of them, Thomas! God will punish them — that is my firm belief."

Twilight was falling as they came up to the Ocean Temple, for the autumn was far advanced. They stood on one of the little chambers facing the bay — it smelled of wood, like the bathing cabins at the Kur, and its walls were scribbled over with mottoes, initials, hearts and rhymes. They stood and looked out over the dripping slope across the narrow, stony strip of beach, out to the turbid, restless sea.

"Great waves," said Thomas Buddenbrook. "How they come on and break, come on and break, one after another, endlessly, idly, empty and vast! And yet, like all the simple, inevitable things, they soothe, they console, after all. I have learned to love the sea more and more. Once, I think, I cared more for the mountains — because they lay farther off. Now I do not long for them. They would only frighten and abash me. They are too capricious, too manifold, too anomalous — I know I should feel myself vanquished in their presence. What sort of men prefer the monotony of the sea? Those, I think, who have looked so long and deeply into the complexities of the spirit, that they ask of outward things merely that they should possess one quality above all: simplicity. It is true that in the mountains one clambers briskly about, while beside the sea one sits quietly on the shore. This is a difference, but a superficial one. The real difference is in the look with which one pays homage to the one and to the other. It is a strong, challenging gaze, full of enterprise, that can soar from peak to peak; but the eyes that rest on the wide ocean and are soothed by the sight of its waves rolling on forever, mystically, relentlessly, are those that are already wearied by looking too deep into the solemn perplexities of life. — Health and illness, that is the difference. The man whose strength is unexhausted climbs boldly up into the lofty multiplicity of the mountain heights. But it is when one is worn out with turning one's eyes inward upon the bewildering complexity of the human heart, that one finds peace in resting them on the wideness of the sea."

Frau Permaneder was silent and uncomfortable, — as simple people are when a profound truth is suddenly expressed in the middle of a conventional conversation. People don't say such things, she thought to herself; and looked out to sea so as not to show her feeling by meeting his eyes. Then, in the silence, to make amends for an embarrassment which she could not help, she drew his arm through hers.

CHAPTER VII

WINTER had come, Christmas had passed. It was January, 1875. The snow, which covered the foot-walks in a firm-trodden mass, mingled with sand and ashes, was piled on either side of the road in high mounds that were growing greyer and more porous all the time, for the temperature was rising. The pavements were wet and dirty, the grey gables dripped. But above all stretched the heavens, a cloudless tender blue, while millions of light atoms seemed to dance like crystal motes in the air.

It was a lively sight in the centre of the town, for this was Saturday, and market-day as well. Under the pointed arches of the Town Hall arcades the butchers had their stalls and weighed out their wares red-handed. The fish-market, however, was held around the fountain in the market-square itself. Here fat old women, with their hands in muffs from which most of the fur was worn off, warming their feet at little coal-braziers, guarded their slippery wares and tried to cajole the servants and housewives into making purchases. There was no fear of being cheated. The fish would certainly be fresh, for the most of them were still alive. The luckiest ones were even swimming about in pails of water, rather cramped for space, but perfectly lively. Others lay with dreadfully goggling eyes and labouring gills, clinging to life and slapping the marble slab desperately with their tails – until such time as their fate was at hand, when somebody would seize them and cut their throats with a crunching sound. Great fat eels writhed and wreathed about in extraordinary shapes. There were deep vats full of black masses of crabs from the Baltic. Once in a while a big flounder gave such a desperate leap that he sprang right off his slab and fell down upon the slippery pavement, among all the refuse, and had to picked up and severely admonished by his possessor.

Broad Street, at midday, was full of life. Schoolchildren with knapsacks on their backs came along the street, filling it with laughter and chatter, snowballing each other with the half-melting snow. Smart young apprentices passed, with Danish sailor caps or suits cut after the English model, carrying their portfolios and obviously pleased with themselves for having escaped from school. Among the crowd were settled, grey-bearded, highly respectable citizens, wearing the most irreproachable national-liberal expression on their faces, and tapping their sticks along the pavement. These looked across with interest to the glazed-brick front of the Town Hall, where the double guard was stationed; for the Senate was in session. The sentries trod their beat, wearing their cloaks, their guns on their shoulders, phlegmatically stamping their feet in the dirty half-melted snow. They met in the centre of their beat, looked at each other, exchanged a word, turned, and moved away each to his own side. Sometimes a lieutenant would pass, his coat-collar turned up, his hands in his pockets, on the track of some grisette, yet at the same time permitting himself to be admired by young ladies of good family; and then each sentry would stand at attention in front of his box, look at himself from head to foot, and present arms. It would be a little time yet before they would perform the same salute before the members of the Senate, the sitting lasted some three quarters of an hour; it would probably adjourn before that.

But one of the sentries suddenly heard a short, discreet whistle from within the building. At the same moment the entrance was illumined by the red uniform of Uhlefeld the beadle, with his dress sword and cocked hat. His air of preoccupation was simply enormous as he uttered a stealthy " Look out " and hastily withdrew. At the same moment approaching steps were heard on the echoing flags within.

The sentries front-faced, inflated their chests, stiffened their necks, grounded their arms, and then, with a couple of rapid motions, presented arms. Between them there had appeared, lifting his top hat, a gentleman of scarcely medium height, with one light eyebrow higher than the other and the pointed ends of his moustaches extending beyond his pallid cheeks. Senator Thomas Buddenbrook was leaving the Town Hall to-day long before the end of the sitting. He did not take the street to his own house, but turned to the right instead. He looked correct, spotless, and elegant as, with the rather hopping step peculiar to him, he walked along Broad Street, constantly saluting people whom he met. He wore white kid gloves, and he had his stick with the silver handle under his left arm. A white dress tie peeped forth from between the lapels of his fur coat. But his head and face, despite their careful grooming, looked rather seedy. People who passed him noticed that his eyes were watering and that he held his mouth shut in a peculiar cautious way; it was twisted a little to one side, and one could see by the muscles of his cheeks and temples that he was clenching his jaw. Sometimes he swallowed, as if a liquid kept rising in his mouth.

"Well, Buddenbrook, so you are cutting the session? That is something new," somebody said unexpectedly to him at the beginning of Mill Street. It was his friend and admirer Stephan Kistenmaker, whose opinion on all subjects was the echo of his own. Stephan Kistenmaker had a full greying beard, bushy eyebrows, and a long nose full of large pores. He had retired from the wine business a few years back with a comfortable sum, and his brother Edouard carried it on by himself. He lived now the life of a private gentleman; but, being rather ashamed of the fact, he always pretended to be overwhelmed with work. "I'm wearing myself out," he would say, stroking his grey hair, which he curled with the tongs. "But what's a man good for, but to wear himself out?" He stood hours on 'Change, gesturing imposingly, but doing no business. He held a number of unimportant offices, the latest one being Director of the city bathing establishments; but he also functioned as juror, broker, and executor, and laboured with such zeal that the perspiration dripped from his brow.

"There's a session, isn't there, Buddenbrook – and you are taking a walk?"

"Oh, it's you," said the Senator in a low voice, moving his lips cautiously. "I'm suffering frightfully – I'm nearly blind with pain."

"Pain? Where?"

"Toothache. Since yesterday. I did not close my eyes last night. I have not been to the dentist yet, because I had business in the office this morning, and then I did not like to miss the sitting. But I couldn't stand it any longer. I'm on my way to Brecht."

"Where is it?"

"Here on the left side, the lower jaw. A back tooth. It is decayed, of course. The pain is simply unbearable. Good-bye, Kistenmaker. You can understand that I am in a good deal of a hurry."

"Yes, of course – don't you think I am, too? Awful lot to do. Good-bye. Good luck! Have it out – get it over with at once – always the best way."

Thomas Buddenbrook went on, biting his jaws together, though it made the pain worse to do so. It was a furious burning, boring pain, starting from the infected back tooth and affecting the whole side of the jaw. The inflammation throbbed like red-hot hammers;

it made his face burn and his eyes water. His nerves were terribly affected by the sleepless night he had spent. He had had to control himself just now, lest his voice break as he spoke.

He entered a yellow-brown house in Mill Street and went up to the first storey, where a brass plate on the door said, "Brecht, Dentist." He did not see the servant who opened the door. The corridor was warm and smelled of beefsteak and cauliflower. Then he suddenly inhaled the sharp odour of the waiting-room into which he was ushered. "Sit down! One moment! " shrieked the voice of an old woman. It was Josephus, who sat in his shining cage at the end of the room and regarded him sidewise out of his venomous little eyes.

The Senator sat down at the round table and tried to read the jokes in a volume of *Fliegende Blätter*, flung down the book, and pressed the cool silver handle of his walking-stick against his cheek. He closed his burning eyes and groaned. There was not a sound, except for the noise made by Josephus as he bit and clawed at the bars of his cage. Herr Brecht might not be busy; but he owed it to himself to make his patient wait a little.

Thomas Buddenbrook stood up precipitately and drank a glass of water from the bottle on the table. It tasted and smelled of chloroform. Then he opened the door into the corridor and called out in an irritated voice: if there were nothing very important to prevent it, would Herr Brecht kindly make haste — he was suffering.

And immediately the bald forehead, hooked nose, and grizzled moustaches of the dentist appeared in the door of the operating-room. "If you please," he said. "If you please," shrieked Josephus. The Senator followed on the invitation. He was not smiling. "A bad case," thought Herr Brecht, and turned pale.

They passed through the large light room to the operating-chair in front of one of the two largest windows. It was an adjustable chair with an upholstered head-rest and green plush arms. As he sat down, Thomas Buddenbrook briefly explained what the trouble was. Then he leaned back his head and closed his eyes.

Herr Brecht screwed up the chair a bit and got to work on the tooth with a tiny mirror and a pointed steel instrument. His hands smelled of almond soap, his breath of cauliflower and beefsteak.

"We must proceed to extraction," he said, after a while, and turned still paler.

"Very well, proceed, then," said the Senator, and shut his eyes more tightly.

There was a pause. Herr Brecht prepared something at his

chest of drawers and got out his instruments. Then he approached the chair again.

"I'll paint it a little," he said; and began at once to apply a strong-smelling liquid in generous quantities. Then he gently implored the patient to sit very still and open his mouth very wide — and then he began.

Thomas Buddenbrook clutched the plush arm-rests with both his hands. He scarcely felt the forceps close around his tooth; but from the grinding sensation in his mouth, and the increasingly painful, really agonizing pressure on his whole head, he was made amply aware that the thing was under way. Thank God, he thought, now it can't last long. The pain grew and grew, to limitless, incredible heights; it grew to an insane, shrieking, inhuman torture, tearing his entire brain. It approached the catastrophe. 'Here we are, he thought. Now I must just bear it.'

It lasted three or four seconds. Herr Brecht's nervous exertions communicated themselves to Thomas Buddenbrook's whole body, he was even lifted up a little on his chair, and he heard a soft, squeaking noise coming from the dentist's throat. Suddenly there was a fearful blow, a violent shaking as if his neck were broken, accompanied by a quick cracking, crackling noise. The pressure was gone, but his head buzzed, the pain throbbed madly in the inflamed and ill-used jaw; and he had the clearest impression that the thing had not been successful: that the extraction of the tooth was not the solution of the difficulty, but merely a premature catastrophe which only made matters worse.

Herr Brecht had retreated. He was leaning against his instrument-cupboard, and he looked like death. He said: "The crown — I thought so."

Thomas Buddenbrook spat a little blood into the blue basin at his side, for the gum was lacerated. He asked, half-dazed: "What did you think? What about the crown?"

"The crown broke off, Herr Senator. I was afraid of it. — The tooth was in very bad condition. But it was my duty to make the experiment."

"What next?"

"Leave it to me, Herr Senator."

"What will you have to do now?"

"Take out the roots. With a lever. There are four of them."

"Four. Then you must take hold and lift four times."

"Yes — unfortunately."

"Well, this is enough for to-day," said the Senator. He started to rise, but remained seated and put his head back instead.

"My dear Sir, you mustn't demand the impossible of me," he said. "I'm not very strong on my legs, just now. I have had enough for to-day. Will you be so kind as to open the window a little?"

Herr Brecht did so. "It will be perfectly agreeable to me, Herr Senator, if you come in to-morrow or next day, at whatever hour you like, and we can go on with the operation. If you will permit me, I will just do a little more rinsing and pencilling, to reduce the pain somewhat."

He did the rinsing and pencilling, and then the Senator went. Herr Brecht accompanied him to the door, pale as death, expending his last remnant of strength in sympathetic shoulder-shruggings.

"One moment, please!" shrieked Josephus as they passed through the waiting-room. He still shrieked as Thomas Buddenbrook went down the steps.

With a lever – yes, yes, that was to-morrow. What should he do now? Go home and rest, sleep, if he could. The actual pain in the nerve seemed deadened; in his mouth was only a dull, heavy burning sensation. Home, then. He went slowly through the streets, mechanically exchanging greetings with those whom he met; his look was absent and wandering, as though he were absorbed in thinking how he felt.

He got as far as Fishers' Lane and began to descend the left-hand sidewalk. After twenty paces he felt nauseated. "I'll go over to the public house and take a drink of brandy," he thought, and began to cross the road. But just as he reached the middle, something happened to him. It was precisely as if his brain was seized and swung around, faster and faster, in circles that grew smaller and smaller, until it crashed with enormous, brutal, pitiless force against a stony centre. He performed a half-turn, fell, and struck the wet pavement, his arms outstretched.

As the street ran steeply down hill, his body lay much lower than his feet. He fell upon his face, beneath which, presently, a little pool of blood began to form. His hat rolled a little way off down the road; his fur coat was wet with mud and slush; his hands, in their white kid gloves, lay outstretched in a puddle.

Thus he lay, and thus he remained, until some people came down the street and turned him over.

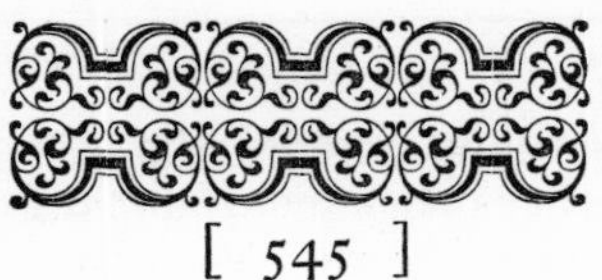

CHAPTER VIII

Frau Permaneder mounted the main staircase, holding up her gown in front of her with one hand and with the other pressing her muff to her cheek. She tripped and stumbled more than she walked; her cheeks were flushed, her capote sat crooked on her head, and little beads stood on her upper lip. . . . Though she met no one, she talked continually as she hurried up, in whispers out of which now and then a word rose clear and audible and emphasized her fear. "It's nothing," she said. "It doesn't mean anything. God wouldn't let anything happen. He knows what he's doing, I'm very sure of that. . . . Oh, my God, I'll pray every day — " She prattled senselessly in her fear, as she rushed up to the second storey and down the corridor.

The door of the ante-chamber opened, and her sister-in-law came toward her. Gerda Buddenbrook's lovely white face was quite distorted with horror and disgust; and her close-set, blue-shadowed brown eyes opened and shut with a look of anger, distraction, and shrinking. As she recognized Frau Permaneder, she beckoned quickly with outstretched arms and embraced her, putting her head on her sister-in-law's shoulder.

"Gerda! Gerda! What is it?" Frau Permaneder cried. "What has happened? What does it mean? They said he fell — unconscious? How is he? — God won't let the worst happen, I know. Tell me, for pity's sake!"

But the reply did not come at once. She only felt how Gerda's whole form was shaken. Then she heard a whisper at her shoulder.

"How he looked," she heard, "when they brought him! His whole life long, he never let any one see even a speck of dust on him. — Oh, it is insulting, it is vile, for the end to have come like that!"

Subdued voices came out to them. The dressing-room door opened, and Ida Jungmann stood in the doorway in a white apron, a basin in her hands. Her eyes were red. She looked at Frau Permaneder and made way, her head bent. Her chin was trembling.

The high flowered curtains stirred in the draught as Tony, followed by her sister-in-law, entered the chamber. The smell of carbolic, ether, and other drugs met them. In the wide mahogany bed, under the red down coverlet, lay Thomas Buddenbrook, on his back, undressed and clad in an embroidered nightshirt. His half-open eyes were rolled up; his lips were moving under the disordered moustaches, and babbling, gurgling sounds came out. Young Dr. Langhals was bending over him, changing a bloody bandage for a fresh one, which he dipped into a basin at the bedside. Then he listened at the patient's chest and felt his pulse.

On the bed-clothes at the foot of the bed sat little Johann, clutching his sailor's knot and listening broodingly to the sounds behind him, which his father was making. The Senator's bemired clothing hung over a chair.

Frau Permaneder cowered down at the bedside, seized one of her brother's hands – it was cold and heavy – and stared wildly into his face. She began to understand that, whether God knew what he was doing or not, he was at all events bent on " the worst "!

" Tom! " she clamoured, " do you know me? How are you? You aren't going to leave us? You won't go away from us? Oh, it *can't* be! "

Nothing answered her, that could be called an answer. She looked imploringly up at Dr. Langhals. He stood there with his beautiful eyes cast down; and his manner, not without a certain self-satisfaction, expressed the will of God.

Ida Jungmann came back into the room, to make herself useful if she could. Old Dr. Grabow appeared in person, looked at the patient with his long, mild face, shook his head, pressed all their hands, and then stood as Dr. Langhals stood. The news had gone like the wind through the whole town. The vestibule door rang constantly, and inquiries after the Senator's condition came up into the sick-chamber. It was unchanged – unchanged. Every one received the same answer.

The two physicians were in favour of sending for a sister of charity – at least for the night. They sent for Sister Leandra, and she came. There was no trace of surprise or alarm in her face as she entered. Again she laid aside her leather bag, her outer hood and cloak, and again she set to work in her gentle way.

Little Johann sat hour after hour on the bed-clothes, watching everything and listening to the gurgling noises. He was to have gone to an arithmetic lesson; but he understood perfectly that what was happening here was something over which the worsted-coats had no jurisdiction. He thought of his lessons only for a moment, and with scorn. He wept, sometimes, when Frau Permaneder came up and pressed him to her; but mostly he sat dry-eyed, with a shrinking, brooding gaze, and his breath came irregularly and cautiously, as if he expected any moment to smell that strange and yet familiar smell.

Toward four o'clock Frau Permaneder took a sudden resolve. She asked Dr. Langhals to come with her into the next room; and there she folded her arms and laid back her head, with the chin dropped.

"Herr Doctor," she said, "there is one thing you can do, and I beg you to do it. Tell me the truth. I am a woman steeled by adversity; I have learned to bear the truth. You may depend upon me. Please tell me plainly: Will my brother be alive to-morrow?"

Dr. Langhals turned his beautiful eyes aside, looked at his finger-nails, and spoke of our human powerlessness, and the impossibility of knowing whether Frau Permaneder's brother would outlive the night, or whether he would be called away the next minute.

"Then I know what I have to do," said she; went out of the room; and sent for Pastor Pringsheim.

Pastor Pringsheim appeared, without his vestments or neckruff, in a long black gown. He swept Sister Leandra with an icy stare, and seated himelf in the chair which they placed for him by the bedside. He asked the patient to recognize and hear him. Then, as this appeal was unsuccessful, he addressed himself at once to God and prayed in carefully modulated tones, with his Frankish pronunciation, with emphasis now solemn and now abrupt, while waves of fanaticism and sanctimony followed each other across his face. He pronounced his *r* in a sleek and oily way peculiar to himself alone, and little Johann received an irresistible impression that he had just been eating rolls and coffee.

He said that he and the family there present no longer importuned God for the life of this dear and beloved sufferer, for they saw plainly that it was God's will to take him to Himself. They only begged Him for the mercy of a gentle death. And then he recited, appropriately and with effect, two of the prayers customary on such occasions. Then he got up. He pressed Gerda Buddenbrook's hand, and Frau Permaneder's, and held little Johann's head for a moment between both his hands, regarding the drooping eyelashes with an expression of the most fervent pity. He saluted Ida Jungmann, stared again at Sister Leandra, and took his leave.

Dr. Langhals had gone home for a little. When he came back there had been no change. He spoke with the nurse, and went again. Dr. Grabow came once more, to see that everything was being done. Thomas Buddenbrook went on babbling and gurgling, with his eyes rolled up. Twilight was falling. There was a pale winter glow at sunset, and it shone through the window upon the soiled clothing lying across the chair.

At five o'clock Frau Permaneder let herself be carried away by her feelings, and committed an indiscretion. She suddenly began to sing, in her throaty voice, her hands folded before her.

"Come, Lord,"

she sang, quite loud, and they all listened without stirring.

"Come, Lord, receive his failing breath;
Strengthen his hands and feet, and lead him unto death."

But in the devoutness of her prayer, she thought only of the words as they welled up from her heart, and forgot that she did not know the whole stanza; after the third line she was left hanging in the air, and had to make up for her abrupt end by the increased dignity of her manner. Everybody shivered with embarrassment. Little Johann coughed so hard that the coughs sounded like sobs. And then, in the sudden pause, there was no sound but the agonizing gurgles of Thomas Buddenbrook.

It was a relief when the servant announced that there was something to eat in the next room. But they had only begun, sitting in Gerda's bedroom, to take a little soup, when Sister Leandra appeared in the doorway and quietly beckoned.

The Senator was dying. He hiccoughed gently two or three times, was silent, and ceased to move his lips. That was the only change. His eyes had been quite dead before.

Dr. Langhals, who was on the spot a few minutes later, put the black stethoscope to the heart, listened, and, after this scientific test, said "Yes, it is over."

And Sister Leandra, with the forefinger of her gentle white hand, softly closed the eyes of the dead.

Then Frau Permaneder flung herself down on her knees by the bed, pressed her face into the coverlet, and wept aloud, surrendering herself utterly and without restraint to one of those refreshing bursts of feeling which her happy nature had always at its command. Her face still streamed with tears, but she was soothed and comforted and entirely herself as she rose to her feet and began straightway to occupy her mind with the announcements of the death – an enormous number of elegant cards, which must be ordered at once.

Christian appeared. He had heard the news of the Senator's stroke in the club, which he had left at once. But he was so afraid of seeing some awful sight that he went instead for a long walk outside the walls, and was not to be found. Now, however, he came in, and on the threshold heard of his brother's death.

"It isn't possible," he said, and limped up the stairs, his eyes rolling wildly.

He stood at the bedside between his sister and his sister-in-law; with his bald head, his sunken cheeks, his drooping moustaches, and his huge beaked nose, he stood there on his bent legs, looking a little like an interrogation-point, and gazed with his little round deep eyes into his brother's face, as it lay so silent, so cold, so detached and inaccessible. The corners of Thomas's mouth were drawn down in an expression almost scornful. Here he lay, at whom once Christian had flung the reproach that he was too heartless to weep at a brother's death. He was dead now himself: he had simply withdrawn, silent, elegant, and irreproachable, into the hereafter. He had, as so often in his life, left it to others to feel put in the wrong. No matter now, whether he had been right or wrong in his cold and scornful indifference toward his brother's afflictions, the "misery," the nodding man, the spirit bottle, the open window. None of that mattered now; for death, with arbitrary and incomprehensible partiality, had singled him out, and taken him up, and given him an awesome dignity and importance. And yet Death had rejected Christian, had held him off, and would not have him at any price – would only keep on making game of him and mocking him with all these tricks and antics which nobody took seriously. Never in his life had Thomas Buddenbrook so impressed his brother as at this hour. Success is so definite, so conclusive! Death alone can make others respect our sufferings; and through death the most pitiable sufferings acquire dignity. "You have won – I give in," Christian thought. He knelt on one knee, with a sudden awkward gesture, and kissed the cold hand on the coverlet. Then he stepped back and moved about the room, his eyes darting back and forth.

Other visitors came – the old Krögers, the Misses Buddenbrook, old Herr Marcus. Poor Clothilde, lean and ashen, stood by the bed; her face was apathetic, and she folded her hands in their worsted gloves. "You must not think, Tony and Gerda," said she, and her voice dragged very much, "that I've no feeling because I don't weep. The truth is, I have no more tears." And as she stood there, incredibly dry and withered, it was evident that she spoke the truth.

Then they all left the room to make way for an elderly female, an unpleasant old creature with a toothless, mumbling jaw, who had come to help Sister Leandra wash and dress the corpse.

Gerda Buddenbrook, Frau Permaneder, Christian, and little Johann sat under the big gas-lamp around the centre-table in the living-room, and worked industriously until far on into the evening. They were addressing envelopes and making a list of people who ought to receive announcements. Now and then somebody thought of another name. Hanno had to help, too; his handwriting was plain, and there was need of haste.

It was still in the house and in the street. The gas-lamp made a soft hissing noise; somebody murmured a name; the papers rustled. Sometimes they looked at each other and remembered what had happened.

Frau Permaneder scratched busily. But regularly once every five minutes she would put down her pen, lift her clasped hands up to her mouth, and break out in lamentations. "I can't realize it! " she would cry – meaning that she was gradually beginning to realize. "It is the end of everything," she burst out another time, in sheer despair, and flung her arms around her sister-in-law's neck with loud weeping. After each outburst she was strengthened, and took up her work again.

With Christian it was as with poor Clothilde. He had not shed a tear – which fact rather mortified him. It was true, too, that his constant preoccupation with his own condition had used him up emotionally and made him insensitive. Now and then he would start up, rub his hand over his bald brow, and murmur, "Yes, it's frightfully sad." He said it to himself, with strong self-reproach, and did his best to make his eyes water.

Suddenly something happened to startle them all: little Johann began to laugh. He was copying a list of names, and had found one with such a funny sound that he could not resist it. He said it aloud and snorted through his nose, bent over, sobbed, and could not control himself. The grown people looked at him in bewildered incredulity; and his mother sent him up to bed.

CHAPTER IX

SENATOR BUDDENBROOK had died of a bad tooth. So it was said in the town. But goodness, people don't die of a bad tooth! He had nad a toothache; Herr Brecht had broken off the crown; and thereupon the Senator had simply fallen in the street. Was ever the like heard?

But however it had happened, that was no longer the point. What had next to be done was to send wreaths – large, expensive wreaths which would do the givers credit and be mentioned in the paper: wreaths which showed that they came from people with sympathetic hearts and long purses. They were sent. They poured in from all sides, from organizations, from families and individuals: laurel wreaths, wreaths of heavily-scented flowers, silver wreaths, wreaths with black bows or bows with the colours of the City on them, or dedications printed in heavy black type or gilt lettering. And palms – simply quantities of palms.

The flower-shops did an enormous business, not least among them being Iwersen's, opposite the Buddenbrook mansion. Frau Iwersen rang many times in the day at the vestibule door, and handed in arrangements in all shapes and styles, from Senator This or That, or Consul So-and-So, from office staffs and civil servants. On one of these visits she asked if she might go up and see the Senator a minute. Yes, of course, she was told; and she followed Frau Permaneder up the main staircase, gazing silently at its magnificence.

She went up heavily, for she was, as usual, expecting. Her looks had grown a little common with the years; but the narrow black eyes and the Malay cheek-bones had not lost their charm. One could still see that she must once have been exceedingly pretty. She was admitted into the salon, where Thomas Buddenbrook lay upon his bier.

He lay in the centre of the large, light room, the furniture of which had been removed, amid the white silk linings of his coffin, dressed in white silk, shrouded in white silk, in a thick and stupefying mingling of odours from the tuberoses, violets, roses, and other flowers with which he was surrounded. At his head, in a half-circle of silver candelabra, stood the pedestal draped in mourning, supporting the marble copy of Thorwaldsen's Christ. The wreaths, garlands, baskets, and bunches stood or lay along the walls, on the floor, and on the coverlet. Palms stood around the bier and drooped over the feet of the dead. The skin of his face was abraded in spots, and the nose was bruised. But his hair was dressed with the tongs, as in life, and his moustache, too, had been drawn through the tongs for the last time by old Herr Wenzel, and stuck out stiff and straight beyond his white cheeks. His head was turned a little to one side, and an ivory cross was stuck between the folded hands.

Frau Iwersen remained near the door, and looked thence, blinking, over to the bier. Only when Frau Permaneder, in deep black, with a cold in her head from much weeping, came from the living-room through the portières and invited Frau Iwersen to come nearer, did she dare to venture a little farther forward on the parquetry floor. She stood with her hands folded across her prominent abdomen, and looked about her with her narrow black eyes: at the plants, the candelabra, the bows and the wreaths, the white silk, and Thomas Buddenbrook's face. It would be hard to describe the expression on the pale, blurred features of the pregnant woman. Finally she said "Yes — " sobbed just once, a brief inarticulate sound, and turned away.

Frau Permaneder loved these visits. She never stirred from the house, but superintended with tireless zeal the homage that pressed about the earthly husk of her departed brother. She read the newspaper articles aloud many times in her throaty voice: those same newspapers which at the time of the jubilee had paid tribute to her brother's merits, now mourned the irreparable loss of his personality. She stood at Gerda's side to receive the visits of condolence in the living-room and there was no end of these; their name was legion. She held conferences with various people about the funeral, which must of course be conducted in the most refined manner. She arranged farewells: she had the office staff come in a body to bid their chief good-bye. The workmen from the granaries came too. They shuffled their huge feet along the parquetry floor, drew down the corners of their mouths to show their respect, and emanated an odour of chewing tobacco, spirits, and physical exertion. They looked at the dead lying in his splendid state, twirled their caps, first admired and then grew restive, until at length one of them found courage to go, and the whole troop followed shuffling on his heels. Frau Permaneder was enchanted.

She asserted that some of them had tears running down into their beards. This simply was not the fact; but she saw it, and it made her happy.

The day of the funeral dawned. The metal casket was hermetically sealed and covered with flowers, the candles burned in their silver holders, the house filled with people, and, surrounded by mourners from near and far, Pastor Pringsheim stood at the head of the coffin in upright majesty, his impressive head resting upon his ruff as on a dish.

A high-shouldered functionary, a brisk intermediate something between a waiter and a major-domo, had in charge the outward ordering of the solemnity. He ran with the softest speed down the staircase and called in a penetrating whisper across the entry, which was filled to overflowing with tax-commissioners in uniform and grain-porters in blouses, knee-breeches, and tall hats: "The rooms are full, but there is a little room left in the corridor."

Then everything was hushed. Pastor Pringsheim began to speak. He filled the whole house with the rolling periods of his exquisitely modulated, sonorous voice. He stood there near the figure of Thorwaldsen's Christ and wrung his hands before his face or spread them out in blessing; while below in the street, before the house door, beneath a white wintry sky, stood the hearse drawn by four black horses, with the other carriages in a long row behind it. A company of soldiers with grounded arms stood in two rows opposite the house door, with Lieutenant von Throta at their head. He held his drawn sword on his arm and looked up at the bow-window with his brilliant eyes. Many people were craning their necks from windows nearby or standing on the pavements to look.

At length there was a stir in the vestibule, the lieutenant's muffled word of command sounded, the soldiers presented arms with a rattle of weapons, Herr von Throta let his sword sink, and the coffin appeared. It swayed cautiously forth of the house door, borne by the four men in black cloaks and cocked hats, and a gust of perfume came with it, wafted over the heads of bystanders. The breeze ruffled the black plumes on top of the hearse, tossed the manes of the horses standing in line down to the river, and dishevelled the mourning hat-scarves of the coachman and grooms. Enormous single flakes of snow drifted down from the sky in long slanting curves.

The horses attached to the hearse, all in black trappings so that only their restless rolling eyeballs could be seen, now slowly got in motion. The hearse moved off, led by the four black servants.

The company of soldiers fell in behind, and one after another the coaches followed on. Christian Buddenbrook and the pastor got into the first; little Johann sat in the second, with a well-fed Hamburg relative. And slowly, slowly, with mournful long-drawn pomp, Thomas Buddenbrook's funeral train wound away, while the flags at half-mast on all the houses flapped before the wind. The office staff and the grain-porters followed on foot.

The casket, with the mourners behind, followed the well-known cemetery paths, past crosses and statues and chapels and bare weeping-willows, to the Buddenbrook family lot, where the military guard of honour already stood, and presented arms again. A funeral march sounded in subdued and solemn strains from behind the shrubbery.

Once more the heavy gravestone, with the family arms in relief, had been moved to one side; and once more the gentlemen of the town stood there, on the edge of the little grove, beside the abyss walled in with masonry into which Thomas Buddenbrook was now lowered to join his fathers. They stood there with bent heads, these worthy and well-to-do citizens: prominent among them were the Senators, in white gloves and cravats. Beyond them was the throng of officials, clerks, grain-porters, and warehouse labourers.

The music stopped. Pastor Pringsheim spoke. While his voice, raised in blessing, still lingered on the air, everybody pressed round to shake hands with the brother and son of the deceased.

The ceremony was long and tedious. Christian Buddenbrook received all the condolences with his usual absent, embarrassed air. Little Johann stood by his side, in his heavy reefer jacket with the gilt buttons, and looked at the ground with his blue-shadowed eyes. He never looked up, but bent his head against the wind with a sensitive twist of all his features.

PART ELEVEN

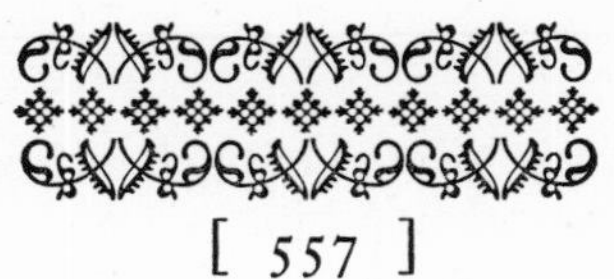

CHAPTER I

IT sometimes happens that we may recall this or that person whom we have not lately seen and wonder how he is. And then, with a start, we remember that he has disappeared from the stage, that his voice no longer swells the general concert — that he is, in short, departed from among us, and lies somewhere outside the walls, beneath the sod.

Frau Consul Buddenbrook, she that was a Stüwing, Uncle Gotthold's widow, passed away. Death set his reconciling and atoning seal upon the brow of her who in her life had been the cause of such violent discord; and her three daughters, Friederike, Henriette, and Pfiffi, received the condolences of their relatives with an affronted air which seemed to say: "You see, your persecutions have at last brought her down to her grave!" As if the Frau Consul were not as old as the hills already!

And Madame Kethelsen had gone to her long rest. In her later years she had suffered much from gout; but she died gently and simply, resting upon a childlike faith which was much envied by her educated sister, who had always had her periodic attacks of rationalistic doubt, and who, though she grew constantly smaller and more bent, was relentlessly bound by an iron constitution to this sinful earth.

Consul Peter Döhlmann was called away. He had eaten up all his money, and finally fell a prey to Hunyadi-Janos, leaving his daughter an income of two hundred marks a year. He depended upon the respect felt in the community for the name of Döhlmann to insure her being admitted into the Order of St. John.

Justus Kröger also departed this life, which was a loss, for now nobody was left to prevent his wife selling everything she owned to send money to the wretched Jacob, who was still leading a dissolute existence somewhere in the world.

Christian Buddenbrook had likewise disappeared from the streets of his native city. He would have been sought in vain within her walls. He had moved to Hamburg, less than a year after his brother's death, and there he united himself, before God and men, with Fräulein Aline Puvogel, a lady with whom he had long stood in a close relationship. No one could now stop him. His inheritance from his mother, indeed, half the interest of which had always found its way to Hamburg, was managed by Herr Stephan Kistenmaker – in so far as it was not already spent in advance. Herr Kistenmaker, in fact, had been appointed administrator by the terms of his deceased friend's will. But in all other respects Christian was his own master. Directly the marriage became known, Frau Permaneder addressed to Frau Aline Buddenbrook in Hamburg a long and extraordinarily violent letter, beginning " Madame! " and declaring in carefully poisoned words that she had absolutely no intention of recognizing as a relative either the person addressed or any of her children.

Herr Kistenmaker was executor and administrator of the Buddenbrook estate and guardian of little Johann. He held these offices in high regard. They were an important activity which justified him in rubbing his head on the Bourse with every indication of overwork and telling everybody that he was simply wearing himself out. Besides, he received two per cent. of the revenues, very punctually. But he was not too successful in the performance of his duties, and Gerda Buddenbrook soon had reason to feel dissatisfied.

The business was to close, the firm to go into liquidation, and the estate to be settled within a year. This was Thomas Buddenbrook's wish, as expressed in his will. Frau Permaneder felt much upset. " And Hanno? And little Johann – what about Hanno? " She was disappointed and grieved that her brother had passed over his son and heir and had not wished to keep the firm alive for him to step into. She wept for hours to think that one should dispose thus summarily of that honourable shield, that jewel cherished by four generations of Buddenbrooks: that the history of the firm was now to close, while yet there existed a direct heir to carry it on. But she finally consoled herself by thinking that the end of the firm was not, after all, the end of the family, and that her nephew might as easily, in a new and different career, perform the high task allotted to him – that task being to carry on the family name and add fresh lustre to the family reputation. It could not be in vain that he possessed so much likeness to his great-grandfather.

The liquidation of the business began, under the auspices of Herr Kistenmaker and old Herr Marcus; and it took a most deplorable course. The time was short, and it must be punctiliously kept to. The pending business was disposed of on hurried and unfavourable terms. One precipitate and disadvantageous sale followed another. The granaries and warehouses were turned into money at a great loss; and what was not lost by Herr Kistenmaker's over-zealousness was wasted by the procrastination of old Herr Marcus. In town they said that the old man, before he left his house in winter warmed not only his coat and hat, but his walking-stick as well. If ever a favourable opportunity arose, he invariably let it slip through his fingers. And so the losses piled up. Thomas Buddenbrook had left, on paper, an estate of six hundred and fifty thousand marks. A year after the will was opened it had become abundantly clear that there was no question of such a sum.

Indefinite, exaggerated rumours of the unfavourable liquidation got about, and were fed by the news that Gerda Buddenbrook meant to sell the great house. Wonderful stories flew about, of the reasons which obliged her to take such a step; of the collapse of the Buddenbrook fortune. Things were thought to look very badly: and a feeling began to grow up in the town, of which the widowed Frau Senator became aware, at first with surprise and astonishment, and then with growing anger. When she told her sister-in-law, one day, that she had been pressed in an unpleasant way for the payment of some considerable accounts, Frau Permaneder had at first been speechless, and then had burst out into frightful laughter. Gerda Buddenbrook was so outraged that she expressed a half-determination to leave the city for ever with little Johann and go back to Amsterdam to play duets with her old father. But this called forth such a storm of protest from Frau Permaneder that she was obliged to give up the plan for the time being.

As was to be expected, Frau Permaneder protested against the sale of the house which her brother had built. She bewailed the bad impression it would make and complained of the blow it would deal the family prestige. But she had to grant it would be folly to continue to keep up the spacious and splendid dwelling that had been Thomas Buddenbrook's costly hobby, and that Gerda's idea of a comfortable little villa outside the wall, in the country, had, after all, much to commend it.

A great day dawned for Siegismund Gosch the broker. His old age was illumined by an event so stupendous that for many hours it held his knees from trembling. It came about that he sat in Gerda Buddenbrook's salon, in an easy-chair, opposite her and discussed tête-à-tête the price of her house. His snow-white locks streamed over his face, his chin protruded grimly, he succeeded for once in looking thoroughly hump-backed. He hissed when he talked, but his manners were cold and businesslike, and nothing betrayed the emotions of his soul. He bound himself to take over the house, stretched out his hand, smiled cunningly, and bid eighty-five thousand marks — which was a possible offer, for some loss would certainly have to be taken in this sale. But Herr Kistenmaker's opinion must be heard; and Gerda Buddenbrook had to let Herr Gosch go without making the bargain. Then it appeared that Herr Kistenmaker was not minded to allow any interference in what he considered his prerogative. He mistrusted Herr Gosch's offer; he laughed at it, and swore that he could easily get much more. He continued to swear this, until at length he was forced to dispose of the property for seventy-five thousand marks to an elderly spinster who had returned from extended travel and decided to settle in the town.

Herr Kistenmaker also arranged for the purchase of the new house, a pleasant little villa for which he paid rather too high a price, but which was about what Gerda Buddenbrook wanted. It lay outside the Castle Gate, on a chestnut-bordered avenue; and thither, in the autumn of the year 1876, the Frau Senator moved with her son, her servants, and a part of her household goods — the remainder, to Frau Permaneder's great distress, being left behind to pass into the possession of the elderly gentlewoman.

As if these were not changes enough, Mamsell Jungmann, after forty years in the service of the Buddenbrook family, left it to return to her native West Prussia to live out the evening of her life. To tell the truth, she was dismissed by the Frau Senator. This good soul had taken up with little Johann when the previous generation had outgrown her. She had cherished him fondly, read him fairy stories, and told him about the uncle who died of hiccoughs. But now little Johann was no longer small. He was a lad of fifteen years, to whom, despite his lack of strength, she could no longer be of much service; and with his mother her relations had not for a long time been on a very comfortable footing. She had never been able to think of this lady, who had entered the family so much later than herself, as a proper Buddenbrook; and of late she had begun, with the freedom of an old servant, to arrogate to herself exaggerated authority. She stirred up dissension in the household by this or that encroachment; the position became untenable; there were disagreements — and though Frau Permaneder made an impassioned plea in her behalf, as for the old house and the furniture, old Ida had to go.

She wept bitterly when the hour came to bid little Johann farewell. He put his arms about her and embraced her. Then, with his hands behind his back, resting his weight on one leg while the other poised on the tips of the toes, he watched her out of sight; his face wore the same brooding, introspective look with which he had stood at his father's death-bed, and his grandmother's bier, witnessed the breaking-up of the great household, and shared in so many events of the same kind, though of lesser outward significance. The departure of old Ida belonged to the same category as other events with which he was already familiar: breakings-up, closings, endings, disintegrations — he had seen them all. Such events did not disturb him — they had never disturbed him. But he would lift his head, with the curling light-brown hair, inflate one delicate nostril, and it was as if he cautiously sniffed the air about him, expecting to perceive that odour, that strange and yet familiar odour which, at his grandmother's bier, not all the scent of the flowers had been able to disguise.

When Frau Permaneder visited her sister-in-law, she would draw her nephew to her and tell him of the Buddenbrook family past, and of that future for which, next to the mercy of God, they would have to thank little Johann. The more depressing the present appeared, the more she strove to depict the elegance of the life that went on in the houses of her parents and grandparents; and she would tell Hanno how his great-grandfather had driven all over the country with his carriage and four horses. One day she had a severe attack of cramps in the stomach because Friederike, Henriette, and Pfiffi had asserted that the Hagenströms were the crême de la crême of town society.

Bad news came of Christian. His marriage seemed not to have improved his health. He had become more and more subject to uncanny delusions and morbid hallucinations, until finally his wife had acted upon the advice of a physician and had him put into an institution. He was unhappy there, and wrote pathetic letters to his relatives, expressive of a fervent desire to leave the establishment, where, it seemed, he was none too well treated. But they kept him shut up, and it was probably the best thing for him. It also put his wife in a position to continue her former independent existence without prejudice to her status as a married woman or to the practical advantages accruing from her marriage.

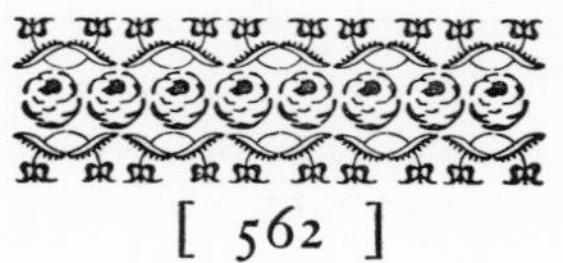

CHAPTER II

THE ALARM-CLOCK went off with cruel alacrity. It was a hoarse rattling and clattering that it made, rather than a ringing, for it was old and worn out; but it kept on for a painfully long time, for it had been thoroughly wound up.

Hanno Buddenbrook was startled to his inmost depths. It was like this every morning. His very entrails rebelled, in rage, protest, and despair, at the onslaught of this at once cruel and faithful monitor standing on the bedside table close to his ear. However, he did not get up, or even change his position in the bed; he only wrenched himself away from some blurred dream of the early morning and opened his eyes.

It was perfectly dark in the wintry room. He could distinguish nothing, not even the hands on the clock. But he knew it was six o'clock, because last night he had set his alarm for six. Last night — And as he lay on his back, with his nerves rasped by the shock of waking, struggling for sufficient resolution to make a light and jump out of bed, everything that had filled his mind yesterday came gradually back into his consciousness.

It was Sunday evening; and after having been maltreated by Herr Brecht for several days on end, he had been taken as a reward to a performance of *Lohengrin.* He had looked forward for a whole week to this evening with a joy which absorbed his entire existence. Only, it was a pity that on such occasions the full pleasure of the anticipation had to be marred by disagreeable commonplaces that went on up to the very last minute. But at length Saturday came, school was over for the week, and Herr Brecht's little drill had bored and buzzed away in the mouth for the last time. Now everything was out of the way and done with — for he had obstinately put off his preparation for Monday until after the opera. What was Monday to him? Was it likely it would ever dawn? Who believes in Monday, when he is to hear *Lohengrin* on Sunday evening? He would get up early on Monday and get the wretched stuff done — and that was all there was to it. Thus he went about free from care, fondled the coming joy in his heart, dreamed at his piano, and forgot all unpleasantness to come.

And then the dream became reality. It came over him with all its enchantment and consecration, all its secret revelations and tremors, its sudden inner emotion, its extravagant, unquenchable intoxication. It was true that the music of the overture was rather too much for the cheap violins in the orchestra; and the fat conceited-looking Lohengrin with straw-coloured hair came in rather hind side foremost in his little boat. And his guardian, Herr Stephan Kistenmaker, had sat in the next box and grumbled about the boy's being taken away from his lessons and having his mind distracted like that. But the sweet, exalted splendour of the music had borne him away upon its wings.

The end had come at length. The singing, shimmering joy was quenched and silent. He had found himself back home in his room, with a burning head and the consciousness that only a few hours of sleep, there in his bed, separated him from dull everyday existence. And he had been overpowered by an attack of the complete despondency which was all too familiar an experience. Again he had learned that beauty can pierce one like a pain, and that it can sing profoundly into shame and a longing despair that utterly consume the courage and energy necessary to the life of every day. His despondency weighed him down like mountains, and once more he told himself, as he had done before, that this was more than his own individual burden of weaknesses that rested upon him: that his burden was one which he had borne upon his soul from the beginning of time, and must one day sink under at last.

He had wound the alarm-clock and gone to sleep — and slept that dead and heavy sleep that comes when one wishes never to awake again. And now Monday was here, and he had not prepared a single lesson.

He sat up and lighted the bedside candle. But his arms and shoulders felt so cold that he lay down again and pulled up the covers.

The hand pointed to ten minutes after six. Oh, it was absurd to get up now! He should hardly have time to make a beginning, for there was preparation in nearly every lesson. And the time he had fixed was already past. Was it as certain, then, as it had seemed to him yesterday that he would be called up in Latin and Chemistry? It was certainly to be expected — in all human probability it would happen. The names at the end of the alphabet had lately been called in the Ovid class, and presumably they would begin again at the beginning. But, after all, it wasn't so absolutely certain, beyond a peradventure — there were exceptions to every rule.

Chance sometimes worked wonders, he knew. He sank deeper and deeper into these false and plausible speculations; his thoughts began to run in together – he was asleep.

The little schoolboy bedchamber, cold and bare, with the copper-plate of the Sistine Madonna over the bed, the extension-table in the middle, the untidy book-shelf, a stiff-legged mahogany desk, the harmonium, and the small wash-hand stand, lay silent in the flickering light of the candle. The window was covered with icy-crystals, and the blind was up in order that the light might come earlier. And Hanno slept, his cheek pressed into the pillow, his lips closed, the eyelashes lying close upon his cheek; he slept with an expression of the most utter abandonment to slumber, the soft, light-brown hair clustering about his temples. And slowly the candle-flame lost its reddish-yellow glow, as the pale, dun-coloured dawn stole into the room through the icy coating on the window-pane.

At seven he woke once more, with a start of fear. He must get up and take upon himself the burden of the day. There was no way out of it. Only a short hour now remained before school would begin. Time pressed; there was no thought of preparation now. And yet he continued to lie, full of exasperation and rebellion against this brutal compulsion that was upon him to forsake his warm bed in the frosty dawning and go out into the world, into contact with harsh and unfriendly people. " Oh, only two little tiny minutes more," he begged of his pillow, in overwhelming tenderness. And then he gave himself a full five minutes more, out of sheer bravado, and closed his eyes, opening one from time to time to stare despairingly at the clock, which went stupidly on in its insensate, accurate way.

Ten minutes after seven o'clock, he tore himself out of bed and began to move about the room with frantic haste. He let the candle burn, for the daylight was not enough by itself. He breathed upon a crystal and, looking out, saw a thick mist abroad.

He was unutterably cold, and a shiver sometimes shook his entire body. The ends of his fingers burned; they were so swollen that he could do nothing with the nail-brush. As he washed the upper parts of his body, his almost lifeless hand let fall the sponge, and he stood a moment stiff and helpless, steaming like a sweating horse.

At last he was dressed. Dull-eyed and breathless, he stood at the table, collected his despairing senses with a jerk, and began to put together the books he was likely to need to-day, murmuring in an anguished voice: " Religion, Latin, chemistry," and shuffling together the wretched ink-spotted paper volumes.

Yes, he was already quite tall, was little Johann. He was more than fifteen years old, and no longer wore a sailor costume, but a light-brown jacket suit with a blue-and-white spotted cravat. Over his waistcoat he wore a long, thin gold chain that had belonged to his grandfather, and on the fourth finger of his broad but delicately articulated right hand was the old seal ring with the green stone. It was his now. He pulled on his heavy winter jacket, put on his hat, snatched his school-bag, extinguished the candle, and dashed down the stair to the ground floor, past the stuffed bear, and into the dining-room on the right.

Fräulein Clementine, his mother's new factotum, a thin girl with curls on her forehead, a pointed nose, and short-sighted eyes, already sat at the breakfast-table.

" How late is it, really? " he asked between his teeth, though he already knew with great precision.

" A quarter before eight," she answered, pointing with a thin, red, rheumatic-looking hand at the clock on the wall. " You must get along, Hanno." She set a steaming cup of cocoa before him, and pushed the bread and butter, salt, and an egg-cup toward his place.

He said no more, clutched a roll, and began, standing, with his hat on and his bag under his arm, to swallow his cocoa. The hot drink hurt the back tooth which Herr Brecht had just been working at. He let half of it stand, pushed away the egg, and with a sound intended for an adieu ran out of the house.

It was ten minutes to eight when he left the garden and the little brick villa behind him and dashed along the wintry avenue. Ten, nine, eight minutes more. And it was a long way. He could scarcely see for the fog. He drew it in with his breath and breathed it out again, this thick, icy cold fog, with all the power of his narrow chest; he stopped his still throbbing tooth with his tongue, and did fearful violence to his leg muscles. He was bathed in perspiration; yet he felt frozen in every limb. He began to have a stitch in his side. The morsel of breakfast revolted in his stomach against this morning jaunt which it was taking; he felt nauseated, and his heart fluttered and trembled so that it took away his breath.

The Castle Gate – only the Castle Gate – and it was four minutes to eight! As he panted on through the streets, in an extremity of mingled pain, perspiration, and nausea, he looked on all sides for his fellow pupils. No, there was no one else; they were all on the spot – and now it was beginning to strike eight. Bells were ringing all over the town, and the chimes of St. Mary's were playing, in celebration of this moment, " now let us all thank God." They played half the notes falsely; they had no idea of rhythm, and they were badly in want of tuning. Thus Hanno, in the madness of despair. But what was that to him? He was late; there was no longer any room for doubt. The school clock was usually a little behind, but not enough to help him this time. He stared hopelessly into people's faces as they passed him. They were going to their offices or about their business; they were in no particular hurry; nothing was threatening them. Some of them looked at him and smiled at his distracted appearance and sulky looks. He was beside himself at these smiles. What were they smiling at, these comfortable, unhurried people? He wanted to shout after them and tell them their smiling was very uncivil. Perhaps *they* would just enjoy falling down dead in front of the closed entrance gate of the school!

The prolonged shrill ringing which was the signal for morning prayers struck on his ear while he was still twenty paces from the long red wall with the two cast-iron gates, which separated the court of the school-building from the street. He felt that his legs had no more power to advance: he simply let his body fall forward, the legs moved willy-nilly to prevent his stumbling, and thus he staggered on and arrived at the gate just as the bell had ceased ringing.

Herr Schlemiel, the porter, a heavy man with the face and rough beard of a labourer, was just about to close the gate. " Well! " he said, and let Buddenbrook slip through. Perhaps, perhaps, he might still be saved! What he had to do now was to slip unobserved into his classroom and wait there until the end of prayers, which were held in the drill-hall, and to act as if everything were in order. Panting, exhausted, in a cold perspiration, he slunk across the courtyard and through the folding doors with glass panes that divided it from the interior.

Everything in the establishment was now new, clean, and adequate. The time had been ripe; and the grey, crumbling walls of the ancient monastic school had been levelled to the ground to make room for the spacious, airy, and imposing new building. The style of the whole had been preserved, and corridors and cloisters were still spanned by the fine old Gothic vaulting. But the lighting and heating arrangements, the ventilation of the classrooms, the comfort of the masters' rooms, the equipment of the halls for the teaching of chemistry, physics and design, all this had been carried out on the most modern lines with respect to comfort and sanitation.

The exhausted Hanno stuck close to the wall and kept his eyes open as he stole along. Heaven be praised, the corridors were empty. He heard distantly the hubbub made by the hosts of masters and pupils going into the drill-hall, to receive there a little spiritual strengthening for the labours of the week. But here everything was empty and still, and his road up the broad linoleum-covered stairs lay free. He stole up cautiously on his tiptoes, holding his breath, straining his ears for sounds from above. His classroom, the lower second of the *Realschule*, was in the first storey, opposite the stairs, and the door was open. Crouched on the top step, he peered down the long corridor, on both sides of which were the entrances to the various classrooms, with porcelain signs above them. Three rapid, noiseless steps forward – and he was in his own room.

It was empty. The curtains of the three large windows were still drawn, and the gas was burning in the chandelier with a soft hissing noise. Green shades diffused the light over the three rows of desks. These desks each had room for two pupils; they were made of light-coloured wood, and opposite them, in remote and edifying austerity, stood the master's platform with a blackboard behind it. A yellow wainscoting ran round the lower part of the wall, and above it the bare white-washed surface was decorated with a few maps. A second blackboard stood on an easel by the master's chair.

Hanno went to his place, which was nearly in the centre of the room. He stuffed his bag into the desk, sank upon the hard seat, laid his arms on the sloping lid, and rested his head upon them. He had a sensation of unspeakable relief. The room was bare, hard, hateful, and ugly; and the burden of the whole threatening forenoon, with its numerous perils, lay before him. But for the moment he was safe; he had saved his skin, and could take things as they came. The first lesson, Herr Ballerstedt's class in religious instruction, was comparatively harmless. He could see, by the vibration of the little strips of paper over the ventilator next the ceiling, that warm air was streaming in, and the gas, too, did its share to heat the room. He could actually stretch out here and feel his stiffened limbs slowly thawing. The heat mounted to his head: it was very pleasant, but not quite healthful; it made his ears buzz and his eyes heavy.

A sudden noise behind him made him start and turn around.

And behold, from behind the last bench rose the head and shoulders of Kai, Count Mölln. He crawled out, did this young man, got up, shook himself, slapped his hands together to get the dust off, and came up to Hanno with a beaming face.

"Oh, it's you, Hanno," he said. "And I crawled back there because I took you for a piece of the faculty when you came in."

His voice cracked as he spoke, because it was changing, which Hanno's had not yet begun to do. He had kept pace with Hanno in his growth, but his looks had not altered, and he still wore a dingy suit of no particular colour, with a button or so missing and a big patch in the seat. His hands, too, were not quite clean; narrow and aristocratic-looking though they were, with long, slender fingers and tapering nails. But his brow was still pure as alabaster beneath the carelessly parted reddish-yellow hair that fell over it, and the glance of the sparkling blue eyes was as keen and as profound as ever. In fact, the contrast was even more striking between his neglected toilette and the racial purity of his face, with its delicate bony structure, slightly aquiline nose, and short upper lip, upon which the down was beginning to show.

"Oh, Kai," said Hanno, with a wry face, putting his hand to his heart. "How can you frighten me like that? What are you doing up here? Why are you hiding? Did you come late too?"

"Dear me, no," Kai said. "I've been here a long time. Though one doesn't much look forward to getting back to the old place, when Monday morning comes around. *You* must know that yourself, old fellow. No, I only stopped up here to have a little game. The deep one seems to be able to reconcile it with his religion to hunt people down to prayers. Well, I get behind him, and I manage to keep close behind his back whichever way he turns, the old mystic! So in the end he goes off, and I can stop up here. But what about you?" he said sympathetically, sitting down beside Hanno on the bench. "You had to run, didn't you? Poor old chap! You look perfectly worn out. Your hair is sticking to your forehead." He took a ruler from the table and carefully combed little Johann's hair with it. "You overslept, didn't you? Look," he interrupted himself, "here I am sitting in the sacred seat of number one — Adolf Todtenhaupt's place! Well, it won't hurt me for once, I suppose. You overslept, didn't you?"

Hanno had put his head down on his arms again. "I was at the opera last night," he said, heaving a long sigh.

"Right — I'd forgot that. Well, was it beautiful?"

He got no answer.

"You are a lucky fellow, after all," went on Kai perseveringly. "I've never been in the theatre, not a single time in my whole life, and there isn't the smallest prospect of my going — at least, not for years."

"If only one did not have to pay for it afterwards," said Hanno gloomily.

"The headache next morning — well, I know how that feels, anyhow." Kai stooped and picked up his friend's coat and hat, which lay on the floor beside the bench, and carried them quietly out into the corridor.

"Then I take for granted you haven't done the verses from the *Metamorphoses?*" he asked as he came back.

"No," said Hanno.

"Have you prepared for the geography test?"

"I haven't done anything, and I don't know anything," said Hanno.

"Not the chemistry nor the English, either? *Benissimo!* Then there's a pair of us — brothers-in-arms," said Kai, with obvious gratification. "I'm in exactly the same boat," he announced jauntily. "I did no work Saturday, because the next day was Sunday; and I did no work on Sunday, because it was Sunday! No, nonsense, it was mostly because I'd something better to do." He spoke with sudden earnestness, and a slight flush spread over his face. "Yes, perhaps it may be rather lively to-day, Hanno."

"If I get only one more bad mark, I shan't go up," said Johann; "and I'm sure to get it when I'm called up for Latin. The letter B comes next, Kai, so there's not much help for it."

"We shall see: What does Caesar say? 'Dangers may threaten me in the rear; but when they see the front of Caesar — '" But Kai did not finish. He was feeling rather out of sorts himself; he went to the platform and sat down in the master's chair, where he began to rock back and forth, scowling. Hanno still sat with his forehead resting on his arms. So they remained for a while in silence.

Then, somewhere in the distance, a dull humming was heard, which quickly swelled to a tumult of voices, approaching, imminent.

"The mob," said Kai, in an exasperated tone. "Goodness, how fast they got through. They haven't taken up ten minutes of the period!"

He got down from the platform and went to the door to mingle with the incoming stream. Hanno, for his part, lifted up his head for a minute, screwed up his mouth, and remained seated.

Stamping, shuffling, with a confusion of masculine voices, treble and falsetto, they flooded up the steps and over the corridor. The classroom suddenly became full of noise and movement. This was the lower second form of the *Realschule*, some twenty-five strong, comrades of Hanno and Kai. They loitered to their places with their hands in their pockets or dangling their arms, sat down, and opened their Bibles. Some of the faces were pleasant, strong, and healthy; others were doubtful or suspicious-looking. Here were tall, stout, lusty rascals who would soon go to sea or else begin a mercantile career, and who had no further interest in their school life; and small, ambitious lads, far ahead of their age, who were brilliant in subjects that could be got by heart. Adolf Todtenhaupt was the head boy. He knew everything. In all his school career he had never failed to answer a question. Part of his reputation was due to his silent, impassioned industry; but part was also due to the fact that the masters were careful not to ask him anything he might not know. It would have pained and mortified them and shaken their faith in human perfectibility to have Adolf Todtenhaupt fail to answer. He had a head full of remarkable bumps, to which his blond hair clung as smooth as glass; grey eyes with black rings beneath them, and long brown hands that stuck out beneath the too short sleeves of his neatly brushed jacket. He sat down next Hanno Buddenbrook with a mild, rather sly smile, and bade his neighbour good morning in the customary jargon, which reduced the greeting to a single careless monosyllable. Then he began to employ himself silently with the class register, holding his pen in a way that was incomparably correct, with the slender fingers outstretched; while about him people yawned, laughed, conned their lessons, and chattered half aloud.

After two minutes there were steps outside. The front rows of pupils rose, and some of those seated farther back followed their example. The rest scarcely interrupted what they were doing as Herr Ballerstedt came into the room, hung his hat on the door, and betook himself to the platform.

He was a man in the forties, with a pleasant *embonpoint*, a large bald spot, a short beard, a rosy complexion, and a mingled expression of unctuousness and sensuality on his humid lips. He took out his notebook and turned over the leaves in silence; but as the order in the classroom left much to be desired, he lifted his head, stretched out his arm over the desk, and waved his flabby white fist a few times powerlessly in the air. His face grew slowly red – such a dark red that his beard looked pale-yellow by contrast. He moved his lips and struggled spasmodically and fruitlessly for half a minute to speak, and finally brought out a single syllable, a short, suppressed grunt that sounded like "Well!" He still struggled after further expression, but in the end gave it up, returned to his notebook, calmed down, and became quite composed once more. This was Herr Ballerstedt's way.

He had intended to be a priest; but on account of his tendency to stutter and his leaning toward the good things of life he had become a pedagogue instead. He was a bachelor of some means, wore a small diamond on his finger, and was much given to eating and drinking. He was the head master who associated with his fellow masters only in working hours; and outside them he spent his time chiefly with the bachelor society of the town — yes, even with the officers of the garrison. He ate twice a day in the best hotel and was a member of the club. If he met any of his elder pupils in the streets, late at night or at two or three o'clock in the morning, he would puff up the way he did in the classroom, fetch out a "Good morning," and let the matter rest there, on both sides. From this master Hanno Buddenbrook had nothing to fear and was almost never called up by him. Herr Ballerstedt had been too often associated with Hanno's Uncle Christian in all too purely human affairs, to make him inclined to conflict with Johann in an official capacity.

"Well," he said, looked about him once more, waved his flabby fist with the diamond upon it, and glanced into his notebook. "Perlemann, the synopsis."

Somewhere in the class, up rose Perlemann. One could hardly see that he had risen; he was one of the small and forward ones. "The synopsis," he said, softly and politely, craning his neck forward with a nervous smile. "The Book of Job falls into three sections. First, the condition of Job before he fell under the chastening of the Lord: Chapter One, Verses one to six: second, the chastening itself, and its consequences, Chapter — "

"Right, Perlemann," interrupted Herr Ballerstedt, touched by so much modesty and obligingness. He put down a good mark in his book. "Continue, Heinricy."

Heinricy was one of the tall rascals who gave themselves no trouble over anything. He shoved the knife he had been playing with into his pocket, and got up noisily, with his lower lip hanging, and coughing in a gruff voice. Nobody was pleased to have him called up after the gentle Perlemann. The pupils sat drowsing in the warm room, some of them half asleep, soothed by the purring sound of the gas. They were all tired after the holiday; they had all crawled out of warm beds that morning with their teeth chattering, groaning in spirit. And they would have preferred to have the gentle Perlemann drone on for the remainder of the period. Heinricy was almost sure to make trouble.

"I wasn't here when we had this," he said, none too respectfully.

Herr Ballerstedt puffed himself up, waved his fist, struggled to speak, and stared young Heinricy in the face with his eyebrows raised. His head shook with the effort he made; but he finally managed to bring out a "Well!" and the spell was broken. He went on with perfect fluency. "There is never any work to be got out of you, and you always have an excuse ready, Heinricy. If you were ill the last time, you could have had help in that part; besides, if the first part dealt with the condition before the tribulation, and the second part with the tribulation itself, you could have told by counting on your fingers that the third part must deal with the condition after the tribulation! But you have no application or interest whatever; you are not only a poor creature, but you are always ready to excuse and defend your mistakes. But so long as this is the case, Heinricy, you cannot expect to make any improvement, and so I warn you. Sit down, Heinricy. Go on, Wasservogel."

Heinricy, thick-skinned and defiant, sat down with much shuffling and scraping, whispered some sort of saucy comment in his neighbour's ear, and took out his jack-knife again. Wasservogel stood up: a boy with inflamed eyes, a snub nose, prominent ears, and bitten finger-nails. He finished the summary in a rather whining voice, and began to relate the story of Job, the man from the land of Uz, and what happened to him. He had simply opened his Bible, behind the back of the pupil ahead of him; and he read from it with an air of utter innocence and concentration, staring then at a point on the wall and translated what he read, coughing the while, into awkward and hesitating modern German. There was something positively repulsive about Wasservogel; but Herr Ballerstedt gave him a large meed of praise. Wasservogel had the knack of making the masters like him; and they praised him in order to show that they were incapable of being led away by his ugliness to blame him unjustly.

The lesson continued. Various pupils were called up to display their knowledge touching Job, the man from the land of Uz. Gottlob Kassbaum, son of the unfortunate merchant P. Phillipp Kassbaum, got an excellent mark, despite the late distressing circumstances of his family, because he knew that Job had seven thousand sheep, three thousand camels, five hundred yoke of oxen, five hundred asses, and a large number of servants.

Then the Bibles, which were already open, were permitted to be opened, and they went on reading. Wherever Herr Ballerstedt thought explanation necessary, he puffed himself up, said " Well! " and after these customary preliminaries made a little speech upon the point in question, interspersed with abstract moral observations. Not a soul listened. A slumberous peace reigned in the room. The heat, with the continuous influx of warm air and the still lighted gas burners, had become oppressive, and the air was well-nigh exhausted by these twenty-five breathing and steaming organisms. The warmth, the purring of the gas, and the drone of the reader's voice lulled them all to a point where they were more asleep than awake. Kai, Count Mölln, however, had a volume of Edgar Allan Poe's *Tales* inside his Bible, and read in it, supporting his head on his hand. Hanno Buddenbrook leaned back, sank down in his seat, and looked with relaxed mouth and hot, swimming eyes at the Book of Job, in which all the lines ran together into a black haze. Now and then, as the Grail *motif* or the Wedding March came into his mind, his lids drooped and he felt an inward soothing; and then he would wish that this safe and peaceful morning hour might go on for ever.

Yet it ended, as all things must end. The shrill sound of the bell, clanging and echoing through the corridor, shook the twenty-five brains out of their slumberous calm.

" That is all," said Herr Ballerstedt. The register was handed up to him and he signed his name in it, as evidence that he had performed his office.

Hanno Buddenbrook closed his Bible and stretched himself, yawning. It was a nervous yawn; and as he dropped his arms and relaxed his limbs he had to take a long, deep breath to bring his heart back to a steady pulsation, for it weakly refused its office for a second. Latin came next. He cast a beseeching glance at Kai, who still sat there reading and seemed not to have remarked the end of the lesson. Then he drew out his Ovid, in stitched covers of marbled paper, and opened it at the lines that were to have been learned by heart for to-day. No, it was no use now trying to memorize any of it: the regular lines, full of pencil marks, numbered by fives all the way down the page, looked hopelessly unfamiliar. He barely understood the sense of them, let alone trying to say a single one of them by heart. And of those in to-day's preparation he had not puzzled out even the first sentence.

"What does that mean—'*deciderant, patula Jovis arbore glandes*'?" he asked in a despairing voice, turning to Adolf Todtenhaupt, who sat beside him working on the register.

"What?" asked Todtenhaupt, continuing to write. "The acorns from the tree of Jupiter—that is the oak; no, I don't quite know myself—"

"Tell me a bit, Todtenhaupt, when it comes my turn, will you?" begged Hanno, and pushed the book away. He scowled at the cool and careless nod Todtenhaupt gave by way of reply; then he slid sidewise off the bench and stood up.

The scene had changed. Herr Ballerstedt had left the room, and his place was taken by a weak enervated little man who stood straight and severe on the platform. He had a sparse white beard and a thin red neck that rose out of a narrow turned-down collar. He held his top hat upside down in front of him, clasped in two small hands covered with white hair. His real name was Professor Hückopp, but he was called "Spider" by the pupils. He was in charge of classrooms and corridors during the recess. "Out with the gas! Up with the blinds! Up with the windows!" he said, and gave his voice as commanding a tone as possible, moving his little arm in the air with an awkward, energetic gesture, as if he were turning a crank. "Everybody downstairs, into the fresh air, as quick as possible!"

The gas went out, the blinds flew up, the sallow daylight filled the room. The cold mist rushed in through the wide-open windows, and the lower second crowded past Professor Hückopp to the exit. Only the head boy might remain upstairs.

Hanno and Kai met at the door and went down the stairs together, and across the architecturally correct vestibule. They were silent. Hanno looked pathetically unwell, and Kai was deep in thought. They reached the courtyard and began to stroll up and down across the wet red tiles, among school companions of all ages and sizes.

A youthful looking man with a blond pointed beard kept order down here: Dr. Goldener, the "dressy one." He kept a *pensionnat* for the sons of the rich landowners from Mecklenburg and Holstein, and dressed, on account of these aristocratic youths, with an elegance not apparent in the other masters. He wore silk cravats, a dandified coat, and pale-coloured trousers fastened down with straps under the soles of his boots, and used perfumed handkerchiefs with coloured borders. He came of rather simple people, and all this elegance was not very becoming—his huge feet, for example, looked absurd in the pointed buttoned boots he wore.

He was vain of his plump red hands, too, and kept rubbing them together, clasping them before him, and regarding them with every mark of admiration. He carried his head laid far back on one side, and constantly made faces by blinking, screwing up his nose, and half-opening his mouth, as though he were about to say: "What's the matter now?" But his refinement led him to overlook all sorts of small infractions of the rules. He overlooked this or that pupil who had brought a book with him into the courtyard to prepare a little at the eleventh hour; he overlooked the fact that one of his boarding-pupils handed money to the porter, Herr Schlemiel, and asked him to get some pastry; he overlooked a small trial of strength between two third-form pupils, which resulted in a beating of one by the other, and around which a ring of connoisseurs was quickly formed; and he overlooked certain sounds behind him which indicated that a pupil who had made himself unpopular by cheating, cowardice, or other weakness was being forcibly escorted to the pump.

It was a lusty, not too gentle race, that of these comrades of Hanno and Kai among whom they walked up and down. The ideals of the victorious, united fatherland were those of a somewhat rude masculinity; its youth talked in a jargon at once brisk and slovenly; the most despised vices were softness and dandyism, the most admired virtues those displayed by prowess in drinking and smoking, bodily strength and skill in athletics. Whoever went out with his coat-collar turned up incurred a visit to the pump; while he who let himself be seen in the streets with a walking-stick must expect a public and ignominious correction administered in the drill-hall.

Hanno's and Kai's conversation was in striking contrast to that which went on around them among their fellows. This friendship had been recognized in the school for a long time. The masters suffered it grudgingly, suspecting that it meant disaffection and future trouble. The pupils could not understand it, but had settled down to regarding it with a sort of embarrassed dislike, and to thinking of the two friends as outlaws and eccentrics who must be left to their own devices. They recognized, it is true, the wildness and insubordination of Kai, Count Mölln, and respected him accordingly. As for Hanno Buddenbrook, big Heinricy, who thrashed everybody, could not make up his mind to lay a finger on him by way of chastisement for dandyism or cowardice. He refrained out of an indefinite respect and awe for the softness of Hanno's hair, the delicacy of his limbs, and his sad, shy, cold glance.

"I'm scared," Hanno said to Kai. He leaned against the wall of the school, drawing his jacket closer about him, yawning and shivering, "I'm so scared, Kai, that it hurts me all over my body. Now just tell me this: is Herr Mantelsack the sort of person one ought to be afraid of? Tell me yourself! If this beastly Ovid lesson were only over! If I just had my bad mark, in peace, and stopped where I am, and everything was in order! I'm not afraid of that. It is the row that goes beforehand that I hate!"

Kai was still deep in thought. "This Roderick Usher is the most remarkable character ever conceived," he said suddenly and abruptly. "I have read the whole lesson-hour. If ever I could write a tale like that!"

Kai was absorbed in his writing. It was to this he had referred when he said that he had something better to do than his preparation, and Hanno had understood him. Attempts at composition had developed out of his old propensity for inventing tales; and he had lately completed a composition in the form of a fantastic fairy tale, a narrative of symbolic adventure, which went forward in the depths of the earth among glowing metals and mysterious fires, and at the same time in the souls of men: a tale in which the primeval forces of nature and of the soul were interchanged and mingled, transformed and refined – the whole conceived and written in a vein of extravagant and even sentimental symbolism, fervid with passion and longing.

Hanno knew the tale well, and loved it; but he was not now in a frame of mind to think of Kai's work or of Edgar Allan Poe. He yawned again, and then sighed, humming to himself a *motif* he had lately composed on the piano. This was a habit with him. He would often give a long sigh, a deep indrawn breath, from the instinct to calm the fluctuating and irregular action of his heart; and he had accustomed himself to set the deep breathing to a musical theme of his own or some one else's invention.

"Look, there comes the Lord God," said Kai. "He is walking in his garden."

"Fine garden," said Hanno. He began to laugh nervously, and could not stop; putting his handkerchief to his mouth the while and looking across the courtyard at him whom Kai called the Lord God.

This was Director Wulicke, the head of the school, who had appeared in the courtyard: an extremely tall man with a slouch hat, a short heavy beard, a prominent abdomen, trousers that were far too short, and very dirty funnel-shaped cuffs. He strode across the flagstones with a face so angry in its expression that he seemed to be actually suffering, and pointed at the pump with outstretched arm. The water was running! A train of pupils ran before him and stumbled in their zeal to repair the damage. Then they stood about, looking first at the pump and then at the Director, their faces pictures of distress; and the Director, meanwhile, had turned to Dr. Goldener, who hurried up with a very red face and spoke to him in a deep hollow voice, fairly babbling with excitement between the words.

This Director Wulicke was a most formidable man. He had succeeded to the headship of the school after the death, soon after 1871, of the genial and benevolent old gentleman under whose guidance Hanno's father and uncle had pursued their studies. Dr. Wulicke was summoned from a professorship in a Prussian high school; and with his advent an entirely new spirit entered the school. In the old days the classical course had been thought of as an end in itself, to be pursued at one's ease, with a sense of joyous idealism. But now the leading conceptions were authority, duty, power, service, the career; " the categorical imperative of our philosopher Kant " was inscribed upon the banner which Dr. Wulicke in every official speech unfurled to the breeze. The school became a state within a state, in which not only the masters but the pupils regarded themselves as officials, whose main concern was the advancement they could make, and who must therefore take care to stand well with the authorities. Soon after the new Director was installed in his office the tearing down of the old school began, and the new one was built up on the most approved hygienic and aesthetic principles, and everything went swimmingly. But it remained an open question whether the old school, as an institution, with its smaller endowment of modern comfort and its larger share of gay good nature, courage, charm, and good feeling, had not been more blest and blessing than the new.

As for Dr. Wulicke himself personally, he had all the awful mystery, duplicity, obstinacy, and jealousy of the Old Testament God. He was as frightful in his smiles as in his anger. The result of the enormous authority that lay in his hands was that he grew more and more arbitrary and moody — he was even capable of making a joke and then visiting with his wrath anybody who dared to laugh. Not one of his trembling creatures knew how to act before him. They found it safest to honour him in the dust, and to protect themselves by a frantic abasement from the fate of being whirled up in the cloud of his wrath and crushed for ever under the weight of his righteous displeasure.

The name Kai had given Dr. Wulicke was known only to himself and Hanno, and they took the greatest pains not to let any of the others overhear it, for they could not possibly understand. No, there was not one single point on which those two stood on common ground with their schoolfellows. Even the methods of revenge, of "getting even," which obtained in the school were foreign to Hanno and Kai; and they utterly distained the current nicknames, which did not in the least appeal to their more subtle sense of humour. It was so poor, it showed such a paucity of invention, to call thin Professor Hückopp "Spider" and Herr Ballerstedt "Cocky." It was such scant compensation for their compulsory service to the state! No, Kai, Count Mölln, flattered himself that he was not so feeble as that! He invented, for his own and Hanno's use, a method of alluding to all their masters by their actual names, with the simple prefix, thus: Herr Ballerstedt, Herr Hückopp. The irony of this, its chilly remoteness and mockery, pleased him very much. He liked to speak of the "teaching body"; and would amuse himself for whole recesses with imagining it as an actual creature, a sort of monster, with a repulsively fantastic form. And they spoke in general of the "Institution" as if it were similar to that which harboured Hanno's Uncle Christian.

Kai's mood improved at sight of the Lord God, who still pervaded the playground and put everybody in a pallid fright by pointing, with fearful rumblings, to the wrapping papers from the luncheons which strewed the courtyard. The two lads went off to one of the gates, through which the masters in charge of the second period were now entering. Kai began to make bows of exaggerated respect before the red-eyed, pale, shabby-looking seminarists, who crossed over to go to their sixth and seventh form pupils in the back court. And when the grey-haired mathematics master, Herr Tietge, appeared, holding a bundle of books on his back with a shaking hand, bent, yellow, cross-eyed, spitting as he walked along, Kai said, "Good-morning, old dead man." He said this, in a loud voice and gazed straight up into the air with his bright, sharp gaze.

Then the bell clanged loudly, and the pupils began to stream through the entrances into the building. Hanno could not stop laughing. He was still laughing so hard on the stairs that his classmates looked at him and Kai with wonder and cold hostility, and even with a slight disgust at such frivolity.

There was a sudden hush in the classroom, and everybody stood up, as Herr Professor Mantelsack entered. He was the Professor *ordinarius*, for whom it was usual to show respect. He pulled the door to after him, bowed, craned his neck to see if all the class were standing up, hung his hat on its nail, and went quickly to the platform, moving his head rapidly up and down as he went. He took his place and stood for a while looking out the window and running his forefinger, with a large seal ring on it, around inside his collar. He was a man of medium size, with thin grey hair, a curled Olympian beard, and short-sighted prominent sapphire-blue eyes gleaming behind his spectacles. He was dressed in an open frock-coat of soft grey material, which he habitually settled at the waist with his short-fingered, wrinkled hand. His trousers were, like all the other masters', even the elegant Dr. Goldener's, far too short, and showed the legs of a pair of very broad and shiny boots.

He turned sharply away from the window and gave vent to a little good-natured sigh, smiling familiarly at several pupils. His mood was obviously good, and a wave of relief ran through the classroom. So much – everything, in fact – depended on whether Dr. Mantelsack was in a good mood! For the whole form was aware that he gave way to the feeling of the moment, whatever that might happen to be, without the slightest restraint. He was most extraordinarily, boundlessly, naïvely unjust, and his favour was as inconstant as that of fortune herself. He had always a few favourites – two or three – whom he called by their given names, and these lived in paradise. They might say almost anything they liked; and after the lesson Dr. Mantelsack would talk with them just like a human being. But a day would come – perhaps after the holidays – when for no apparent reason they were dethroned, cast out, rejected, and others elevated to their place. The mistakes of these favourites would be passed over with neat, careful corrections, so that their work retained a respectable appearance, no matter how bad it was; whereas he would attack the other copy-books with heavy, ruthless pen, and fairly flood them with red ink, so that their appearance was shocking indeed. And as he never troubled to count the mistakes, but distributed bad marks in proportion to the red ink he had expended, his favourites always emerged with great credit from these exercises. He was not even aware of the rank injustice of this conduct. And if anybody had ever had the temerity to call his attention to it, that person would have been for ever deprived of even the chance of becoming a favourite and being called by his first name. There was nobody who was willing to let slip the chance.

Now Dr. Mantelsack crossed his legs, still standing, and began to turn over the leaves of his notebook. Hanno Buddenbrook wrung his hands under the desk. B, the letter B, came next. Now he would hear his name, he would get up, he would not know a line, and there would be a row, a loud, frightful catastrophe – no matter how good a mood Dr. Mantelsack might be in. The seconds dragged out, each a martyrdom. "Buddenbrook" – Now he would say "Buddenbrook." "Edgar," said Dr. Mantelsack, closing his notebook with his finger in it. He sat down, as if all were in the best of order.

What? Who? Edgar? That was Lüders, the fat Lüders boy over there by the window. Letter L, which was not next at all! No! Was it possible? Dr. Mantelsack's mood was so good that he simply selected one of his favourites, without troubling in the least about whose turn it was.

Lüders stood up. He had a face like a pug dog, and dull brown eyes. He had an advantageous seat, and could easily have read it off, but he was too lazy. He felt too secure in his paradise, and answered simply, "I had a headache yesterday, and couldn't study."

"Oh, so you are leaving me in the lurch, Edgar," said Dr. Mantelsack with tender reproach. "You cannot say the lines on the Golden Age? What a shocking pity, my friend! You had a headache? It seems to me you should have told me before the lesson began, instead of waiting till I called you up. Didn't you have a headache just lately, Edgar? You should do something for them, for otherwise there is danger of your not passing. Timm, will you take his place?"

Lüders sat down. At this moment he was the object of universal hatred. It was plain that the master's mood had altered for the worse, and that Lüders, perhaps in the very next lesson, would be called by his last name. Timm stood up in one of the back seats. He was a blond country-looking lad with a light-brown jacket and short, broad fingers. He held his mouth open in a funnel shape, and hastily found the place, looking straight ahead the while with the most idiotic expression. Then he put down his head and began to read, in long-drawn-out, monotonous, hesitating accents, like a child with a first lesson-book: "*Aurea prima sata est ætas!*"

It was plain that Dr. Mantelsack was calling up quite at random, without reference to the alphabet. And thus it was no longer so imminently likely that Hanno would be called on, though this might happen through unlucky chance. He exchanged a joyful glance with Kai and began to relax somewhat.

But now Timm's reading was interrupted. Whether Dr.

Mantelsack could not hear him, or whether he stood in need of exercise, is not to be known. But he left his platform and walked slowly down through the room. He paused near Timm, with his book in his hand; Timm meanwhile had succeeded in getting his own book out of sight, but was now entirely helpless. His funnel-shaped mouth emitted a gasp, he looked at the *Ordinarius* with honest, troubled blue eyes, and could not fetch out another syllable.

" Well, Timm," said Dr. Mantelsack. " Can't you get on? "

Timm clutched his brow, rolled up his eyes, sighed windily, and said with a dazed smile: " I get all mixed up, Herr Doctor, when you stand so close to me."

Dr. Mantelsack smiled too. He smiled in a very flattered way and said " Well, pull yourself together and get on." And he strolled back to his place.

And Timm pulled himself together. He drew out and opened his book again, all the time apparently wrestling to recover his self-control and staring about the room. Then he dropped his head and was himself again.

" Very good," said the master, when he had finished. " It is clear that you have studied to some purpose. But you sacrifice the rhythm too much, Timm. You seem to understand the elisions; yet you have not been really reading hexameters at all. I have an impression as if you had learned the whole thing by heart, like prose. But, as I say, you have been diligent, you have done your best – and whoever does his best – ; you may sit down."

Timm sat down, proud and beaming, and Dr. Mantelsack gave him a good mark in his book. And the extraordinary thing was that at this moment not only the master, but also Timm himself and all his classmates, sincerely felt that Timm was a good industrious pupil who had fully deserved the mark he got. Hanno Buddenbrook, even, thought the same, though something within him revolted against the thought. He listened with strained attention to the next name.

" Mumme," said Dr. Mantelsack. " Again: *aurea prima* – "

Mumme! Well! Thank Heaven! Hanno was now in probable safety. The lines would hardly be asked for a third time, and in the sight-reading the letter B had just been called up.

Mumme got up. He was tall and pale, with trembling hands and extraordinary large round glasses. He had trouble with his eyes, and was so short-sighted that he could not possibly read standing up from a book on the desk before him. He had to learn, and he had learned. But to-day he had not expected to be called up; he was, besides, painfully ungifted; and he stuck after the first few words. Dr. Mantelsack helped him, he helped him again in a sharper tone, and for the third time with intense irritation. But when Mumme came to a final stop, the *Ordinarius* was mastered by indignation.

" This is entirely insufficient, Mumme. Sit down. You cut a disgraceful figure, let me tell you, sir. A *cretin!* Stupid and lazy both — it is really too much."

Mumme was overwhelmed. He looked the child of calamity, and at this moment everybody in the room despised him. A sort of disgust, almost like nausea, mounted again in Hanno Buddenbrook's throat; but at the same time he observed with horrid clarity all that was going forward. Dr. Mantelsack made a mark of sinister meaning after Mumme's name, and then looked through his notebook with frowning brows. He went over, in his disgust, to the order of the day, and looked to see whose turn it really was. There was no doubt that this was the case: and just as Hanno was overpowered by this knowledge, he heard his name — as if in a bad dream.

" Buddenbrook! " Dr. Mantelsack had said " Buddenbrook." The scale was in the air again. Hanno could not believe his senses. There was a buzzing in his ears. He sat still.

" Herr Buddenbrook! " said Dr. Mantelsack, and stared at him sharply through his glasses with his prominent sapphire-blue eyes. " Will you have the goodness? "

Very well, then. It was to be. It had to come. It had come differently from his expectations, but still, here it was, and he was none the less lost. But he was calm. Would it be a very big row? He rose in his place and was about to utter some forlorn and absurd excuse to the effect that he had " forgotten " to study the lines, when he became aware that the boy ahead of him was offering him his open book.

This boy, Hans Hermann Kilian, was a small brown lad with oily hair and broad shoulders. He had set his heart on becoming an officer, and was so possessed by an ideal of comradeship that he would not leave in the lurch even little Buddenbrook, whom he did not like. He pointed with his finger to the place.

Hanno gazed down upon it and began to read. With trembling voice, his face working, he read of the Golden Age, when truth and justice flourished of their own free will, without laws or compulsions. " Punishment and fear did not exist," he said, in Latin. " No threats were graven upon the bronze tablets, nor did those who came to petition fear the countenance of the judges. . . ."

He read in fear and trembling, read with design badly and disjointedly, purposely omitted some of the elisions that were marked with pencil in Kilian's book, made mistakes in the lines, progressed with apparent difficulty, and constantly expected the master to discover the fraud and pounce upon him. The guilty satisfaction of seeing the open book in front of him gave him a pricking sensation in his skin; but at the same time he had such a feeling of disgust that he intentionally deceived as badly as possible, simply to make the deceit seem less vulgar to himself. He came to the end, and a pause ensued, during which he did not dare look up. He felt convinced that Dr. Mantelsack had seen all, and his lips were perfectly white. But at length the master sighed and said:

"Oh, Buddenbrook! *Si tacuisses!* You will permit me the classical thou, for this once. Do you know what you have done? You have conducted yourself like a vandal, a barbarian. You are a humourist, Buddenbrook; I can see that by your face. If I ask myself whether you have been coughing or whether you have been reciting this noble verse, I should incline to the former. Timm showed small feeling for rhythm, but compared to you he is a genius, a rhapsodist! Sit down, unhappy wretch! You have studied the lines, I cannot deny it, and I am constrained to give you a good mark. You have probably done your best. But tell me — have I not been told that you are musical, that you play the piano? How is it possible? Well, very well, sit down. You have worked hard — that must suffice."

He put a good mark down in his book, and Hanno Buddenbrook took his seat. He felt as Timm, the rhapsodist had felt before him — that he really deserved the praise which Dr. Mantelsack gave him. Yes, at the moment he was of the opinion that he was, if rather a dull, yet an industrious pupil, who had come off with honour, comparatively speaking. He was conscious that all his schoolmates, not excepting Hans Hermann Kilian, had the same view. Yet he felt at the same time somewhat nauseated. Pale, trembling, too exhausted to think about what had happened, he closed his eyes and sank back in lethargy.

Dr. Mantelsack, however, went on with the lesson. He came to the verses that were to have been prepared for to-day, and called up Petersen. Petersen rose, fresh, lively, sanguine, in a stout attitude, ready for the fray. Yet to-day, even to-day, was destined to see his fall. Yes, the lesson hour was not to pass without a catastrophe far worse than that which had befallen the hapless, short-sighted Mumme.

Petersen translated, glancing now and then at the other page of his book, which should have had nothing on it. He did it quite cleverly: he acted as though something there distracted him – a speck of dust, perhaps, which he brushed with his hand or tried to blow away. And yet – there followed the catastrophe.

Dr. Mantelsack made a sudden violent movement, which was responded to on Petersen's part by a similar movement. And in the same moment the master left his seat, dashed headlong down from his platform, and approached Petersen with long, impetuous strides.

"You have a crib in your book," he said as he came up.

"A crib – I – no," stammered Petersen. He was a charming lad, with a great wave of blond hair on his forehead and lovely blue eyes which now flickered in a frightened way.

"You have no crib in your book?"

"A crib, Herr Doctor? No, really, I haven't. You are mistaken. You are accusing me falsely." Petersen betrayed himself by the unnatural correctness of his language, which he used in order to intimidate the master. "I am not deceiving you," he repeated, in the greatness of his need. "I have always been honourable, my whole life long."

But Dr. Mantelsack was all too certain of the painful fact.

"Give me your book," he said coldly.

Petersen clung to his book; he raised it up in both hands and went on protesting. He stammered, his tongue grew thick. "Believe me, Herr Doctor. There is nothing in the book – I have no crib – I have not deceived you – I have always been honourable – "

"Give me your book," repeated the master, stamping his foot.

Then Petersen collapsed, and his face grew grey.

"Very well," said he, and delivered up his book. "Here it is. Yes, there is a crib in it. You can see for yourself; there it is. But I haven't used it," he suddenly shrieked, quite at random.

Dr. Mantelsack ignored this idiotic lie, which was rooted in despair. He drew out the crib, looked at it with an expression of extreme disgust, as if it were a piece of decaying offal, thrust it into his pocket, and threw the volume of Ovid contemptuously back on Petersen's desk.

"Give me the class register," he said in a hollow voice.

Adolf Todtenhaupt dutifully fetched it, and Petersen received a mark for dishonesty which effectually demolished his chances of being sent up at Easter. "You are the shame of the class," said Dr. Mantelsack.

Petersen sat down. He was condemned. His neighbour avoided

contact with him. Every one looked at him with a mixture of pity, aversion, and disgust. He had fallen, utterly and completely, because he had been found out. There was but one opinion as to Petersen, and that was that he was, in very truth, the shame of the class. They recognized and accepted his fall, as they had the rise of Timm and Buddenbrook and the unhappy Mumme's mischance. And Petersen did too.

Thus most of this class of twenty-five young folk, being of sound and strong constitution, armed and prepared to wage the battle of life as it is, took things just as they found them, and did not at this moment feel any offence or uneasiness. Everything seemed to them to be quite in order. But one pair of eyes, little Johann's, which stared gloomily at a point on Hans Hermann Kilian's broad back, were filled, in their blue-shadowed depths, with abhorrence, fear, and revulsion. The lesson went on. Dr. Mantelsack called on somebody, anybody—he had lost all desire to test any one. And after Adolf Todtenhaupt, another pupil, who was but moderately prepared, and did not even know what "*patula Jovis arbore*" meant, had been called on, Buddenbrook had to say it. He said it in a low voice, without looking up, because Dr. Mantelsack asked him, and he received a nod of the head for the answer.

And now that the performance of the pupils was over, the lesson had lost all interest. Dr. Mantelsack had one of the best scholars read at his own sweet will, and listened just as little as the twenty-four others, who began to get ready for the next class. This one was finished, in effect. No one could be marked on it, nor his interest or industry judged. And the bell would soon ring. It did ring. It rang for Hanno, and he had received a nod of approbation. Thus it was.

"Well!" said Kai to Hanno, as they walked down the Gothic corridor with their classmates, to go to the chemistry class, "what do you say now about the brow of Caesar? You had wonderful luck!"

"I feel sick, Kai," said little Johann, "I don't like that kind of luck. It makes me sick." Kai knew he would have felt the same in Hanno's place.

The chemistry hall was a vaulted chamber like an amphitheatre with benches rising in tiers, a long table for the experiments, and two glass cases of phials. The air in the classroom had grown very hot and heavy again; but here it was saturated with an odour of sulphuretted hydrogen from a just-completed experiment, and smelled abominable. Kai flung up the window and then stole

Adolf Todtenhaupt's copy-book and began in great haste to copy down the lesson for the day. Hanno and several others did the same. This occupied the entire pause till the bell rang, and Dr. Marotzke came in.

This was the " deep one," as Kai and Hanno called him. He was a medium-sized dark man with a very yellow skin, two large lumps on his brow, a stiff smeary beard, and hair of the same kind. He always looked unwashed and unkempt, but his appearance probably belied him. He taught the natural sciences, but his own field was mathematics, in which subject he had the reputation of being an original thinker. He liked to hold forth on the subject of metaphysical passages from the Bible; and when in a good-natured or discursive mood, he would entertain the boys of the first and second forms with marvellous interpretations of mysterious passages. He was, besides all this, a reserve officer, and very enthusiastic over the service. As an official who was also in the army, he stood very well with Director Wulicke. He set more store by discipline than any of the other masters: he would review the ranks of sturdy youngsters with a professional eye, and he insisted on short, brisk answers to questions. This mixture of mysticism and severity was not, on the whole, attractive.

The copy-books were shown, and Dr. Marotzke went around and touched each one with his finger. Some of the pupils who had not done theirs at all, put down other books or turned this one back to an old lesson; but he never noticed.

Then the lesson began, and the twenty-five boys had to display their industry and interest with respect to boric acid, and chlorine, and strontium, as in the previous period they had displayed it with respect to Ovid. Hans Hermann Kilian was commended because he knew that $BaSO_4$, or barytes, was the metal most commonly used in counterfeiting. He was the best in the class, anyhow, because of his desire to be an officer. Kai and Hanno knew nothing at all, and fared very badly in Dr. Marotzke's notebook.

And when the tests, recitation, and marking were over, the interest in chemistry was about exhausted too. Dr. Marotzke began to make a few experiments; there were a few pops, a few coloured gases; but that was only to fill out the hour. He dictated the next lesson; and then the third period, too, was a thing of the past.

Everybody was in good spirits now — even Petersen, despite the blow he had received. For the next hour was likely to be a jolly one. Not a soul felt any qualms before it, and it even promised occasion for entertainment and mischief. This was English, with Candidate Modersohn, a young philologian who had been for a few weeks on trial in the faculty – or, as Kai, Count Mölln, put it, he was filling a limited engagement with the company. There was little prospect, however, of his being re-engaged. His classes were much too entertaining.

Some of the form remained in the chemistry hall, others went up to the classroom; nobody needed to go down and freeze in the courtyard, because Herr Modersohn was in charge up in the corridors, and he never dared send any one down. Moreover, there were preparations to be made for his reception.

The room did not become in the least quieter when it rang for the fourth hour. Everybody chattered and laughed and prepared to see some fun. Count Mölln, his head in his hands, went on reading Roderick Usher. Hanno was audience. Some of the boys imitated the voices of animals; there was the shrill crowing of a cock; and Wasservogel, in the back row, grunted like a pig without anybody's being able to see that the noise came from his inside. On the blackboard was a huge chalk drawing, a caricature, with squinting eyes, drawn by Timm the rhapsodist. And when Herr Modersohn entered he could not shut the door, even with the most violent efforts, because there was a thick fir-cone in the crack; Adolf Todtenhaupt had to take it away.

Candidate Modersohn was an undersized, insignificant looking man. His face was always contorted with a sour, peevish expression, and he walked with one shoulder thrust forward. He was frightfully self-conscious, blinked, drew in his breath, and kept opening his mouth as if he wanted to say something if he could only think of it. Three steps from the door he trod on a cracker of such exceptional quality that it made a noise like dynamite. He jumped violently; then, in these straits, he smiled exactly as though nothing had happened and took his place before the middle row of benches, stooping sideways, in his customary attitude, and resting one palm on the desk in front of him. But this posture of his was familiar to everybody; somebody had put some ink on the right spot, and Herr Modersohn's small clumsy hand got all inky. He acted as though he had not noticed, laid his wet black hand on his back, blinked, and said in a soft, weak voice: "The order in the classroom leaves something to be desired."

Hanno Buddenbrook loved him in that moment, sat quite still, and looked up into his worried, helpless face. But Wasservogel grunted louder than ever, and a handful of peas went rattling against the window and bounced back into the room.

"It's hailing," somebody said, quite loudly. Herr Modersohn appeared to believe this, for he went without more ado to the platform and asked for the register. He needed it to call the names from, for, though he had been teaching the class for five or six weeks, he hardly knew any of them by name.

"Feddermann," he said, "will you please recite the poem?"

"Absent," shouted a chorus of voices. And there sat Feddermann, large as life, in his place, shooting peas with great skill and accuracy.

Herr Modersohn blinked again and selected a new name. "Wasservogel," he said.

"Dead," shouted Petersen, attacked by a grim humour. And the chorus, grunting, crowing, and with shouts of derision, asseverated that Wasservogel was dead.

Herr Modersohn blinked afresh. He looked about him, drew down his mouth, and put his finger on another name in the register. "Perlemann," he said, without much confidence.

"Unfortunately, gone mad," uttered Kai, Count Mölln, with great clarity and precision. And this also was confirmed by the chorus amid an ever-increasing tumult.

Then Herr Modersohn stood up and shouted in to the hubbub: "Buddenbrook, you will do me a hundred lines imposition. If you laugh again, I shall be obliged to mark you."

Then he sat down again. It was true that Hanno had laughed. He had been seized by a quiet but violent spasm of laughter, and went on because he could not stop. He had found Kai's joke so good – the "unfortunately" had especially appealed to him. But he became quiet when Herr Modersohn attacked him, and sat looking solemnly into the Candidate's face. He observed at that moment every detail of the man's appearance: saw every pathetic little hair in his scanty beard, which showed the skin through it; saw his brown, empty, disconsolate eyes; saw that he had on what appeared to be two pairs of cuffs, because the sleeves of his shirt came down so long; saw the whole pathetic, inadequate figure he made. He saw more: he saw into the man's inner self. Hanno Buddenbrook was almost the only pupil whom Herr Modersohn knew by name, and he availed himself of the knowledge to call him constantly to order, give him impositions, and tyrannize over him. He had distinguished Buddenbrook from the others simply because of his quieter behaviour – and of this he took advantage to make him feel his authority, an authority he did not dare exert upon the real offenders. Hanno looked at him and reflected that Herr Modersohn's lack of fine feeling made it almost impossible even to pity him! "I don't bully you," he addressed the Candidate, in his thoughts: "I don't share in the general tormenting like the others — and how do you repay me? But so it is, and so will it be, always and everywhere," he thought; and fear, and that sensation almost amounting to physical nausea, rose again in him. "And the most dreadful thing is that I can't help seeing through you with such disgusting clearness!"

At last Herr Modersohn found some one who was neither dead nor crazy, and who would take it upon himself to repeat the English verse. This was a poem called "The Monkey," a poor childish composition, required to be committed to memory by these growing lads whose thoughts were already mostly bent on business, on the sea, on the coming conflicts of actual life.

"Monkey, little, merry fellow,
Thou art nature's punchinello . . ."

There were endless verses — Kassbaum read them, quite simply, out of his book. Nobody needed to trouble himself about what Herr Modersohn thought. The noise grew worse and worse, the feet shuffled and scraped on the dusty floor, the cock crowed, the pig grunted, peas filled the air. The five-and-twenty were drunk with disorder. And the unregulated instincts of their years awoke. They drew obscene pictures on pieces of paper, passed them about, and laughed at them greedily.

All at once everything was still. The pupil who was then reciting interrupted himself; even Herr Modersohn got up and listened. They heard something charming: a pure, bell-like sound, coming from the bottom of the room and flowing sweetly, sensuously, with indescribably tender effect, on the sudden silence. It was a music-box which somebody had brought, playing "*Du, du, liegst mir am Herzen*" in the middle of the English lesson. But precisely at that moment when the little melody died away, something frightful ensued. It broke like a sudden storm over the heads of the class, unexpected, cruel, overwhelming, paralyzing.

Without anybody's having knocked, the door opened wide with a great shove, and a presence came in, high and huge, growled, and stood with a single stride in front of the benches. It was the Lord God.

Herr Modersohn grew ashy pale and dragged down the chair from the platform, dusting it with his handkerchief. The pupils had sprung up like one man. They pressed their arms to their sides, stood on their tip-toes, bent their heads, and bit their tongues in the fervour of their devotion. The deepest silence reigned. Somebody gasped with the effort he made — then all was still again.

Director Wulicke measured the saluting columns for a while with his eye. He lifted his arm with its dirty funnel-shaped cuff, and let it fall with the fingers spread out, as if he were attacking a keyboard. " Sit down," he said in his double-bass voice.

The pupils sank back into their seats. Herr Modersohn pulled up the chair with trembling hands, and the Director sat down beside the dais. " Please proceed," he said. That was all, but it sounded as frightful as if the words he uttered had been " Now we shall see, and woe to him who – "

The reason for his coming was clear. Herr Modersohn was to give evidence of his ability to teach, to show what the lower second had learned in the six or seven hours he had been with them. It was a question of Herr Modersohn's existence and future. The Candidate was a sorry figure as he stood on the platform and called again on somebody to recite " The Monkey." Up to now it had been only the pupils who were examined, but now it was the master as well. Alas, it went badly on both sides! Herr Director Wulicke's appearance was entirely unexpected, and only two or three of the pupils were prepared. It was impossible for Herr Modersohn to call up Adolf Todtenhaupt for the whole hour on end; after " The Monkey " had been recited once, it could not be asked for again, and so things were in a bad way. When the reading from Ivanhoe began, young Count Mölln was the only person who could translate it at all, he having a personal interest in the novel. The others hemmed and hawed, stuttered, and got hopelessly stuck. Hanno Buddenbrook was called up and could not do a line. Director Wulicke gave utterance to a sound that was as though the lowest string of his double-bass had been violently plucked, and Herr Modersohn wrung his small, clumsy, inky hands repeating plaintively over and over. " And it went so well – it always went so well! "

He was still saying it, half to the pupils and half to the Director, when the bell rang. But the Lord God stood erect with folded arms before his chair and stared in front of him over the heads of the class. Then he commanded that the register be brought, and slowly marked down for laziness all those pupils whose performances of the morning had been deficient – or entirely lacking – six or seven marks at one fell swoop. He could not put down a mark for Herr Modersohn, but he was much worse than the others. He stood there with a face like chalk, broken, done for. Hanno Buddenbrook was among those marked down. And Director Wulicke said besides, " I will spoil all your careers for you." Then he went.

The bell rang; class was over. It was always like that. When you expected trouble it did not come. When you thought all was well – then, the catastrophe. It was now impossible for Hanno to go up at Easter. He rose from his seat and went drearily out of the room, seeking the aching back tooth with his tongue.

Kai came up to him and put his arm across his shoulders. Together they walked down to the courtyard, among the crowd of excited comrades, all of whom were discussing the extraordinary event. He looked with loving anxiety into Hanno's face and said, "Please forgive, Hanno, for translating. It would have been better to keep still and get a mark. It's so cheap – "

"Didn't I say what '*patula Jovis arbore*' meant?" answered Hanno. "Don't mind, Kai. That doesn't matter. One just mustn't mind."

"I suppose that's true. Well, the Lord God is going to ruin your career. You may as well resign yourself, Hanno, because if it is His inscrutable will –. Career – what a lovely word 'career' is! Herr Modersohn's career is spoilt too. He will never get to be a master, poor chap! There are assistant masters, you may know, and there are head masters; but never by any chance a plain master. This is a mystery not to be revealed to youthful minds; it is only intended for grown-ups and persons of mature experience. An ordinary intelligence might say that either one is a master or one is not. I might go up to the Lord God or Herr Marotzke and explain this to him. But what would be the result? They would consider it an insult, and I should be punished for insubordination – all for having discovered for them a much higher significance in their calling than they themselves were aware of! No, let's not talk about them – they're all thick-skinned brutes!"

They walked about the court; Kai made jokes to help Hanno forget his bad mark, and Hanno listened and enjoyed.

"Look, here is a door, an outer door. It is open, and outside there is the street. How would it be if we were to go out and take a little walk? It is recess, and we have still six minutes. We could easily be back in time. But it is perfectly impossible. You see what I mean? Here is the door. It is open, there is no grating, there is nothing, nothing whatever to prevent us. And yet it is impossible for us to step outside for even a second – it is even impossible for us to think of doing so. Well, let's not think of it, then. Let's take another example: we don't say, for instance, that it is nearly half-past twelve. No, we say, 'It's nearly time for the geography period'! You see? Now, I ask, is this any sort of a life to lead?

Everything is wrong. Oh, Lord, if the institution would just once let us out of her loving embrace! "

"Well, and what then? No, Kai, we should just have to do something then; here, at least we are taken care of. Since my Father died Herr Stephan Kistenmaker and Pastor Pringsheim have taken over the business of asking me every day what I want to be. I don't know. I can't answer. I can't be anything. I'm afraid of everything — "

"How can anybody talk so dismally? What about your music? "

"What about my music, Kai? There is nothing to it. Shall I travel round and give concerts? In the first place, they wouldn't let me; and in the second place, I should never really know enough. I can play very little. I can only improvise a little when I am alone. And then, the traveling about must be dreadful, I imagine. It is different with you. You have more courage. You go about laughing at it all — you have something to set against it. You want to write, to tell wonderful stories. Well, that *is* something. You will surely become famous, you are so clever. The thing is, you are so much livelier. Sometimes in class we look at each other, the way we did when Petersen got marked because he read out of a crib, when all the rest of us did the same. The same thought is in both our minds — but you know how to make a face and let it pass. I can't. I get so tired of things. I'd like to sleep and never wake up. I'd like to die, Kai! No, I am no good. I can't want anything. I don't even want to be famous. I'm afraid of it, just as much as if it were a wrong thing to do. Nothing can come of me, that is perfectly sure. One day, after confirmation-class, I heard Pastor Pringsheim tell somebody that one must just give me up, because I come of a decayed family."

"Did he say that? " Kai asked with deep interest.

"Yes; he meant my Uncle Christian, in the institution in Hamburg. One must just give me up — oh, I'd be so happy if they would! I have so many worries; everything is so hard for me. If I give myself a little cut or bruise anywhere, and make a wound that would heal in a week with anybody else, it takes a month with me. It gets inflamed and infected and makes me all sorts of trouble. Herr Brecht told me lately that all my teeth are in a dreadful condition — not to mention the ones that have been pulled already. If they are like that now, what will they be when I am thirty or forty years old? I am completely discouraged."

"Oh, come," Kai said, and struck into a livelier gait. "Now you must tell me something about your playing. I want to write something marvellous – perhaps I'll begin it to-day, in drawing period. Will you play this afternoon? "

Hanno was silent a moment. A flush came upon his face, and a painful, confused look.

" Yes, I'll play – I suppose – though I ought not. I ought to practise my sonatas and études and then stop. But I suppose I'll play; I cannot help it, though it only makes everything worse."

" Worse? "

Hanno was silent.

" I know what you mean," said Kai after a bit, and then neither of the lads spoke again.

They were both at the same difficult age. Kai's face burned, and he cast down his eyes. Hanno looked pale and serious; his eyes had clouded over, and he kept giving sideways glances.

Then the bell rang, and they went up.

The geography period came next, and an important test on the kingdom of Hesse-Nassau. A man with a red beard and brown tail-coat came in. His face was pale, and his hands were very full of pores, but without a single hair. This was " the clever one," Dr. Mühsam. He suffered from occasional haemorrhages, and always spoke in an ironic tone, because it was his pose to be considered as witty as he was ailing. He possessed a Heine collection, a quantity of papers and objects connected with that cynical and sickly poet. He proceeded to mark the boundaries of Hesse-Nassau on the map that hung on the wall, and then asked, with a melancholy, mocking smile, if the gentlemen would indicate in their books the important features of the country. It was as though he meant to make game of the class and of Hesse-Nassau as well; yet this was an important test, and much dreaded by the entire form.

Hanno Buddenbrook knew next to nothing about Hesse-Nassau. He tried to look on Adolf Todtenhaupt's book; but Heinrich Heine, who had a penetrating observation despite his suffering, melancholy air, pounced on him at once and said: " Herr Buddenbrook, I am tempted to ask you to close your book, but that I suspect you would be glad to have me do so. Go on with your work."

The remark contained two witticisms. First, that Dr. Mühsam addressed Hanno as Herr Buddenbrook, and, second, that about the copy-book. Hanno continued to brood over his book, and handed it in almost empty when he went out with Kai.

The difficulties were now over with for the day. The fortunate ones who had come through without marks, had light and easy consciences, and life seemed like play to them as they betook themselves to the large well-lighted room where they might sit and draw under the supervision of Herr Drägemüller. Plaster casts from the antique stood about the room, and there was a great cupboard containing divers pieces of wood and doll-furniture which served as models. Herr Drägemüller was a thick-set man with a full round beard and a smooth, cheap brown wig which stood out in the back of the neck and betrayed itself. He possessed two wigs, one with longer hair, the other with shorter; if he had had his beard cut he would don the shorter wig as well. He was a man with some droll peculiarities of speech. For instance, he called a lead pencil a " lead." He gave out an oily-alcoholic odour; and it was said of him that he drank petroleum. It always delighted him to have an opportunity to take a class in something besides drawing. On such occasions he would lecture on the policy of Bismarck, accompanying himself with impressive spiral gestures from his nose to his shoulder. Social democracy was his bugbear – he spoke of it with fear and loathing. " We must keep together," he used to say to refractory pupils, pinching them on the arm. " Social democracy is at the door! " He was possessed by a sort of spasmodic activity: would sit down next a pupil, exhaling a strong spirituous odour, tap him on the forehead with his seal ring, shoot out certain isolated words and phrases like " Perspective! Light and shade! The lead! Social democracy! Stick together! " – and then dash off again.

Kai worked at his new literary project during this period, and Hanno occupied himself with conducting, in fancy, an overture with full orchestra. Then school was over, they fetched down their things, the gate was opened, they were free to pass, and they went home.

Hanno and Kai went the same road together as far as the little red villa, their books under their arms. Young Count Mölln had a good distance farther to go alone before he reached the paternal dwelling. He never wore an overcoat.

The morning's fog had turned to snow, which came down in great white flocks and rapidly became slush. They parted at the Buddenbrook gate; but when Hanno was half-way up the garden Kai came back to put his arm about his neck. " Don't give up – better not play! " he said gently. Then his slender, jaunty figure disappeared in the whirling snow.

Hanno put down his books on the bear's tray in the corridor and went into the living room to see his mother. She sat on the sofa reading a book with a yellow paper cover, and looked up as he crossed the room. She gazed at him with her brown, close-set, blue-shadowed eyes; as he stood before her, she took his head in both her hands and kissed him on the brow.

He went upstairs, where Fräulein Clementine had some luncheon ready for him, washed, and ate. When he was done he took out of his desk a packet of little biting Russian cigarettes and began to smoke. He was no stranger to their use by now. Then he sat down at the harmonium and played something from Bach: something very severe and difficult, in fugue form. At length he clasped his hands behind his head and looked out the window at the snow noiselessly tumbling down. Nothing else was to be seen; for there was no longer a charming little garden with a plashing fountain beneath his window. The view was cut off by the grey side-wall of the neighbouring villa.

Dinner was at four o'clock, and Hanno, his mother, and Fräulein Clementine sat down to it. Afterward Hanno saw that there were preparations for music in the salon, and awaited his mother at the piano. They played the Sonata Opus 24 of Beethoven. In the adagio the violin sang like an angel; but Gerda took the instrument from her chin with a dissatisfied air, looked at it in irritation, and said it was not in tune. She played no more, but went up to rest.

Hanno remained in the salon. He went to the glass door that led out on the small verandah and looked into the drenched garden. But suddenly he took a step back and jerked the cream-coloured curtains across the door, so that the room lay in a soft yellow twilight. Then he went to the piano. He stood for a while, and his gaze, directed fixed and unseeing upon a distant point, altered slowly, grew blurred and vague and shadowy. He sat down at the instrument and began to improvise.

It was a simple *motif* which he employed — a mere trifle, an unfinished fragment of melody in one bar and a half. He brought it out first, with unsuspected power, in the bass, as a single voice: indicating it as the source and fount of all that was to come, and announcing it, with a commanding entry, by a burst of trumpets. It was not quite easy to grasp his intention; but when he repeated and harmonized it in the treble, with a timbre like dull silver, it proved to consist essentially of a single resolution, a yearning and painful melting of one tone into another — a short-winded, pitiful invention, which nevertheless gained a strange, mysterious, and significant value precisely by means of the meticulous and solemn precision with which it was defined and produced. And now there began more lively passages, a restless coming and going of syncopated sound, seeking, wandering, torn by shrieks like a soul in unrest and tormented by some knowledge it possesses and cannot conceal, but must repeat in ever different harmonies, questioning, complaining, protesting, demanding, dying away. The syncopation increased, grew more pronounced, driven hither and thither by scampering triplets; the shrieks of fear recurred, they took form and became melody. There was a moment when they dominated, in a mounting, imploring chorus of wind-instruments that conquered the endlessly thronging, welling, wandering, vanishing harmonies, and swelled out in unmistakable simple rhythms—a crushed, childlike, imposing, imploring chorale. This concluded with a sort of ecclesiastical cadence. A *fermate* followed, a silence. And then, quite softly, in a timbre of dull silver, there came the first *motif* again, the paltry invention, a figure either tiresome or obscure, a sweet, sentimental dying-away of one tone into another. This was followed by a tremendous uproar, a wild activity, punctuated by notes like fanfares, expressive of violent resolve. What was coming? Then came horns again, sounding the march; there was an assembling, a concentrating, firm, consolidated rhythms; and a new figure began, a bold improvisation, a sort of lively, stormy hunting song. There was no joy in this hunting song; its note was one of defiant despair. Signals sounded through it; yet they were not only signals but cries of fear; while throughout, winding through it all, through all the writhen, bizarre harmonies, came again that mysterious first *motif*, wandering in despair, torturingly sweet. And now began a ceaseless hurry of events whose sense and meaning could not be guessed, a restless flood of sound-adventures, rhythms, harmonies, welling up uncontrolled from the keyboard, as they shaped themselves under Hanno's labouring fingers. He experienced them, as it were; he did not know them beforehand. He sat a little bent over the keys, with parted lips and deep, far gaze, his brown hair covering his forehead with its soft curls. What was the meaning of what he played? Were these images of fearful difficulties surmounted, flames passed through and torrents swum, castles stormed and dragons slain? But always—now like a yelling laugh, now like an ineffably sweet promise—the original *motif* wound through it all, the pitiful phrase with its notes melting into one another! Now the music seemed to rouse itself to new and gigantic efforts: wild runs in octaves followed, sounding like shrieks; an irresistible mounting, a chromatic upward struggle, a wild relentless longing, abruptly broken by startling, arresting pianissimi which gave a sensation as if the ground were disappearing from beneath one's feet, or like a sudden abandonment and sinking into a gulf of desire.

Once, far off and softly warning, sounded the first chords of the imploring prayer; but the flood of rising cacophonies overwhelmed them with their rolling, streaming, clinging, sinking, and struggling up again, as they fought on toward the end that must come, must come this very moment, at the height of this fearful climax — for the pressure of longing had become intolerable. And it came; it could no longer be kept back — those spasms of yearning could not be prolonged. And it came as though curtains were rent apart, doors sprang open, thorn-hedges parted of themselves, walls of flame sank down. The resolution, the redemption, the complete fulfilment — a chorus of jubilation burst forth, and everything resolved itself in a harmony — and the harmony, in sweet *ritardando*, at once sank into another. It was the *motif*, the *first motif!* And now began a festival, a triumph, an unbounded orgy of this very figure, which now displayed a wealth of dynamic colour which passed through every octave, wept and shivered in tremolo, sang, rejoiced, and sobbed in exultation, triumphantly adorned with all the bursting, tinkling, foaming, purling resources of orchestral pomp. The fanatical worship of this worthless trifle, this scrap of melody, this brief, childish harmonic invention only a bar and a half in length, had about it something stupid and gross, and at the same time something ascetic and religious — something that contained the essence of faith and renunciation. There was a quality of the perverse in the insatiability with which it was produced and revelled in: there was a sort of cynical despair; there was a longing for joy, a yielding to desire, in the way the last drop of sweetness was, as it were, extracted from the melody, till exhaustion, disgust, and satiety supervened. Then, at last; at last, in the weariness after excess, a long, soft arpeggio in the minor trickled through, mounted a tone, resolved itself in the major, and died in mournful lingering away.

Hanno sat still a moment, his chin on his breast, his hands in his lap. Then he got up and closed the instrument. He was very pale, there was no strength in his knees, and his eyes were burning. He went into the next room, stretched himself on the chaise-lounge, and remained for a long time motionless.

Later there was supper, and he played a game of chess with his mother, at which neither side won. But until after midnight he still sat in his room, before his harmonium, and played — played in thought only, for he must make no noise. He did this despite his firm intention to get up the next morning at half-past five, to do some most necessary preparation.

This was one day in the life of little Johann.

CHAPTER III

CASES of typhoid fever take the following course.

The patient feels depressed and moody – a condition which grows rapidly worse until it amounts to acute despondency. At the same time he is overpowered by physical weariness, not only of the muscles and sinews, but also of the organic functions, in particular of the digestion – so that the stomach refuses food. There is a great desire for sleep, but even in conditions of extreme fatigue the sleep is restless and superficial and not refreshing. There is pain in the head, the brain feels dull and confused, and there are spells of giddiness. An indefinite ache is felt in all the bones. There is blood from the nose now and then, without apparent cause. – This is the onset.

Then comes a violent chill which seizes the whole body and makes the teeth chatter; the fever sets in, and is immediately at its height. Little red spots appear on the breast and abdomen, about the size of a lentil. They go away when pressed by the finger, but return at once. The pulse is unsteady; there are about a hundred pulsations to the minute. The temperature goes up to 104°. Thus passes the first week.

In the second week the patient is free from pain in the head and limbs; but the giddiness is distinctly worse, and there is so much humming in the ears that he is practically deaf. The facial expression becomes dull, the mouth stands open, the eyes are without life. The consciousness is blurred, desire for sleep takes entire possession of the patient, and he often sinks, not into actual sleep, but into a leaden lethargy. At other intervals there are the loud and excited ravings of delirium. The patient's helplessness is complete, and his uncleanliness becomes repulsive. His gums, teeth, and tongue are covered with a blackish deposit which makes his breath foul. He lies motionless on his back, with distended abdomen. He has sunk down in the bed, with his knees wide apart. Pulse and breathing are rapid, jerky, superficial and laboured; the pulse is fluttering, and gallops one hundred and twenty to the minute. The eyelids are half closed, the cheeks are no longer glowing, but have assumed a bluish colour. The red spots on breast and abdomen are more numerous. The temperature reaches 105.8°.

In the third week the weakness is at its height. The patient raves no longer: who can say whether his spirit is sunk in empty night or whether it lingers, remote from the flesh, in far, deep, quiet dreams, of which he gives no sound and no sign? He lies in total insensibility. This is the crisis of the disease.

In individual cases the diagnosis is sometimes rendered more difficult; as, for example, when the early symptoms – depression, weariness, lack of appetite, headache and unquiet sleep – are nearly all present while the patient is still going about in his usual health; when they are scarcely noticeable as anything out of the common, even if they are suddenly and definitely increased. But a clever doctor, of real scientific acumen – like, for example, Dr. Langhals, the good-looking Dr. Langhals with the small, hairy hands – will still be in a position to call the case by its right name; and the appearance of the red spots on the chest and abdomen will be conclusive evidence that his diagnosis was correct. He will know what measures to take and what remedies to apply. He will arrange for a large, well-aired room, the temperature of which must not be higher than 70°. He will insist on absolute cleanliness, and by means of frequent shifting and changes of linen will keep the patient free from bedsores – if possible; in some cases it is not possible. He will have the mouth frequently cleansed with moist linen rags. As for treatment, preparations of iodine, potash, quinine, and antipyrin are indicated – with a diet as light and nourishing as possible, for the patient's stomach and bowels are profoundly attacked by the disease. He will treat the consuming fever by means of frequent baths, into which the patient will often be put every three hours, day and night, cooling them gradually from the foot end of the tub, and always, after each bath, administering something stimulating, like brandy or champagne.

But all these remedies he uses entirely at random, in the hope that they may be of some use in the case; ignorant whether any one of them will have the slightest effect. For there is one thing which he does not know at all; with respect to one fact, he labours in complete darkness. Up to the third week, up to the very crisis of the disease, he cannot possibly tell whether this illness, which he calls typhoid, is an unfortunate accident, the disagreeable consequence of an infection which might perhaps have been avoided, and which can be combated with the resources of medical science; or whether it is, quite simply, a form of dissolution, the garment, as it were, of death. And then, whether death choose to assume this form or another is all the same—against him there is no remedy.

Cases of typhoid take the following course:

When the fever is at its height, life calls to the patient: calls out to him as he wanders in his distant dream, and summons him in no uncertain voice. The harsh, imperious call reaches the spirit on that remote path that leads into the shadows, the coolness and peace. He hears the call of life, the clear, fresh, mocking summons to return to that distant scene which he had already left so far behind him, and already forgotten. And there may well up in him something like a feeling of shame for a neglected duty; a sense of renewed energy, courage, and hope; he may recognize a bond existing still between him and that stirring, colourful, callous existence which he thought he had left so far behind him. Then, however far he may have wandered on his distant path, he will turn back—and live. But if he shudders when he hears life's voice, if the memory of that vanished scene and the sound of that lusty summons make him shake his head, make him put out his hand to ward off as he flies forward in the way of escape that has opened to him—then it is clear that the patient will die.

CHAPTER IV

"It is not right, it is not right, Gerda," said old Fräulein Weichbrodt, perhaps for the hundredth time. Her voice was full of reproach and distress. She had a sofa place to-day in the circle that sat round the centre-table in the drawing-room of her former pupil. Gerda Buddenbrook, Frau Permaneder, her daughter Erica, poor Clothilde, and the three Misses Buddenbrook made up the group. The green capstrings still fell down upon the old lady's childish shoulders; but she had grown so tiny, with her seventy-five years of life, that she could scarcely raise her elbow high enough to gesticulate above the surface of the table.

"No, it is not right, and so I tell you, Gerda," she repeated. She spoke with such warmth that her voice trembled. "I have one foot in the grave, my time is short – and you can think of leaving me – of leaving us all – for ever! If it were just a visit to Amsterdam that you were thinking of – but to leave us for ever – !" She shook her bird-like old head vigorously, and her brown eyes were clouded with her distress. "It is true, you have lost a great deal – "

"No, she has not lost a great deal, she has lost everything," said Frau Permaneder. "We must not be selfish, Therese. Gerda wishes to go, and she is going – that is all. She came with Thomas, one-and-twenty years ago; and we all loved her, though she very likely didn't like any of us. – No, you didn't, Gerda; don't deny it! – But Thomas is no more – and nothing is any more. What are we to her? Nothing. We feel it very much, we cannot help feeling it; but yet I say, go, with God's blessing, Gerda, and thanks for not going before, when Thomas died."

It was an autumn evening, after supper. Little Johann (Justus, Johann, Kaspar) had been lying for nearly six months, equipped with the blessing of Pastor Pringsheim, out there at the edge of the little grove, beneath the sandstone cross, beneath the family arms. The rain rustled the half-leafless trees in the avenue, and sometimes gusts of wind drove it against the window-panes. All eight ladies were dressed in black.

The little family had gathered to take leave of Gerda Buddenbrook, who was about to leave the town and return to Amsterdam, to play duets once more with her old father. No duties now restrained her. Frau Permaneder could no longer oppose her decision. She said it was right, she knew it must be so; but in her heart she mourned over her sister-in-law's departure. If the Senator's widow had remained in the town, and kept her station and her place in society, and left her property where it was, there would still have remained a little prestige to the family name. But let that be as it must, Frau Antoine was determined to hold her head high while she lived and there were people to look at her. Had not her grandfather driven with four horses all over the country?

Despite the stormy life that lay behind her, and despite her weak digestion, she did not look her fifty years. Her skin was a little faded and downy, and a few hairs grew on her upper lip – the pretty upper lip of Tony Buddenbrook. But there was not a white hair in the smooth coiffure beneath the mourning cap.

Poor Clothilde bore up under the departure of her relative, as one must bear up under the afflictions of this life. She took it with patience and tranquillity. She had done wonders at the supper table, and now she sat among the others, lean and grey as of yore, and her words were drawling and friendly.

Erica Weinschenk, now thirty-one years old, was likewise not one to excite herself unduly over her aunt's departure. She had lived through worse things, and had early learned resignation. Submission was her strongest characteristic: one read it in her weary light-blue eyes – the eyes of Bendix Grünlich – and heard it in the tones of her patient, sometimes plaintive voice.

The three Misses Buddenbrook, Uncle Gotthold's daughters, wore their old affronted and critical air; Friederike and Henriette, the eldest, had grown leaner and more angular with the years; while Pfiffi, the youngest, now fifty-three years old, was much too little and fat.

Old Frau Consul Kröger, Uncle Justus' widow, had been asked too, but she was rather ailing – or perhaps she had no suitable gown to put on: one couldn't tell which.

They talked about Gerda's journey and the train she was to take; about the sale of the villa and its furnishings, which Herr Gosch had undertaken. For Gerda was taking nothing with her – she was going away as she had come.

Then Frau Permaneder began to talk about life. She was very serious and made observations upon the past and the future –

though of the future there was in truth almost nothing to be said.

"When I am dead," she declared, "Erica may move away if she likes. But as for me, I cannot live anywhere else; and so long as I am on earth, we will come together here, we who are left. Once a week you will come to dinner with me — and we will read the family papers." She put her hand on the portfolio that lay before her on the table. "Yes, Gerda, I will take them over, and be glad to have them. Well, that is settled. Do you hear, Tilda? Though it might exactly as well be you who should invite us, for you are just as well off as we are now. Yes — so it goes. I've struggled against fate, and done my best, and you have just sat there and waited for everything to come round. But you are a goose, you know, all the same — please don't mind if I say so — "

"Oh, Tony," Clothilde said, smiling.

"I am sorry I cannot say good-bye to Christian," said Gerda, and the talk turned aside to that subject. There was small prospect of his ever coming out of the institution in which he was confined, although he was probably not too bad to go about in freedom. But the present state of things was very agreeable for his wife. She was, Frau Permaneder asserted, in league with the doctor; and Christian would, in all probability, end his days where he was.

There was a pause. They touched delicately and with hesitation upon recent events, and when one of them let fall little Johann's name, it was still in the room, except for the sound of the rain, which fell faster than before.

This silence lay like a heavy secret over the events of Hanno's last illness. It must have been a frightful onslaught. They did not look in each other's eyes as they talked; their voices were hushed, and their words were broken. But they spoke of one last episode — the visit of the little ragged count who had almost forced his way to Hanno's bedside. Hanno had smiled when he heard his voice, though he hardly knew any one; and Kai had kissed his hands again and again.

"He kissed his hands?" asked the Buddenbrook ladies.

"Yes, over and over."

They all thought for a while of this strange thing, and then suddenly Frau Permaneder burst into tears.

"I loved him so much," she sobbed. "You don't any of you know how much — more than any of you — yes, forgive me, Gerda — you are his mother. — Oh, he was an angel."

"He is an angel, now," corrected Sesemi.

"Hanno, little Hanno," went on Frau Permaneder, the tears flowing down over her soft faded cheeks. "Tom, Father, Grandfather, and all the rest! Where are they? We shall see them no more. Oh, it is so sad, so hard! "

"There will be a reunion," said Friederike Buddenbrook. She folded her hands in her lap, cast down her eyes, and put her nose in the air.

"Yes – they say so. – Oh, there are times, Friederike, when that is no consolation, God forgive me! When one begins to doubt – doubt justice and goodness – and everything. Life crushes so much in us, it destroys so many of our beliefs – ! A reunion – if that were so – "

But now Sesemi Weichbrodt stood up, as tall as ever she could. She stood on tip-toe, rapped on the table; the cap shook on her old head.

"It *is so!* " she said, with her whole strength; and looked at them all with a challenge in her eyes.

She stood there, a victor in the good fight which all her life she had waged against the assaults of Reason: hump-backed, tiny, quivering with the strength of her convictions, a little prophetess, admonishing and inspired.

The Principal Works of Thomas Mann

First Editions in German

DER KLEINE HERR FRIEDEMANN
[Little Herr Friedemann]. Tales
Berlin, S. Fischer Verlag. 1898

BUDDENBROOKS
Novel *Berlin, S. Fischer Verlag.* 1901

TRISTAN
Contains *Tonio Kröger*. Tales *Berlin, S. Fischer Verlag.* 1903

FIORENZA
Drama *Berlin, S. Fischer Verlag.* 1905

KÖNIGLICHE HOHEIT
[Royal Highness]. Novel *Berlin, S. Fischer Verlag.* 1909

DER TOD IN VENEDIG
[Death in Venice]. Short novel *Berlin, S. Fischer Verlag.* 1913

DAS WUNDERKIND
[The Infant Prodigy]. Tales *Berlin, S. Fischer Verlag.* 1914

BETRACHTUNGEN EINES UNPOLITISCHEN
Autobiographical reflections *Berlin, S. Fischer Verlag.* 1918

HERR UND HUND
[A Man and His Dog]. Idyll
Contains also *Gesang vom Kindchen*, an idyll in verse
Berlin, S. Fischer Verlag. 1919

WÄLSUNGENBLUT
Tale *München, Phantasus Verlag.* 1921

BEKENNTNISSE DES HOCHSTAPLERS FELIX KRULL
Fragment of a novel *Stuttgart, Deutsche Verlags-Anstalt.*

BEMÜHUNGEN
Essays *Berlin, S. Fischer Verlag.* 1922

REDE UND ANTWORT
Essays *Berlin, S. Fischer Verlag.* 1922

DER ZAUBERBERG
[The Magic Mountain]. Novel *Berlin, S. Fischer Verlag.* 1924

UNORDNUNG UND FRÜHES LEID
[Disorder and Early Sorrow]. Short novel
Berlin, S. Fischer Verlag. 1926

KINO
Fragment of a novel *Berlin, S. Fischer Verlag.* 1926

PARISER RECHENSCHAFT
Travelogue *Berlin, S. Fischer Verlag.* 1926

DEUTSCHE ANSPRACHE
Ein Appell an die Vernunft *Berlin, S. Fischer Verlag.* 1930

DIE FORDERUNG DES TAGES
Essays *Berlin, S. Fischer Verlag.* 1930

MARIO UND DER ZAUBERER
[Mario and the Magician]. Short novel
Berlin, S. Fischer Verlag. 1930

GOETHE ALS REPRÄSENTANT DES BÜRGERLICHEN ZEITALTERS
Lecture *Berlin, S. Fischer Verlag.* 1932

JOSEPH UND SEINE BRÜDER
[Joseph and His Brothers]. Novel
I. Die Geschichten Jaakobs. 1933.
II. Der junge Joseph. 1934.
III. Joseph in Ägypten. 1936.
IV. Joseph, der Ernährer. 1943.
I, II, Berlin, S. Fischer Verlag.
III, Vienna, Bermann-Fischer Verlag.
IV, Stockholm, Bermann-Fischer Verlag.

LEIDEN UND GRÖSSE DER MEISTER
Essays *Berlin, S. Fischer Verlag.* 1935

FREUD UND DIE ZUKUNFT
Lecture *Vienna, Bermann-Fischer Verlag.* 1936

EIN BRIEFWECHSEL
[An Exchange of Letters]
Zürich, Dr. Oprecht & Helbling AG. 1937

DAS PROBLEM DER FREIHEIT
Essay *Stockholm, Bermann-Fischer Verlag.*

SCHOPENHAUER
Essay *Stockholm, Bermann-Fischer Verlag.*

ACHTUNG, EUROPA!
Manifesto *Stockholm, Bermann-Fischer Verlag.*

DIE SCHÖNSTEN ERZÄHLUNGEN
Contains *Tonio Kröger, Der Tod in Venedig, Unordnung und frühes Leid, Mario und der Zauberer*
Stockholm, Bermann-Fischer Verlag. 1938

LOTTE IN WEIMAR
[The Beloved Returns]. Novel
Stockholm, Bermann-Fischer Verlag. 1939

DIE VERTAUSCHTEN KÖPFE
Eine indische Legende [The Transposed Heads]
Stockholm, Bermann-Fischer Verlag. 1940

DEUTSCHE HÖRER
[Listen, Germany!] Broadcasts
Stockholm, Bermann-Fischer Verlag. 1942

DAS GESETZ
[The Tables of the Law]
Stockholm, Bermann-Fischer Verlag. 1944

DOKTOR FAUSTUS: DAS LEBEN DES DEUTSCHEN TONSETZERS ADRIAN LEVERKÜHN, ERZÄHLT VON EINEM FREUNDE
Novel *Stockholm, Bermann-Fischer Verlag.* 1947

DER ERWÄHLTE
[The Holy Sinner]. Novel
Frankfurt am Main, S. Fischer Verlag. 1951

DIE BETROGENE
[The Black Swan]. Short Novel
Frankfurt am Main, S. Fischer Verlag. 1953

BEKENNTNISSE DES HOCHSTAPLERS FELIX KRULL: DER MEMOIREN ERSTER TEIL [Confessions of Felix Krull]. Novel
Frankfurt am Main, S. Fischer Verlag. 1954

American Editions in Translation

published by ALFRED A. KNOPF, *New York*

ROYAL HIGHNESS: A NOVEL OF GERMAN COURT LIFE
Translated by A. Cecil Curtis 1916

BUDDENBROOKS
Translated by H. T. Lowe-Porter 1924

DEATH IN VENICE AND OTHER STORIES
Translated by Kenneth Burke. Contains Der Tod in Venedig, Tristan, *and* Tonio Kröger (*out of print*)* 1925

THE MAGIC MOUNTAIN
Translated by H. T. Lowe-Porter. Two volumes 1927

CHILDREN AND FOOLS
Translated by Herman George Scheffauer. Nine stories, including translations of Der kleine Herr Friedemann *and* Unordnung und frühes Leid (*out of print*)* 1928

THREE ESSAYS
Translated by H. T. Lowe-Porter. Contains translations of Friedrich und die grosse Koalition *from* Rede und Antwort, *and of* Goethe und Tolstoi *and* Okkulte Erlebnisse *from* Bemühungen 1929

EARLY SORROW
Translated by Herman George Scheffauer (*out of print*)* 1930

A MAN AND HIS DOG
Translated by Herman George Scheffauer (*out of print*)* 1930

DEATH IN VENICE
A new translation by H. T. Lowe-Porter, with an Introduction by Ludwig Lewisohn. 1930

MARIO AND THE MAGICIAN
Translated by H. T. Lowe-Porter (*out of print*)* 1931

PAST MASTERS AND OTHER PAPERS
Translated by H. T. Lowe-Porter (*out of print*) 1933

JOSEPH AND HIS BROTHERS
I. Joseph and His Brothers (The Tales of Jacob) 1934
II. Young Joseph 1935
III. Joseph in Egypt 1938
IV. Joseph the Provider 1944
The complete work in 1 volume 1948
Translated by H. T. Lowe-Porter

STORIES OF THREE DECADES
Translated by H. T. Lowe-Porter. Contains all of Thomas Mann's fiction prior to 1940 except the long novels 1936

---

* Included in *Stories of Three Decades*, translated by H. T. Lowe-Porter.

AN EXCHANGE OF LETTERS
Translated by H. T. Lowe-Porter † 1937

FREUD, GOETHE, WAGNER
Translated by H. T. Lowe-Porter and Rita Matthias-Reil. Three essays 1937

THE COMING VICTORY OF DEMOCRACY
Translated by Agnes E. Meyer † 1938

THIS PEACE
Translated by H. T. Lowe-Porter † 1938

THIS WAR
Translated by Eric Sutton † 1940

THE BELOVED RETURNS
[Lotte in Weimar]
Translated by H. T. Lowe-Porter 1940

THE TRANSPOSED HEADS
Translated by H. T. Lowe-Porter 1941

ORDER OF THE DAY
Political Essays and Speeches of Two Decades
Translated by H. T. Lowe-Porter, Agnes E. Meyer, and Eric Sutton 1942

LISTEN, GERMANY!
Twenty-five Radio Messages to the German People over BBC 1943

THE TABLES OF THE LAW
Translated by H. T. Lowe-Porter 1945

ESSAYS OF THREE DECADES
Translated by H. T. Lowe-Porter 1947

DOCTOR FAUSTUS: THE LIFE OF THE GERMAN COMPOSER ADRIAN LEVERKÜHN AS TOLD BY A FRIEND
Translated by H. T. Lowe-Porter 1948

THE HOLY SINNER
Translated by H. T. Lowe-Porter 1951

THE BLACK SWAN
Translated by Willard R. Trask 1954

CONFESSIONS OF FELIX KRULL, CONFIDENCE MAN: THE EARLY YEARS
Translated by Denver Lindley 1955

---

† Also included in *Order of the Day*.

The book was set on the Linotype in Janson, a recutting made direct from the type cast from matrices (now in possession of the Stempel foundry, Frankfurt am Main) made by Anton Janson some time between 1660 and 1687.

Of Janson's origin nothing is known. He may have been a relative of Justus Janson, a printer of Danish birth who practised in Leipzig from 1614 to 1635. Some time between 1657 and 1668 Anton Janson, a punch-cutter and type-founder, bought from the Leipzig printer Johann Erich Hahn the type-foundry which had formerly been a part of the printing house of M. Friedrich Lankisch. Janson's types were first shown in a specimen sheet issued at Leipzig about 1675. Janson's successor, and perhaps his son-in-law, Johann Karl Edling, issued a specimen sheet of Janson types in 1689. His heirs sold the Janson matrices in Holland to Wolffgang Dietrich Erhardt, of Leipzig.

Composed, printed, and bound by The Plimpton Press, Norwood, Mass.

Typography and binding are based on original designs by W. A. Dwiggins.